A GUIDE TO OBESITY AND THE METABOLIC SYNDROME

A GUIDE TO OBESITY AND THE METABOLIC SYNDROME

ORIGINS AND TREATMENT

GEORGE A. BRAY
Louisiana State University, Baton Rouge, USA

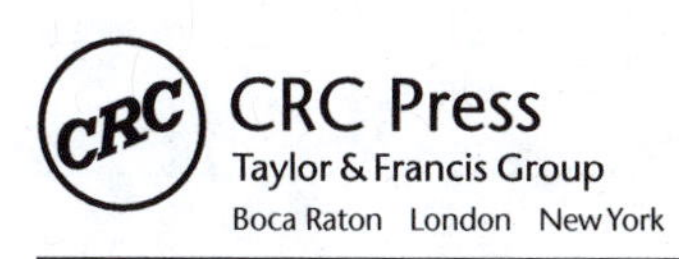

CRC Press is an imprint of the
Taylor & Francis Group, an **informa** business

CRC Press
Taylor & Francis Group
6000 Broken Sound Parkway NW, Suite 300
Boca Raton, FL 33487-2742

Printed in the United States of America on acid-free paper
10 9 8 7 6 5 4 3 2 1

International Standard Book Number: 978-1-4398-1457-4 (Hardback)

Library of Congress Cataloging-in-Publication Data

Bray, George A.
A guide to obesity and the metabolic syndrome : origins and treatment / by George A. Bray.
p. ; cm.
Includes bibliographical references and index.
ISBN 978-1-4398-1457-4 (hardcover : alk. paper)
1. Obesity. 2. Metabolic syndrome. I. Title.
[DNLM: 1. Obesity--etiology. 2. Metabolic Syndrome X--etiology. 3. Metabolic Syndrome X--therapy. 4. Obesity--therapy. WD 210]

RC628.B6529 2011
616.3'98--dc22 2010033565

Visit the Taylor & Francis Web site at
http://www.taylorandfrancis.com

and the CRC Press Web site at
http://www.crcpress.com

This book is dedicated to my wife, Marilyn, and to my children, both biological and scientific

Contents

Preface

OBESITY: ORIGINS AND SOLUTIONS

How Did Americans Get So Fat?

If you have been to your local shopping mall recently and are older than 20 years of age, you have witnessed the growing girth of many Americans. The United States is now the fattest country in the world! The U.S. government regularly surveys the American public to put numbers on the face of fatness. These surveys are called the National Health and Nutrition Examination Surveys (NHANES). Between 1960 and 1976, there was a slow rise in the number of Americans who were overweight. This rise was similar to the slow increase in overweight that occurred from the time of the Civil War (in 1860) through 1976 (Bray 1976a). Between 1976 and today, however, there has been a big jump in the number of overweight and obese Americans. The number has more than doubled between 1980 to 2002 (from 14.5% to 33.5% obese) (Ogden et al. 2007). The increased rate at which people are becoming fat has led some to label this an "epidemic" (the World Health Organization [WHO], the National Heart, Lung, and Blood Institute [NHLBI]).

Figure 1 shows this pattern of increase for three levels of body weight. The upper limit of normal is 25 body mass index (BMI) units, a number we will describe in more detail in Chapter 2. People above a normal BMI of 25 have increased from 45% of the population to over 60% today—a rise of more than one-third. A BMI of 30 in Figure 1 is the dividing line for obesity. The number of adults above a BMI of 30 has grown from 14% in 1960 to over 30% today—a 100% increase. The final line at a BMI of 40 defined the dividing line for the very obese. Very obese people were uncommon in 1960 but are now more than 5%—a more than 400% increase.

Nearly 40 years ago, even before the "obesity epidemic" began in earnest, the plight of fat Americans became my life's work. Much of my office practice of medicine dealt with obese adolescents and young adults. Back in the 1960s, I was saddened and dismayed by the young people

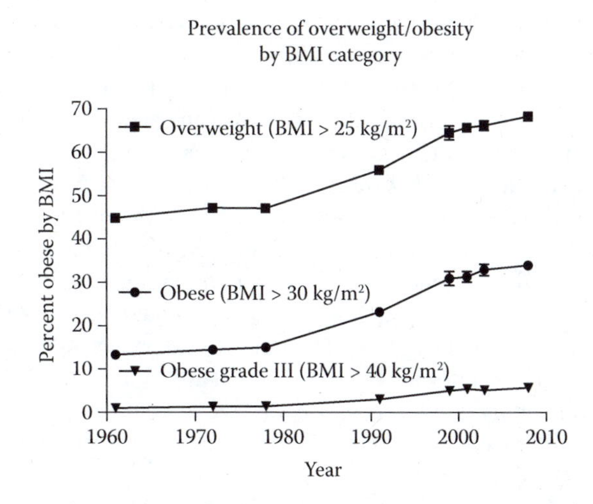

FIGURE 1. The increasing number of Americans who are labeled as overweight (■), obese (●), or very obese (▼) by U.S. government surveys from 1980 to 2004. (Drawn from data in Ogden, C.L., et al., *Gastroenterology* 132, 2087–2102, 2007.)

weighing more than 300 pounds who came to my office for help. The problem is much worse now. In the 1960s, the group with a body weight greater than 300 lbs was less than 0.1% of the American population. Now it is over 5% and growing rapidly. Thirty years ago, I published my first book on obesity, (Bray 1976a) followed by an update in 2007 (Bray 2007b). Twenty-five years ago, I published my first treatment program to help people manage their weight problem (Bray 1982). Many things have changed in the intervening years. Preparation of this book has been strongly influenced by my experiences at the Pennington Biomedical Research Center in Baton Rouge, Louisiana. When I became director of this center in 1989, the current obesity epidemic was in full swing. As director of this magnificent nutrition research facility, I had additional resources to tackle the problem that has been my life's work. This book incorporates many new ideas about weight management that I have learned through the help of many patients and professional colleagues.

Let me put my strategy of weight management forward for you and then fill in the details about how this approach came about. First, we know that in famines, and when food is in short supply, people don't gain weight—indeed, they lose weight (Ravelli et al. 1999; Franco et al. 2007). No food—no fatness. This means that food plays a key part in the problem (Swinburn et al. 2009).

Focusing on food and how its intake is regulated is the first step toward understanding the epidemic of obesity. Reasoning that some foods are playing a bigger role than others, we examined the data from the U.S. Department of Agriculture about changes in food supply during the twentieth century. One of the striking findings was that the epidemic of overweight occurred in parallel with the introduction of high fructose corn syrup (HFCS) into the American food supply (Bray 2004). The association between the rapid rise in obesity and the introduction of HFCS doesn't prove that HFCS is the *cause* of obesity—obesity clearly has a number of causes, many of which are related to eating more food than we need. But the evidence is growing that the fructose that comes from HFCS or sucrose (table sugar) may be one contributor to the rise in obesity rates (Vartanian et al. 2007; Malik et al. 2010).

Along with a major shift in the supply of caloric sweeteners in the American diet, a number of other changes have occurred over recent decades that impact the epidemic of obesity. These trends can be summed up under the five "Bs": Beverages, Burgers, Behavior, Being Active, Buyer Beware.

Beverages: I have already introduced you to beverages sweetened with fructose from either HFCS or sugar. There are a number of potentially harmful effects of fructose on body weight (Malik et al. 2010; Bray 2009). Thus, reducing fructose intake makes sense to me and soft drinks and sweetened fruit drinks that contain this sugar are easy targets. Several studies reviewing scientific publication (meta-analyses) have shown that soft drink consumption predicts energy intake and often weight gain and obesity (Vartanian et al. 2007; Olsen and Heitmann, 2009; Malik et al. 2009). Get as much of your fluid and beverage needs as you can from water, tea, or coffee—at least six to eight 8-ounce glasses a day and avoid beverages that have fructose in them.

Burgers: Everyone, or nearly everyone, has eaten at one of the fast food restaurants. They are ubiquitous in the United States and around the world. Burgers tend to be loaded with fat —but they are "tasty." Over the past 50 years, the size of most burgers has ballooned. A single large burger meal can provide 1000 calories or more, which is 50% or more of the calories needed by many Americans each day. These are problem foods for some people who want to lose weight and keep it off, as well as for people who do not want to gain weight. This threat to a healthy weight was shown dramatically in the documentary movie, *Supersize Me*. The director, Morgan Spurlock, gained over 25 pounds in 1 month while supersizing his meal every time it was offered. Grilling burgers at home without the "special" sauce is good advice.

Behavior: Eating and drinking are behaviors. One view has it that we become overweight because we have "faulty" behaviors. Whether true or not, this idea has been helping people plan what they eat, and with whom and where they eat, to get better control over their own personal eating. The Internet is one of the most striking developments of the past decade (Winett et al. 2005). The power of the Internet is being harnessed to use in behavioral weight management, and offers promise for the future. One of the most important concepts has been the control of portion size using "portion-controlled" foods. I will explore behavioral techniques in Chapter 6 and focus on the types of foods and beverages to include in a diet plan.

Be as active as you can to counteract the tendency to be inactive. Society no longer requires much strenuous activity, unless we choose to do so. Television, video games, and comfortable automobiles all make the United States one of the most inactive societies on earth. Inactivity is the norm. We know that overweight people sit an average of 2 hours more per day than do thinner people. Standing up while talking on your cell phone uses more energy. The beauty of the cell phone is that you can talk anywhere and walk while doing so, all of which burns more energy. A step counter to count the steps you take, described in Chapter 6 is one way to set a goal of becoming more active.

Buyer Beware: We are all influenced by the prices of the things we buy, including food. Price reductions and sale items get our attention. Food pricing works the same way. Special deals, such as "two-for-the-price-of-one" and "supersizing" are ways of selling more for a "better deal"—a better deal for the seller maybe, but not necessarily a better deal for you. Buy healthy foods, not necessarily the cheap ones. Remember, you don't have to clean your plate. Put the waste in the garbage bin rather than on your own waist. Avoid combinations of fructose from HFCS or sugar and fat.

Isn't Obesity Just a Recent Problem?

Overweight was a problem long before I finished medical school 50 years ago. I found this out when I came across a short book from the nineteenth century that traced the origins of obesity. Although it was written in French by an American who was studying in Paris—something lots of young physicians did in the nineteenth century—it opened my eyes to the long history of overweight that is described in Chapter 1 (Worthington 1875). It is hard to believe that there was enough to fill an obesity book that far back. Yet there was, and this book stimulated me to learn more about the history of obesity and when it began (Bray 2007a).

Treatment for overweight people has been described for more than 5000 years (Bray 2007a). These descriptions can be found in medical writings from the Egyptian, Babylonian, Chinese, Indian, Meso-American, and Greco-Roman cultures. Many causes were proposed and many treatments suggested long before we had any modern medicines. In spite of this long history, the problem is still with us—and getting worse—meaning that we neither understand it well nor have completely effective treatments. We have greatly increased our knowledge and have much more to offer people working to manage their weight, yet, at this writing, the problem continues to worsen—we haven't even yet contained it—to use a firefighter's phrase.

The first English-language books devoted solely to the subject of obesity or corpulence as it was called were written in the eighteenth century, well before the American Revolution (Short 1727; Flemyng 1760). These were followed during the next two hundred years by books in many languages (Bray 2007a). The first American book dealing with the medical side of obesity was published in 1940, just prior to World War II. By the time Rony (1940) wrote this book, the basic concepts of energy balance and metabolism had been well established. Scientific studies at the time of the French Revolution (Lavoisier 1789; Boyle 1764) had clearly shown that metabolism was similar to burning a candle. Some 50 years later, the law of conservation of energy (von Helmholtz 1847; von Mayer 1842) was clearly stated by two German scientists. This work in Germany stimulated Americans to develop equipment that could measure human metabolism (Atwater and Rosa 1899). With this equipment, they showed that the idea of energy balance applied to human beings just as it did to other animals. We were metabolically part of the same evolutionary animal kingdom.

While the basic science behind fatness was developing, the first popular weight reduction "diet" was published in London in 1863 (Banting 1864). William Banting, its author, was a layman. The first edition of his small pamphlet, titled *Letter on Corpulence Addressed to the Public* was published because Banting was thrilled with the success he achieved using a diet given to him by his doctor (Harvey 1872). It was high in protein and low in carbohydrate, and it aroused the same fervor in England at the time of our Civil War as have some of the modern popular diet books.

We made a major step forward when we recognized that overweight had many causes—a major achievement in the twentieth century. One type of overweight, although rare, is due to brain tumors that are often associated with impaired vision and glandular disturbances (Frohlich 1901; Babinski 1900). Shortly after this discovery, a famous American neurosurgeon, Dr. Harvey Cushing, showed in 1912 that a tumor in the "master gland" (the pituitary) could also produce overweight (Cushing 1912).

For more than half of the twentieth century, the life insurance industry did its best to convince Americans that being overweight was dangerous to health and tended to shorten lifespan (The Association of Life Insurance Medical Directors 1913). Industry leaders knew this from the money they had to pay out to settle death-benefit claims for insurance on people who were overweight. We now know that even modest increases in excess weight are associated with shortened lifespan (Adams et al. 2007; Whitlock et al. 2009).

Two other observations in the twentieth century were key to understanding obesity. The first was the discovery in 1994 of leptin, a peptide produced in fat that is involved in the regulation of food intake and other functions when calorie intake is reduced during starvation, and possibly to predict weight gain. The second was the publication of two articles that showed that losing weight prolongs life (Sjostrom et al. 2007; Adams et al. 2007). This had been predicted from the improvements in risk factors for diabetes and heart disease that occur with weight loss. The direct demonstration that voluntary weight loss prolongs life, however, was a necessary step forward.

Lessons Learned about Obesity in the Past 30 Years

Overweight as a problem came of age in the 1970s. The National Institutes of Health (NIH) are funded by American taxpayers to support basic research aimed at curing heart disease, diabetes, arthritis, cancer, and other diseases. In the late 1960s, the Fogarty International Center for Preventive Diseases at the National Institutes of Health was established to honor Congressman John E. Fogarty (1913–1967), a US Congressional Representative from the State of Rhode Island, who had been a long-time and vocal supporter of expanded research at the NIH. One of the first activities of the new Fogarty Center was to organize a Conference on Prevention of Obesity. "Obesity" was perceived, even in the 1970s, to be a major public health issue. This Conference was held at NIH in 1973 (Bray 1976b).

The impetus for the study of overweight given by the Fogarty Center Conference on Obesity was followed by the first in a series of International Congresses on Obesity. The first was held in London in 1974 (Howard 1975) Along with the development of these international meetings came the publication in 1976 of the first journal devoted specifically to obesity—the *International Journal of Obesity.* Tucked away at the same time was the first edition of my first book about obesity, *The Obese Patient*, published in 1976 (Bray 1976a).

The most important advance in obesity in recent years was the discovery of leptin (Zhang et al. 1994). This peptide hormone is made predominantly in the fat cells. When leptin is absent, massive overweight occurs in human beings and in research animals. Defects in the leptin receptor, the "lock" that the leptin molecule "key" fits into, are also responsible for a small number of massively overweight people (Farooqi and O'Rahilly 2007). In addition to derangements in the leptin genes, defects in other genes can produce obesity in human beings. One of these genes, called the melanocortin-4 receptor gene, is defective in up to 5% of markedly overweight youngsters (Farooqu and O'Rahilly 2007). This is one of the most frequent genetic causes for a chronic human disease. Yet, collectively, these individuals are only a tiny fraction of all obese people.

Behavior modification could be used to treat overweight subjects (Stuart and Davis 1972). As this technique was developed in detail (Chapter 6), it became one of the "three pillars," along with diet and exercise, for the treatment of obesity. Efforts have been made to adapt these behavioral techniques to prevent development of weight gain in large groups of people, but they have often been disappointing. Behavioral strategies are cognitive strategies, that is to say, they require you to do something active, such as dieting, exercising, or modifying the way you live. We are slowly learning that these cognitive strategies do not translate into the prevention of overweight, and the weight that people initially lose using them is often regained. The alternative to "cognitive" approaches are the "noncognitive" approaches, that is, ways of dealing with obesity that do not require much active individual involvement. An analogy in the prevention of dental caries ("cavities") can be used to make this distinction. Tooth-brushing and flossing regularly will reduce dental disease. These procedures are "cognitive" strategies since the individual has to remember to do them and actually do them. The addition of fluoride to the water supply is a noncognitive strategy that accomplished the same end. When our water was fluoridated, dental caries were dramatically reduced, without our volitional activity.

Several things may help prevent obesity and don't require much effort. Taking more calcium may be one of them. People with higher intakes of calcium have lower body weight in some, but not all, studies. The use of low fat dairy products, which are a good source of calcium, lower blood pressure, and are part of one of the diets I describe in Chapter 6.

Less sleep is associated with higher body weights. Children who sleep less gain more weight in their preschool years (Bray 2007b) (Chapter 3). This also applies to adults, and there is now a potential explanation for this effect in the changes of sleep on hormones.

Another low-effort strategy for weight loss would be to buy foods for "health," not for "price." Turning off that natural desire to get more for your money when buying food may be hard, but what you get for your money when you buy cheap food may be fat and fructose and added sugar, which may simply become "waste on your waist." It is better to eat well than to eat cheaply.

The fat cell is much more than where fat is stored (Flier 2004). It is a cell that plays a part in the daily orchestra of life. It makes music through the chemicals it produces. Sometimes the notes are beautiful, but they can also be discordant. With the discovery that leptin is made almost entirely in the fat cell, it has become clear that the fat cell has very significant functions besides storing fat. Fat cells are part of the largest glandular (endocrine) tissue in the body. They produce numerous products that are released into the circulation and that act on other cells. Among these are molecules that cause inflammation, molecules that are involved in controlling blood pressure or influencing cell growth, and molecules that regulate fat metabolism and blood clotting (Chapter 3).

The past 30 years have seen the development of a plethora of new drugs for the treatment of many diseases. Some of these medications produce weight gain (Chapters 3 and 5). Switching to alternative medications that do not cause weight gain is one approach the physician can take to this problem.

The commonly observed "beer-belly" in men or "apple shape" in women is medically termed "central adiposity." We have learned that central adiposity is a risk to health. This was first noted nearly 100 years ago, but it wasn't until the early 1980s (Larsson et al. 1984) that it became widely appreciated that people with central adiposity were at high risk for diabetes and heart disease. Waist circumference has become the standard way to measure central adiposity. It is also one of a group of signs and symptoms related to heart disease and diabetes, including high blood pressure, high blood sugar, low levels of HDL-cholesterol, and high levels of triglycerides.

Diets can reduce your risk of disease and provide a way to treat some of them effectively. This was shown elegantly in a study comparing the effects of three different dietary patterns on blood pressure (Appel et al. 1997; Sacks et al. 2001). The first diet, the reference diet, was a standard American diet or Western-type of diet, with plenty of fat, meat, and normal amounts of fruits and vegetables. The second diet, one of the two experimental diets, was called the fruits and vegetable diet because it was enriched with fruits and vegetables. The aim was to increase dietary intake of magnesium and potassium from fruits and vegetables to the seventy-fifth percentile of normal, that is, a level above what three out of four people would normally get in their diet. The third diet—the Combination or DASH Diet—was enriched to the same degree as the second diet with fruits and vegetables. In addition, it had more low fat dairy products to increase calcium intake and also had lowered total fat intake (27% vs. 33% in the control diet), more fiber, higher protein (18%) from the extra 3% from vegetable sources, and reduced intake of calorically sweetened beverages and other sweets. Blood pressure was significantly reduced in people eating the fruits and vegetables diet and reduced even more in the people eating the Combination (fruits, vegetables, low fat dairy products) or DASH diet (Appel et al. 1997; Sacks et al. 2001).

Another large clinical trial, called the Diabetes Prevention Program, showed that weight loss through reduced intake of calories and fat plus more physical activity could significantly reduce the risk of diabetes mellitus in people at high risk for this disease (The DPP Research Group) (Chapter 4). Modest weight loss can have important health benefits for people at risk for diabetes and other chronic metabolic diseases.

Obesity is a stigmatized condition. That is, there is prejudice against and dislike for the obese. The efforts, particularly among women, to lose weight and avoid this stigma cost billions of dollars per year.

In addition to the health benefits from weight loss, including prolonging life (Sjostrom et al. 2007; Adams et al. 2007), there is an improvement in the quality of life. Weight loss improves the ability to move and to get around. When weight loss is not sufficient to give a cosmetic benefit and improvements in quality of life people may not be willing to continue the effort needed to maintain a program of weight management. Set goals that you can accomplish and take small steps toward these goals.

Surgical treatment for obesity began in the 1960s. The current popularity of these procedures is the result of the lowered risk from surgery with the use of newer, so-called laparoscopic surgeries. Using laparoscopic techniques reduces the risk and has increased the number of treated patients. It is estimated that more than 200,000 people had this surgery in 2010. This approach to obesity is discussed in detail in Chapter 8.

This book has been divided into two parts:

Part I. Origins of Obesity

The Introduction and Chapter 1 put the ideas behind the development of current theories of obesity into an historical context. The Introduction covers the period from the Old Stone Age to the onset of scientific science in the beginning of the 1500s. Chapter 1 covers the period from the sixteenth through the nineteenth century. With Chapters 2 through 5, we move into the twentieth century and provide definitions of obesity and establish the prevalence of obesity and the mechanisms involved in the energy imbalance that produces obesity. The ill-consequences to health associated with increasing body fat, and the evaluation and prevention of obesity that are essential for trying to deal with the problem, are also discussed.

Part II. Treatment of Obesity

Effective treatments for obesity have been slow in developing. Prior to the twentieth century, diet and physical activity had been mainstays of advice for those with weight problems dating back 2500 years or more. The idea that obesity might reflect a maladaptive behavior leads to the concept of modifying this lifestyle with a set of techniques that are now part of most treatment programs (Chapter 6). With the dawn of the twentieth century, drugs developed by organic chemists based on the concept of a "lock and key" fit were introduced for the treatment of many diseases, including obesity (Chapter 7). Chapter 8 deals with surgery, which dates its introduction to the ideas of surgeons after World War II. With the introduction of fiber optic instruments that allowed laparoscopic surgery, the number of patients receiving surgical treatment for obesity ballooned to well over 200,000 per year (Chapter 8).

This book could not have been written without input over the years from many people, and the particular help of those now working with me. I am grateful to CRC Press for inviting me to write this monograph some 35 years after I wrote my first monograph in 1976. Dr. Greenway, a long term colleague from my years in Los Angeles, has provided input to the text as has my colleague Dr. Donna Ryan who has worked with me for the 20 years that I have been at the Pennington Biomedical Research Center. Preparation of the manuscript has been under the careful supervision of my editorial assistant Ms. Robin Post, to whom I acknowledge my debt of gratitude.

Introduction

HISTORICAL ORIGINS OF OBESITY

From Paleolithic Times to the Introduction of Printing

"We do not live in our own time alone; we carry our history within us."

Gaarder (1995)

Key Points:

- Artifacts showing obesity date from the Paleolithic era, more than 30,000 years ago, and are scattered across Eurasia.
- The Venus of Willendorf in the Vienna Museum of Natural History is the best known of these artifacts.

Many new artifacts showing obesity from the Neolithic period, just after the beginning of agriculture 10,000 years ago, have appeared around the Mediterranean.

- Obesity is also evident in artifacts from the Mayan culture prior to the discovery of America in 1492.
- Obese patients and their treatment are described in all medical traditions.
- Diet and exercise were the mainstays of treatment by Hippocrates, the Greek father of medicine, and by Galen, the leading Roman physician.

Origins of Obesity before Recorded History

Obesity in the Paleolithic (Old) Stone Age

A key message from a study of Stone Age records is that obesity has always been with us. This is evident in artifacts from the Old Stone Age. The cultural significance of the obese figures that we find in this period is still unknown but we may conclude that human beings had the genetic and physiological make-up for obesity from the time of the first revolution in communication nearly 50,000 years ago.

Imagine your surprise when your spade comes upon a small statue of a fat woman when you are digging for a construction project on the outskirts of a small town. A curious mind would want to know more about this statue and about the times from which it came. The statue I am referring to is called the Venus of Willendorf after the town in Austria where it was found in 1908 during excavations along the Danube River by archeologist Josef Szombathy (Angell 1989; Witcombe 2005). It is a small limestone statuette measuring a little over 4 inches (11 cm) in height (Figure 1). The arms are small and there are no feet or facial features, but there is clear-cut abdominal obesity and pendulous breasts. This is not the only statue of its kind. Although it has been in our possession for nearly 100 years, we still do not know what it represents. We do not know its role in the culture at the time it was made. This statue has been the subject of research for over 100 years and still many questions remain. We can conclude some things, however. First, this statue tells us that obesity has been a human issue for a very long time. Second, it has raised boundless speculation about whether this statue represented some kind of good or bad omen, or whether it was a fertility rite.

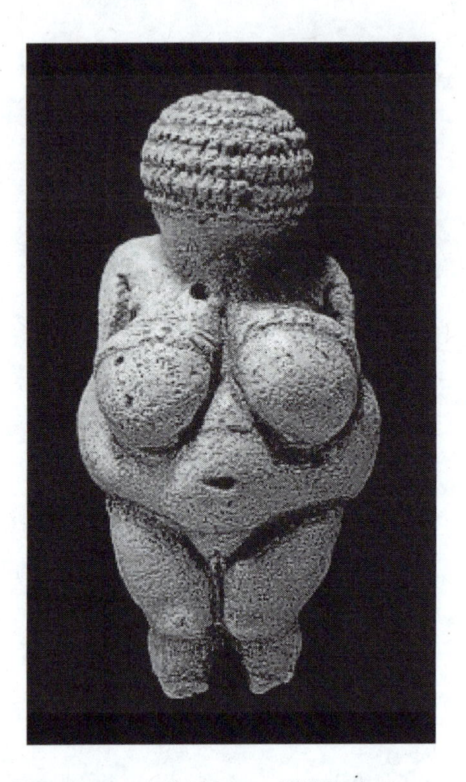

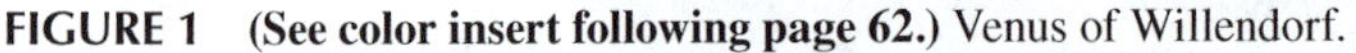

FIGURE 1 **(See color insert following page 62.)** Venus of Willendorf.

The Venus of Willendorf is the best known of the Stone Age statuettes depicting an obese woman, but is it is not the oldest. Almost a century after the Venus of Willendorf was found, Nicholas Conrad discovered an even older ivory figurine that he has called the Venus of Hohle Fels, after the cave where he discovered it in 2008. Carbon dating estimated its age at 35,000 years, about 10,000 years before any of the other figurines (Conrad 2009). It is a short squat statue with large breasts and exaggerated vulva suggesting the importance of this figure in fertility rites. It was designed to be worn around the neck and was found in several small pieces that were close together. Its length was 5.97 cm or about half the height of the Venus of Willendorf. Its discovery will reopen the interpretation of early art.

Learning about disease and medicine prior to written history can be done using artifacts such as the Venus of Hohle Fels, the Venus of Willendorf, or other artistic representations, skeletal finds, and related objects from archeological excavations. From these artifacts it is clear that our forefathers and foremothers suffered many illnesses, including obesity, and that they tried to do something about them. Treatment in prehistoric times was aimed at the relief of fevers and burns, attempts to relieve pain, to stop bleeding, and to repair broken bones. Injury, burns, fevers, and infections took a major human toll before our era of anesthetics, antibiotics, and modern medicine and surgery. Indeed, it is hard for us to imagine life and medicine in the times before anesthesia, antibiotics, and antisera.

Almost all of the statues showing obesity from the Paleolithic or Old Stone Age are women (Stephen-Chauvet 1936; Gimbutas 1999). These artifacts were found in Europe from southwestern France to north of the Black Sea in Russia, as well as in the Middle East (Bray 2004, 2007; Clark 1967). Most of these figures were produced over a 2000-year period, 23,000 to 25,000 years ago in the so-called Upper Perigordian or Gravettian part of the Paleolithic era, although the recent discovery of the Venus of Hohle Fels from 35,000 years ago may require modification of this thesis. They were probably carved between the development of speech about 50,000 years ago and the development of agriculture about 10,000 years ago (Gamble 1986). A 2000-year period (two millennia) may be an accurate estimate of the time during which most of them were created, or it may reflect the limits in our ability to date objects more precisely. These statues are distributed over more than 5000 km (3000 miles) from west to east and have been found either by lucky individuals or as part of systematic archeological excavations. In the Stone Age, the artisans' tools were stone, which limited the types of materials used to make these statues to ivory, limestone, or baked clay (terracotta). Statuettes have been found in southern France (Lespegue), in Italy at Savignano, in the Czech Republic of the former Austro-Hungarian Empire, in Germany (Venuses of Willendorf and Hohle Fels), and in the Ukraine (Gamble 1986). The similarity in design of these statues suggests that there may have been communication across Europe during the Ice Age in the Paleolithic period. The height of these statues varies from about 2 cm (1 inch) to more than 25 cm (10 inches). The Venuses called Gagarino and Kostienki were found along the Volga River (Clark 1967). Both the Venus of Willendorf (Figure 1) and the Dolni Vestonice were found along the Danube River in middle Europe. The five limestone reliefs discovered at Laussel in the southern Dordogne region of France depict four obese women and an obese man (Stephen-Chauvet 1936). Obese men are rare among these statues.

Several of these female statues had an additional feature. They have very large buttocks called steatopygia. At Brassempouy in France, three carved ivory statues were found in 1892 showing obese or steatopygic women. The statuettes carved in soapstone found at Grimaldi near Menton were also obese and steatopygic (Stephen-Chauvet 1936). The Venus of Lespegue, made of ivory, found near Haute Garonne in France in 1922, is one of the most perfect of this group (Stephen-Chauvet 1936). The most distant member of this group is a fat plaster figure found at Tin Hinan in the Sahara Desert in Tunisia (Stephen-Chauvet 1936).

The meaning of these statues to their owners and to the culture has been the subject of intense controversy (Stephen-Chauvet 1936; Gimbutas 1999; Goodison and Morris 1998). A French physician, Dr. Stephen-Chauvet, suggested that these obese figures with prominent buttocks might be "clinical" illustrations of endocrine, or glandular, disease that was present in Stone Age people (Stephen-Chauvet 1936). Hautin, another Frenchman writing in 1939, interpreted these statues differently. He concluded that they proved the existence of obesity in Paleolithic times and that they also symbolized the expression and possible esthetic ideals of the period (Hautin 1939). Beller, in her book titled *Fat and Thin*, agrees with Hautin. She says, "The women immortalized in Stone Age sculpture were fat; there is no other word for it . . . [O]besity was already a fact of life for Paleolithic man—or at least for Paleolithic woman" (Beller 1977). Beller also reached three other conclusions from these statues. First, the genes necessary for the development of corpulence were already present in the Paleolithic period of human development when the major event was likely to be food shortages rather than a surfeit of food. For people who had to hunt and gather their food, obesity could be an advantage in allowing them to store up food energy as fat for times when food was in short supply. In contrast, obesity would be a disadvantage for nomadic tribes who had to move from one place to another. The burden of carrying extra weight, as fat slows an individual down, limits the amount of weight he or she can carry, and the distance it can be carried. Second, the wide geographic distribution of these figurines shows that adiposity could develop in many different regions of the world eating diets that depended on the available plant and animal sources. This means that development of obesity did not require special foods or an agricultural society or the presence of cities. Finally, the paucity of corpulent male figures would fit with the present-day difference in the prevalence of obesity between men and women.

Another view of both the Paleolithic and Neolithic female figurines is that they were primordial female deities, reflecting the bounty of the earth (Gimbutas 1999; Husain 1997; Neuman 1972). In modern parlance, they are part of the view of obesity as a "feminist issue" (Ohrbach 1978). This view of these "goddesses" has several proponents, including Melaart (1965) and Gimbutas (1989, 1999). Their central idea is that a peaceful, goddess-centered culture existed in many places in the distant past, especially in "Old Europe," Greece, Malta, Egypt, and the Near East. The end of the story tells of the takeover of this matriarchal society by warlike Indo-European males about 3500 BC and carries a strong moral subtext with women as the "goodies" and men as the "baddies" (Gimbutas 1999). Lumping together the Paleolithic figures, which were primarily located across middle Europe and separated by 15,000 years, with the Neolithic figures, located primarily in the Middle East, requires a major simplification that may lose important contexts for newer interpretations of the data, particularly with the recent and much older Venus of Hohle Fels (Conrad 2009). These contrasting views are nicely summarized in a book of contributions to this problem by female archeologists (Goodison 1998). Although there is clear evidence that obesity existed in the Old (Paleolithic) Stone Age, there is no evidence of how or if there was any effort to control obesity or whether it was looked at as a survival advantage.

Obesity in the Neolithic and Bronze Ages

After an interval of nearly 15,000 years from the Paleolithic period 25,000 years ago to the Neolithic period 8,000–10,000 years ago, when agriculture was first appearing, a new wave of sculptures depicting obesity appeared. Why this long 15,000-year interval? Did climatic and survival conditions in the Ice Age eliminate corpulent individuals, thus removing the "model" for the artists? Did artistic preferences change or have examples from this intervening period just not been found? We do not have the answer to these questions. However, in the Neolithic Stone Age, which spans the time from 8000 BC to approximately 5500 BC, corpulent figures appeared around the globe.

People in Neolithic times introduced agriculture and established the first human settlements in Europe, Asia, and Meso-America. The Neolithic Age and the Copper (Chalcolithic) Age that followed, about 3000 BC, were notable for numerous corpulent statues or again labeled as "mother goddesses" by some writers (Gimbutas 1999; Husain 1997; Neumann 1972; Melaart 1965). One famous New Stone Age figure is made of clay and is called "Pazardzik." This figure was found in Thrace and dates from about 4000 BC. She has very large hips and abdomen and is sitting on a throne. Other artifacts showing obesity were found around the Mediterranean region, and particularly in Anatolia (currently Turkey) and Malta (Kulacoglu 1992; Seton 1967; Meskell 1998; Malone 1998). Finally, examples of corpulent figures from Meso-American cultures indicate that obesity or corpulence was worldwide even before the New World was discovered by Columbus in 1492.

Anatolia The region of Anatolia covers much of modern Turkey and has some of the richest finds of obese female statues (Kulacoglu 1992; Seton 1967; Meskell 1998; Malone 1998). Probably the best known were from the excavations at Çatalhöyük and the later ones from nearby Hacilar. These two cities were inhabited from about 6500 to 5600 BCE (Melaart 1965). The 32 acres of excavations at Çatalhöyük make it one of the largest in Turkey. Most of the figurines found there are made of clay (terracotta), but a few are made of limestone or alabaster. Their corpulence is evident in the pendulous breasts and large fat deposits on the abdomen and hips.

These statues cover a wide range of sizes. Some are as short as 2.5 cm (1 inch), while others are more than 24 cm (10 inches) tall. Figure 2 shows a copy of a statue from Çatalhöyük (author's collection) that stands about 20 cm (9 inches) tall, which depicts a woman sitting on a throne with two lions serving as arm rests (Kulacoglu 1992; Meskell 1998). It is a very powerful image of a large imperial woman flanked by two lions. Most of the figurines from this period show exaggerated hips, belly, and breasts. The genital area is typically indicated by triangular decoration, possibly symbolizing fertility and motherhood.

Again, one interpretation of these figures is that they are mother goddesses representing a matrilineal society. This proposition has been expounded upon in detail by Gimbutas (1989, 1999). Additional findings in the Çatalhöyük area in the 1990s have softened this interpretation. First, the places where these figures have been found are generally not in buildings associated with rituals. Second, whether these figures are women or men is sometimes in doubt. There is also recent evidence that the hunter–gatherer role was more important in this culture than had been previously recognized. That is, the agricultural transition continued to depend in significant measure on

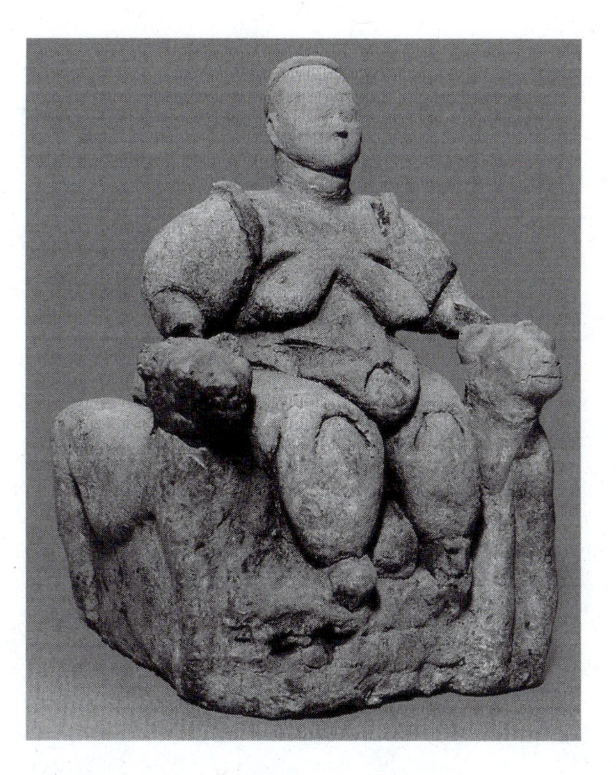

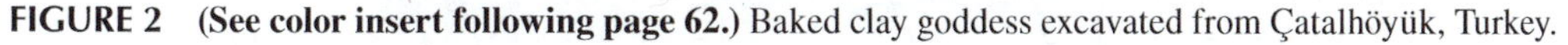

FIGURE 2 (See color insert following page 62.) Baked clay goddess excavated from Çatalhöyük, Turkey.

hunting and gathering of food. Thus, the one clear conclusion that we can draw from these Neolithic Age figures is that obesity was evident in the Neolithic (New) Stone Age culture, just as it had been in the Paleolithic (Old) Stone Age, 15,000 years earlier. Agriculture may have extended the degree and amount of obesity, but was in no way essential for it to occur. This implies, as Beller (1977) noted, that the genes needed for development of obesity were present from the earliest human history. From the available evidence, it is not possible to establish a religious or "goddess" identity for these statues since they were distributed throughout villages with and without religious reference (Kulacoglu 1992).

Malta The settlers of Malta arrived from Sicily about 5000 BC and contact continued for up to 1500 years (Malone 1998). Corpulent figurines from Malta are abundant and occur in several sizes. The smaller clay figures were found in family areas, not religious ones. Larger, almost life-sized, figures of clay or stone measuring up to 2 m (6 ft) in height were found in public areas and were clearly intended for some visible function in the society. However, we do not yet know what the nature of the relationship was between these statues and society. Many of them are larger than the ones found in Turkey and the Middle East. Stone is a common material used in sculpture from this area (Malone 1998). Making such large figures took a great deal of time and effort since the tools they used were also stone, copper, or bronze, and suggests that they were important to the culture in some yet poorly understood way.

The Sleeping Lady of Malta is important because it was found in a residential area of Malta and shows an obese female figure (Figure 3). This statuette is 12 cm in length, made of clay, and depicts a figure with a pleated skirt lying on a couch. It was found at the Hypogeum of Hal-Saflieni and is dated at around 3300 BCE. There is an abundance of flesh. Malta possesses the oldest known standing megalithic structures in the world, some of which are believed to date from 4000 BCE, a time before the Egyptian pyramids were built.

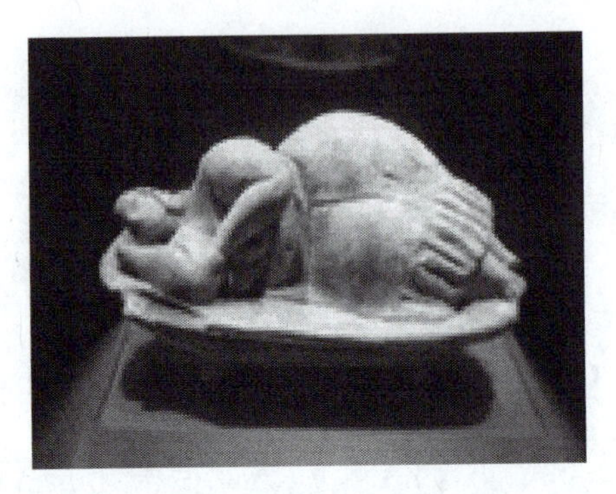

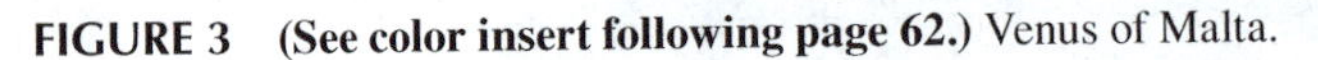

FIGURE 3 **(See color insert following page 62.)** Venus of Malta.

Crete and the Eastern Mediterranean The Neolithic period in Crete has left us with a number of statuettes of corpulent women. As with most of the other New Stone Age cultures, we have no clear idea of whether these figures were secular or religious in origin. These statues were part of the island or Cycladic culture in the Aegean (Goodison 1998).

Middle East Neolithic pottery from around 10,000 years ago, near the Tigris and Euphrates Rivers, has left many examples of obesity. One artifact found at Ain Ghazal near Amman, Jordan, was made of pottery and stands about 15 cm (6 inches) in height (Bienkowski 1991). They do not appear to represent pregnancy nor have they been associated with the cult of the female goddesses. Other Stone Age statues, such as the one from the museum at Aleppo representing a corpulent woman from the latter part of the Neolithic Age, indicate the wide dissemination of the idea of obesity, but do not help us to discern their precise cultural meaning.

Indus River Civilizations of South Asia The Neolithic Age in the Indus Valley, in what is now Pakistan, also shows the presence of obesity in clay figures. Wheeler (1966) describes the makers of these obese terracotta figurines as "enjoying a sense of humor." In his book, there is a picture of a "fat woman" with a large abdomen and hips (Wheeler 1966). The interpretation of obesity as a humorous subject has been a recurring one (Haslam 2009). Whether these early cultures disapproved of obesity, or disliked the people who were obese, is unknown.

Meso-American Neolithic Artifacts Prior to the "discovery" of the New World by Columbus in 1492, there were three high cultures in the Meso-American world (Moll 1998; Bernal 1999; Coe 1995). The Incas occupied the highlands along the west coast of South America, including much of what is now Peru. The Mayan culture occupied areas in what is now Honduras, Guatemala, Belize, Southern Mexico, and the Yucatan Peninsula. The Aztecs controlled the high plateaus of Mexico and Central America. When Columbus, Cortez, Pizarro, and their fellow explorers and plunderers arrived in the New World, they brought several devastating diseases, including measles, smallpox, and chickenpox, that were more lethal than the military might of the invaders. The Pre-Columbian Americans were Stone Age peoples. However, they were highly sophisticated in their knowledge of mathematics, astronomy, written language, and medicine. The New World proved to be a rich source of new foods and medicines for Europe. Columbus and other explorers brought back corn, tomatoes, potatoes, and useful plants for treating disease, including *Cinchona* bark, the source of quinine that was used to treat fevers, including malaria. At this time, diseases were believed to be caused by supernatural and magical forces, and treatment was directed at removing or calming these natural and supernatural causes. Sculptured artifacts are one of the sources of information about disease in Pre-Columbian societies. These figurines represent malnutrition, deformity, and physical illness. In addition to various diseases and conditions such as spinal defects, endemic goiter, eye diseases, and skin ailments, there is also evidence of obesity.

In Meso-America, the major evidence for obesity comes from pottery statues from the so-called "Formative" or "Preclassic" period (1600 BC to AD 200). By the beginning of this period, corn-based agriculture was widespread. Small, sedentary, and self-sufficient communities were well established. Human skeletal remains from this period show that human beings were short—the average man was only 164 cm (5 ft 4 in) tall and the average woman was even shorter at 153 cm (5 ft). Numerous pottery finds from the early Preclassic Mayan culture show marked enlargement of the thighs, what we would call lower segment or pear-shaped obesity. Women with abdominal fat are also abundantly represented.

Examples are also found in other cultures. The Gulf Coast Olmec and Huasteca cultures produced many examples of corpulent people. From the preclassic Olmec period, an 18-cm tall pottery figurine referred to as "baby face" has fat legs and a fat abdomen. The Huasteca culture also provided several examples of obesity in pottery figures that are about the size and shape of the Venus of Willendorf (11 cm tall). There are also several examples of women with large thighs standing 4 to 10 cm tall.

What these Meso-American figurines tell us is that both central (apple-shaped) and peripheral (pear-shaped) forms of obesity were well known in the agricultural societies at the beginning of the cultural expansion in Central America. Even in the Classic period of Mayan culture, from AD 650 to 800, obesity is evident. In the Classic period, the arts reached a high level. A statue in the Art Institute of Chicago from this period shows an obese, round-bellied man. The statue is beautifully sculpted with headdress and ornaments. The bare bulging belly and the lifelike features suggest that it may be a portrait in pottery of one of the more affluent individuals, in whom we might expect more obesity because food was more available.

Conclusions about Obesity in the Prehistoric Period

We have traveled from the Old Stone Age more than 35,000 years ago when the Venus of Hohle Fels and then the Venus of Willendorf were made, down through the New Stone Age and Copper Age, and ended in the agricultural communities of early prehistory. In addition to showing that corpulence has a history as long as mankind, this survey of obesity in the Old and New Stone Ages also shows some other important things. First, almost all of the figures were female or of indeterminate sex. Only one male, from Laussel in France, was noted in this survey. Although these figures have been touted as examples of "mother goddesses," others interpret them as examples of glandular or endocrine disease evident before recorded history. Beller (1977) goes further, suggesting that these figures tell us that human beings knew about obesity and that the genetic basis for its development, independent of the type of diet or location, was present in early human cultures. Finally, these figures are distributed worldwide and in all cultures except Africa. The reason for the lack of such figures from Africa is unknown. It could be that obesity didn't appear in these cultures because of increased heat. It may be that artists had other things to represent. The high prevalence of obesity in the Pre-Columbian statues from Central and South America is consistent with the high prevalence of this problem among the descendents of these Pre-Columbian peoples of North and South America. In careful surveys, the prevalence of obesity in Latinos, many of whom are descendants of these early indigenous American peoples, is higher than in those of European ancestry. Although this survey shows us that obesity has a long history, we have no information on how or if it was treated in these early periods.

Origins of Obesity from the Beginnings of Recorded History to the Development of the Printing Press

In the historical record there is abundant evidence that obesity was a medical and health concern as long as medicine has been practiced. Moreover, treatment for obesity has a similarly long history, although the number of people who might need it was smaller than today. The obese probably came from the upper class of society, where obesity seems to accompany increased wealth, leisure time, and easier access to food. It is also clear that the type of diet is irrelevant to the development of obesity, since it is evident worldwide.

When you are "sick," you want help. For us, this means calling the doctor, going to an emergency room, seeking information on the Internet, or getting advice from a myriad of popular magazines. It has not always been so. Although medical traditions have developed in all cultures, we know much more than our forebears, even as recently as 50 to 100 years ago (Castiglioni 1941; Sigerist 1961; Mettler 1947; Major 1954; Garrison 1929; Duffin 1999). To understand how obesity has developed at various times in history, we need to have some understanding of these various medical traditions, several of which are described below (Bray 2007; Haslam 2009).

We find obesity in all medical traditions and geographic regions, which suggests that independent of diet, the potential to turn food into excess fat evolved even before we have a historical record documenting this fact (Beller 1977; Hautin 1939; Martinie 1934; Bray 2007; Haslam 2009).

The development of agriculture, metallurgy, writing systems, and political structures all influence the level of cultural sophistication. Several of the most sophisticated cultures have developed between two great river systems, the so-called two rivers hypothesis of cultural development. This hypothesis implies that we should look for higher levels of cultural sophistication where two rivers parallel each other. Some of these river pairs are the Yellow River and the Yangtse or Chiang Jang River in China, the Ganges and Indus Rivers in India, the Amu Darya and Syr Darya Rivers in Central Asia, and the Tigris and Euphrates Rivers in the Fertile Crescent of the Middle East.

Mesopotamian Medicine

The Tigris and Euphrates river basin was a land of healers and astrologers. Cuneiform writing, libraries, sanitation, and medical knowledge were evident by 3600 BC. Of the 30,000 clay tablets with cuneiform writing that were recovered in the library at Nineveh from approximately 2000 BC, 800 are related to medical matters. The medical armamentarium of Sumerian physicians consisted of more than 120 minerals and 250 herbs including cannabis, mustard, mandragora, belladonna, and henbane (Garrison 1929). In this advanced culture, we find one of the best known examples of a nude corpulent figure. This clay statuette showing enormously fat thighs and arms is an example of this problem. It was found at Susa in the twelfth century BC, middle Elamite period (Contenau 1938; Spycket 1995). A figure found in Syria also indicates the continuing representation of obesity in artifacts of the female body.

Egyptian Medicine

Egyptian medicine paralleled the Mesopotamian medical tradition from 3000 to 1000 BC. The physicians in Egypt were often priests and many priests were physicians. For example, Imhotep, who became the god of healing, began as a vizier or trusted adviser to King Zoser in 2900 BCE. Imhotep was a man of great accomplishment who, in addition to being a physician, was also an architect, a poet, and a statesman. Two major archeological finds, the Edwin Smith papyrus (Smith 1930), written between 2500 and 2000 BC, and the Ebers papyrus, written approximately 1550 BCE, provide our major knowledge about medicine in Egypt.

Obesity was known to the Egyptians and there may well have been attempts to treat it, particularly among the ruling classes. A study of royal mummies from the upper classes showed that both stout women (queens Henut-Tawy and Inhapy) and stout men were not uncommon in Egypt. Culturally, "obesity was regarded as objectionable" (Darby 1977) since the ideal depicted in their art was the thin stylized body shown in the side view. Several examples of obesity can be seen in stone reliefs, which were the principal artistic medium: a doorkeeper in one temple of Amon-Ra Khor-en-Khonsu complex; a cook in another tomb of Ankh-ma-Hor complex (sixth dynasty of the Middle Kingdom 2613–2181 BCE) (Nunn 1996); a fat man enjoying food presented to him by his lean servants in Mereruka's tomb; the local yeoman, the famed Sheikh et Balad (Darby 1977); and the grossly obese harpist playing before the prince Aki of the Middle Kingdom (Reeves 1992). Studies of the skinfold thickness of mummies using x-rays showed that Amenophis III and Ramses III were both fat (Reeves 1992; Filer 1995).

Chinese and Tibetan Medicine

The early Chinese believed that disease was sent by the gods or by demons. From the examination of bone fragments from Chinese graves, we know that the Chinese suffered from leprosy, typhoid fever, cholera, and plague. Although anatomic dissection was not permitted in China because of ancestor worship, the Chinese nonetheless developed a vigorous medical tradition. Herbal medicines were very important to the ancient, as well as modern, Chinese. Their physicians could select from at least 365 herbal medicines. The principal source of early medical teachings was the *The Yellow Emperor's Classic of Internal Medicine* (Huang Ti 1966), which dates from 200 BCE and is a dialogue on bodily functions and disease. The father of Chinese medicine is Zhang Zhongjing, who is considered the Chinese equivalent of the Greek Hippocrates in Western civilization. Zhang described symptoms and treatment for many diseases. Hua Toh (third century AD) is the only known surgeon from early China. Acupuncture, the art of treatment by inserting sharp needles into the body, was developed in China and reached its zenith there. An acupuncture site on the earlobe is said to reduce appetite and may have been a treatment for obesity.

Obesity was common among the upper classes in the Tang dynasty (AD 618–907). During the first half of the Tang dynasty, female courtesans were physically active and were particularly skillful on horseback. During the second half of this dynasty, they lost interest in physical activity and horseback riding by the women was largely abandoned. Obesity followed. This is nicely illustrated in a series of beautiful porcelain figures of women at court (Archeological Catalogue of China). These elegantly painted porcelain figures, nearly 50 cm (20 in) tall, clearly show "portly" or "plump" women dressed in long flowing gowns with well-coiffed hairstyles (Figure 4).

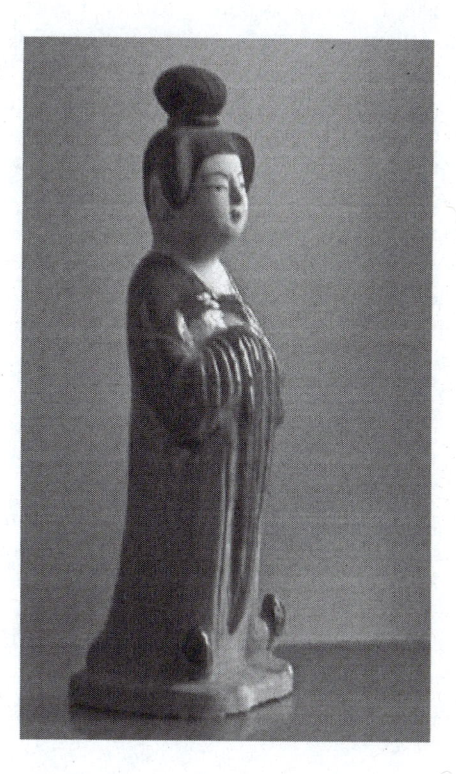

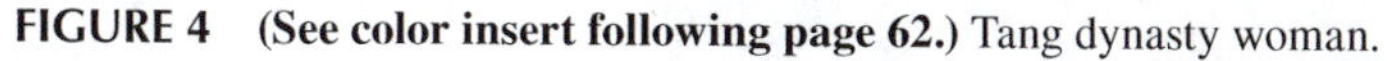

FIGURE 4 (See color insert following page 62.) Tang dynasty woman.

The Tibetan offspring of the Chinese medical tradition is beautifully illustrated in the seventeenth-century treatise entitled "The Blue Beryl," composed by Sangye Gyamtso, the scholar and regent of Tibet. It is an erudite yet practical commentary on the ancient text entitled *The Four Tantras* (Parfionovitch and Dorje 1992). In this text, obesity is described as a condition requiring catabolic treatment (breaking down fat tissue) documenting that there was an approach to treating obesity in this medical tradition:

> [O]vereating . . . causes illness and shortens life span. It is a contraindication to the use of compresses or mild enemas. For treatment of obesity two suggestions are made . . . The vigorous massage of the body with pea flour counteracts phlegm diseases and obesity . . . The gullet hair compress and flesh of a wolf remedy [to treat] goiters, dropsy and obesity (Parfionovitch and Dorje 1992).

Indian Medicine

A fourth great medical tradition is that of India (Alphen 1996). In the sacred medical texts of Ayurvedic medicine, sin was viewed as the cause of disease and medical knowledge was closely interwoven with religion and magic. The *Caraka Samhita* was the first book on Indian medicine and the *Susruta Samhita* was the second great Indian [Sanskrit] medical text. These texts describe many aspects of medical practice. For example, the *Caraka Samhita* describes an operating table and 20 sharp and 101 blunt instruments used in surgery. For nonsurgical treatment, at least 500 drugs are listed along with 700 medical herbs. Included in this list are cinnamon, borax, castor oil, ginger, and sodium carbonate. A tactic for treating obesity is mentioned in the Ayurveda and consists of administrating testicular tissue (organotherapy) as a cure for impotence as well as a treatment for corpulence (Iason 1946). Indian sculpture has many corpulent figures that demonstrate the presence of obesity.

Greco-Roman Medicine

From the vantage point of Western civilization, Greco-Roman medicine has been the major source of our medical tradition, and Hippocrates the "father of medicine." Greco-Roman medicine also provides lessons for treating obesity. The health hazards associated with obesity were clearly noted in the medical writings of Hippocrates who stated that "sudden death is more common in those who are naturally fat than in the lean" (Lloyd 1978; Hippocrates 1839). The Greeks also noted that obesity was a cause of infertility in women and that the frequency of menses was reduced in the obese.

Sleep apnea is a condition with snoring at night that obstructs breathing, with occasional periods with no breaths and a compensatory sleepiness during the daytime. Sleep apnea is particularly likely to occur in very obese people. The first descriptions of this complication associated with obesity date from Roman times. Dionysius, the tyrant of Heracleia of Pontius who reigned about 360 BCE, is one of the first historical figures afflicted with obesity and somnolence. When this enormously fat man frequently fell asleep, his servants would insert long needles through his skin and fat to the muscle beneath to jolt him into wakefulness. Kryger cites a second case of Magas, King of Cyrene, who died in 258 BC. He was a man "weighted down with monstrous masses of flesh in his last days; in fact he choked himself to death" (Kryger 1983, 1985).

Galen was the leading physician of Roman times. His influence on medicine and medical teaching lasted more than 1500 years. He identified two types of obesity, one he called "moderate," and the other "immoderate." The former is regarded as natural and the other as morbid. By this he meant it was associated with the development of other serious diseases.

Being overweight was often associated with the upper classes in Roman culture as it has been in other cultures throughout history. In a letter by Pliny the Younger written to the Roman historian Tacitus describing the eruption of Mount Vesuvius that destroyed Pompei in AD 79, he describes both his corpulent uncle, Pliny the Elder who was Admiral of the Fleet, and his mother who was also fat:

> .... Mount Vesuvius was blazing in several places with spreading and towering flames, whose refulgent brightness the darkness of the night set in high relief. But my uncle [Pliny the Elder—Admiral of the Fleet], in order to soothe apprehensions, kept saying that some fires had been left alight by the terrified country people, and what they saw were only deserted villas on fire in the abandoned district. After this he retired to rest, and it is most certain that this rest was a most genuine slumber: for his breathing, which, as he was pretty fat, was somewhat heavy and sonorous, was heard by those who attended at his chamber-door (Leppmann 1968).

This "sonorous and heavy breathing" is evidence of sleep apnea. Further on, Pliny the younger says about his mother as she urged him to flee: "My mother began to beseech, exhort, and command me to escape as best I might: a young man could do it: she, burdened with age and corpulency, would die easy if only she had not caused my death" (Leppmann 1968).

The approach of the modern physician to the treatment of obesity can be traced to fifth-century Greek and Roman times. From the time of Hippocrates 2500 years ago (Precope 1952), and Galen at the height of the Roman Empire nearly 2000 years ago (Green 1951), diet and exercise were an integral part of the therapeutic regimen for obese patients. To treat obesity, Hippocrates, the "father of medicine," suggested:

> [o]bese people and those desiring to lose weight should perform hard work before food. Meals should be taken after exertion and while still panting from fatigue and with no other refreshment before meals except only wine, diluted and slightly cold. Their meals should be prepared with sesame or seasoning and other similar substances and be of a fatty nature as people get thus, satiated with little food. They should, moreover, eat only once a day and take no baths and sleep on a hard bed and walk naked as long as possible (Precope 1952).

Galen's system of disease evolved from the humoral ideas of Hippocrates and the four elements—fire, air, earth, and water. This idea provided a way of looking at health and disease. Good health was a proper balance between the humors. Ill-health was a loss of this balance and it was the physician's job was to restore it. This concept served as the basis for concepts about disease for over 2000 years.

Bleeding was important in the therapeutic armamentarium of Galen. Galen also believed strongly in the use of diet as an approach to treating obesity (see Chapter 20 in Green 1951). Galen, nearly 2000 years ago, outlined his approach to treatment of obesity as follows:

> I have made any sufficiently stout patient moderately thin in a short time, by compelling him to do rapid running, then wiping off his perspiration with very soft or very rough muslin and then massaging him maximally with diaphoretic inuctions, which the younger doctors customarily call restoratives, and after such massage leading him to the bath after which I give him nourishment immediately but bade him rest for a while or do nothing to which he was accustomed, then lead him to a second bath and then gave him abundant food of little nourishment so as to fill him up but distribute little of it to the entire body (Green 1951).

Claudius Galen (AD 131–201?) is included here because he was one of the most influential physicians of Western history and provided a description of how he treated obesity. Galen was born in Pergamon on the western coast in what is now modern Turkey, probably in AD 131. This was at the height of the Roman Empire, and Galen became its most famous physician. Osler captured his lofty medical standing with these words:

No other physician has ever occupied the commanding position of Claudius Galen. For fifteen centuries he dominated medical thought powerfully as did Aristotle in the school of the day. Not until the Renaissance did daring spirits begin to question the infallibility of this medical Pope. He was the last, and, in many ways, the greatest of the Greeks—a man very much of our own type, who, could he visit this country today, might teach us many lessons. (Osler 1921)

Galen was born into an affluent family at a time of relative peace in the Roman Empire. His father spared no expense on his son's education, sending him to study in Greece at the School of the Stoics, the School of the Academicians, the School of the Peripatetics, and, finally, the School of the Epicureans. He had many of the famous physicians of his time as mentors, but he outshone all of them. He was appointed physician to the gladiators, which provided him with considerable clinical exposure to traumatic wounds. He spent at least two periods of his life in Rome. Periodically, he returned to Pergamon, the city of his birth in Turkey. His published output was prodigious and speaks to an unquenchable internal drive to write. We can account for more than 400 works on medicine, and there were books on other subjects as well. However, only 83 works survive (Castiglioni 1941).

Galen could be called a "teleologic dogmatist" since he believed that, "Nature acts with perfect wisdom and does nothing uselessly" (Castiglioni 1941). Although he did many experiments, his teleologic approach to understanding medicine left no experimental heritage for the future.

His ego matched his scholarly output. As Professor Selwyn-Brown observed about Galen in his book on great medical personalities, "His style was forceful and persuasive, but it was also pugnacious . . . Galen's enthusiasm and conceit led him to class all writers who disagreed with him as fools, and this unfortunate capacity for making enemies kept him continually embroiled with his fellow doctors" (Selwyn-Brown 1928). Another medical historian, Castiglioni, noted that "[h]e often magnified in exaggerated terms his diagnostic and therapeutic successes" (Castiglioni 1941). He is reputed to have said, "No one before me has given the true method of treating diseases." Galen considered himself the greatest of all physicians, just as his contemporary, the Emperor Trajan, considered himself the greatest of all Roman emperors. Galen's scholarly impact is clear from the fact that his work was still used in European medical education into the seventeenth century (Garrison 1914).

Arabic Medicine

With the decline of Roman influence and the rise of Constantinople after AD 400, scholarly activity shifted from Rome to Byzantium and then to the broader Arabic world following the rise of Islam in the seventh century. Two great figures stand out from this middle period of medicine—AD 500 to 1500. One of them was Maimonides and the other leading figure of this medical tradition was Abu Ali Ibn Sina, or Avicenna, in its Westernized form. Like Galen, he was an influential scholarly author who published more than 40 medical works and 145 works on philosophy, logic, theology, and other subjects. Obesity was well known to this Arabic physician.

From the Greco-Roman beginning, dietary treatment of obesity can be traced to the Arabic tradition in medicine. In the first book of Avicenna's five-volume *Canon*, he describes how to reduce the overweight individual:

> The regimen which will reduce obesity. (Gaarder 1995) 1) Produce a rapid descent of the food from the stomach and intestines, in order to prevent completion of absorption by the mesentery. (Castiglioni 1941) 2) Take food which is bulky but feebly nutritious. (Sigerist 1961) 3) Take the bath before food, often. (Major 1954) 4) Hard exercise. . . (Gruner 1930).

As we can see, the idea of diet and exercise are bulwarks in the fight against obesity in history from the time of Hippocrates to the sixteenth century—a span of 2000 years. Had they accomplished what their authors intended, we would have effective strategies, and the current quest might not have been needed. However, the fact that we have an epidemic of obesity today that is covering

Abu- "Ali al-Husayn ibn-"Abd-allah ibn-Sina (Latinized as Avicenna) [980–1037] was born in Afshana near Bokhara in what is now the central Asian country of Uzbekistan. The Arab lands of those days extended from Spain in the west to central Asia in the east. The time of Avicenna's birth was one of intellectual ferment in Bokhara in Central Asia that saw a flowering of talent in many fields. According to Avicenna's "self-conscious" autobiography, written at the age of 18, he had memorized the Koran by age 10 and was a practicing doctor by age 16. He is alleged to have successfully treated Amir Nuh ibn-Mansur Al-Samani, prince of Khorasan, the ruler of Bokhara. His success gave him access to the Amir's library that was reputed to be the second best in the world. Avicenna's scholarship extended into many areas, including religion, law, metaphysics, mathematics, astronomy, and medicine. The instability of the local governments in central Asia led him to take up arms to fight in military campaigns. His military life resulted in riotous living followed by a long severe illness and his eventual death at the age of 57, in 1037.

Avicenna's masterpiece is his five-volume work on medicine called the *Canon* on medicine (*Kitab al-Qanun*) that was translated into Latin in the eleventh century by Gerard of Cremona and used in Western medical education until at least the seventeenth century. The *Canon* contains no personal experiences and no new ideas, but was rather a summary of existing knowledge. The first book deals with theoretical medicine, including physiology, etiology, symptomatology, disease classification (nosology), and the principles of therapy. The second book is largely about hygiene and hygienic matters. The third book is on localized diseases and their treatment, and the fourth book is about generalized diseases and their treatment. The final book deals with herbal treatments called "materia medica" and is a dispensary and an apothecary's book.

Avicenna surpassed both Aristotle and Galen in his dialectical subtlety (Campbell 1926; Ullmann 1978). By some estimates, he published more than 100 medical books, as well as many volumes in other areas. Avicenna's attempt to reconcile the doctrines of Galen with those of Aristotle is similar to the effort of the intellectual Catholic scholar, St. Thomas Aquinas, to reconcile these authors with the teachings of the Roman Catholic Church some two centuries later. The influence of the *Canon* on Western medicine was on the whole bad, for "it confirmed physicians in the pernicious idea that the use of syllogisms and logic is a better way to solve problems than first-hand observation and investigation" of Nature (Garrison 1914). Albrecht van Haller in the eighteenth century referred to the *Canon* as a "methodic inanity." Fielding Garrison, the twentieth-century historian of medicine, called Avicenna's *Canon* "a huge, unwieldy storehouse of learning."

the globe suggests that the strategically simple ideas of eating less and exercising more, ideas that require commitment and personal involvement by the individual, have not been very successful. As we move forward in trying to understand this problem, we need to be alert to strategies and tactics that may not require individual motivation and commitment—history has shown that they do not work well.

A second major medical figure of the Arabian world is Maimonides. In contrast with Avicenna, who was prominent in Baghdad and the Eastern Arab world, Maimonides had his base in the western Arabian world of Spain.

With increasing trade and travel from the twelfth to the sixteenth centuries, European culture gradually reestablished contact with Arabian medicine and the Roman traditions that it absorbed. Both the Crusades in the Middle Ages (AD 1000–1200) and the invasions by the Arabs of the Peloponnesus and southern Spain brought an infusion of classical knowledge from which came the Renaissance and the beginning of the scientific era in the fifteenth and sixteenth centuries (Castiglioni 1941; Ullmann 1978).

Maimonides was the great twelfth-century Jewish physician in the era of Arabic medicine. Rabi Moses ben Maimon or Maimonides (1135–1204) is sometimes called the "second Moses." He was born into a medical family in Cordoba, Spain, in AD 1135 and lived nearly 70 years, dying in Cairo in AD 1204. In addition to being a physician, he was a theologian and philosopher who influenced the thinking of many other great philosophers, from St. Thomas Aquinas to Immanuel Kant and Spinoza. One of his goals was to reconcile the thought of the Jewish people with the great traditions of classical philosophy as well as with more recent philosophy. His openness struck responsive chords among Jewish intellectuals of the time, but it aroused opposition from the strongly orthodox Rabbis. Maimonides in Spain was a recipient of the teachings of his Arab contemporaries in the Caliphates in Baghdad, Damascus, and Egypt.

In this introduction, I have explored obesity from the beginnings of recorded history to the opening of the sixteenth century. We find obesity and its treatment in all medical traditions in this historic period. Treatments date from the beginning of written language. We can conclude that obesity was worldwide from the earliest recorded medical traditions. Quantitatively we are ahead in the absolute number of obese people, but the problem existed from historic times and treatment is evident from early historical records more than 25,000 years ago. Changes in diet and the use of vigorous exercise were major recommendations of early physicians to their obese patients. It has developed in cultures eating widely divergent diets, meaning that specific foods are neither necessary nor causative, nor do specific diets prevent it. Finally, the genes for enlargement of fat cells that predispose us to obesity were present in the earliest Stone Age cultures and continued through the period of written history.

Part I

Origins of Obesity

1 Origins of Obesity in the Scientific Era
AD 1500 to the Present

"The history of truth is neither linear nor monotone."

Canguilhem (1988)

KEY POINTS

- The sixteenth century was one of discovery and this included, for obesity, the initial dissections of the human body.
- The seventeenth century was the century of physics, discovery of the circulation of blood, and the use of beam balances to weigh the intake of food in human beings. It was also the time of the first microscopic studies.
- The landmark for obesity in the eighteenth century was the discovery of oxygen and the demonstration that metabolism was like the burning of a candle.
- The nineteenth century saw the formulation of the laws of thermodynamics and their application to humans, the introduction of the body mass index, and the first popular diet book.

INTRODUCTION

This chapter moves us into the third revolution in communication. The first revolution in communication was the development of speech, which occurred around 50,000 years ago. The second revolution in communication was the development of writing that occurred in China, in the Middle East, and in Central America, some 5000 years ago. The third major revolution in communication, and the beginning point of this chapter, was the introduction of printing with movable type. In the twentieth century, we entered a fourth revolution in communication—the electronic and Internet revolution that has already dramatically sped up the way information about obesity and other subjects is transmitted.

In this chapter, we will follow the emergence of obesity from the time when printing presses were widely distributed around Europe (around 1500) and the New World was undergoing exploration following its discovery through the voyages of Christopher Columbus in 1492, to the early twentieth century (Bray 1990, 2007, 2009). The evolution and treatment of obesity in the twentieth century will occupy the rest of this book.

Table 1.1 gives a brief summary of events related to the development of obesity that have occurred during these five centuries, alongside other historical and scientific landmarks (Taylor 1949). The increasing pace of discovery is evident and will be a central theme of this chapter.

The story begins with Gutenberg, the famous German who invented movable type and used it to print Bibles in Mainz, Germany, in the middle of the fifteenth century. Thus began the third revolution in communication.

TABLE 1.1
Short Summary of Events in the History of Science and Obesity since AD 1500

	World Scene	Science and Technology	Biology and Medicine	Obesity
15th century		Printing		
16th century		Copernicus (heliocentric theory)	Vesalius (anatomy)	Benvieni (fat dissection)
17th century		Galileo (telescope)	Harvey (blood circulation)	Santorio (metabolic balance)
		Boyle (laws of temperature and pressure)	Malpighi (pulmonary circulation)	
	1649 English Civil War	Watt (steam engine)	Hooke (micrographia)	
18th century		Photography	Morgagni (first pathology text)	1727 Short (first monograph on corpulency)
		Electrical cell	Lind (*On Scurvy*)	1760 Flemyng (second monograph)
		Atomic theory	Cullen (classification)	1780s Lavoisier (oxygen theory of metabolism)
		Electromagnetism	Oxygen and hydrogen discovered	
	1776 American Revolution			
	1789 French Revolution			
19th century		Wohler (urea synthesized from inorganic molecules)	Jenner (vaccination)	1810 Wadd (*On Corpulency*)
	Napoleon	Mendeleev (periodic table of elements)	Laennec (stethoscope)	1826 Brillat-Savarin (*Physiologie du Gout*)
		Bernard (liver glycogen)	Schwann (cell theory)	1835 Quetelet (body mass index)
	1861–1865 U.S. Civil War	Morphine, cocaine, quinine, amphetamine	Morton (ether anesthesia)	1848 von Helmholtz (conservation of energy)
		Ions hypothesized	Von Helmholtz (ophthalmoscope)	1849 Hassal describes fat cell
		Internal combustion engine	Darwin (*Origin of the Species*)	1863 Banting (first diet book)
			Semmelweis (puerperal fever)	1866 Sleep apnea described
			Lister (antiseptic surgery)	1870 Fat cell identified
		Salvarsan to treat syphilis	Mendelian genetics	1896 Atwater (room calorimeter)
			Sherrington and reflex arc	
20th century		Wright brothers' flight		1900 Babinski
				1901 Frohlich describes hypothalamic obesity

(*continued*)

TABLE 1.1 (Continued)
Short Summary of Events in the History of Science and Obesity since AD 1500

	World Scene	Science and Technology	Biology and Medicine	Obesity
		Vacuum tube	Secretin—first hormone	1912 Cushing's syndrome
	Spanish-American War	Theory of relativity	Pavlov identified conditioned reflexes	1914 Gastric contractions and hunger
		Sulfonamides		
		Nylon		1932 Garrod and Inborn errors
		DDT		
		Vitamins		Family study of obesity
	World War I	$E = mc^2$—atomic bomb	1921 Banting isolates insulin	Genetically obese animals
		Quantum physics	1928 Fleming finds penicillin	Amphetamines used to treat obesity
		Rockets	Operant conditioning	CT/MRI scans for visceral fat
		Transistor		
	World War II	Laser	Salk/Sabin polio vaccine	DXA and density for body fat
		Computed tomography	Watson/Crick DNA hypothesis	Doubly labeled water
	Vietnam War	Magnetic resonance imaging scans	AIDS	1994 Leptin
			Genetic engineering	Laparoscopic surgery
			Humane genome	Combination therapy
21st century	Iraq War		Genome-wide scans	
			Functional brain imaging	

Source: Adapted from Bray, G.A., *Obesity Science to Practice*, Wiley-Blackwell, Chichester, 2009.

Printing was a driving force in the expansion of knowledge from that time onward. It provided a rapid means of communicating new ideas. It informed us of our progress and our failures. It helped scientists communicate and it provided a way for good and bad advice to be widely distributed. The electronic age has dramatically changed this. The way scientific information is now communicated, retrieved, and distributed has changed from paper to electronic devices, which will impact future scientific communication as surely as printing did 500 years ago. All of these revolutions in communication have changed our understanding of the problem of obesity and have provided ever more rapid means of disseminating knowledge about it and how to treat it.

In the 50 years following the development of the printing press—from around AD 1450 to 1500—printing presses and printing shops gradually spread throughout Europe. By 1500, large numbers of classical texts from Greek, Roman, and Arabic times had been printed and widely circulated. In addition, a smattering of original books began to appear in print as well.

As the amount of scientific literature has grown since Gutenberg, so have the complaints about it. Scientific literature has a doubling time of about 20 years or so (Price 1961). This means that nearly 75% of all scientific literature ever published will be published during the lifetime of a scientist. The frustration engendered by the rapid growth of scientific literature, both books and journals, has been reflected in quotations from scholars beginning in the seventeenth century and continuing to the present (Ziman 1976). The following are a few examples of these complaints.

A seventeenth-century comment from Barnaby Rich:

> One of the diseases of this age is the multiplicity of books; they doth so overcharge the world that it is not able to digest the abundance of idle matter that is every day hatched and brought forth into the world. (Price 1961, p. 63)

From the great eighteenth-century encyclopedist Diderot, we have the following statement of the problem (he did not know that Google was coming):

> The number of books will grow continually, and one can predict that a time will come when it will be almost as difficult to learn anything from books as from the direct study of the whole universe. It will be almost as convenient to search for some bit of truth concealed in nature as it will be to find it hidden away in an immense multitude of bound volumes. (Price 1961, p. 63)

In the early nineteenth century, Thomas Beddoes, a leading physician, made these comments about the problem:

> You must needs hang your heavy head, and role your blood shot eyes over thousands of pages weekly. Of their contents at the week's end you will know about as much of a district through which you have been whirled night and day in the mail coach. (Beddoes 1802)

In the twentieth century, as the volume of scientific literature continued to increase, even more concerns were raised:

> Scientists have always felt themselves to be awash in a sea of scientific literature that augments in each decade as much as in all times before (Price 1961).
> Like beach bums, new journals appear in crops overnight . . . There are too many of them, they are published too often, they stare from the racks and reproach us for sloth (Weissmann 1990).
> . . . it has been apparent for the past couple of centuries, that like books, the making of journals is endless (Bynum and Wilson 1992).
> Today, when the excessive number of medical journals is a common source of complaint it is salutary to realize that even by the end of the eighteenth century some were voicing the same concern (Loudon and Loudon 1992).

From the beginnings in the seventeenth century, there has been a steady logarithmic growth in knowledge and information. The epidemic of obesity expands around us, as does the scientific literature from which solutions will eventually come. To provide some order for the journey through this ever increasing scientific knowledge, I have prepared five timelines, beginning in 1500. Each timeline consists of 11 separate lines. They show the developments in science and technology, anatomy and histology, physiology, chemistry/biochemistry, genetics, pharmacology, neuroscience, and clinical medicine. If one wanted a demarcation line for the beginning of modern medicine, it might well be the time of the American and French Revolutions, which occurred between 1776 and 1789. To these timelines, I have added the American presidents, beginning with George Washington in 1789. These timelines provide a framework for relating the medical and scientific advances in each century to the progress in understanding obesity. As a historical anchor, I have also included some of the key historical events that were occurring at the same time. These other events are intended to put the scientific achievements in a broader historical framework. The rate of scientific progress over these five centuries is evident from the increasing number of entries in each category. The rapidity of scientific progress is particularly clear from the beginning of the nineteenth century through the twentieth century.

Most of the major contributions to science in the sixteenth and seventeenth centuries appeared in the form of monographs, syllabuses, pamphlets, and textbooks. As the number of scientists increased during the seventeenth century, early scientific societies were formed in England, France, and Italy. These scientific societies became a focal point for meetings and correspondence about new scientific discoveries.

Application of the experimental method to obesity has come as it has come to all other areas, but progress has been slow. From the beginning of the "scientific era" (AD 1500) to the beginning of "modern medicine" (around 1800), only a small number of scientific dissertations or theses resulting from academic scholarship with obesity as the subject matter had been published (see Appendix for an alphabetical list of the dissertations written in the sixteenth, seventeenth, and eighteenth centuries). In general, these early scholarly dissertations reflected the medical traditions that originated 1000 to 1500 years earlier in the writings of Hippocrates (460–370 BCE) (1839–1861), Galen (AD 131–201) (1531), or Avicenna (980–1037) (1984).

Obesity is, in one sense, in the eye of the beholder. In Chapter 2, we will examine the ways it can be defined and measured. One concept of this book is that obesity is a disease in the same sense that diabetes and hypertension are diseases (Bray 2004). From ancient times to the beginning of the nineteenth century, disease was viewed from the Greco-Roman perspective as an imbalance in the four humors (Duffin 1999). The goal of the physician is to restore the imbalances that may have occurred. This concept was only effectively displaced when the germ theory of disease emerged in the nineteenth century (Pasteur [1822–1895] 1822–1839; Koch [1834–1913] 1884; Lister [1827–1912] 1870).

SIXTEENTH CENTURY

Exploration was a central theme of the sixteenth century. Exploration of the solar system led to the publication by Copernicus (1543) of his ideas that the sun was the center of the planetary system with the earth revolving around the sun. Exploration of the earth followed the discovery of the Americas in 1492 by Christopher Columbus and exploration of the human body followed the publication of *The Fabric of the Human Body* by Vesalius (1514–1564) in 1543.

The sixteenth century also saw the introduction of quantitative methods for the study of health and disease Figure 1.1. Both normal anatomy and pathologic anatomy had their modern beginnings at this time.

The revolution in communication provided by printing ushered in the age of anatomy at the beginning of the sixteenth century. Before then, the writings of Galen in Roman times and the *Canon of Avicenna* from Arabic medicine in the tenth century (Gruner 1930) had been the main sources of information about anatomy, physiology, and clinical medicine. These sources had come down through handwritten texts. Although there is no clear evidence that either Galen or Avicenna ever dissected a human cadaver, their influence over the teaching of anatomy was profound and it only diminished by the application of direct dissection of human bodies and by the dissemination of these findings in printed books that occurred in the sixteenth century.

Anatomy was a central theme for obesity in the sixteenth century. The year was 1543, the year when Andreas Vesalius (1514–1564) published his treatise on human anatomy (Vesalius 1543). Andreas Vesalius was only 28 years old when he published his masterpiece. In his accurate and careful dissections, Vesalius showed that the human body could be directly explored by dissection rather than reading from Galen's anatomy.

Advances in normal anatomy were accompanied by the first pathological descriptions of obese individuals are attributed to Benivieni (1443–1502) (1507, 1954). One of the earliest descriptions of the treatment and cure of obesity was presented in his book published posthumously in 1507.

In the sixteenth century, there were only two dissertations (disputations) known to this author that dealt with obesity or nutrition. One of these discussed how fat is formed. It was presented in 1580 as a disputation in Heidelberg between a young student named Thomas Erastus and a

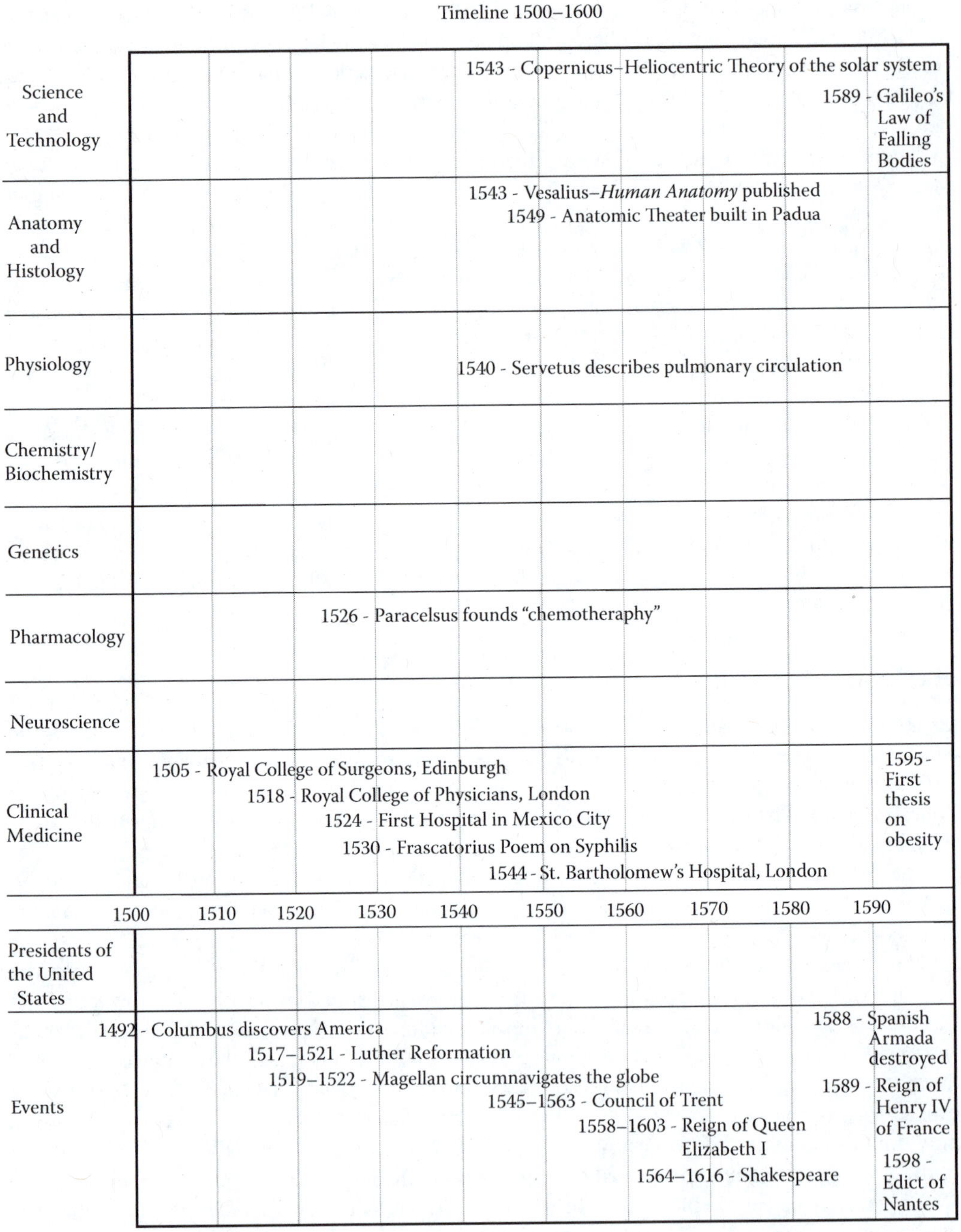

Timeline 1500–1600

	1500 – 1590
Science and Technology	1543 - Copernicus–Heliocentric Theory of the solar system 1589 - Galileo's Law of Falling Bodies
Anatomy and Histology	1543 - Vesalius–*Human Anatomy* published 1549 - Anatomic Theater built in Padua
Physiology	1540 - Servetus describes pulmonary circulation
Chemistry/ Biochemistry	
Genetics	
Pharmacology	1526 - Paracelsus founds "chemotheraphy"
Neuroscience	
Clinical Medicine	1505 - Royal College of Surgeons, Edinburgh 1518 - Royal College of Physicians, London 1524 - First Hospital in Mexico City 1530 - Frascatorius Poem on Syphilis 1544 - St. Bartholomew's Hospital, London 1595 - First thesis on obesity
	1500 1510 1520 1530 1540 1550 1560 1570 1580 1590
Presidents of the United States	
Events	1492 - Columbus discovers America 1517–1521 - Luther Reformation 1519–1522 - Magellan circumnavigates the globe 1545–1563 - Council of Trent 1558–1603 - Reign of Queen Elizabeth I 1564–1616 - Shakespeare 1588 - Spanish Armada destroyed 1589 - Reign of Henry IV of France 1598 - Edict of Nantes

FIGURE 1.1 Timeline for the sixteenth century. The key events in several categories including politics, science, and obesity are shown.

renowned professor, M. Michael Schenkius. However, it was not published until 1595 in a collection of disputations. The humoral perspective originated in the Greco-Roman times still dominated this disputation. It raised the question of whether fat congeals as a result of cold—a Galenic idea—or whether it would congeal from heat. The latter idea is a logical deduction of another basic Galenic idea—that along with milk and sperm, fat is merely the result of an excess of nutritive matter

Antonio di Paolo Benivieni (1443–1502) is known for his description of the treatment of obesity in his collected work on pathology was one of the first publications of the scientific era (1507). Benivieni was born in Florence. He was the oldest of five children born into an ancient Florentine family. As a child at the onset of the Renaissance, he studied Greek and Latin. He was both a man of letters and a physician. He attended both the University of Pisa and the University of Siena. Although he was 12 when Gutenberg printed his bible, he had acquired a substantial library of more than 169 titles, covering a wide range of subjects, by his early 40s. Of these, some 70 related to medicine. Leonardo da Vinci performed some of his anatomic dissections at the Santa Maria Nuova hospital where Benivieni may have worked, but there is no definitive record of their association. His single publication *De Abditis Nonnullis ac Mirandis Morborum et Sanationum Causis* was edited by Giovanni Rosati, a Florentine physician, from his case records and published soon after his death. Case LXIX is "A man apparently dying of excessive obesity, cured by blood letting only" (Garrison 1914, p. 165; Mettler 1947, p. 249).

converted from the blood by heat (see *Classics of Obesity*) (Albala 2005). The other was by Pierre Forrest (from Regneller) and dealt with undernutrition.

The paradigm for treatment of any disease in the sixteenth, seventeenth, and even the eighteenth century was largely derived from the idea of the four humors theory that originated in Greco-Roman medicine. The four humors are illustrated in Figure 1.2. Diet, exercise, purgatives, diuretics, sweating agents, and blood-letting were among the major approaches used to readjust the ill-humors. Treatment was thus aimed at realigning these four humors.

Diet was one way to rebalance this system. It has been used for treatment of obesity since the time of Hippocrates and Galen more than 2000 years ago. Chaucer, the great fourteenth-century poet, echoed the advice of Hippocrates when he said against gluttony, the remedy is abstinence, or in his Middle English, "Agonys glotonye, the remedie is abstinence." From the twelfth century onward, the *Regimen Sanitatis* (Harington 1920), written in the School of Medicine at Salerno, Italy and translated into many languages, provided guidance for the use of diet and nutrition for achieving and maintaining good health. Although it went through many editions over several hundred

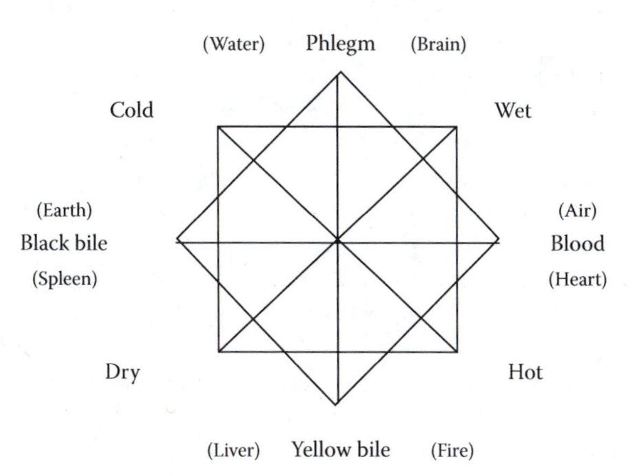

FIGURE 1.2 Diagram of the four humors.

Luigi Cornaro (1467–1566) is known for his small monograph on "the sober life" was so widely disseminated as a way of dealing with the problem of obesity in his time. Cornaro was born in Padua and during his youth indulged himself freely in matters of eating and drinking. He married and had one child. By the age of 25, his "intemperance" began to catch up with him, and he suffered from colic and gout. Cornaro came from a distinguished Venetian family held in high honor from the fifteenth to the eighteenth century. As his health problems mounted, he was advised by the medical men he sought to change his life and renounce his old ways. This book is a description of the triumphs of the changes in his personal hygiene (*Trattato della vita sobria* or *Discourses on the Sober Life*), which was published in Padua in 1558. It was one of the bestselling books on personal hygiene of the time. He was described as having an "infirm constitution till about 40 years of age." He had originally been a fat man, but through a sort of spiritual conversion, he adopted the "simple life" and recovered to a state of "perfect health." He did this by reducing his intake of solid food to 12 ounces and his wine intake to 14 ounces. It took less than a year for him to be entirely free from all of his complaints. He published his book at age 80 and lived to his 99th year, seeing a third and fourth edition of his book published. Cornaro's advice from his doctor was to eat or drink nothing that was not wholesome and that only in small quantities. With this advice, Cornaro lost his excess weight and then became a zealot for moderation in dieting (Cornaro 1916).

years, the *Regimen* did not specifically provide advice for treating obesity, which was relatively infrequent during the Middle Ages.

The idea of abstinence from food as a strategy for treatment of corpulence goes back centuries. A now famous Italian layman named Luigi Cornaro railed against the consequences of gluttony in a widely published and translated monograph (Cornaro 1558, 1737). At the beginning of his book he says, "O wretched, miserable Italy! Does not though plain see, that gluttony deprives [us] of more soul years, than either war, or the plague itself could have done?"

Diets have been used for centuries. The use of a stringent diet, one which limits food choices and amounts, was popularized again in the seventeenth century by an Italian layman named Luigi Cornaro (1467–1566). In a short book, he championed dietary moderation after he successfully conquered his own obesity (Cornaro 1737).

SEVENTEENTH CENTURY

Experimentation is a scientific tradition that has its origins in the sixteenth and seventeenth centuries. The scientist has a question, for example, "How do we become obese?" He designs an experiment to ask whether an animal or a human being can become obese when food intake is limited. The results of this experiment will either support or not support the original idea. As Hans Popper, one of great philosophers of the scientific method, has defined it, experimentation is a method of verification and falsification (Miller 1985). That is, progress was made by designing experiments to test hypotheses and applying mathematical analysis, where appropriate, to the results. If the experimental results are incompatible with the hypothesis, the hypothesis has been falsified and the search is on for a new hypothesis. The fruitfulness of this tradition is all around us. For example, cellular telephones, the Internet, in vitro fertilization, and the new drugs to fight human diseases including obesity.

The sixteenth century was an age of exploration and also an age of colonization—a time when intellectual genius flowered. Galileo Galilei (1564–1642) in Italy studied gravity and the solar system. Isaac Newton (1642–1727) in England developed the laws of motion. Their concepts of a mechanical universe were soon applied to medicine and the so-called medico-physical theories of health and disease abounded.

Several scientific themes in the seventeenth century expanded the scientific base for understanding obesity. First was the application of a balance scale for weighing human beings and their food intake and output and applying it to the study of metabolism. This was the life work of Santorio Santorio (1561–1636) in Padua (1624, English translations 1676 and 1720), who might be called the "father of metabolism." A second theme was the beginning of anatomic description of diseased bodies. A third theme was the introduction of the microscope and the earliest description of microscopic structures. The final theme of the seventeenth century was the beginning of human physiology, personified in the work of William Harvey (1578–1657) who described the circulation of the blood. Although thinking about medicine was influenced by the rapid growth of physics and the application of mechanical principles to the operation of the body, ideas about treatment of disease and about obesity in particular remained relatively in the dark ages and classical Greco-Roman tradition. The only new addition was the reduction of the four humors to three by Paracelsus, a free-thinking, itinerant seventeenth-century physician (Figure 1.3).

From the perspective of obesity, the work of Santorio Santorio (1624; 1676; 1720) at the University of Padua where he was a contemporary of Galileo. Santorio defined health as the maintenance of a normal body weight. With the use of a weighing chair on which he could weigh his intake and excreta, he was thus able to calculate the difference between the weight of food eaten and the urine and feces produced. The missing part he defined as "insensible perspiration." From his 30 years of recording his intake and output, he concluded that insensible perspiration through the skin and breath makes up the greater proportion of bodily waste. If a healthy man, for example, consumed 4 kg of food in one day, more than 2 kg would be excreted through insensible loss. Perspiration was a sign that the body had properly refined and assimilated the nutritive matter of food and drink. Excess perspiration indicated that the body was beginning to waste away. On the other hand, too little perspiration was a sign that crude deposits were being left in the body. "Health continues firm as long as the body returns daily to the same weight by insensible perspiration . . ." Following Santorio, many writers would naturally assume that increased perspiration itself serves to slim the body (Albala 2005).

What is perhaps even stranger is that Santorio insisted that the accumulation of fat was not a simple matter of eating too much. "He who eats more than he can digest, is nourished less than he ought to be, and [becomes] consequently emaciated" (Albala 2005). Just because food is eaten does not mean it is digested or offers nutrition, a way of thinking totally foreign to our sensibilities, and one that would be abandoned along with many of the ideas of Galen in the coming generations.

Anatomic dissections of diseased people were a second theme of the seventeenth century. The first anatomic dissections of obese individuals, after Benvieni, are attributed to Théophile Bonet (latinized *Bonetus*) (1620–1689). Bonet was a physician as well as an anatomist. His work included the practice of medicine and the use of anatomic dissections to examine some aspects of pathologic anatomy (Bonetus 1700).

A summary of some approaches to the treatment of obesity in the seventeenth century are found in Bonet's book, in the section called "Obesitas or Corpulency" where he describes six examples of the treatment of obesity:

I. Chiapinius Vitellius, Camp Master-General, a middle aged man, grew so fat, that he was forced to sustain his belly by a swathe, which came about his neck: And observing that he was every day more unfit for the Wars than other, he voluntarily abstained from Wine, and continued to drink vinegar as long as he lived; upon which his Belly fell, and his Skin hung loose, with which he could wrap himself as with a Doublet. It was observed that he lost 87 pounds of weight.

II. Lest any great mischief should follow, we must try to subtract by medicine, what a spare diet will not; because it has been observed, that a looseness either natural, or procured by

Timeline 1600–1700

Science and Technology	1620 - Bacon's *Organum Novum*; 1662 - Descartes' *De Homine*; 1662 - Newton and Leibniz develop calculus; 1665 - Newton's Law of Gravity; 1687 - Newton's *Principia*
Anatomy and Histology	1610 - Galileo devises microscope; 1658 - Swammerdam describes red corpuscles; 1661 - Malpighi publishes *Pulmonary Circulation*; 1665 - Hooke's *Micrographia*; 1672 - DeGraaf ovarian follicle; 1675 - Leeuwenhoek protozoa
Physiology	1614 - Santorio, father of Metabolic Obesity, describes metabolic scale, pulse counting, thermometer.; 1628 - Harvey publishes *Circulation of Blood*; 1665 - Lower-transfuses blood in dogs
Chemistry/ Biochemistry	1661 - Boyle defines Chemical Element; 1674 - Mayow–Animal heat in muscles
Genetics	
Pharmacology	
Neuroscience	
Clinical Medicine	1639 - First hospital in Canada; 1642 - Jacob Bontius describes beri-beri; 1650 - Glisson describes rickets; 1656 - Wharton publishes *Adenographia*; 1659 - Willis describes Puerperal Fever; 1670 - Willis describes "sweet" urine in diabetes; 1683 - Sydenham treatise on gout
	1600 1610 1620 1630 1640 1650 1660 1670 1680 1690
Presidents of the United States	
Events	1607 - Jamestown, VA, settled; 1618–1648 - 30 Years War; 1620 - Plymouth, MA, settled; 1636 - Harvard College founded; 1640–1688 - Reign of Frederick the Great Elector; 1642–1661 - English Civil War and Cromwell Rule; 1654–1715 - Reign of Louis XIV; 1660–1689 - Reign of Charles II of England; 1666 - London Fire; 1682–1725 - Reign of Peter the Great of Russia; 1690 - Locke publishes *On Human Under-standing*; 1692 - Salem Witch-Hunt

FIGURE 1.3 Timeline for the seventeenth century. The key events in several categories including politics, science, and obesity are shown.

Santorio Santorio (1561–1636), or *Sanctorius* in Latin, is known for his application of quantitative methods to studying human metabolism and his identification of "insensible perspiration." Santorio was born March 29, 1561, in Capodistria, the capital of Istria. He and his brother and two sisters were raised in an aristocratic family. After his initial education in Capodistria, his father took him to Venice, where he was tutored by many of the best minds of his time. In 1575, he began his university education in Padua at age 14. After 7 years of education he received his medical degree in 1582 at the age of 21. After graduation he practiced medicine in Poland for 14 years before returning to Venice, where he practiced medicine and joined the intellectual circle that included the astronomer and physicist Galileo (1564–1642), the surgeon and anatomist Hieronymous Fabricius (1537–1619), and the theologian and philosopher Fra Paolo Sarpi (1552–1623). His first book, *Methodus Vitandorum Errorum Omnium qui in Arte Medica Contigunt*, was published in Venice in 1602 at age 41, and 9 years later he was invited to be professor of theoretical medicine in Padua from 1611 to 1624. He left academic medicine to practice medicine in Venice. His most famous work, *Ars de Statica medicina*, was published in 1614. This work was translated into Italian, English, German, and French and went through 28 editions. Santorio Santorio never married and died in Venice in 1636. In the copy of his work that he presented to Galileo he claims to have studied more than 10,000 subjects in the span of 25 years, but sadly the records of these studies have been lost. Although the idea of insensible perspiration had been recognized by the Greeks and by Galen, it was Sanctorius who brought the concept of quantitation and experimentation to this problem. His work on insensible perspiration probably began about 1582 when he graduated from medical school. As one of the leading figures of the early scientific revolution, with many imaginative inventions to his credit, Sanctorius might appropriately be called the "father of metabolic obesity" (Figure 1.4) (Castiglione 1931; Eknoyan 1999; Talbot 1970, p. 87; Garrison 1914, p. 191; Mettler 1947, p. 117; Bray 2007; Major 1954, p. 484).

Theophile Bonet (1620–1689) is attributed with describing the presence of fat in dissections of diseased bodies. Bonet was born in Geneva to a long line of physicians. He was the son of Andre Bonet, a physician refugee from the counterrevolution. Bonet's brother and two sons were both doctors. He received his MD from Bologna, Italy in 1643. He began his medical practice at Neuchatel at the age of 23 as physician to the city, before becoming physician to Prince Henri II d'Orleans-Longueville. He attracted the enmity of his colleagues by his prescription of exercise as "medicine." He returned to Geneva in 1652. He became deaf around the age of 50 and spent much of his remaining years editing medical works. He published his first book at age 48 (1668) shortly before he became deaf and had to give up his practice of medicine in Geneva, a Protestant enclave to which he had returned. His greatest book was the *Sepulchretum*, published in 1679, which contains a compendium of over 3000 postmortem protocols and runs to a length of 1700 pages. The autopsies are classified by symptoms or diseases. The book contains a famous autopsy by William Harvey on Thomas Parr who is said to have died at age 152. This important book set the stage for the work of Morgagni a century later. (Talbot 1970, p. 117; Garrison 1914, p. 211; Mettler 1947, p. 252; Bray 2007).

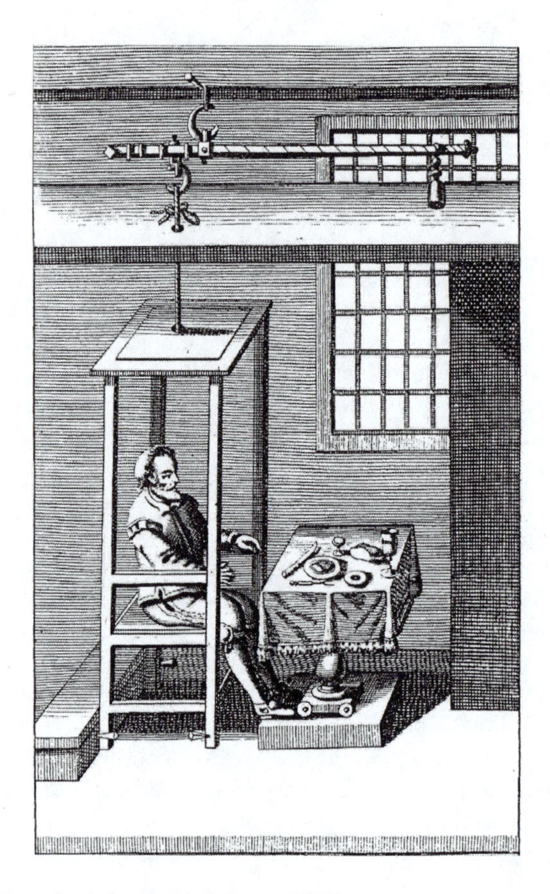

FIGURE 1.4 Santorio Santorio sitting on his balance (1676).

Art, does not a little good. But this must be done by degrees and slowly, since it is not safe to disturb so much matter violently, lest it should come all at once. Therefore the best way of Purging is by Pills, of Rheubarb, *Aloes* each 2 drachms*, Agarick 1 drachm, Cinnamon, yellow Sanders, each half a drachm. Make them up with Syrup of Cichory. They must be taken in this manner; First, 1 Scruple+ must be given an hour and a half before Meal; then two or three days afterwards, take half a drachm or two scruples before Meal. Thus purging must be often repeated at short intervals, till you think all the cacochymie is removed. *(1 draghm = an eighth ounce or 60 grains; thus 1 ounce = 8 draghms or 48 grains) + (1 scruple = 20 grains)

III. A certain Goldsmith, who was extreme fat, so that he was ready to be choaked, took the following Powder in his Meat, and so he was cured; Take of Tartar two ounces, Cinnamon three ounces, Ginger one ounce, Sugar four ounces. Make a Powder.

IV. *Horstius* found the things following to take down Fat men; especially onions, Garlick, Cresses, Leeks, Seed of Rue, and especially Vinegar of Squills: Let them purge well: Let them Sweat, and purge by Urine: Let them use violent exercise before they eat: Let them induce hunger, want of Sleep and Thirst: Let them Sweat in a Stove and continue in the Sun. Let them abstain from Drink between Dinner and Supper: for to drink between Meals makes Men fat.

V. I knew a Nobleman so fat, that he could scarce sit on Horse-back, but he was asleep; and he could scarce stir a foot. But now he is able to walk, and his body is come to it self, onely by chewing of Tobacco Leaves, as he affirmed to me. For it is good for Phlegmatick and cold Bodies.

VI. Let *Lingua Avis*, or Ash-Keyes be taken constantly about one drachm in Wine. According to *Pliny* it cures Hydropical persons, and makes fat people lean. (Bonetus 1700)

Besides the contributions of Theophile Bonet to the anatomy of obesity and disease, we also have important contributions to the anatomy of disease (pathology) during the seventeenth century by Giovanni Morgagni (1682–1771), and the eighteenth century by Albrecht van Haller (1708–1777) (Morgani 1761; Haller 1756, 1757).

The seventeenth century also saw the use of simple microscopes to expand anatomic exploration to the inner structure of the body. The invention of the microscope in the seventeenth century moved anatomy to the next level. Three great seventeenth-century anatomists, Robert Hooke (1635–1703) working in England, Antoni Leeuwenhoek (1632–1723) working in The Netherlands, and Marcello Malpighi (1628–1694) working in Italy might be described as "three who made a microscopic revolution" (Hooke 1655–1657; Leeuwenhoek 1800; Malpighi 1686). In the middle decades of the seventeenth century, these early microscopists began to publish the results of their investigations with breathtaking pictures of everything from insects, to plants, blood cells, and sperm and ova.

Physiological chemistry can also be traced to the seventeenth century and the Oxford physiologists, which included Robert Boyle (1627–1691), Richard Lower (1631–1691), and Robert Mayow (1643–1679) (Boyle 1764; Lower 1669; Mayow 1674; Frank 1980). The work of Robert Boyle established the concept of chemical elements (Partington 1951). By the late seventeenth century, Boyle and his students recognized that when a lighted candle went out in a bell jar without an outside source of air, a mouse living in the same jar rapidly died (Boyle 1764). It was clear that some important element was present in the air that was essential for life and for a candle to burn, but it was another century before oxygen—that missing substance—was discovered. Lower also performed the first blood transfusion into a human being (Lower 1666).

Each era has its clinical scholars and the seventeenth century was no exception (Celsus 1951). Thomas Willis (1621–1675) was one of the leading seventeenth-century physicians in England (Willis 1681; Talbot 1970, p. 122). He is noted particularly for his work on the nervous system. The circulatory connection between the right and left halves of the brain carries his name, the Circle of Willis. Willis also detected the "sweetness" of urine from diabetic patients.

Thomas Sydenham (1624–1689) is a second physician noted for clinical acumen (Sydenham 1676; Talbot 1970, p. 125). He believed that direct observation by the physician was the primary basis for knowledge of disease. Direct clinical observation was the basis for the important work of Richard Morton (1635–1698), who described anorexia nervosa (Morton 1689).

The number of scholarly dissertations in the seventeenth century in which obesity was a subject increased modestly. During this time period, I have been able to identify five dissertations,

Richard Morton (1637–1698) is described by the *Dictionary of National Biography* as an "ejected minister and physician". His initial education led him to Oxford, where he received an MA in 1659 when he was serving as chaplain to the family of Philip Foley of Prestwood. With the Reformation, he was unable to comply with the requirement of the Act of Uniformity and was ejected from his livelihood as a minister in 1662. He then turned his attention to medicine and received an MD in 1670 on nomination of the Prince of Orange. He subsequently moved to London and became a member and then fellow of the Royal College of Physicians in 1679. His most important work for us is his *Phthisiologia: seu Exercitationes de Phthisi*, published in 1689. This work follows the principles of clinical observation espoused by Thomas Sydenham. His book describes all of the conditions of "wasting" that he personally saw. It was Sir William Osler who noted that one of Morton's cases was probably "anorexia nervosa" (Osler 1904).

compared to two in the sixteenth century (see Appendix) (Bray 1990; Worthington 1876; Regneller 1839).

EIGHTEENTH CENTURY

The eighteenth century saw a marked expansion in the public interest in science and a growing base of knowledge about obesity (Uglow 2002) (Figure 1.5). Five themes in the eighteenth century characterize this progress toward understanding obesity. The first was the discovery of oxygen and the use of the first calorimeter to measure energy expenditure in living animals. The second theme consisted of advances in the understanding of how food is digested. The third was the discovery of percussion, which began a revolution in the clinical examination of the chest. The fourth was the use of a binary classification for diseases similar to the system of genus and species used to classify plants and animals. This system reached its zenith during this century. Obesity was included in this system under a term called "polysarcie." The fifth was the transition of medical education from southern Europe to northern Europe.

At the beginning of the eighteenth century, the phlogiston theory was King. Georg Stahl (1660–1734), its leading proponent, postulated that phlogiston was given off as objects burned (Stahl 1708). It was not until Joseph Priestley (1733–1804) and Carl Wilhelm Scheele (1742–1786) simultaneously discovered what we now call oxygen that the phlogiston theory began to fade (Priestley 1775; Scheele 1777). However, it was Antoine-Laurent Lavoisier (1743–1794) who put the final nails in the coffin of the phlogiston theory of combustion and replaced it with the oxygen theory of combustion (Lavoisier 1789; Holmes 1985). By Lavoisier's theory, oxygen was used up rather than phlogiston being given off. Lavoisier's oxygen theory recognized that oxidation meant combining with oxygen, which accounted for the increase in weight when the metals were heated (Lavoisier 1782; Lavoisier 1785). He introduced the animal calorimeter to show that metabolism was similar to a slow combustion (Figure 1.6). Lavoisier's death at the hands of the revolutionary French government in 1794 deprived humanity of one of its great intellects (Hartog 1941; Holmes 1985).

Another group of eighteenth physiological studies that relate to obesity describe how the gastrointestinal track digests and absorbs food. In 1752, R. A. F. de Reaumur (1683–1757) succeeded in isolating gastric juice from his pet bird by putting a sponge into the stomach attached to a string that he could withdraw (de Reaumur 1756). When he put the gastric juices in contact with food, the juices digested the food. Later in the eighteenth century, Abate Lazaro Spallanzani (1729–1799) showed that gastric juice outside the body would both digest food and prevent putrefaction (Spallanzani 1776, 1796).

In the second half of the eighteenth century, an Austrian named Leopold Auenbrugger (1722–1809) applied the wine maker's technique of determining the fullness of a barrel by tapping on it to the concept of clinical diagnosis by percussing the chest (Auebrugger 1761). Like so many other important discoveries, this one was not widely recognized for more than 40 years after it was published. Recognition of percussion largely came after the translation of Auenbrugger's work from German into French by Corvisart (1755–1821) in 1808 (Corvisart 1984).

The French Revolution (1789–1794), like the slightly earlier American Revolution of 1776–1781, was a watershed for obesity and for almost everything else. During the French Revolution, the existing system of medical education in Europe was upended along with the monarchy. The citizens' government in France believed that all citizens could be their own doctors and that medical education in the classical sense was no longer needed (Ackerknecht 1967). However, this view didn't last long. With the military campaigns of 1795–1797 that followed the ascent of Napoleon as first Consul and then Emperor, it became clear that the care of military casualties required trained physicians and surgeons, and medical schools were reborn. However, these reborn postrevolution medical schools were radically different from those in France prior to the revolution. Two important changes were introduced that altered the future of medical education. First, medicine and surgery were brought together in the same medical faculty, ending forever the barber-surgeon status of surgery.

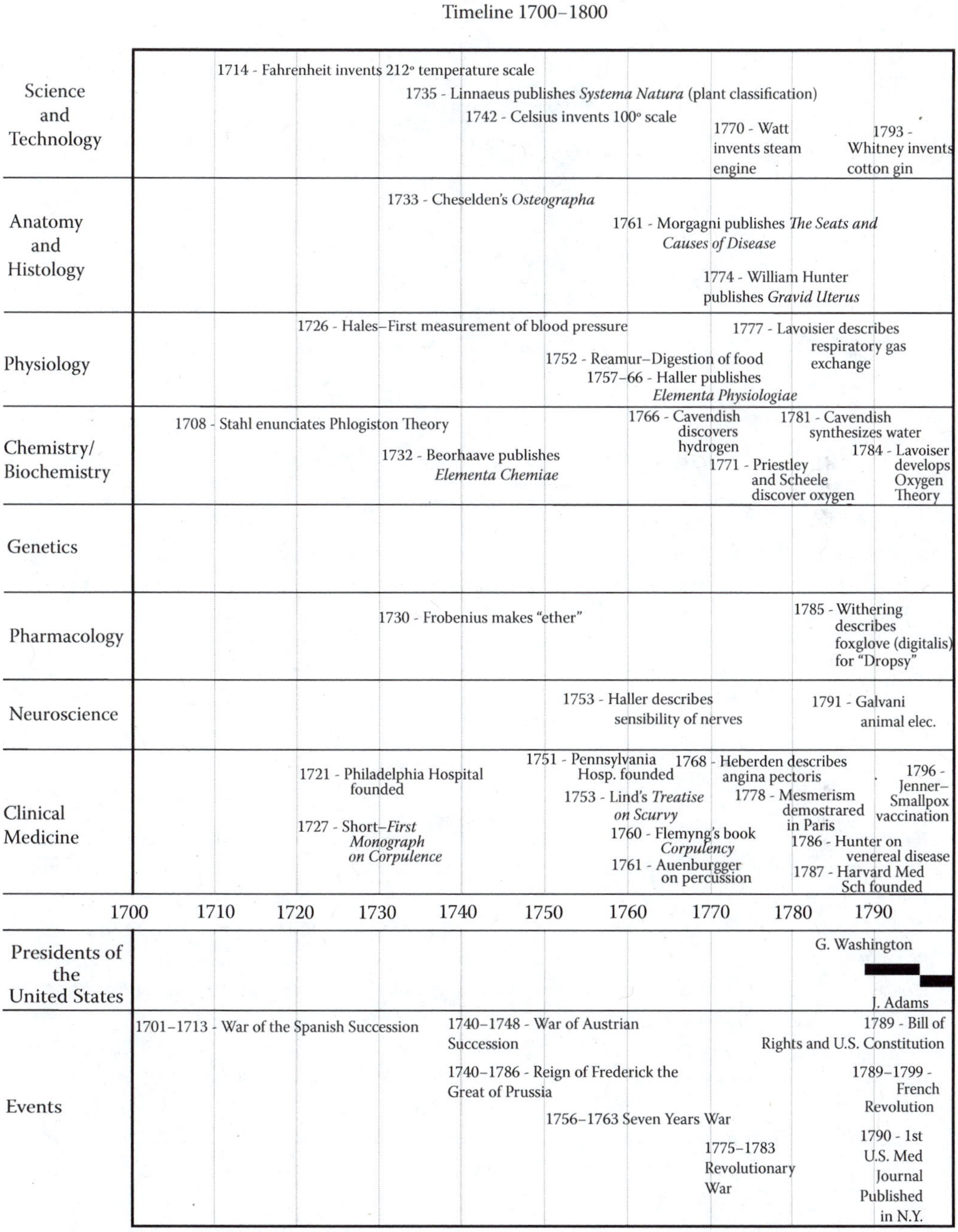

Timeline 1700–1800

Science and Technology	1714 - Fahrenheit invents 212° temperature scale; 1735 - Linnaeus publishes *Systema Natura* (plant classification); 1742 - Celsius invents 100° scale; 1770 - Watt invents steam engine; 1793 - Whitney invents cotton gin
Anatomy and Histology	1733 - Cheselden's *Osteographa*; 1761 - Morgagni publishes *The Seats and Causes of Disease*; 1774 - William Hunter publishes *Gravid Uterus*
Physiology	1726 - Hales–First measurement of blood pressure; 1752 - Reamur–Digestion of food; 1757–66 - Haller publishes *Elementa Physiologiae*; 1777 - Lavoisier describes respiratory gas exchange
Chemistry/ Biochemistry	1708 - Stahl enunciates Phlogiston Theory; 1732 - Beorhaave publishes *Elementa Chemiae*; 1766 - Cavendish discovers hydrogen; 1771 - Priestley and Scheele discover oxygen; 1781 - Cavendish synthesizes water; 1784 - Lavoiser develops Oxygen Theory
Genetics	
Pharmacology	1730 - Frobenius makes "ether"; 1785 - Withering describes foxglove (digitalis) for "Dropsy"
Neuroscience	1753 - Haller describes sensibility of nerves; 1791 - Galvani animal elec.
Clinical Medicine	1721 - Philadelphia Hospital founded; 1727 - Short–*First Monograph on Corpulence*; 1751 - Pennsylvania Hosp. founded; 1753 - Lind's *Treatise on Scurvy*; 1760 - Flemyng's book *Corpulency*; 1761 - Auenburgger on percussion; 1768 - Heberden describes angina pectoris; 1778 - Mesmerism demostrared in Paris; 1786 - Hunter on venereal disease; 1787 - Harvard Med Sch founded; 1796 - Jenner–Smallpox vaccination
	1700 1710 1720 1730 1740 1750 1760 1770 1780 1790
Presidents of the United States	G. Washington; J. Adams
Events	1701–1713 - War of the Spanish Succession; 1740–1748 - War of Austrian Succession; 1740–1786 - Reign of Frederick the Great of Prussia; 1756–1763 Seven Years War; 1775–1783 Revolutionary War; 1789 - Bill of Rights and U.S. Constitution; 1789–1799 - French Revolution; 1790 - 1st U.S. Med Journal Published in N.Y.

FIGURE 1.5 Timeline for the eighteenth century. The key events in several categories including politics, science, and obesity are shown.

Second, medical teaching shifted from the lofty atmosphere of amphitheaters where the professor pontificated from the writings of Hippocrates, Galen, or Avicenna to the hospitals where the sick and injured awaited care. As chemistry came of age in the eighteenth and nineteenth century, a chemical view and interpretation of medicine and disease arose—a view that is referred to as the "iatro-chemical" theory of disease.

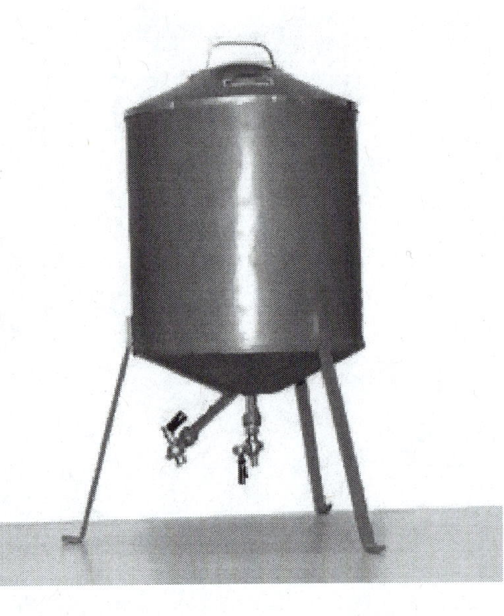

FIGURE 1.6 The ice calorimeter that Lavoisier used to measure the heat given off by a guinea pig calculated from the amount of ice that was melted and the amount of melted ice when a candle was burned to produce heat. When the heat production was similar to the amount of fixed air (carbon dioxide) produced for a guinea pig or a candle, this lead to the conclusion that metabolism was like a slow combustion.

Antoine-Laurent Lavoisier (1743–1794) is known for his seminal studies that established the oxygen theory of combustion and metabolism. Lavoisier was born in 1743, the son of well-to-do parents. He had all the advantages that education in upper-class France could provide (Foster 1926). He entered the College of Mazarin, where he received a law degree. His passion, however, was for science. He received training in mathematics and astronomy, and studied botany, mineralogy, geology, and chemistry. In his scientific training, he came in contact with some of the most distinguished scientists in France and, by the age of 20, he began making barometric observations that he continued throughout his life. At the age of 25, he became a junior member of the Academy of Sciences. He remained closely associated with the Academy until it was abolished, near the end of his life. I quote again from Lavoisier: "It is easy to see that from the year 1772, I had conceived the whole doctrine of combustion which I have since published" (Hartog 1941). The events that led to his political persecution and death during the Revolution occurred when he became a member of the Ferme Générale, a semiprivate corporation that collected tax revenues. Being involved with the Ferme Générale was an unpardonable sin to the leaders of the Reign of Terror, which ruled France from 1793. After a mockery of a trial, Lavoisier was guillotined on May 8, 1794 (Holmes 1985; Talbot 1970, p. 278; Garrison 1914, p. 258; Mettler 1947, p. 138; Bray 2007). To slightly paraphrase Whitehead:

> The progress of science had reached a turning point. The stable foundations of physics have broken up . . . the old foundations of scientific thought all require reinterpretation.

This is what Lavoisier did (Hartog 1941).

TABLE 1.2
Some Early Monographs on Obesity

English	French	German
18th Century		
Short, T.		
Flemyng M.		
19th Century		
Wadd, Wm.	Regneller, G.	Kisch, E.H.
Chambers, T.	Maccaray, A.	Ebstein, W.
Harvey, J.	Dancel, J.F.	
Harvey, Wm.	Worthington, L.S.	

As interest in obesity increased in the eighteenth century, a much larger number of disputations and dissertations with obesity as their subject were published—34 in the eighteenth century versus 5 in the seventeenth century (see Appendix). The first monographs devoted entirely to obesity were also published in the eighteenth century (Short 1727; Flemyng 1760). Table 1.2 lists the English, French, and German books about obesity that were published between 1700 and 1900.

The eighteenth century saw a second major transition in medical education. In the seventeenth century, the dominant medical schools and places for medical education were found in Italy and France. Two of the most prominent schools were at Padua, Italy and Montpellier, France. During the eighteenth century, the dominant schools were to be found in The Netherlands and in Scotland in northern Europe. The seat of greatness in medicine shifted to Leiden in the first half of the eighteenth century, where Hermann Boerhaave (1668–1738), a professor of medicine, chemistry, and botany, attracted students from all over Europe (Boerhaave 1757; Burton 1743). His eminence as a teacher was expanded by the introduction of hospital beds that were specially designed for teaching. With Boerhaave's death, the center for clinical medicine in the last half of the eighteenth century shifted further north to Edinburgh, where many American physicians studied.

In contrast to the advances on the scientific front, ideas about disease did not progress very far. Nosology, the classification of diseases, took a major step backward, if anything. This was the time of productive ideas for classifying plants and animals by their genus and species. Classification of obesity is part of the more general efforts to classify diseases. Although many classifications of disease exist, one of the most unusual was the effort to classify disease based on the binary classification of plants and animals introduced by Karl von Linne (Linnaeus) (1707–1778). His system involved giving each individual a genus and species name and categorizing the genera into classes, orders, and phyla (Linnaeus 1753). Although Thomas Sydenham (1624–1689) began such a systematic classification of disease (Sydenham 1676), the two best-known efforts to classify diseases in this way were published by Bossier de Sauvages (1706–1767) in France and William Cullen (1710–1790) in Edinburgh (Sauvages 1768; Cullen 1810). In both, obesity was called "polysarcie," meaning "too much tissue." In the English translation of Cullen's work, Polysarcie (obesity) is in Class III, called The Cachexieas, which refers to changes in body composition. It is listed under the second order called Intumescentiae (swelling) with a genus name of Polysarcia (Corporis pinguedinosa intumescentia molesta). Obesity, as a word to describe increased fatness, gradually replaced polysarcie, the French word embonpoint, and the English word corpulence during the nineteenth century.

Thomas Short (?1690–1772) is known as the author of the first monograph related to obesity published in the English language. Thomas Short was born in southern Scotland. After graduating in medicine, he settled and began to practice medicine in Sheffield. In 1713, William Steel communicated a secret idea (although later published) of making cerated glass of antimony, a cure for dysentery. Short made several journeys to visit the mineral springs of Yorkshire and other parts of England. In 1725, he published *A Rational Discourse on the Inward Uses of Water.* This was followed in 1727 with his book on corpulency and, in 1730, by *A Dissertation upon Tea.* In 1750, he published *New Observations on the Bills of Mortality* in which he added something to the remarks of Graunt and Sir William Petty, and treated the whole subject in relation to a book published anonymously by him the year before, *A General Chronological History of the Air*, in two volumes dedicated to Dr. Mead. In 1767, near the end of his life, he published *A Comparative History of the Increase and Decrease of Mankind* in which he advocated early marriages, denounced alcohol as a "Stygian poison," and collected much historical and medical information (Bray 2007).

The attempt to apply this idea to medicine reached its peak in the work of Sauvages (1768) and of Cullen (1793). This is the way that Cullen, a leading professor at the University of Edinburgh classified obesity:

> The only disease to be mentioned in this chapter, I have, with other nosologists, named Polysarca; and in English it may be named Corpulency, or, more strictly Obesity; as it is placed here upon the common supposition of its depending chiefly upon the increase of oil in the cellular texture of the body. This corpulency or obesity, is in very different degrees in different persons, and is often considerable without being considered as a disease. There is, however, a certain degree of it, which will be generally allowed to be a disease; as, for example, when it renders persons, from a difficult respiration, uneasy in themselves, and, from the inability of exercise, unfit for discharging the duties of life to others: and for that reason I have given such a disease a place here (Cullen 1793).

From our perspective, Dr. George Cheyne (1671–1743) is one of the most interesting clinical practitioners of the eighteenth century (Guerrini 2000; Talbot 1990, p. 500; Garrison 1914, p. 301; *Dictionary of National Biography*; Mettler 1947, p. 551). He was born in Scotland and obtained a medical degree from Edinburgh when it was one of the leading schools of medical education. Along with many others at the turn of the eighteenth century, he made his way to London in 1701. Over the ensuing few years, his profligate life style and familial tendency to corpulence became evident as his weight increased to 448 pounds. In 1705, he had a medical and emotional crisis and he stopped clinical practice. He returned to Scotland and then migrated to Bath and Bristol in the west of England. He developed a spiritual side to his life that became an important part of his medical practice. With continuing efforts, he brought his weight under control with periodic ups and downs over the rest of his life. Two books, *The Essay of Health and Long Life* (1724) and *The English Malady* (1733), are the most relevant. In *The English Malady*, Cheyne includes a number of medical cases including his own medical biography. Moderation was the key to his weight control. In his dietary approach, Cheyne replaced meat, particularly red meat, with milk. Temperance and exercise were important and he recommended 2 pints of water and one of wine in 24 hours (Guerrini 2000). In *The English Malady*, he elaborated on his themes of the relationship between mind, body, and spirit. The success of these two books is evident from the fact that they went through a number of editions and were translated into other languages.

Diets were important ways to helping patients with their weight during the eighteenth century. J. Tweedie, in his book entitled *Hints on Temperance and Exercise, Shewing Their Advantage in the Cure of Dyspepsia, Rheumatism, Polysarcia, and Certain States of Palsy*, provided one summary of dietary treatment for obesity from the eighteenth century.

> The diet should be sparing. They [the overweight] should abstain from spirits, wines and malt liquors, drinking in their stead, either spring water, toast and water or else water agreeably acidulated by any pure vegetable acids. . . . In attempting its cure, when the habit is threatened with any morbid effects, from the plethora existing either in the head or lungs, this must be removed by a bleeding or two; and as corpulent people do not bear blood-letting well, purging is most to be depended upon for the removal of the plethora (Tweedie 1799).

Finally, Tweedie recommends a gradual increase in exercise.

NINETEENTH CENTURY

Several themes related to obesity emerged in the nineteenth century (Figure 1.7). The first theme was the introduction of the first law of thermodynamics, stating that energy is neither created nor destroyed. A second theme was the measurement of body size and shape and introduction to the concept of the body mass index. A third theme was developing the concept of the cell and recognizing that the cell was the basis for life and that fat was stored in cells. The fourth theme was the publication of the first "popular" diet book for obesity based on the newer ideas about the source of blood glucose.

The early nineteenth century was a period of enormous excitement with the restructuring of medical education. The intellectual ferment in France led to a period of unprecedented medical and scientific advances, with major new contributions stemming from clinical medicine. A young man named François Xavier Bichat (1771–1802) expounded a pathology of disease based in tissues rather than organs that developed in the eighteenth century (Bichat 1801; Morgagni 1761). This was the beginning of the overthrow of the concept of a humoral-based pathology of disease in which an imbalance in one of the four humors (fire, air, water, and earth) was thought to cause disease (Figure 1.2). It was followed mid-century with the concept of cellular pathology for disease, a concept that survived well into the twentieth century (Virchow 1858).

In the early nineteenth century, René Théophile Hyacinthe Laennec (1781–1826) invented the stethoscope in 1816 to examine the chest of an overweight girl (Laennec 1819). He then expanded this technique for use in examining the chests of all kinds of people. This expanded the information obtained from the clinical examination of the patient beyond Auenbrugger's eighteenth-century technique of percussing the chest. The stethoscope became a key instrument for clinical diagnosis for nearly two centuries. Using the clinical discoveries he made with the stethoscope, Laennec wrote the first modern textbook of medicine where diseases of the chest were diagnosed by percussion and auscultation (Laennec 1819).

During this period of excitement in French medicine, morphine was isolated and quinine was extracted from *Cinchona* bark. Physiologic science was established through the genius of François Magendie (1783–1855), the teacher of the famous Claude Bernard (1813–1878) (Magendie 1816; Bernard 1855; Holmes 1974). Thus, Paris medicine, as it has been called because of its focus on clinical diagnosis at the bedside, was the center for the teaching of clinical medicine in the first part of the nineteenth century (Ackerknecht 1927). The stagnation of French medicine later in the nineteenth century stemmed in part from the failure of French scientists to recognize the importance of the microscope as a tool to investigate nature and the failure to pursue chemical and laboratory medicine.

Paris medicine had an important impact on British and American medicine by providing training for many of their clinicians. The list includes many nineteenth century luminaries whose names were synonymous with diseases. Included were Thomas Hodgkin (1798–1866), who described the lymphatic tumors known as Hodgkin's disease, Richard Bright (1789–1858), who identified the form of kidney failure called Bright's disease, Thomas Addison (1793–1860), who identified failure of the adrenal glands (called Addison's disease) as the basis for a wasting disease, and William Jenner (1749–1823) who introduced vaccination for smallpox at the end of the eighteenth century (Hodgkin 1832; Bright 1827; Addison 1855; Jenner 1801). All of these men, having been taught in Paris, were steeped in the clinical tradition.

Timeline 1800–1900

Science and Technology	1800 - Electrical cell; 1803 - Fulton's steamboat; 1814 - First locomotive; 1825 - Erie Canal; 1827 - First photograph; 1834 - Babbage's analytical engine; 1860 - Internal combustion engine; 1876 - Telephone; 1877 - Photograph; 1880 - Edison electric light; 1886 - Kodak camera; 1887 - Arrhenius–Ion theory; 1895 - Motion picture camera
Anatomy and Histology	1800 - Bichat's *Tissue Pathology*; 1801 - Bell System of Anatomy; 1830 - Lister–Achromatic microscope; 1835 - Quetelet describes body mass index; 1838 - Schwann and Schleden propose cell theory; 1849 - Hassall's fat cell; 1858 - Vicchow publishes *Cellular Pathology*; 1858 - Gray's *Anatomy*
Physiology	1821 - Magendie–Food absorption; 1833 - Beaumont on digestion; 1833 - Müller's Physiology text; 1842 - Mayer on conservation of energy; 1846 - Bernard–Digestive function of pancreas; 1847 - Ludwig–Kymograph; 1849 - Ludwig–Urinary secretion; 1867 - Helmholtz–physiological optics
Chemistry/ Biochemistry	1825 - Wohler synthesizes urea; 1847 - Helmholtz–conservation of energy; 1848 - Bernard isolates glycogen; 1863 - Voit and Pettenkoffer–Metabolism; 1896 - Atwater makes calorimeter
Genetics	1859 - Darwin–*Origin of the Species*; 1865 - G. Mendel–Plant breeding genetics
Pharmacology	1805 - Pelletier isolates morphine; 1819 - Pelletier and Caventon isolate quinine; 1822 - Magendie's *Pharmacopoeia*; 1833 - Atropine isolated; 1834 - Chloroform discovered; 1856 - Cocaine extracted; 1893 - Thyroid to treat obesity
Neuroscience	1811 - Bell–Spinal nerve function; 1854 - Bernard–vasodilator nerves; 1863 - Helmholtz–book of hearing
Clinical Medicine	1809 - McDowell–Ovariotomy; 1810 - Wadd *On Corpulence*; 1819 - Laennec–Stethoscope; 1840 - Basedow goiter; 1846 - Ether anesthesia; 1847 - Semmekweis-Puerperal fever; 1849 - Addison & Pernicicus Anemia & puprarenal disease; 1850 - Chambers *On Obesity*; 1851 - Helmholtz-Ophthalmoscope; 1854 - Laryngoscope; 1863 - Banting *Letter On Corpulence*; 1865 - Antiseptic surgery; 1866 - Russel-sleep apnea; 1873 - Gull–Myxedenia; 1882 - Koch isolates tubercle bacillus; 1895 - Roentgen discovers x-rays
	1800 · 1810 · 1820 · 1830 · 1840 · 1850 · 1860 · 1870 · 1880 · 1890
Presidents of the United States	T. Jefferson; J. Madison; J. Monroe; J.Q. Adams; Jackson; Van Buren; W. Harrison; Tyler; Polk; Taylor; Fillmore; Pierce; Buchanan; Lincoln; Johnson; U. Grant; Hayes; Garfield; Arthur; Cleveland; Harrison; Cleveland; McKinley
Events	1804–1815 - Napoleon emperor; 1805 - Battle of Trafalgar; 1812 - War of 1812; 1830 - Reign of Louis Phillipe; 1839 - R. Hill–Postage stamps introduced; 1848–1849 - California Gold Rush; 1848–1852 - Second French Republic; 1861–1865 - Civil War; 1863 - Emancipation Proclamation; 1866 - Seven Weeks' war; 1870–1871 - Franco-Prussian War; 1886 - Statue of Liberty; 1898 - Spanish-American War

FIGURE 1.7 Timeline for the nineteenth century. The key events in several categories including politics, science, and obesity are shown.

If the first half of the century can be described by its focus on clinical medicine in France, the second half of the nineteenth century belongs to the German laboratory school, so called for the numerous contributions to chemical and laboratory studies. A date for the transition between the French clinical school and the German laboratory school can be set at 1850. The German laboratory school of medicine grew in large measure from two eminent scientists, Johannes Müller (1801–1858) and his students and Justus Liebig (1803–1873) and his followers (Müller 1834; Liebig

1842). Müller recognized the importance of the microscope as a tool for studying life and, unlike his French colleagues, encouraged his students to use it. Liebig established the first laboratory for chemistry and agricultural science.

The sophistication of the microscope improved in the nineteenth century and the early simple lenses were replaced by microscopes with two lenses. This was followed by the introduction of achromatic lenses in the early nineteenth century, which made microscopes sufficiently powerful to define the structures inside of cells. With the achromatic microscope, Theodor Schwann (1810–1882) and Matthias Schleiden (1804–1881), two students of Johannes Mueller, recognized the unifying principles of the cell wall, the nucleus, and the area of structures surrounding the nucleus as the basic elements of the cell (Schwann 1839; Schleiden 1839). Shortly afterward, the first substantial textbooks of microscopic anatomy were published (Henle 1841; Hassall 1849a) and, a few years later, the fat cell was recognized as a member of this group. In his early observations on the development of the fat vesicle, Arthur Hassall (1817–1894) suggested that certain types of obesity might result from an increased number of fat cells (Hassall 1849b). A description of the growth and development of fat cells was published in 1879 by Hoggan and Hogan (1879).

In addition to microscopy, Müller also trained students as physiologists to explore the function of the human body. Hermann von Helmholtz (1821–1894) was among the most famous (Koenigsberger 1906). From our perspective, his publication showing that energy is neither made nor lost—the conservation of energy, which is referred to as the First Law of Thermodynamics—is a central dogma for understanding obesity (Helmholtz 1847). He also invented the ophthalmoscope in 1851 (Helmholtz 1851, 1867), which allows physicians to see the back of the eye and to gain clues about the diseases that might be occurring in blood vessels, including some consequences of obesity. He developed a modern theory of hearing and of how the ear works (Helmholtz 1863).

Other outstanding members of the German school of laboratory science were Robert Koch (1843–1910), who discovered bacteria as causes of specific diseases, and Wilhelm Roentgen (1845–1923), who discovered x-rays in 1895 (Koch 1884; Roentgen 1895). As we shall see, x-rays have played an important role in our understanding of obesity in the latter part of the twentieth century.

Pharmacology, the study of drugs and their biological effects, grew in the nineteenth century from a base in chemistry. Its early successes in the first half of the nineteenth century included the isolation from various plants of morphine, strychnine, emetine, and quinine, and the publication in 1822 by François Magendie (1783–1855) of the first pharmacopeia of drugs for use by physicians (Magendie 1828). The discovery of anesthesia in the middle of the nineteenth century was one of the major advances of the century. It was discovered almost simultaneously by three Americans. Crawford Long (1815–1878) was a native of Georgia who first used ether anesthesia to remove a tumor in 1842, but did not publish this finding until many years later, and William T. G. Morton (1819–1868) and Horace Wells (1815–1848) were both dentists (Long 1849; Warren 1847; Wells 1847). Wells pioneered the use of nitrous oxide, or laughing gas, in anesthesia, but when he demonstrated his technique during surgery at the Massachusetts General Hospital in Boston, it failed because the patient was not adequately anesthetized (Davy 1800). Morton was the one with the first successful public demonstration of the use of ether anesthesia. This occurred in October of 1846 in a room now appropriately called the "ether dome" at Massachusetts General Hospital in Boston, MA. At the end of the operation, the elderly but distinguished surgeon John Warren (1778–1856) said, "This is no humbug." Morton's patient had remained unconscious throughout the surgical procedure. The subsequent publication of this event brought anesthesia to worldwide attention (Bigelow 1846; Bowditch 1848).

The risk of infection is a major hazard during surgery and this was all the more so before sterile techniques were introduced (Wangensteen and Wangensteen 1978). In 1865, shortly after the discovery of anesthesia and the introduction of the ideas that "germs" could cause disease, Joseph Lister (1827–1912) introduced the use of carbolic acid sprays in the operating room to reduce infection during surgery (Lister 1870, 1909).

The replacement in the eighteenth century of the phlogiston theory with the oxygen theory of metabolism by Lavoisier was followed by the development of the laws of the conservation of mass

Arthur Hill Hassall (1817–1894) published one of the early textbooks of histology describing the fat cell and because he was active in the effort to prevent water pollution. Hassall was born in Teddington, England (Visscher 1971; Garrison 1914, p. 593; Bray 2007). He was the son of a general practitioner and is remembered for the unique thymic corpuscles that bear his name. Hassall received his medical training under Sir James Murray in Dublin, Ireland where he was indentured as an apprentice. Upon returning to England, he developed a great interest in botany through his association with Sir William Hooker who was then director of Kew Gardens. His work on a history of British freshwater algae is a classic. He received his fellowship in the Royal College of Surgeons in 1839 and obtained a diploma from the Apothecaries Hall in 1841. In 1851, he obtained membership in the Royal College of Physicians of London and later received an MD from the University of London. Based on his work in the postmortem room at St. George's Hospital where he studied the microscopical structure of tissues, he published the first complete book of histology in the English language in 1849 entitled *The Microscopic Anatomy of the Human Body* (1849a). Using his microscope, he next examined a large number of samples of foods. His seminal studies on food and its adulteration resulted in a book, *Adulteration in Food and Medicine* (1855). This work was instrumental in establishing parliamentary legislation to control adulteration of food and drink. His next book dealt with urine in health and disease and was published in 1863. After he developed tuberculosis in 1866, he was instrumental in establishing the Ventnor Tuberculosis Hospital in London as a result of his experience with this disease. Under his portrait in the hospital are his words "*Non omnis moriar*." His life of great activity was summarized by the titles of his autobiography, *The Narrative of a Busy Life*. It begins:

> There are but few persons who have long passed the mid-day of their lives, who do not from time to time look back and recall the chief events and circumstances of their careers to determine there from how far these lives have been well or ill spent; what lessons are to be learned from the experience gained, what opportunities lost, what faults and sins committed; in fine, to judge whether they have been of any benefit to their fellow creatures, their country or the world (Hassall 1893).

The conclusion a century later is that Arthur Hill Hassall did indeed benefit his fellow creatures, his country, and the world.

and energy in the middle of the nineteenth century, which formed the basis for the work on metabolism during the latter half of the nineteenth and twentieth centuries (Helmholtz 1847). Although Helmholtz (1847) and Mayer (1842) nearly simultaneously described the laws of conservation of mass and energy, it was Max Rubner (1854–1932), Carl Voit (1831–1908), and Max Pettenkofer (1818–1901) in Germany and the American Wilbur Olin Atwater (1849–1907) who demonstrated that the law of conservation of energy proposed by Helmholtz and Mayer applied to human beings (Rubner 1902, 1982; Voit 1860; Pettenkofer 1862–1863; Atwater 1899, 1900–1902). This final major piece of work was done in the United States at Wesleyan College by Atwater and the physicist Edward B. Rosa, who constructed the first functional human calorimeter in 1896. This instrument served as a tool for extensive studies on metabolic requirements during food intake and on the effects of starvation by Atwater and subsequently by Francis Gano Benedict (1870–1957) (Benedict 1915, 1919).

Following its construction, this singularly valuable instrument was put into operation by Atwater and Rosa. Its first subject was a 29-year-old Swede who was a laboratory janitor (Atwater 1899). With this instrument they confirmed that the laws of conservation of mass and energy applied to human beings.

Biological chemistry in the mid-nineteenth century was dominated by three main figures. The first was François Magendie (1783–1855) in France (Magendie 1816). At the beginning of the nineteenth century, he was a leader in the application of the experimental method to the study of living animals. He was succeeded by his outstanding pupil, Claude Bernard (1813–1878) in the middle of the nineteenth century (Holmes 1974). Bernard discovered liver glycogen as the source of blood glucose and showed that damage (*piqure*) to the hypothalamus could produce glycosuria, a loss of glucose in the urine (Bernard 1848, 1855). Bernard's scientific philosophy was one of "gradualism," that is, that scientific theory would naturally lead to step-by-step progress, a concept that was a dominant element in the nineteenth century philosophy of science (Bernard 1865). This concept of gradualism is in sharp contrast to the concept of paradigm shifts and scientific revolutions that moved science in big leaps as opposed to many small steps (Kuhn 1962).

The third major figure in the nineteenth century in physiology related to obesity was a German named Justus Liebig (1803–1873). He headed one of the most productive laboratories in the nineteenth century on chemistry, food chemistry, and agricultural chemistry (Liebeg 1842). His ultimately flawed concept that carbohydrates, proteins, and fats were all that were needed for human nutrition, however, served as the basis for nutritional science during much of the nineteenth century.

Hermann von Helmholtz (1821–1894) was among the masters of medicine in the second half of the nineteenth century. He is included here because he articulated the first law of thermodynamics (1847), invented the ophthalmoscope, and formulated modern theories about vision and hearing. He was preeminent in the physics related to optics and sound, and is responsible for articulation of the law of conservation of energy. Von Helmholtz was born in Potsdam and educated as a surgeon for the Prussian Army. While studying in Berlin, he came under the influence of Johannes Muller, MD, professor of physiology. Muller influenced Helmholtz and a whole generation of German physician-scientists. His inaugural dissertation dealt with the origin of nerve fibers from leeches and crabs that he had studied with a rudimentary compound microscope. In 1847, while serving in the army, Helmholtz published his first masterpiece on the conservation of energy (*Ueber die Erhaltung der Kraft*). His academic appointments included professor of physiology and pathology at the University of Königsberg (1849–1855), professor of physiology and anatomy at the University of Bonn (1855–1858), professor of physiology at the University of Heidelberg (1858–1871), and professor of physics at the University of Berlin (1871–1894). Among his scientific contributions is the observation that muscle is the major source of animal heat (1848), the measurement of the velocity of the nervous impulse (1850–1852), and the invention of the ophthalmoscope (1851). His two other great works were the *Handbook of Physiological Optics* published in 1865–1867 and his acoustical masterpiece *Der Tonenfindungen* (1863). Although his contributions to physical medicine were extraordinary, he never forgot he was a physician. He once said, "Medicine was once the intellectual home in which I grew up; and even the emigrant best understands and is best understood by his native land." (Garrison 1914, p. 478; Mettler 1947, p. 157; Bray 2007; Koenigsberger 1906).

What matter titled? Helmholtz is a name
That challenges alone the award of fame!
When Emperors, Kings, Pretenders, shadows all,
Leave not a dust-trace on our sterling ball,
Thy work, oh grave-eyed searcher, shall endure,
Unmarred by faction, from low passion pure.

Punch, London, 1894

The discovery of vitamins at the turn of the twentieth century gave birth to a new and broader concept of nutrition (McCollum 1957).

Like preceding centuries, the nineteenth century made clinical contributions to obesity. One of these is a small monograph written in 1810 by the surgeon William Wadd entitled *Cursory Remarks on Corpulence: By a Member of the Royal College of Surgeons* (Wadd 1829). In it he describes clinical cases of obese individuals and how they fit into the ideas of obesity. This book is a very readable account of obesity viewed from 200 years ago (Bray 2007, pp. 663–671 for transcript). In the last edition of this book, published in 1829, Wadd described several cases, and using his skills as a draughtsman, drew graphic pictures of some of them. Most of the cases in this last book were from his medical correspondence, a characteristic way of evaluating patients by consulting physicians since the physical examination was not a part of the usual medical evaluation in the early 1800s. Of

Wilbur Olin Atwater (1849–1907) is known for his demonstration that human beings obeyed the laws of conservation of energy completed the work begun by Lavoisier and Helmholtz. Atwater was the son of a Methodist minister. He began his collegiate education at the University of Vermont, but transferred to the Methodist-dominated Wesleyan University in Middletown, CT, where he graduated in 1865. He earned his PhD 4 years later from the Sheffield Scientific School at Yale University. Following 2 years of study at German universities in Leipzig and Berlin, Atwater returned to begin an academic career in the United States. After two initial appointments, he was recruited in 1873 to be professor of chemistry at his alma mater, Wesleyan University. He remained there until his death in 1907 (Maynard 1962; Potts 1992).

The first agricultural experiment station was established at Wesleyan College in 1875 as the result of two activities, effective lobbying by Atwater and Professor Johnson, his former instructor at Yale, and a contribution of $1000 from Orange Judd, a wealthy philanthropist from Hartford, CT. Two years later, due to lobbying by Yale University, the scientific station was moved to Yale University under the direction of Professor Johnson. Following the lead of Connecticut, the federal government, through the Hatch Act of 1887, established the USDA Office of Experiment Stations. Funds for Connecticut were allocated between Yale University and a newly established agricultural college at Storrs, CT. Although 40 miles from Wesleyan University, Atwater served as director of the program at Storrs while remaining professor of chemistry at Wesleyan. The studies on research with fertilizers and crops were gradually moved to the new agricultural experiment station, where Professor Atwater maintained research direction of this program over the next 14 years. However, his interest shifted slowly from agricultural nutrition to human nutrition and energy expenditure.

Atwater's interest in energy expenditure had been reignited by a tour of Europe in 1882 and 1883. During the 19th century, Munich was a leading center for studies in nutritional science. Professor Justus von Liebig, one of the giants of nutrition and agriculture in the first half of the nineteenth century, eventually became a professor at the University of Munich. This university also counted Carl von Voit as professor of physiology and Max-Joseph Pettenkofer as professor of hygiene. As Kirkland says, "[F]or the devout nutritionist, Munich became a sort of Mecca" (Kirkland 1974).

With his background in nutrition and his political skills in raising money, Atwater launched "big science" at Wesleyan College. At the physiological institute in Munich in 1882–83, Atwater had seen the respiration calorimeter invented by Professor Pettenkofer. With the availability of new funds from the state of Connecticut after 1887, Professors Atwater and E. B. Rosa, a new professor of physics, started to build a respiration calorimeter in 1892. The construction and operation costs were more than $10,000 per year, a figure that exceeded the salary of a professor at Wesleyan by more than fivefold (Garrison 1914, p. 500; Maynard 1962; Bray 2007).

Claude Bernard (1813–1878) discovered glycogen and that the liver is a major source of glucose, as well as establishing the concept that the body defends the internal milieu to which its tissues communicate through the bloodstream. Along with Helmholtz and Ludwig, he stands as one of the leading scientific figures of physiology in the nineteenth century. He was born into a vintner's family at St. Julien in the Beaujolais region of France on July 12, 1813. Because of financial difficulties, he became a pharmacist's assistant in Lyons, France. The young Bernard at first turned his attention to writing plays, one of which, a vaudeville comedy, met with some success. Armed with two plays, one of which had been performed, he went to Paris where the critic Girardin advised him that medicine was a better choice to make a living. Bernard completed his 7-year medical curriculum in 1841 at the age of 28. Under the tutelage of Magendie, the leading French physiologist of the time, Bernard matured to be a better scientist than his master. Bernard was a genius at the experimental method and founded experimental medicine by which disease states were induced by chemical or physical manipulation. His discovery that the liver released glucose into the circulation revolutionized the concept of metabolism. His idea of the "internal milieu" as a buffer against the outside world is still an important concept. His mastery of the entire range of physiology is shown in the series of lectures that were published between 1855 and 1879. In February of 1878, he died a lonely death from acute nephritis as his wife and two daughters lived away from him because they felt distaste for his life's work (Garrison 1914, p. 490–4). His genius, however, was recognized with the pomp and circumstance of the public funeral held at state expense (Mayer 1951; Holmes 1974; Garrison 1914, p. 491; Talbot 1970, p. 606; Mettler 1947, p. 142; Bray 2007).

the 12 cases in his book, all but one were men. Weights were noted in five cases and ranged from 106 kg (16 st 10 lb or 234 pounds) to 146 kg (23 st 2 lb or 324 pounds). Two of the cases examined at postmortem had enormous accumulations of fat. Although autopsy observations of obese individuals had been made previously by Benivieni, Bonet, Morgagni, and Haller, this is the first instance in which they are included in a monograph devoted to obesity and leanness.

Wadd (1829) notes that sudden death is not uncommon in the corpulent, thus validating a concept from Hippocrates. Wadd states, "A sudden palpitation excited in the heart of a fat man has often proved as fatal as a bullet through the thorax." In several of Wadd's cases, corpulent patients asked him for pills to treat their obesity, although nothing of pharmacological value was available then. Wadd makes a distinction between the therapeutic activists and those favoring less aggressive therapy, with the homeopathists being at the far extreme with minimal dosages of medication. As Wadd said, "Truly it has been said—some Doctors let the patient die, for fear they should kill him; while others kill the patient, for fear he should die."

One important lesson from the study of massively obese individuals was the association of obesity with sleep apnea, a disease often referred to as the Pickwickian Syndrome, referring to "Joe," the fat nineteenth-century boy in *The Pickwick Papers* by Charles Dickens (Burwell 1956; Bray 2007). Patients with this syndrome snore at night and have periods when breathing briefly stops. During the daytime, they are often sleepy (Kryger 1983, 1985). One of the early published medical reports of sleep apnea and the hypoventilation and its consequences may be that by Russell (1866) although Wadd (1810) also noted this clinical response.

Besides the lessons learned from individual patients, the nineteenth century also introduced the concept of studies in populations. In the mid-nineteenth century, Lambert-Adolph-Jacques Quetelet (1796–1874) was a leader in developing mathematical methods to evaluate populations (Quetelet 1835). He developed the concept of the "average man" and used the ratio of weight divided by the square of stature (height) (kg/m^2) as a measure of an individual's fatness. This unit, the body mass index, might be termed the Quetelet Index (QI) in honor of the man who developed what has become a widely used way of evaluating weight status.

Justus von Liebig (1803–1873) is known for his ideas about protein, fat, and carbohydrate being the only major nutrients needed. They were a central theme of nineteenth century nutrition and impacted the view of obesity. Liebig was born in Darmstedt, Germany. After receiving his doctoral degree in 1822, he went to Paris to continue his work in chemistry with Gay-Lussac, one of the leading chemists of the day. He returned to Germany and became professor within 4 years—a clear example of his intellectual prowess. He was founder, in 1832, of *Liebig's Annalen,* a scientific journal that survived until 1874. Liebig began as a chemist, but his interests shifted to the chemistry of plants and animals. His analytical techniques facilitated his studies of body tissues and fluids. He emphasized the importance of protein in human nutrition. He contributed both to human nutrition and to the development of agriculture. He introduced the use of fertilizers that helped increase agricultural output. He discovered the amino acid tyrosine and he also isolated hippuric acid and chloroform. He studied uric acid, so important in gout, and developed a method to measure urea (Garrison 1914, p. 413; Mettler 1947, p. 162).

The small book by the nineteenth-century physician Thomas King Chambers (1817–1889) titled *On Corpulence* published in 1850 serves as a convenient dividing line between Paris medicine (1800–1850) in the first half of the nineteenth century and German laboratory medicine (1850–1920) in the second half of the century (Chambers 1850). In his Gulstonian lecture of 1850, Chambers describes the state of knowledge about fat and how it gets deposited at a time when the cell theory of biology had just come into existence. He said, "For the formation of fat it is necessary that the materials be digested in a greater quantity than is sufficient to supply carbon for respiration" (Chambers

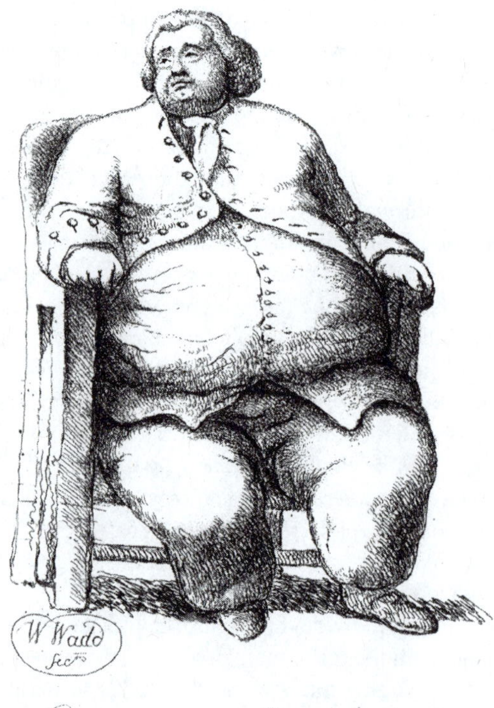

FIGURE 1.8 Etching from the writings of William Wadd (1829).

William Wadd (1776–1829) is known for his enjoyable book on obesity by a surgeon (Figure 1.8). Wadd was the eldest son of Solomon Wadd, a surgeon, who lived and practiced for more than half a century in Basinghall Street, London. He was born on June 21, 1776, and was entered at Merchant Taylors' school late in 1784. He was apprenticed to Sir James Earle in 1797, and thus became one of the privileged class of surgeon's pupils at St. Bartholomew's Hospital. He was admitted as a member of the Royal College of Surgeons on Dec. 18, 1801, and in 1816 he contested the post of assistant-surgeon to St. Bartholomew's Hospital, to which John Painter Vincent was elected. Wadd was appointed one of the surgeons extraordinary to the Prince Regent on August 19, 1817, and surgeon extraordinary to George IV on March 30, 1821. Wadd was chosen a member of the council of the College of Surgeons in 1824, and was appointed a member of the court of examiners in succession to John Abernethy on August 3, 1829. A life-size half-length in oils painted by John Jackson is in the Royal College of Surgeons in Lincoln's Inn Fields, London. Dr. Wadd was killed on August 29, 1829, by jumping off a runaway railway car on the road from Killarney to Mitchelstown while he was making a holiday tour of Ireland. At the time of his death, he was a fellow of the Linnean Society and an associate of the Société de Médecine of Paris. A man of high talents, Wadd had a rich fund of anecdotes. He was an excellent draughtsman, and learned etching to such good effect that the illustrations in his works are all the products of his own needle. He married Caroline Mackenzie, who survived him, on July 8, 1806. They had two children, a son who was drowned at Mauritius and a daughter (Power 1935–1938; Bray 2007; Haslam 2009).

1850). This early statement of the concept of a positive energy balance as the basis of adiposity has been amply confirmed.

Chambers goes on to note that the overweight individual "is prone to heart disease, to apoplexy (stroke) and congestions. While if a person is much above or below the standard weight, it is not necessary to discover any other bad symptom to pronounce the insurance of his life as 'above the ordinary risk'" (Chambers 1850). This insurance approach to assessing risk in relation to obesity has been a major stimulus to the study of this field from the time of Chambers through most of the twentieth century. Chambers' book goes farther and provides a table of weights in relation to height that had only been published 3 years earlier.

The hereditary disposition to obesity, which had become a major focus for research at the end of the twentieth century and has continued into the twenty-first century, can clearly be dated as far back as Chambers in 1850. He points out the familial basis of obesity through a series of 38 cases in which he notes the strong familial history. Chambers was also one of the first to note that "obese girls often menstruate at an unusually early age" (Chambers 1850). He noted the predisposing effects of sedentary occupations, of marriage, and of decreased exercise as important components in the increase of fat as individual's age. "Birth of a first child appears as a proximate cause of obesity for many women" (Chambers 1850). Thus, in his understanding of the natural history and development of obesity, Chambers is a truly modern physician.

Diet and exercise play a role in Chambers' treatment of obesity. He says, "The first thing indicated in all cases, is to cut off as far as possible, the supply of material (food). Fat, oil and butter should be rigorously interdicted in the diet." He goes on to say that "Very light meals should be taken at times most favorable to rapid digestion," and he then proceeds to describe a number of components of three meals (Chambers 1850).

Chambers also noted the importance of physical activity for overweight people. He said, "As respects exercise, a distinction requires to be made. The young and vigorous, whose obesity does not prevent their use of their legs, cannot employ them more usefully than in walking as long as they are able. The greater number of hours per diem that can be devoted to this exercise, the quicker will be the diminution of bulk" (Chambers 1850). This is a very modern notion indeed—the more you exercise,

Thomas King Chambers (1817–1889) was a senior physician in the mid-nineteenth century who placed obesity into perspective for us. Chambers was the fifth son of Robert Joseph Chambers. He received his medical training at Christ Church, Oxford where he graduated with honors in classics. He studied medicine at St. George's Hospital in London and received his bachelor of medicine in 1842 from Oxford. He became one of the first physicians at St. Mary's Hospital, London, and later a consulting physician to the Lock Hospital. As a result of a popliteal aneurism, one of his legs was amputated. Dr. Chambers was a censor with the Royal College of Physicians and delivered the Gulstonian Lectures in 1850, the Lumleian Lectures in 1863, and the Harveian Oration in 1871. He was one of the earliest advocates of medicine as a career for women. One of his chief hobbies was painting in watercolors. He was also an accomplished woodcarver (Munks 1955; Mettler 1947, p. 910).

the more quickly you will lose weight, providing that your joints hold up. He also notes, "It is very convenient for a patient to wear a band round the abdomen which may be tightened gradually" (Chambers 1850). The concept of using a band to reflect changes in weight thus has a long tradition.

In contrast to these relatively modern pronouncements about obesity, Chambers' discussion of treatment is steeped in the traditional scientific base of the mid-nineteenth century and earlier. In addition to diet and exercise, it includes bleeding, purging, and the use of soap or vinegar. It is, however, his insights into pathogenesis, physiology, and pathology that make his book a landmark for the transition to modern concepts of obesity in the mid-nineteenth century.

Cases of massive obesity have been noted since antiquity and these individuals have often been subjected to public curiosity. These individuals were frequently noted for their "odd" or "monstrous" appearance. The outlook for this group was particularly bleak, both from a clinical and social perspective (Willis 1681; Gould 1956; Kryger 1983, 1985; Russell 1866). In the nineteenth century, Dubourg discussed 25 such cases, Schindler identified another 17 individuals, and Maccary described 11 more (Dubourg 1864; Schindler 1871; Maccary 1811). Individual cases of very overweight individuals have also been reported by many other authors (Glais 1875; Dupytren 1806; Anonymous 1818; Barkhausen 1843; Coe 1751–1752; Don 1859; Eschenmeyer 1815; Gordon 1862; McNaughton 1829; Wood 1785).

There are always people eager to make money from the obese by selling them "shady" remedies. For people who are obese, the associated stress prompts many people to try dubious treatments if they promise a successful treatment for obesity. The nineteenth century saw its share of shady remedies as the patent medicine man plied his wares. Among these were the use of hydrotherapy and various laxatives and purgatives. Thyroid extract was also initially used to treat obesity in 1893 as the nineteenth century was drawing to a close.

The aniline dyes used in dyeing fabrics had a major impact on the entire field of pharmacology in the late nineteenth and early twentieth centuries (Canguilhem 1988). Developed by the chemical industry, the aniline chemical dyes served as the base for synthesizing numerous drugs in the twentieth century and for the "magic bullet" concept of Paul Ehrlich (1854–1915). Ehrlich reasoned that there should be a molecular structure like a key that would fit into a lock and be an effective treatment (Ehrlich 1910). His discovery of salvarsan, a drug that was moderately effective for the treatment of syphilis, bore out his concept.

The nineteenth century began the proliferation of popular books about obesity and how to treat it. One of the best known and most interesting is a book entitled *The Physiology of Taste: Or Meditations on Transcendental Gastronomy* by Jean Anthelme Brillat-Savarin (1755–1826), published in 1825—two months before his death—and republished and translated many times throughout the nineteenth and twentieth centuries. One of the most attractive versions of this masterpiece was illustrated by Wayne Thibeault, a California artist whose paintings of food look so good that you think you could eat them right off of the canvas (Brillat-Savarin 1826, 1970, 1994). Brillat-Savarin attributes obesity to two causes:

Jean Anthelme Brillat-Savarin (1755–1826) came from a family of lawyers and was neither an academic nor a cook. Born in the town of Belley, his studies took him into the family profession of the law. At one point prior to his appointment in 1802 as a judge in the Supreme Court of Appeals in Paris, he had been mayor of Belley. He survived the French Revolution, but barely, escaping France and ending up in New York where for some time he supported himself as a pianist. In 1789, he was the representative of Belley to the Third Estate. He narrowly escaped the guillotine in 1793 and fled to Switzerland and then to America, where he spent 3 years before returning to France. Compiling his masterpiece took 30 years (Von Helmholtz 1851; Brillat-Savarin 1970; Rossner 2007).

> The first is the natural temperament of the individual. . . The second principal cause of obesity lies in the starches and flours which man uses as the base for his daily nourishment . . . A double cause of obesity results from too much sleep combined with too little exercise. . . . The final cause of obesity is excess, whether in eating or drinking (Brillat-Savarin 1826, 1970, 1994).

In his discussion of treatment for obesity, Brillat-Savarin says, "Any cure of obesity must begin with the three following and absolute precepts: discretion in eating, moderation in sleeping, and exercise on foot or on horseback" (Brillat-Savarin 1826, 1970, 1994). Having said this much he goes on to say, "Such are the first commandments which science makes to us: nevertheless I place little faith in them" (Brillat-Savarin 1994). He then goes on to recommend a diet low in grains and starches. The book by Brillat-Savarin covered not only obesity, but many other areas of taste and food as well. It has continued to be a best seller, but never in the sense of the popular diet books that began only a few years later.

As the nineteenth century closed, the relation of the brain to obesity came into view for the first time. A neural basis for some kinds of obesity became evident at the beginning of the twentieth century. Two widely known case reports, one by Joseph Babinski (1871–1953) and the other by Alfred Frohlich (1857–1932) described single individuals who developed obesity due to a tumor at the base of the brain (Babinski 1900; Frohlich 1901).

Four dietary themes have occupied the nineteenth and twentieth centuries. The first is the low-carbohydrate diet, with various degrees of carbohydrate deprivation that began with Banting's diet. The second is the low-calorie or balanced-deficit diet in which total calories are reduced and all of the macronutrients are reduced. The third theme is the low-fat diet that comes in both low-fat, about 25% of energy from fat, and very low-fat, where the goal is 10% of energy from fat. The fourth is starvation and semistarvation.

TWENTIETH CENTURY: AN AGE OF SPECIALIZATION IN SCIENCE AND MEDICINE

By the beginning of the twentieth century, the ground had been laid for the concepts of energy balance and multiple causes of obesity occurring on a familial background and increasing the risk for ill-health. The twentieth century saw a sharpening of focus in each of these areas, and the birth of many new themes. Central themes for obesity in the twentieth century include the discovery of leptin, sophisticated developments in fat cell biology, the use of human calorimeters and double-labeled water to measure energy expenditure, improvements in methods for measuring body fat and recognizing that not all fat deposits have the same implications for health, identifying neurotransmitters that regulate feeding, identifying the gut as an important source of endocrine and neural messages to the brain, expanding the number of specific causes of obesity, understanding the genetic code and using this information to explore genetic causes of obesity, the introduction of lifestyle changes as a way to treat obesity, a plethora of diets, the application of pharmacological

Timeline 1900–2000

Science and Technology	1903 - Wright brothers' flight; 1915 - Theory of Relativity; 1926 - Liquid-fueled rocket; 1927 - Lindbergh's flight; 1933 - Television demonstrated; 1939 - DDT synthesized; 1939 - Polyethylene invented; 1945 - Atomic bomb dropped; 1947 - Transistor invented; 1956 - Birth control pill tested; 1957 - Spuntik launched; 1969 - Armstrong walks on moon; 1975 - Wilson–Sociobiology; 1980 - Transgenic mouse; 1989 - Human genome project
Anatomy and Histology	1928 - Ramon y Cajal; 1932 - Knoll & Ruskin–Electron microscope; 1951 - Hyperplastic obesity; 1973 - CT scan; 1982 - CT of visceral fat
Physiology	1902 - Bayliss–Secretin; 1912 - Cannon and Carlson–Gastric contraction and hunger; 1918 - Starling–Law of the heart; 1929 - Hayman–Carotid sinus reflex; 1932 - Cannon- *Wisdom of the Body*; 1946 - Hydrostatic weight; 1946 - Fat cells metabolize; 1949 - Lipostatic theory; 1953 - Glucostatic theory; 1963 - Doubly labeled water; 1975 - Fat cells cultured; 1978 - BAT/SNS; 1978 - Adrenalectomy prevents obesity; 1982 - NPY stimulated F.I.
Chemistry/ Biochemistry	1912 - Hopkins–Vitamins; 1921 - Banting isolates insulin; 1928 - Warburg broken cells respire; 1937 - Krebs–Citric acid cycle; 1946 - Lippmann-Coenzyme; 1953 - Insulin sequenced; 1958 - Sutherland cyclic Amp; 1960 - RIA for insulin; 1965 - Holley transfer RNA; 1972 - Releasing factor; 1995 - Cpe-gene Leptin-receptor gene
Genetics	1909 - Garrod–*Inborn Errors*; 1924 - Davenport–familial association of obesity; 1944 - Avery–DNA; 1950 - Obese mouse described; 1953 - Watson and Crick–double helix; 1956–Prader-Willi syndrome; 1992 - Yellow gene cloned; 1994 - Leptin gene cloned
Pharmacology	1901 - Adrenaline isolated; 1909 - Ehrlich invents Salvarsan; 1912 - Vitamin coined; 1922 - Insulin therapy; 1928 - Fleming discovers penicillin; 1932 - Domagk discovers sulfonamide; 1937 - Lesses & Myerson–Amphetamine to treat obesity; 1944 - Quinine synthesized; 1954 - Salk–Polio vaccine; 1973 - Fenfluramine approved; 1992 - Weintraub combined Rx
Neuroscience	1900–1901-Frohlich-Babinski syndrome; 1902 - Pavlov–Conditioned reflexes; 1912 - Cushing's syndrome; 1940 - Hetherington VMH lesion; 1953 - Eccles–Nerve transmission; 1962 - ME stimulates feeding; 1967 - Behavior modification; 1992 - Glucocorticoid obesity transgene
Clinical Medicine	1901 - Life insurance companies show risk of obesity; 1903 - Einthoven–Electrocardiograph; 1928 - Very-low-calorie diets; 1947 - Risk of peripheral fat; 1951 - Heart-lung machine; 1953 - Bypass surgery for obesity; 1963 - Socioeconomic status and obesity; 1968 - Vermont overfeeding study; 1978 - First test tube baby; 1981 - First AIDS diagnosis; 1986 - Twin overfeeding study
	1900 1910 1920 1930 1940 1950 1960 1970 1980 1990
Presidents of the United States	T. Roosevelt; W. Taft; Wilson; Harding; Coolidge; Hoover; F. D. Roosevelt; Truman; Eisenhower; Kennedy; L.B. Johnson; Nixon; Ford; Carter; Reagan; Bush; Clinton; Bush
Events	1914–1918 - WWI; 1919 - Prohibition; 1920 - U.S. women get to vote; 1929 - The Great Depression; 1939–1945 - WWII; 1941 - Pearl Harbor attack; 1945 - United Nations founded; 1950–1953 - Korean conflict; 1961 - Berlin Wall; 1962 - Cuban Missile Crisis; 1962 – 1976 - Vietnam War; 1963 - Kennedy assassinated; 1968 - MLK assassinated; 1974 - Nixon resigns; 1989 - Berlin Wall falls; 1991 - Desert Storm; 1991- Soviet Union dissolves

FIGURE 1.9 Timeline for the twentieth century. The key events in several categories including politics, science, and obesity are shown.

science to the development of new drugs to treat obesity, and the introduction and development of bariatric surgery as an important therapeutic strategy for treating obesity and reversing diabetes. These themes are the subjects of the remaining chapters in this book and the twentieth century. These themes and the related science are summarized in the sixth timeline, shown in Figure 1.9.

2 Definition, Measurement, and Prevalence

KEY POINTS

- Body composition is described at the whole body level, organ and tissue level, cellular, molecular, and atomic levels.
- Obesity is an increase in body fat, but is often defined operationally by the body mass index (BMI).
- Central adiposity can be assessed clinically with the waist circumference.
- Other measures of body fat and visceral fat are more precise but do not improve much on the clinical value of BMI and waist circumference.
- The overweight population increased slowly during most of the 20th century, but showed a rise of 50% or more between 1984 and 2010.
- Children are also becoming obese at a rapid rate.
- Women have a higher prevalence of obesity than men.
- Ethnic differences exist in the prevalence of obesity.
- Central adiposity measured by the waist circumference is a key element in the diagnosis of metabolic syndrome.

INTRODUCTION

In this chapter, we will explore how we define and measure obesity and then use these definitions to explore the prevalence of obesity and the factors that modify it. I will begin with the use of a five-level model that reflects the historical development of methods used to describe the body and its composition. With this background I will define obesity and central adiposity and then use these definitions to explore the prevalence of obesity. The rising prevalence of obesity that is evident all around us affects children and adults, affects some ethnic groups more than others, and is worldwide in its scope.

DEFINITIONS

According to *Merriam's Collegiate Dictionary*, "Obesity is a condition characterized by excessive bodily fat." For "overweight" the dictionary says, "Exceeding the bodily weight normal for one's age, height, and build." Since overweight is more easily measured, it has become a surrogate for "obesity," both clinically and epidemiologically. Central adiposity refers to the location of fat in the abdominal area as opposed to hips, thighs, or arms. Metabolic syndrome is a collection of measurements: an enlarged waist, increased blood pressure, abnormal blood lipids (high triglycerides and low HDL-cholesterol), and elevated fasting plasma glucose.

DESCRIBING BODY COMPOSITION

The human body can be analyzed from many perspectives. I prefer the five-level model developed by Wang et al. (1992) and shown in Figure 2.1. These five levels reflect improvements over the past

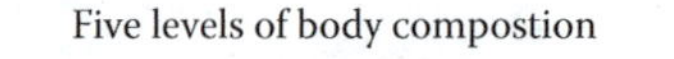

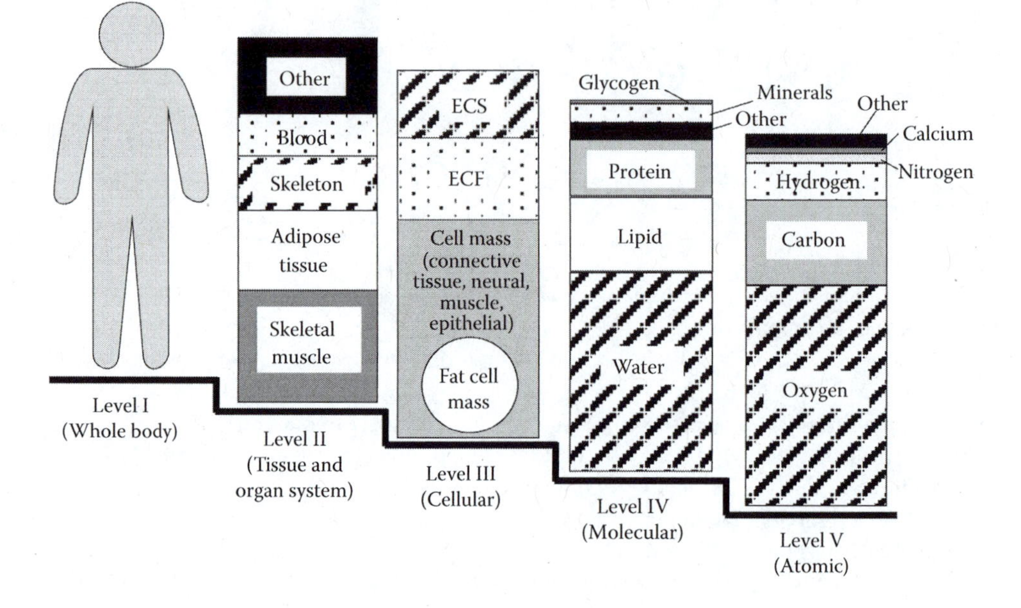

FIGURE 2.1 A five-level model depicting the whole body as Level I, the tissue and organ systems as Level II, the divisions of the body cell mass as Level III, the molecules that compose the body as Level IV, and the atomic composition of those molecules as Level V. (Adapted from Wang et al., *Am. J. Clin. Nutr.* 56(1), 19–28, 1992.)

five centuries in the methods of examining the human body. The initial anatomic studies of the human body during the Renaissance were done for artistic purposes, which required studies of the underlying anatomic structure.

Vesalius published the first modern anatomy of the human body in 1543 (Vesalius 1543). When the microscope was invented in the seventeenth century, it allowed exploration at the tissue (Level II) and cellular levels (Level III) of the human body. This was followed in the nineteenth and twentieth centuries by improvements in chemistry and physics that allowed for exploration of the molecular (Level IV) and atomic (Level V) levels for understanding body composition. A similar progression occurred in the study of human disease or pathology. It began with descriptions of illness in the "whole" patient and, as techniques improved, the diseases were gradually identified as affecting organs (organ pathology), then tissues (tissue pathology), and, finally, cellular and subcellular structures gave rise to cellular and molecular pathology.

Whole Body (Level I)

The first level of analysis of body composition is the whole body (Level I). Wang et al. (1992) identified at least 10 different measurable components, including stature (height), length of limbs, various circumferences including waist and hips, skinfold thickness at various sites (e.g., triceps, subscapular), body surface area, body volume, body mass index (BMI), and body density (Wang 1992; Heymsfield 2004). This whole body level of analysis got its impetus from the great anatomy book published in 1543 by Andreas Vesalius (1514–1564).

Andreas Vesalius (1514–1564) wrote a monumental book that opened up anatomic dissection to the medical profession. His feat was made possible by the printing press and movable type that were developed by Gutenberg less than a century earlier. Andreas Vesalius was born into a medical family in Brussels where he was a fourth generation physician. He began his studies in Brussels and moved to Paris to work with Jacobus Sylvius, one of the leading physicians of the sixteenth century. From there he moved to Padua, Italy and was elected to the chair of anatomy at age 25. He published his first set of anatomical dissections, the *Tabulae anatoamicae sex* within a year. By the age of 30, he had completed his masterpiece on the anatomy of the human body (*De fabrica humani corporis*). Published in 1543, with a second and somewhat more elegant version published in 1555, he achieved stardom in the history of medicine. In contrast to the accolades one might expect from this work, Vesalius was persecuted by the authorities and was forced to end his scientific activities. He left Padua and became the court physician to Emperor Charles V in Madrid where he lived a relatively quiet life. He died in 1564 as he was returning to resume his chair in Padua following a pilgrimage to Jerusalem (Garrison 1929, pp. 217–220; Talbot 1972; Osler 1921; Cushing 1943).

Organ and Tissue Composition (Level II)

The division of the body into organs and tissues is the next obvious subdivision. Five major tissues are shown in Figure 2.1, including skeletal muscle, adipose tissue, skeleton, blood or hematopoietic tissues, and others. The amount and location of adipose tissue is most important to our discussion. As much as 80% of body fat is subcutaneous; however, fat also surrounds many organs and accumulates around the abdominal organs. Intra-abdominal fat may produce more pathology than in other locations because the adipokines (inflammatory and other peptides) produced by fat cells from intra-abdominal locations enter the portal vein and then flow directly to the liver before entering the systemic circulation. Visceral fat in this latter category is most difficult to measure accurately except with expensive imaging techniques (Gallagher et al. 2005).

Marie Francois Xavier Bichat (1771–1802) pioneered the transition from an organ-based view of disease to one with tissues as the basis for disease and pathology. He lived a relatively short life, dying at the age of 31, but in that short time he revolutionized the view of disease by focusing on tissues rather than organs. Bichat was born in 1771 into a medical family where his father was a doctor of medicine at the University of Montpellier. The French Revolution began when he was a teenager and he sought refuge in the clinic of Professor Desault, one of the leading French surgeons. He came to the professor's attention and he befriended him, took him into his home, and treated him as an adopted son. When Desault died suddenly in 1795, near the end of the French Revolution, Bichat, then age 26, became a teacher and anatomist at the Hotel Dieu hospital. Over the next 6 years, he was extremely productive, collecting enough pathological material to write four major books and performing more than 600 autopsies in one year. His concept of disease and its pathology focused on the tissues that made up organs rather than the organs themselves. He was thus an intermediate between the organ-based pathology of Morgagni in the mid-eighteenth century and the cell-based pathology of Virchow in the mid-nineteenth century. As Talbot says, "Only a few medical scientists have been able to compress into a few years of maturity the quantity of investigation, teaching, and writing of . . . Bichat" (Garrison 1929, pp. 444–445; Talbot 1972).

Cellular Composition (Level III)

The third level in the analysis of body composition is its cellular components. Before we could think about body composition in terms of cells, we had to have an idea of a "cell." This concept developed in the early nineteenth century and required the availability of microscopes that could clearly see intracellular structures. With this type of microscope, Theodor Schwann (1839) identified the nucleus, cell membrane, and other structures and came up with the synthesis of a "cell" as a unit that would be similar in different tissues and different animals. Once this concept was established for animals by Schwann, and plants by a contemporary named Schlieden (1838), both students of Johannes Muller in Germany, the way was open to cells as the basis of biology.

Cells have properties that differentiate them. Potassium is the major intracellular cation where 95% of it is located. There is a naturally occurring radioactive form of potassium that occurs in all cells. This isotope, ^{40}K, can be used to determine the "cell mass" of the human body (Forbes 1987; He et al. 2003). Figure 2.2 lists two major cellular categories. Group 1 includes connective-tissue cells, neural cells, muscle cells, and epithelial cells, and group 2 includes fat cells, which we are most concerned about in obesity. Total body weight is the sum of all tissues, including muscle cells, connective-tissue cells, epithelial cells, and neural cells. The metabolically active tissues, such as bone, adipose tissue, blood cells, and muscle make up 75% of body weight (Sjostrom et al. 1986; Heymsfield 2004).

Molecular Composition (Level IV)

This part of the model is most widely used in clinical medicine. Water constitutes 60% or more of body weight in males, and 50% or more in females. Of this 60%, approximately 26% is extracellular and 34% intracellular. Lipids range from less than 10% of body weight in well-trained athletes to slightly more than 50% in very obese patients. Of these lipids, 2% to 3% are essential structural components and the remainder is nonessential fat stores. Protein constitutes 15% of normal body composition and minerals constitute 5.3%. Thus, water, lipids, protein, and minerals account for 99.3% of the molecular constituents of the body.

Theodor Schwann (1810–1882) developed the concept of a cell. The Schwann cell, which surrounds many axonal neurons, is named after him. Schwann was born near Dusseldorf in 1810. His father was a jeweler and printer, and it is possible that Schwann's mechanical skill was learned at his father's side. Schwann began his advanced studies toward a degree in theology at the University of Bonn. It was there that he came under the influence of Johannes Müller, the professor of anatomy. This changed Schwann's life. He was granted an MD degree in 1834 from the University of Berlin. Schwann served as an assistant in experimental physiology for his first five postdoctoral years. Although his cell theory is his dominant legacy, he contributed three other important discoveries. He found that pepsin, an enzyme from the stomach, could convert albumen into peptones. He also described the organic nature of yeast and the production of alcohol by fermentation. And finally, he showed that the particulate matter in air might be responsible for putrefaction, since it could be destroyed by heat. All of these discoveries were completed by the age of 29. He was then appointed professor at the Catholic University of Louvain in Belgium and was awarded the Copley Medal of the Royal Society of London in 1845. In 1848, at the age of 38, he moved for the last time to become chair of anatomy at Liege in Belgium, where he remained until his death at age 72 (Talbot 1992).

Several formulas can be used to describe body weight by dividing it into some of the compartments described above. Two compartment models measure fat and the fat-free mass and are the most widely used (Levitt et al. 2007; Lee and Gallagher 2008).

1. *Two-Compartment Models*

$$\text{Body weight} = \text{fat} + \text{fat-free mass (FFM)}$$

   Body density, the Bod Pod, bioelectrical impedance, and single-isotope dilution provide data for two-compartment models.
2. *Three-Compartment Models*
   Three-compartment models, including fat, lean body mass, and bone mineral can be obtained from dual energy x-ray absorptiometry.

$$\text{Body weight} = \text{fat} + \text{bone mineral mass} + \text{lean body mass}$$

3. *Four-Compartment Models*
   Four-compartment models provide more precise estimates of body fat.

$$\text{Body weight} = \text{fat} + \text{water} + \text{protein} + \text{bone mineral}$$

For laboratory purposes, a four-compartment model, including body weight, body water, body density, and bone mineral content provides the best way to estimate fat (Bray 2002; Heymsfield et al. 2004).

The amount of fat in the body varies more widely than any other single component. Table 2.1 shows the percent of body fat for men and women for three ethnic groups at three levels of the BMI. Several things are obvious. First, at any level of BMI, women have more fat than men. At a designated BMI of 25 kg/m^2 (overweight), women have 12% more fat than men. Ethnicity and age differences are also evident. Asian men and women at the same BMI are generally fatter than blacks or whites. Body fat rises by 1% to 2% for each additional 20 years of age in each gender and in all three ethnic groups (Gallagher et al. 2000).

Women have a higher percentage of body fat than do men. Values of body fat below 10% have been reported in highly trained long-distance runners, but as the values get lower, the precision of the measurement worsens and the reliability of these numbers is sometimes questionable. At the

TABLE 2.1
Ethnic Differences in Body Fat at Three Levels of the Body Mass Index in Caucasian, African-American, and Asian Men and Women

	Females			Males		
BMI	**African-American**	**Asian**	**Caucasian**	**African-American**	**Asian**	**Caucasian**
Ages 20–39						
18.5	20	25	21	8	13	8
25	32	35	33	20	23	21
30	38	40	39	26	28	26
Ages 40–59						
18.5	21	25	23	9	13	11
25	34	36	35	22	24	23
30	39	41	41	27	29	29

Source: Adapted from Gallagher, D., et al., *Am. J. Clin. Nutr.* 72(3), 694–701, 2000.

other extreme, body fat can rise to more than 50% of total body weight, but rarely above 60%. The very large majority of this fat is stored in droplets in the 40 to 90 billion adipocytes in the adult human body. The size of fat cells is larger in obese people and they may also have an increased number of fat cells (Salans et al. 1967). A small quantity of lipids is associated with membrane structures and is considered essential.

Proteins provide the structural and functional components of the body. Approximately 15% of the body is protein, but this varies with age, degree of physical training, and with a variety of clinical and hormonal states. Minerals of many kinds constitute the remainder of the body's molecular structure. Water, lipids, protein, and minerals account for more than 99% of the molecular constituents of the body.

Atomic Composition (Level V)

The final level in Figure 2.1 partitions the human body into its atomic components. If the standard or reference man weighs 70 kg, this individual's weight would be 60% oxygen, 23% carbon, 10% hydrogen, 2.6% nitrogen, 1.4% calcium, and less than 1% assigned to all of the other atoms in the body, such as chloride, copper, fluoride, chromium, magnesium, potassium, phosphorus, sodium, sulfur, nickel, zinc, and others. Eleven elements thus account for more than 99.5% of body weight, and five of them—oxygen, carbon, hydrogen, nitrogen, and calcium—account for more than 98% of total body mass. Less than 2% is attributable to the other atomic elements. The atomic components of clinical interest are nitrogen, calcium, magnesium, sodium, potassium, and chloride (Wang et al. 1992).

METHODS OF MEASURING BODY WEIGHT AND BODY FAT

Methods for determining body composition, including the fraction that is fat, and the standards to define degrees of overweight and central adiposity have greatly improved over the past 50 years, increasing the accuracy and ease of measuring body compartments and defining the degree of "overweight" in patients (Heymsfield et al. 2004; Lohman 1992; Gallagher and Song 2003). For children, many of the same methods can be used, except those involving radiation (Veldhuis et al. 2005).

Weight, Height, and Body Mass Index

Weight should be determined with a calibrated scale and height with a stadiometer. Electronic scales have largely replaced mechanical ones. Height and weight can be measured accurately and can be used to determine the BMI. The BMI is defined as the body weight divided by the square of the height (wt/ht^2), and is usually expressed in metric terms (kg/m^2). Although called the Body Mass Index, it could more appropriately be called the Quetelet Index after the man who developed the concept (Quetelet 1835, 1869). Table 2.2 contains the BMI values for various heights and weights in pounds and inches as well as in kilograms and meters. It can also be calculated using pounds and inches if the following formula is used. BMI = 703 × {weight (lbs) / [height (inches)]^2}.

To put the BMI in some perspective, I have used information on several prominent Americans published in the Wall Street Journal (July 23, 2002). The actresses Demi Moore and Rebecca Lobo have BMIs of 22 kg/m^2, as does the tennis star, Venus Williams; all are in the middle of the normal range. At the thin end of the scale is Julia Roberts with a BMI of 18 kg/m^2, Nicole Kidman and Madonna with BMIs of 17 kg/m^2, and Gwynneth Paltrow with a BMI of 16 kg/m^2, which is below the normal range. For men, BMIs tend to be higher. Sylvester Stallone has a BMI of 34 kg/m^2, which puts him in the "obese" category. Arnold Schwarzenegger, movie star and governor of California, has a BMI of 33 kg/m^2, and the baseline players Sammy Sosa and Mike Piazza have BMIs

Lambert-Adolph-Jacques Quetelet (1796–1874) developed the concept of the body mass index. This measurement is now widely used as a surrogate measure of obesity. He introduced this concept in 1835 based on his statistical evaluation of changes in people's weights (Quetelet 1835). Quetelet was born in Belgium in 1796 and died in Brussels in 1874 (Freudenthal 1975). Following graduation from the Lycée in Ghent, he worked for a year as a teacher. In 1815, at the age of 19, he was appointed professor of mathematics at the college in Ghent and in 1819 received a doctorate from the newly established University of Ghent, with a dissertation on geometry. The same year he received his doctoral degree, Quetelet was appointed professor of mathématiques élémentaires at the Athenee in Brussels. Quetelet was a man of many talents. He wrote an opera with his friend G. P. Dandelin and also published poems and essays. He was a teacher of mathematics, physics, and astronomy, and a major force in the development of the Belgian Observatory. His interest in probability theory may well be due to the influence of the French scientists LaPlace and Fourier. From 1832 onward, he lived at the Observatory where his work on meteorology, astronomy, and geophysics was conducted with its strong statistical focus. Following publication in 1825 of his famous work "*On Man . . .* " (*Sur l'Homme*) (Quetelet 1835), he rose to international stature throughout Europe and spent a great deal of his activity organizing international cooperative activities in astronomy, meteorology, geophysics, and statistics. He was the driving force of the first International Statistical Congress that met in Brussels in 1853 (Walker 1929). He was a member of more than 100 learned societies and wrote prodigiously on subjects covering the gamut from astronomy and meteorology to anthropometry and morals. In 1855 at the age of 59, he suffered a stroke, which impaired his subsequent work, although a second edition of "*On Man . . .* " (*Sur l'Homme*) was published in 1869. He died in 1874 and his work has not been republished since (Bray 2007, pp. 102–108; Garrison 1929, p. 674; Haslam 2009, pp. 200–201). Quetelet's contributions to mathematical statistics have been captured in the closing quote.

"Statistics will not make any progress until it is trusted to those who have created profound mathematical theories."

—Fourier (Walker 1929)

Quetelet was one of the creators of profound theories.

of 30 kg/m^2 and 27 kg/m^2, respectively. The actors Harrison Ford and George Clooney tip in at the overweight BMI of 29 kg/m^2, and Brad Pitt has a modest 27 kg/m^2. The basketball great Michael Jordan has a reported BMI of 25 kg/m^2, which is at the top of the normal range.

The accuracy of the body mass index in diagnosing obesity in the adult general population has been examined using data from the Third National Health and Nutrition Examination Survey (NHANES) where there was also a measure of body fat using impedance analysis (Romero-Corral et al. 2008). The authors conclude that the accuracy is limited for individuals in the BMI 25–29 kg/m^2 range, in men, and in the elderly. A BMI cutoff of ≥30 kg/m^2 has good specificity, but misses more than half of people with excess fat. However, as an estimate of risk for disease, the BMI provides valuable information (see Chapter 4).

One concern with the use of the BMI is that it does not account for people with increased muscle mass, such as football players, weight lifters, and other people who use weight lifting as part of their exercise program. This is indeed a fair concern, but in the field of obesity, which is the subject of this book, this is not a problem. For most Americans, the BMI is a reasonably good reflection of their degree of excess weight but it needs to be interpreted in ethnic and gender terms. The BMI has a positive association between height and adiposity among children and is better than other height–weight relationships for this group as well as for adults (Freedman et al. 2004).

TABLE 2.2
Body Mass Index Using English (lb and in) or Metric (kg and cm) Units

	Body Mass Index (kg/m²)																						
Inches	19	20	21	22	23	24	25	26	27	28	29	30	31	32	33	34	35	36	37	38	39	40	Cm
58	*91*	*95*	*100*	*105*	*110*	*115*	*119*	*124*	*129*	*134*	*138*	*143*	*148*	*153*	*158*	*162*	*167*	*172*	*177*	*181*	*186*	*191*	
	41	**43**	**45**	**48**	**50**	**52**	**54**	**56**	**58**	**61**	**63**	**65**	**67**	**69**	**71**	**73**	**76**	**78**	**80**	**82**	**84**	**86**	**147**
59	*94*	*99*	*104*	*109*	*114*	*119*	*124*	*128*	*133*	*138*	*143*	*148*	*153*	*158*	*163*	*168*	*173*	*178*	*183*	*188*	*193*	*198*	
	43	**45**	**47**	**50**	**52**	**54**	**56**	**59**	**61**	**63**	**65**	**68**	**70**	**72**	**74**	**77**	**79**	**81**	**83**	**86**	**88**	**90**	**150**
60	*97*	*102*	*107*	*112*	*118*	*123*	*128*	*133*	*138*	*143*	*148*	*153*	*158*	*164*	*169*	*174*	*179*	*184*	*189*	*194*	*199*	*204*	
	44	**46**	**49**	**51**	**53**	**55**	**58**	**60**	**62**	**65**	**67**	**69**	**72**	**74**	**76**	**79**	**81**	**83**	**85**	**88**	**90**	**92**	**152**
61	*100*	*106*	*111*	*116*	*121*	*127*	*132*	*137*	*143*	*148*	*153*	*158*	*164*	*169*	*174*	*180*	*185*	*190*	*195*	*201*	*206*	*211*	
	46	**48**	**50**	**53**	**55**	**58**	**60**	**62**	**65**	**67**	**70**	**72**	**74**	**77**	**79**	**82**	**84**	**86**	**89**	**91**	**94**	**96**	**155**
62	*104*	*109*	*115*	*120*	*125*	*131*	*136*	*142*	*147*	*153*	*158*	*164*	*169*	*175*	*180*	*186*	*191*	*196*	*202*	*207*	*213*	*218*	
	47	**50**	**52**	**55**	**57**	**60**	**62**	**65**	**67**	**70**	**72**	**75**	**77**	**80**	**82**	**85**	**87**	**90**	**92**	**95**	**97**	**100**	**158**
63	*107*	*113*	*118*	*124*	*130*	*135*	*141*	*146*	*152*	*158*	*163*	*169*	*175*	*180*	*186*	*192*	*197*	*203*	*208*	*214*	*220*	*225*	
	49	**51**	**54**	**56**	**59**	**61**	**64**	**67**	**69**	**72**	**74**	**77**	**79**	**82**	**84**	**87**	**90**	**92**	**95**	**97**	**100**	**102**	**160**
64	*110*	*116*	*122*	*128*	*134*	*140*	*145*	*151*	*157*	*163*	*169*	*174*	*180*	*186*	*192*	*198*	*203*	*209*	*215*	*221*	*227*	*233*	
	50	**52**	**55**	**58**	**60**	**63**	**66**	**68**	**71**	**73**	**76**	**79**	**81**	**84**	**87**	**89**	**92**	**94**	**97**	**100**	**102**	**105**	**162**
65	*114*	*120*	*126*	*132*	*138*	*144*	*150*	*156*	*162*	*168*	*174*	*180*	*186*	*192*	*198*	*204*	*210*	*216*	*222*	*228*	*234*	*240*	
	52	**54**	**57**	**60**	**63**	**65**	**68**	**71**	**74**	**76**	**79**	**82**	**84**	**87**	**90**	**93**	**95**	**98**	**101**	**103**	**106**	**109**	**165**
66	*117*	*124*	*130*	*136*	*142*	*148*	*155*	*161*	*167*	*173*	*179*	*185*	*192*	*198*	*204*	*210*	*216*	*223*	*229*	*235*	*241*	*247*	
	54	**56**	**59**	**62**	**65**	**68**	**71**	**73**	**76**	**79**	**82**	**85**	**87**	**90**	**93**	**96**	**99**	**102**	**104**	**107**	**110**	**113**	**168**
67	*121*	*127*	*134*	*140*	*147*	*153*	*159*	*166*	*172*	*178*	*185*	*191*	*198*	*204*	*210*	*217*	*223*	*229*	*236*	*242*	*248*	*255*	
	55	**58**	**61**	**64**	**66**	**69**	**72**	**75**	**78**	**81**	**84**	**87**	**90**	**92**	**95**	**98**	**101**	**104**	**107**	**110**	**113**	**116**	**170**

68	*125*	*131*	*138*	*144*	*151*	*158*	*164*	*171*	*177*	*184*	*190*	*197*	*203*	*210*	*217*	*223*	*230*	*236*	*243*	*249*	*256*	*263*	
	57	**60**	**63**	**66**	**69**	**72**	**75**	**78**	**81**	**84**	**87**	**90**	**93**	**96**	**99**	**102**	**105**	**108**	**111**	**114**	**117**	**120**	**173**
69	*128*	*135*	*142*	*149*	*155*	*162*	*169*	*176*	*182*	*189*	*196*	*203*	*209*	*216*	*223*	*230*	*237*	*243*	*250*	*257*	*264*	*270*	
	58	**61**	**64**	**67**	**70**	**74**	**77**	**80**	**83**	**86**	**89**	**92**	**95**	**98**	**101**	**104**	**107**	**110**	**113**	**116**	**119**	**123**	**175**
70	*132*	*139*	*146*	*153*	*160*	*167*	*174*	*181*	*188*	*195*	*202*	*209*	*216*	*223*	*230*	*236*	*243*	*250*	*257*	*264*	*271*	*278*	
	60	**63**	**67**	**70**	**73**	**76**	**79**	**82**	**86**	**89**	**92**	**95**	**98**	**101**	**105**	**108**	**111**	**114**	**117**	**120**	**124**	**127**	**178**
71	*136*	*143*	*150*	*157*	*165*	*172*	*179*	*186*	*193*	*200*	*207*	*215*	*222*	*229*	*236*	*243*	*250*	*258*	*265*	*272*	*279*	*286*	
	62	**65**	**68**	**71**	**75**	**78**	**81**	**84**	**87**	**91**	**94**	**97**	**100**	**104**	**107**	**110**	**113**	**117**	**120**	**123**	**126**	**130**	**180**
72	*140*	*147*	*155*	*162*	*169*	*177*	*184*	*191*	*199*	*206*	*213*	*221*	*228*	*235*	*243*	*250*	*258*	*265*	*272*	*280*	*287*	*294*	
	64	**67**	**70**	**74**	**77**	**80**	**84**	**87**	**90**	**94**	**97**	**100**	**104**	**107**	**111**	**114**	**117**	**121**	**124**	**127**	**131**	**134**	**183**
73	*144*	*151*	*159*	*166*	*174*	*182*	*189*	*197*	*204*	*212*	*219*	*227*	*234*	*242*	*250*	*257*	*265*	*272*	*280*	*287*	*295*	*303*	
	65	**68**	**72**	**75**	**79**	**82**	**86**	**89**	**92**	**96**	**99**	**103**	**106**	**110**	**113**	**116**	**120**	**123**	**127**	**130**	**133**	**137**	**185**
74	*148*	*155*	*163*	*171*	*179*	*187*	*194*	*202*	*210*	*218*	*225*	*233*	*241*	*249*	*256*	*264*	*272*	*280*	*288*	*295*	*303*	*311*	
	67	**71**	**74**	**78**	**81**	**85**	**88**	**92**	**95**	**99**	**102**	**106**	**110**	**113**	**117**	**120**	**124**	**127**	**131**	**134**	**138**	**141**	**188**
75	*152*	*160*	*168*	*176*	*184*	*192*	*200*	*208*	*216*	*224*	*232*	*240*	*247*	*255*	*263*	*271*	*279*	*287*	*295*	*303*	*311*	*319*	
	69	**72**	**76**	**79**	**83**	**87**	**90**	**94**	**97**	**101**	**105**	**108**	**112**	**116**	**119**	**123**	**126**	**130**	**134**	**137**	**141**	**144**	**190**
76	*156*	*164*	*172*	*180*	*189*	*197*	*205*	*213*	*221*	*230*	*238*	*246*	*254*	*262*	*271*	*279*	*287*	*295*	*303*	*312*	*320*	*328*	
	71	**74**	**78**	**82**	**86**	**89**	**93**	**97**	**101**	**104**	**108**	**112**	**115**	**119**	**123**	**127**	**130**	**134**	**138**	**142**	**145**	**149**	**193**
BMI	**19**	**20**	**21**	**22**	**23**	**24**	**25**	**26**	**27**	**28**	**29**	**30**	**31**	**32**	**33**	**34**	**35**	**36**	**37**	**38**	**39**	**40**	**BMI**

Source: © 1999 George A. Bray

Notes: The Body Mass Index is shown as **bold underlined** numbers at the top and bottom.

To determine your BMI, select your height in either inches or cm and move across the row until you find your weight in pounds or inches. Your BMI can be read at the top or bottom.

Pounds and inches in italics; **kilograms and centimeters in bold**.

TABLE 2.3
Waist Circumference Cut-Points by Gender and Ethnicity

	Waist Circumference Cut-Points	
Group	**Men**	**Women**
American	102 cm (40 in)	88 cm (35 in)
European (IDF)	94 cm (37 in)	80 cm (31 in)
Chinese and South Asian	90 cm (35 in)	80 cm (31 in)
Japanese	85 cm (33 in)	90 cm (35 in)

Note: IDF = International Diabetes Federation

Central Adiposity

Body fat is located subcutaneously and around various internal organs. In women, about 90% of body fat is subcutaneous and about 80% in men. Measurement of fat distribution, and particularly the internal or visceral fat, is a second important element of assessing body composition clinically because it has a strong relationship to future risk of developing cardiometabolic diseases. Several techniques have been proposed. Skinfold thickness estimates the subcutaneous distribution of fat, but does not estimate the visceral or intraabdominal fat. The adipomuscular index proposed by Jean Vague adds the circumferences of arms to the subcutaneous fat. The first widely used method was the waist circumference divided by the hip circumference or Waist to Hip Ratio (WHR). The waist circumference divided by the height or waist to height ratio (WHtR) is a second, and the waist circumference itself is a third. Both the waist circumference and the WHtR have similar predictive powers for the risk of cardiometabolic disease (Browning et al. 2010). All three methods provide predictive estimates of future risk from cardiovascular disease that are relatively close, and often independent of the BMI (Browning et al. 2010).

Waist circumference is, thus, a second essential anthropometric measurement in evaluating a patient and is preferred because it is a single measure and as good as any other. It can be determined by using a nonextensible tape measure (metal or plastic) that is placed around the abdomen at the waist. At least three definitions of "waist" have been used. One method places the tape at the level of the umbilicus. The problem with this one is that in very overweight people the "umbilicus" may be quite low. Another places the tape measure halfway between the last rib and the suprailiac crest, which is my preferred method because it uses stable landmarks. A third is to measure it at the iliac crest. Currently in the United States, a waist circumference greater than 102 cm (40 in) in men or greater than 88 cm (35 in) in women is one criterion for increased waist circumference (Shen et al. 2006).

Professor Jean Vague (1911–2002) is noted for his proposal that android or central adiposity is associated with increased risk for developing diabetes and heart disease. Jean Vague received his undergraduate education in Aix-en-Provence and his medical education at the University of Marseilles. Following an internship at the Hôtel Dieu Conception in Marseilles, he began his medical practice and research in endocrinology and rose through the ranks at the university to become professor in 1957. He served in the French army during World War II and was decorated with the Legion of Honor. Among many other distinctions, he is a member of the French Academy of Medicine (Bray 2007, p. 323; Haslam 2009, pp. 17–18; Jaffiol 2004).

Ethnic differences for waist circumference have been identified, and several recommended ones are shown in Table 2.3 (Alberti et al. 2006). A lower waist circumference is used for many populations.

The idea that central distribution of body fat is unhealthy had its beginnings in the late nineteenth and early twentieth centuries, but it was the work of Jean Vague in Marseille France that began to raise the consciousness of the medical profession about this problem (Vague 1947, 1956).

INSTRUMENTS USED TO MEASURE BODY COMPOSITION

In many settings, it is desirable to quantify body fat or fat distribution. This usually requires some kind of sophisticated instrument. Instruments used for measuring body composition have improved greatly over the past 25 years (Heymsfield et al. 2004; Sjostrom et al. 1986). Some of them are expensive and used primarily in research settings. Others, particularly dual-x-ray absorptiometry and bioelectric impedance, have found wider clinical and epidemiological use (Table 2.4).

DUAL X-RAY ABSORPTIOMETRY

Dual x-ray absorptiometry (DXA) instruments were developed to determine the bone mineral content in osteoporotics, but can measure body fat as well. The method requires the subject to lie supine on a table. Two very low-energy x-ray beams of different intensity are passed through the body. The x-ray beams are analyzed by computer to estimate lean body mass, body fat, and bone mineral content (Heymsfield et al. 2004; Laforgia 2009). DXA has replaced underwater weighing in many laboratories as the gold standard for determining body fat and lean body mass (Behnke 1942; Bray et al. 2002). The advantages of DXA are that it can be safely applied to individuals weighing up to 150 kg (300 lb) and it is easy to use, and with appropriate standards, it is very accurate. The instruments are expensive, costing between $40,000 and $100,000, and must be calibrated regularly. The weight limits of the table prevent measurement for individuals weighing more than 150 kg. The reproducibility of DXA is 0.8% for bone, 1.3% for density, 1.7% for fat, and 2.0% for body weight.

TABLE 2.4
Instrumental Methods of Measuring Body Composition

Method	Cost	Ease of Use	Can Measure Regional Fat	External Radiation
Hydrodensitometry	$$	Easy	No	
Air displacement plethysmography	$$$$	Easy	No	
Dual x-ray absorptiometry (DXA)	$$$	Easy	+	tr
Isotope dilution	$$	Moderate	No	
Impedance (BIA)	$$	Easy	+	
^{40}K counting	$$$$	Difficult	No	
Conductivity (TOBEC)	$$$	Difficult	±	
CT scan	$$$$	Difficult	++	++
MRI scan	$$$$	Difficult	++	
Neutron activation	$$$$+	Difficult	No	+++
Ultrasound	$$	Moderate	+	

Note: * Special Equipment; $=Inexpensive; $$=Some Expense; $$$=Expensive; $$$$=Very Expensive; tr+trace

Wilhelm Konrad Roentgen (1845–1923) discovered x-rays in 1895 that have been used to measure body composition. His discovery provided a fundamental technique that has made current quantitative study of body composition so precise and that provided the technique that lies behind computed tomograhic scans. Roentgen was born in 1845 to a German farmer and a Dutch mother. He was only a modest student during his education at Utrecht. His path was set when he met Rudolf Clausius (1822–1888). It was during his studies at Würzburg in 1895, while working with the radiation from a Crooke's tube, that he discovered a greenish fluorescent light produced on a distant barium screen with platinum that would pass through most substances, particularly soft tissue, so that the bones of the hand were easily visible. His discovery was published in 1895 and he won the Nobel Prize in 1901. He was troubled by World War I and died in relative isolation in 1922 (Garrison 1929, pp. 121–122; Bray 2007, p. 117; Koenigsberger 1906).

The radiation exposure with this procedure is barely higher than normal background radiation, and well below that of a chest x-ray (DeLany et al. 2002).

Underwater Weight (Hydrodensitometry)

Partitioning body density into fat and nonfat compartments, based on the fact that fat floats and nonfat components sink, was the gold standard of body composition until the advent of DXA (Gallagher and Song 2003). Its advantages are that it is highly reproducible, easy to perform, and requires only a good scale. Its disadvantage is that some individuals are unable or unwilling to completely submerge in water. Measurement of pulmonary residual volume at the time of the test is an important secondary method required to increase the accuracy of this procedure.

Whole Body Plethysmography (Bod Pod)

Air displacement using body plethysmography is similar in principle to hydrodensitometry or underwater weighing, but does not require submersion in water. One instrument is a life-size capsule with a see-through door that lets the subject in and out and that can be tightly sealed. In a comparison of air plethysmography using the Bod Pod Instrument versus water displacement (underwater weighing), Ginde et al. (2005) found that the underwater weighing and air displacement were highly

Albert R. Behnke Jr. (1903–1992) pioneered the quantitative use of hydrodensitometry to measure body fat—the technique Archimedes used to ascertain the amount of gold in his king's crown—to determine how much body fat people had. Dr. Behnke was born in Chicago in 1903 and received his MD from Stanford University in 1930. He served his internship at the U.S. Naval Hospital of Vallejo, CA, following which he was a research fellow in the Department of Physiology in the Harvard School of Public Health from 1932 through 1935. Most of Behnke's career was spent in the U.S. Naval Medical Service, which he entered in 1929. He was an instructor from 1937 to 1942, scientific director of the Naval Medical Research Institute from 1943 to 1950, and medical director at the U.S. Navy Radiological Defense Laboratory from 1953 to 1959, when he retired from active service in the Navy. After his military retirement, Behnke did extensive work on body composition and worked for awhile at the University of California School of Public Health in Berkeley. He died in January 1992 (ABMS 1990; Bray 2007, p. 117).

correlated ($r = 0.94$) with a standard error for the estimate of 0.0073. Bland–Altman analysis showed no significant bias between the two methods. Thus, air displacement appears to be an important new instrument for measurement of body fat.

Isotope Dilution

Estimating body water by injecting a tracer amount of isotopic water (D2O, $H_2{}^{18}O$, or ^3H_2O) or some other chemical that mixes completely in body water, such as thiocyanate, makes it possible to calculate body fat and thus partition body weight into fat and fat-free compartments. Body fat can then be calculated by assuming a value of the percent of water in lean tissue. For adults this figure is 73%, but it is lower in children. This method, density, and DXA have comparable accuracy (Bray et al. 2002).

Bioelectrical Impedance

Measurement of the resistance and impedance of the body between predetermined points on the leg and arm or between feet and arms has been widely used to determine the content of water in the body. It is available in some home scales that have two metallic foot pads. With proper training and careful placement of electrodes, highly reproducible measurements can be obtained. The instruments for this procedure cost between $2000 are $3000 and are portable. The advantages of this method are its relatively low cost and its ease of performance from the subject's point of view, and the ability to compare with other centers that use similar instrumentation (Völgyi et al. 2008; Fakhrawi et al. 2009). The disadvantages are that impedance only adds a small amount of extra information to the data on height and age, required for the equations. Second, the method is indirect because it only measures body water, which is used to estimate body fat. Several precautions are needed to obtain valid information from bioelectrical impedance (BIA). First, the instrumentation must be reliable. Second, the procedures must be standardized by using the same time of the day, the same ambient temperature, and standard placement of electrodes. Third, the subject should be similar to the populations from which the standard values are derived. Finally, the subject's water status should be stable because BIA measures water.

Infrared Reactance

This technique involves the application of an infrared signal over the biceps, where reflectance is read and acts as a signal for underlying fatness. No commercially acceptable instruments using this approach are known to the author.

Total Body Electrical Conductivity

Two instruments, one for adults and one for children, have been developed that use total body conductivity (TOBEC) to measure body composition. The principle is similar to the methods of evaluating the fat content of meat through changes in electromagnetic fields that depend on the relation of fat and water. TOBEC instruments are expensive, but may be useful in a research setting, particularly for children since no ionizing radiation is involved (Heymsfield et al. 2004).

INSTRUMENTAL METHODS FOR MEASURING VISCERAL FAT

Patterns of body fat distribution between subcutaneous and internal or visceral compartments can be reliably determined by either computed tomography (CT) or magnetic resonance imaging (MRI) (Heymsfield et al. 2004; Shen et al. 2004). The most common procedure is to obtain a single

TABLE 2.5
NHLBI Classification of Obesity by BMI and Waist Circumference

	BMI (kg/m²)	Obesity Class	Disease Risk* Relative to Normal Weight and Waist Circumference: Men <102 cm Women <88 cm	>102 cm >88 cm
Underweight	<18.5		—	—
Normal +	18.5–24.9		—	—
Overweight	25.0–29.9		Increased	High
Obesity	30.0–34.9	1	High	Very High
	35.0–39.9	2	Very High	Very High
Extreme Obesity	≥40.0	3	Extremely High	Extremely High

Source: National Institutes of Health, *Obes. Res.* 6(Suppl. 2), 51S-209S, September 1998.
* Disease risk for type 2 diabetes, hypertension and CVD
+ Increased waist can also be a marker for increased risk in normal weight individuals

cross-sectional slice at the interspace between the fourth and fifth lumbar vertebrae, which does not differ significantly from a cross-sectional area at the second and third lumbar vertebral space (Bray et al. 2008). This slice can then be divided into the area above the abdominal muscles and the intraabdominal fat and the amount of each quantitated.

A second procedure involves taking several slices, often eight, with two below and five above the L 4–5 lumbar vertebrae and calculating the volume of visceral adipose tissue. This volumetric method reduces the error of measurement considerably because variations in gas patterns within the abdomen have less influence on the volume of fat than on a single slice (Smith et al. 2005; Shen et al. 2004). Because of the expense, these techniques are not used for routine clinical determination of visceral fat. In a recent comparison of methods as predictors for the development of diabetes, it was found that the waist circumference was as good an index of fat distribution as the visceral or subcutaneous fat determined by computed tomography (Bray et al. 2006).

Clinical Recommendations: Careful measurement of height, weight, and waist circumference are the essential measurements and can be considered part of the vital signs needed to begin evaluation of an overweight patient. This will provide the BMI, which is a measure of the risk associated with weight status and a measure of central adiposity, which is needed to make the diagnosis of metabolic syndrome. If the clinician is concerned about whether lean body mass is increased, DXA may be considered. Although impedance measurements are used in many clinical settings they often underestimate fat. Most other techniques are for research use. The criteria for obesity recommended by the World Health Organization and the National Heart Lung and Blood Institute are shown in Table 2.5. It includes the various categories of body mass index and the current divisions of waist circumference. The waist to height ratio is similar to waist in its prediction of cardiometabolic disease and has the virtue of a simple number of a waist to height ratio < 0.5 as a useful dividing line. If the waist/height is less than 0.5, the individual is at higher risk (Browning et al. 2010).

BODY FAT THROUGH THE LIFE SPAN

Body fat changes with age and is modified by several factors including gender, age, level of physical activity, and hormonal status. The percentage of body fat steadily increases with age in both men and women. Women have a higher percentage of body fat than do men for a comparable height and weight at all ages after puberty. Visceral fat is about 10% of total fat in women and 20% in men. Visceral fat in women is lower during the reproductive years, but rises rapidly to nearly male levels in the postmenopausal years, at a time when risk for cardiovascular disease and other diseases in women also increase sharply. Indeed, when differences in body fat distribution are considered, almost all of the differences in excess mortality of men over women disappear, suggesting that the underlying factors leading to differences in fat distribution are major contributors to the risk of diabetes, heart disease, high blood pressure, and stroke. Some elderly people are characterized by a relative decrease in muscle mass, called sarcopenia. The reduction in muscle mass and retention of body fat can predict functional capacity in older people (Dey et al. 2009; Baumgartner et al. 2004). In a study using DXA in 45 elderly people, four groups were defined (normal or obese with or without sarcopenia) using DXA. An assessment of the hypothalamic-pituitary axis showed that the obese had reduced growth and the sarcopenic showed increased cortisol and leptin relative to their lean mass.

Ethnic background also influences body fat and its distribution. African Americans have less visceral fat and more subcutaneous fat than Caucasians. Asians have more visceral fat (Gallagher et al. 2000; Fernandez et al. 2003).

BODY FAT AND BODY ENERGY STORES

Using the methods described earlier, we can compare body composition and its energetic equivalent in men and women of two different body weights. This is presented in Figure 2.2, which shows the effect of a 30-kg increase in weight for the standard 70-kg man and the standard 56-kg woman. More than two-thirds of this increase in weight in men, and up to 90% in women, is accounted for by increased fat. The remainder is lean tissue that supports the extra fat. Because the extra stored triglycerides are energy-rich, the 30-kg increase in weight nearly doubles body energy stores. The therapeutic challenge for treating overweight patients is to reduce this excess energy stored in body fat without a disproportionate loss in lean tissue associated with fat storage.

CRITERIA FOR THE METABOLIC SYNDROME

The work of Vague in France, beginning after World War II, pointed to a relationship between fat distribution and the risk for cardiometabolic disease. He pointed out that women with android or male-like patterns of fat distribution were more likely to get diabetes and heart disease. It was two key studies, one by Kissebah et al. (1982) in the United States and by Bjorntorp and his colleagues

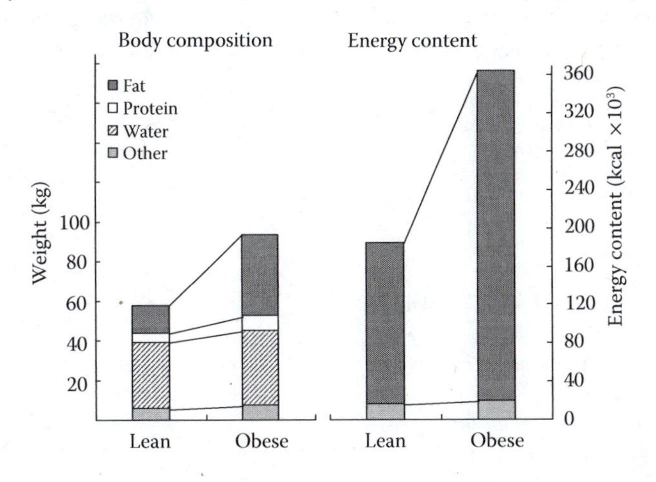

FIGURE 2.2 Relation of energy stores to body compartments. A 30-kg increase in body weight occurs mainly as an increase in body fat with a small increase in protein and water (lean body mass). Since most body energy is stored in fat, the 30-kg (50%) increase in body weight produces a near doubling of body energy stores.

Per Björntorp (1931–2003) is known for his work on the metabolic syndrome and its relationship to the hypothalamic-pituitary axis. Björntorp was born in Linköping on May 25, 1931. He received his undergraduate and graduate medical education at Gothenburg University, in Gothenburg, Sweden. After completing his medical degree, he did a graduate fellowship at the Oklahoma Research Foundation in Oklahoma City, where his work on studies of adipose tissue began. He returned to Gothenburg, and as is usual in Europe, he spent most of his academic life there, rising through the ranks to become professor and head of the Department of Medicine. However, he was always a research scholar at heart. He recruited and worked with some of the brightest young minds in Europe. His work covered many areas of human obesity. He chaired the Third International Congress of Obesity in Rome, Italy and served as Editor-in-Chief of the *International Journal of Obesity* between 1983 and 1989. In the early 1950s, Björntorp had studied cello at the Gothenburg Conservatory of Music and found playing the cello a form of relaxation when coming home in the evening. Summers were a time for him to exercise his interest in sailing his boat, which he launched with relish each spring. He was an inveterate sailor. Finally, he was a chef who enjoyed cooking. Following a period of illness, he died October 10, 2003 at the age of 72 (Sjostrom 2004; Rossner 2010).

(Lapidus 1984; Larsson 1984) that brought this concept to the wider public. They showed that central adiposity predicted heart disease, diabetes, and increased mortality. In a key lecture to the American Diabetes Association in 1988, Reaven coined the term Syndrome-X to bring together the group of findings that included high blood pressure, abnormal lipids, diabetes, and central adiposity. It has since become known as the metabolic syndrome. It predicts the risk for diabetes and cardiovascular disease, although it may not be better than its individual components. The features of the metabolic syndrome often reflect insulin resistance, a measurement that is difficult to do clinically. Thus, efforts began to identify components that might lead to a diagnosis of the metabolic syndrome without requiring measurement of insulin resistance. Several proposals have been made to provide criteria for identifying the metabolic syndrome. They include those of the National Cholesterol Education Program, Adult Treatment Panel III, the International Diabetes Federation, and the World Health Organization. One of the most widely used is the proposal from the United States National Cholesterol Education Program (NCEP) when they published their Adult Treatment Panel III recommendations in 2001 (Grundy et al. 2001). These criteria required that three of the five measures be abnormal to make the diagnosis. A recent international conference has proposed

TABLE 2.6
International Criteria for the Metabolic Syndrome

Measure	Categorical Cut-Points
Elevated waist circumference	Population- and country-specific definitions
Elevated triglycerides (drug treatment for this condition is an alternative indicator criterion)	≥150 mg/dl
Reduced HDL-cholesterol (drug treatment for reduced HDL is an alternate indicator criterion)	Males <40 mg/dL Females <50 mg/dl
Elevated blood pressure (drug treatment for elevated blood pressure is an alternate criterion)	>130 mm Hg systolic and/or >85 mm Hg diastolic
Elevated fasting blood glucose (treatment for an elevated blood glucose is an alternate criterion)	>100 mg/dL

Source: From Alberti, K.G., et al., *Circulation*, 120(16), 1640–1645, 2009.

a widely accepted set of criteria to make the diagnosis. The diagnosis requires that three of the five measures listed in Table 2.6 be abnormal (Alberti et al. 2009).

PREVALENCE OF OBESITY

Prevalence in Adults in the United States

Obesity in the United States has been called an epidemic. It has received this appellation because it now affects nearly one-third of the adult population and a large number of children (Hedley et al. 2004; Ogden 2006, 2007; Jolliffe 2004; Ogden et al. 2008). The World Health Organization has also called obesity an epidemic because worldwide it may affect more than 300 million people (WHO 2000; James 2004).

Using the BMI, we can divide the population into groups, compare these groups across national boundaries, and examine time trends. The percentage of Americans with a BMI above 25 kg/m^2 or 30 kg/m^2 has been determined in several surveys (Flegal et al. 2002; Ogden et al. 2007; Flegal et al. 2010). The data have been collected in two different ways. One uses telephone surveys and is conducted by state departments of health in collaboration with the Centers for Disease Control and Prevention in Atlanta, GA. These surveys are now done annually and are called the Behavioral Risk Factor Surveillance System (BRFSS). The other approach is to take a direct measurement of height and weight in a stratified sample of the population. This is the approach used in the field surveys by the NHANES that began in 1960. A comparison of the results from these two surveys is shown in Figure 2.3.

It can be seen that the BRFSS data give a prevalence that is about two-thirds that of the NHANES. This could be because people underreport their weight, overreport their height, or both during the telephone surveys. Data would suggest that they do a bit of both. When reading the literature on the prevalence of overweight in the U.S., however, it is important to identify which method has been used. In the survey of 1988–1994 the percentage increase was 8% compared to 1976–1980. The rise continued through the survey of 1999–2000. For the period 1999–2008, there was not a significant further increase in women who had an obesity rate in 2007–08 of 35.5% (BMI ≥ 30 kg/m^2). For men there was a significant trend upward over the years from 2003–2004 to 2007–2008, but no pairs were significantly different. The percent of obese men with a BMI ≥ 30 kg/2 was 32.2% in 2007–08. The conclusion from this analysis by Flegal et al. (2010) is that the weight gain has slowed or ceased, but at an unsatisfactorily high level (Figure 2.4).

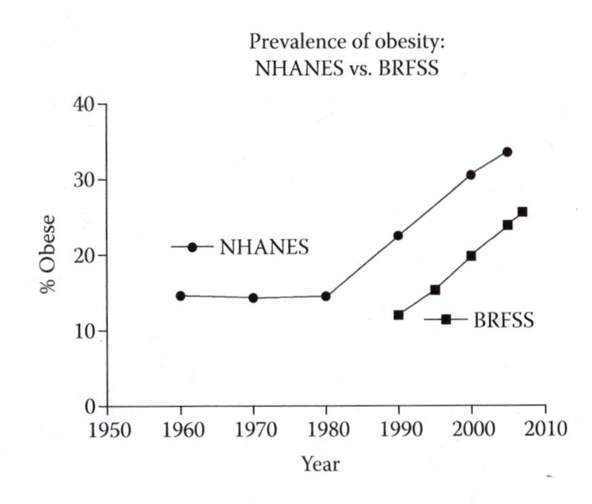

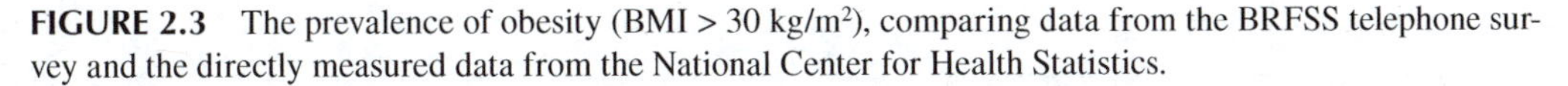
FIGURE 2.3 The prevalence of obesity (BMI > 30 kg/m^2), comparing data from the BRFSS telephone survey and the directly measured data from the National Center for Health Statistics.

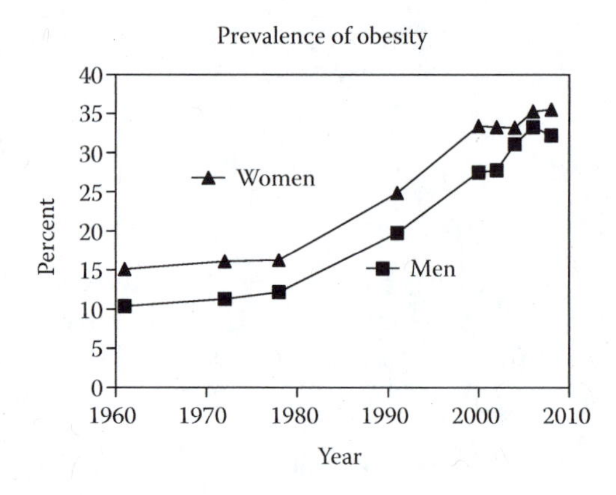

FIGURE 2.4 The prevalence of overweight (BMI > 25 kg/m²) and obesity Class I (BMI > 30 kg/m²) or Class III (BMI > 40 kg/m²) from 1960 to 2004 based on the U.S. National Center for Health Statistics surveys (Flegal et al. 2010; Ogden et al. 2008).

The measurements from the Framingham Study provide the long-term perspective from a single community. This is a study that has followed over 5000 residents of Framingham, Massachusetts since 1948, and showed the increasing prevalence rates between the 1950s and the 1990s (see Table 2.7). The category from 30–35 has gone up threefold for men, but not for women; whereas, the group with the highest BMI category (30 kg/m²) has risen 20-fold in men and 2.5-fold in women (Parikh et al. 2007).

The maps in Figure 2.5 graphically show the increase in the BMI from 1991 to 2008 by the state using the BRFSS telephone interview technique. Ezzati et al. (2006) have examined quantitatively the differences between the NHANES and BRFSS data sets and find that on average, women underreported their weight, but men did not. Young and middle-aged (<65 years) adult men overreported their height more than women of the same age. The data from telephone surveys can be corrected for these errors and shows that for men, Mississippi (31%) and Texas (30%) had the highest prevalence of obesity and, in women, several states (Alabama, District of Columbia, Louisiana, Mississippi, and Texas had similar rates of 37%).

TABLE 2.7
Prevalence of Obesity in the Framingham Study Population in the 1950s and 1990s

BMI Category	1950s	1990s
	Men	
25–30 kg/m²	21.8%	35.2%
30–35 kg/m²	5.8%	14.8%
>35	0.2%	5.4%
	Women	
25–30	15.0%	33.1%
30–35	14.0%	14.0%
>35	1.7%	4.4%

Source: Adapted from Parikh, N.I., et al., *Am. J. Med.*, 120, 242–252, 2007.

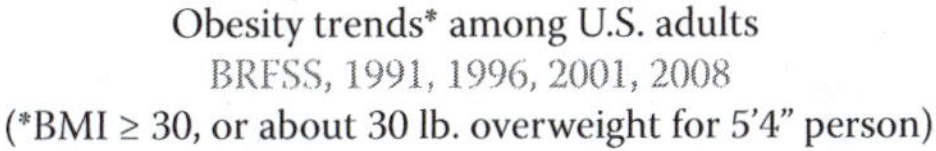

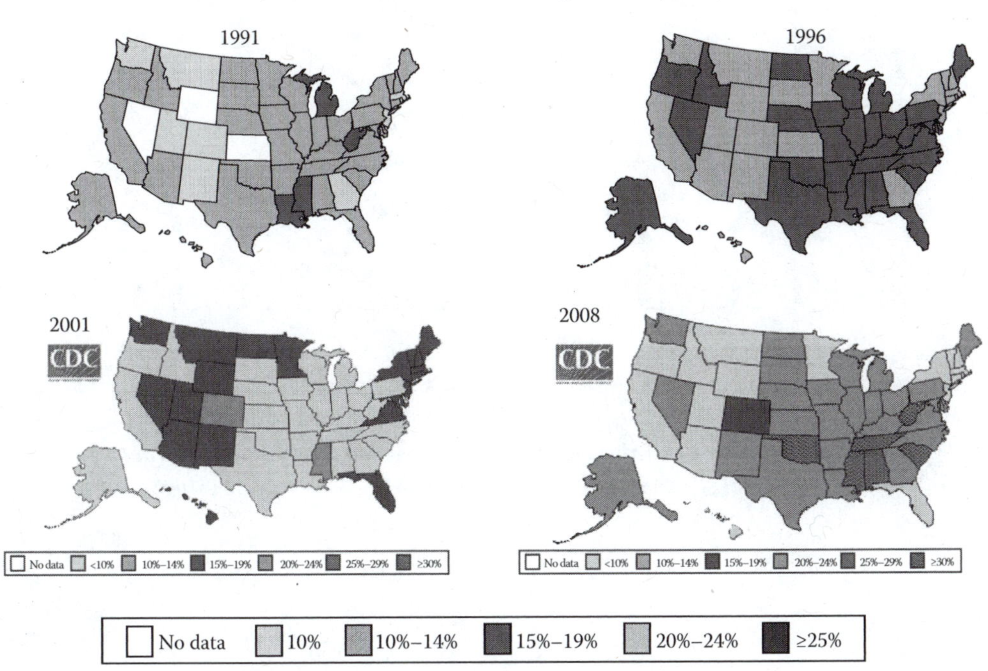

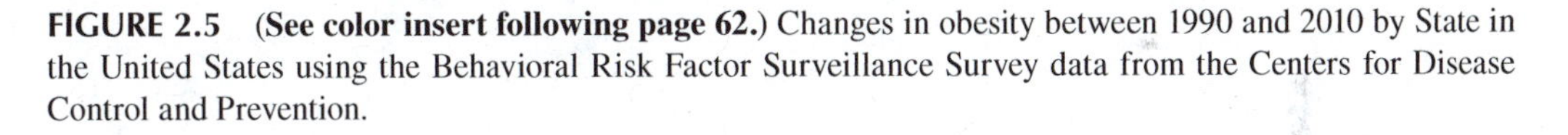

FIGURE 2.5 **(See color insert following page 62.)** Changes in obesity between 1990 and 2010 by State in the United States using the Behavioral Risk Factor Surveillance Survey data from the Centers for Disease Control and Prevention.

Between 1960 and 2002, the percentage of men with a BMI above 30 kg/m^2 more than doubled, and the percentage of women with a BMI above 30 kg/m^2 rose by more than 50%. The rise in body weight relative to height is not new (Bray 1976), but it has accelerated. Figure 2.6 shows that the body weights of American men for a given height have been rising since the Civil War. What is new in the NHANES and BRFSS data is the rate of this rise (Figure 2.6).

The lifetime risk of developing overweight in the United States is significant. Using the data from the Framingham Heart Study, Vasan et al. (2005) have calculated the 4-year risk and the 10- to 30-year risk of becoming overweight. They examined the effects for men and women at ages 30, 40, and 50 who had a normal BMI at each age. The 4-year risk of becoming overweight, that is developing a BMI > 25 kg/m^2, was 14% to 19% in women, and 26% to 30% in men. The 4-year risk for developing a BMI > 30 kg/m^2 if your BMI was normal was 5% to 7% for women and 7% to 9% for men. Over the longer 30-year interval, the risks were similar in men and women, and varied somewhat with age, being lower if you were under 50 years of age. The 30-year risk was 1 in 2 (50%) of developing overweight (BMI > 25 kg/m^2), and was 1 in 4 (25%) of developing a BMI > 30 kg/m^2 and 1 in 10 (10%) of developing a BMI > 35 kg/m^2. Because most pre-overweight people will become overweight, it is important to have as much insight as possible into the risk factors (Vasan et al. 2005). The transition from normal weight to overweight and then to obesity has been depicted for men and women in Figure 2.7. By ages 20–39, 64% of the men and 59.4% of women were either overweight (middle panel) or obese (top panel). Over the remaining intervals, there was an increase in the percent that were obese and a decline in the number that were normal weight. These life trends show that a substantial amount of the obesity we have occurs in the early years and that the shift in later years is relatively slow.

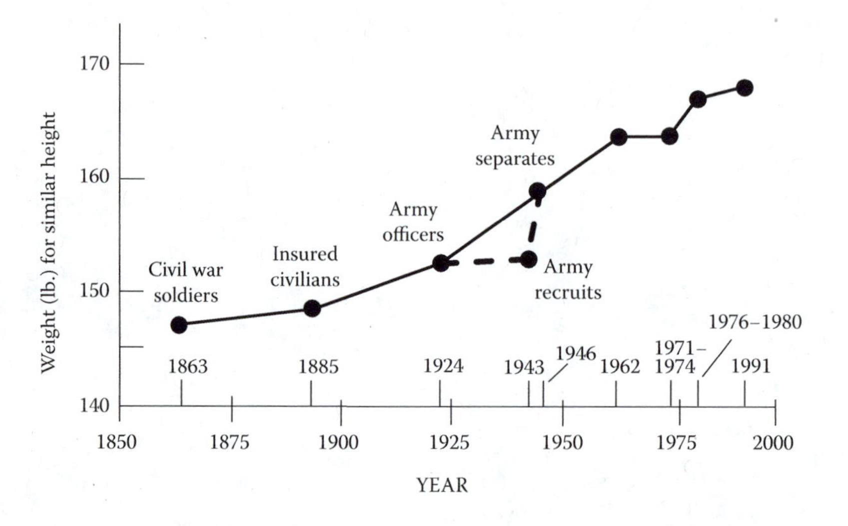

FIGURE 2.6 Changes in the body weight of males since the Civil War (From Bray, G.A., *The Obese Patient: Major Problems in Internal Medicine*. Philadelphia: W.B. Saunders Co., 1976. With permission.)

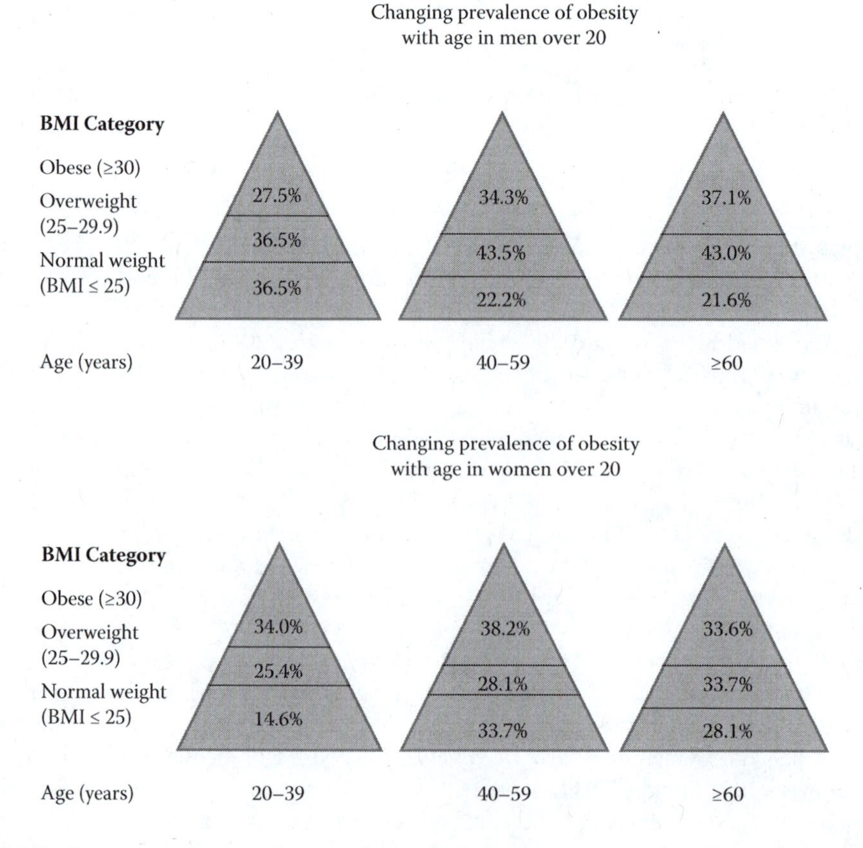

FIGURE 2.7 Percentage of men and women in the normal weight, overweight (BMI = 25–29.9) and obese (BMI > 30 kg/m^2) categories by age group (From Flegal, K.M., et al., *JAMA* 303, 235–241, 2010.).

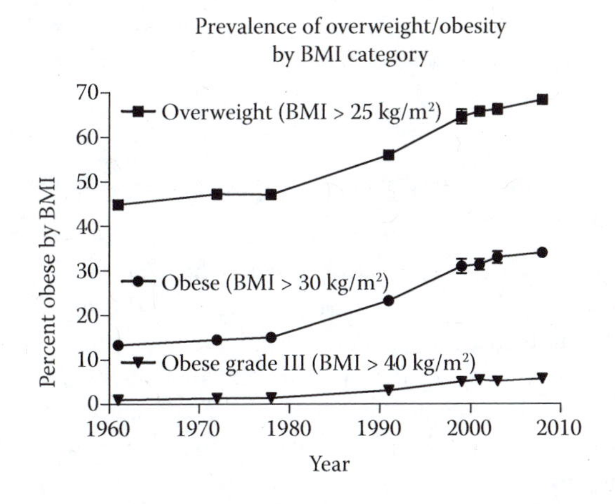

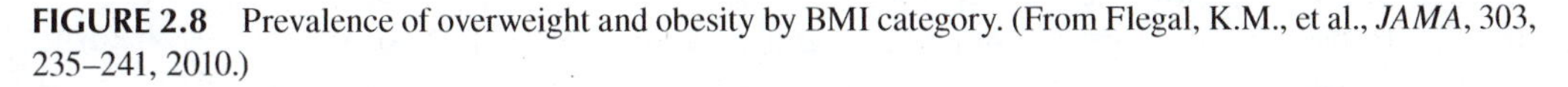

FIGURE 2.8 Prevalence of overweight and obesity by BMI category. (From Flegal, K.M., et al., *JAMA*, 303, 235–241, 2010.)

Class III obesity, which is a BMI > 40 kg/m^2, is a particular problem because it is one of the fastest growing groups of obese individuals. This is shown in Figure 2.8. Individuals with a BMI > 40 are often considered for bariatric surgery (see Chapter 8). In the most recent NCHS survey, this group accounted for 5.7% of the adult population (Flegal et al. 2010). In men, 4.2% fell in this category compared to 7.2% of women over 20 years of age. The prevalence of a BMI > 40 kg/m^2 was highest in the non-Hispanic Black population (9.0%), with much of this being non-Hispanic Black (10.8%). More non-Hispanic Black women were obese than any other group with a prevalence of 14.2% (Flegal et al. 2010).

Prevalence of Overweight in Women: Effects of Ethnicity and Poverty Level

The distribution of body weight and obesity is affected by gender, race, and economic status (Flegal et al. 2002; Baskin et al. 2005; Flegal et al. 2010). Table 2.8 shows the percentages of whites, blacks, and Mexican-Americans in the United States with a BMI above 30 kg/m^2. Both Mexican-Americans and Black women in particular have high percentages of obesity (BMI ≥ 30 kg/m^2). Using the National Health Interview Survey with self-reported height and weight, the prevalence of a BMI ≥ 30 kg/m^2 was 16% among immigrants and 22% among U.S.-born individuals. The prevalence was 8% among immigrants living in the U.S. for less than 1 year, and 19% for those in the U.S. for at least 15 years. These differences were not accounted for by sociodemographic characteristics, illness burden, BMI, or access to health care among some subgroups of immigrants (Goel et al.

TABLE 2.8
Prevalence of Obesity (BMI > 30 kg/m^2) in Men and Women from Different Ethnic Groups

Group	Men	Women
White—Non-Hispanic	31.9%	33.0%
Black—Non-Hispanic	37.3%	49.6%
Hispanic	34.3%	43.0%
Mexican-American	35.9%	45.1%

Source: Data from Flegal, K.M., et al., *JAMA*, 303, 235–241, 2010.

2004). Adolescents aged 15–17 years from families below the poverty level had a higher prevalence of obesity than those above the poverty level. These differences were less clear in those aged 12–14 years (Miech et al. 2006; Ogden et al. 2007).

Prevalence of Obesity around the World

The epidemic of overweight is not confined to the United States, but can be identified in data from all over the world (Berghofer et al. 2008; James 2004) and the data from several countries are shown in Table 2.9. The prevalence of overweight clearly is increasing in both the Eastern and Western hemispheres, and above and below the equator. Despite the wide range, all data suggest that most populations have increased the percentage of people who are overweight over the past 20 years. In Europe, there is a gradient for increasing obesity in eastern and southern Europe compared with the north and west regions. Obesity is increasing in most countries in the world. Several recent reviews have focused on specific regions. As a rapidly developing country, China is an interesting case. In China, a BMI of 24 kg/m^2 is the upper limit for normal, with 28 kg/m^2 as the cut-point for obesity. In 2002, the prevalence of overweight was 22.8% and obesity was 7.1%. These have increased 40.7% and 97.2% since 1992 (Chen 2007).

Waist circumference may also be increasing. Using data on cardiovascular disease and diabetes, criteria for waist circumference and BMI have been established for the Asia-Pacific region. The BMI showed a continuous positive association between baseline BMI and the risks of ischemic stroke, hemorrhagic stroke, and ischemic heart disease (IHD), with each 2 kg/m^2 lower BMI associated with a 12% lower risk of ischemic stroke, 8% lower risk of hemorrhagic stroke, and 11% lower risk of IHD (Asia Pacific Cohort Studies Collaboration 2004). Using the relationships of waist circumference, WHR, and BMI, a working group found that, for a given level of BMI, waist

TABLE 2.9
Prevalence of Overweight (BMI > 30kg/m^2) in Several Countries

		Prevalence of BMI > 30 kg/m^2	
Country	**Years**	**Men**	**Women**
Belgium (Ghent)	1989–96	10	11
Germany (Augsburg)	1989–96	21	22
Italy (Friuli)	1989–96	17	19
United Kingdom (Glasgow)	1989–96	23	23
Poland (Warsaw)	1989–96	22	28
Russia (Moscow)	1989–96	8	21
Argentina	1997	28	25
Mexico	1995	11	23
India	1988–90	0.5	0.5
Malaysia	1990	8	6
Saudi Arabia	1996	16	24
Tunisia	1997	7	23
China	1992	1	2
Japan	1990–94	2	3
Philippines	1993	3	2
South Africa (Cape Town)	1990	14	49
Western Cape (White)	1990	18	20
Durban (Indian)	1990	4	18

Source: Adapted from Seidell, J.C., and A.M. Rissanen, *The Handbook of Obesity*, Marcel Dekker, Inc., New York, 2002.

circumference, or WHR, the absolute risk of diabetes and hypertension tended to be higher among Asians than Caucasians, supporting the use of lower cut-points in Asian populations (Huxley et al. 2007).

Prevalence of Obesity and Overweight in Children

In children, obesity is defined as a weight above the ninety-fifth percentile for height and is comparable to an adult BMI of >30 kg/m^2. "Overweight" is the term used in children for a weight between the eighty-fifth and ninety-fifth percentile and corresponds to an adult BMI range of 25–30 kg/m^2. The prevalence of overweight in children is rising (see Figure 2.9). Strauss and Pollack showed that the yearly rate of increase in overweight children (BMI > ninety-fifth percentile) in the National Longitudinal Survey of Youth was 3.23% in non-Hispanic Whites, 4.3% in Hispanics, and 5.85% in African-American youth (Strauss and Pollack 2001).

In data from the 2003–2006 NHANES, Ogden et al. found that there was a high prevalence of obesity and overweight, but that there was no upward trend detectable between 1999 and 2006. Combining the years 2003–2006, 11.3% (95% CI 9.7, 12.9%) of children age 2–19 years were at or above the ninety-seventh percentile, 16.3% (95% CI 14.5, 18.1%) were at or above the ninety-fifth percentile, and 31.9% (29.4, 34.4%) were at or above the eighty-fifth percentile (Ogden et al. 2008). African-American and Mexican-American children had a higher percentage in almost all categories than non-Hispanic Whites. The most recent data show a prevalence of 18% (Anderson and Whitaker 2009), but some data suggest that the rising rate in children and adolescents may be reaching a peak (Ogden et al. 2008).

The prevalence of overweight and obesity in school-aged children from 34 countries (Janssen et al. 2005) showed that the two countries with the highest prevalence were Malta (25.4% and 7.9%) and the United States (25.1% and 6.8%). Lithuania (5.1% and 0.4%) and Latvia (5.9% and 0.5%) had the lowest prevalence. Television viewing time and levels of physical activity were generally higher in overweight than in normal weight youth. Overweight, in this study, was not associated with intake of fruits, vegetables, or soft drinks, or with the time spent on a computer.

Weight status in childhood predicts weight later in life. In a review of 24 studies on the relationship of weight status in infancy and childhood to weight later in life, Baird et al. (Baird et al. 2005; Kinra et al. 2005) found that in most studies, infants that were obese or at the higher end

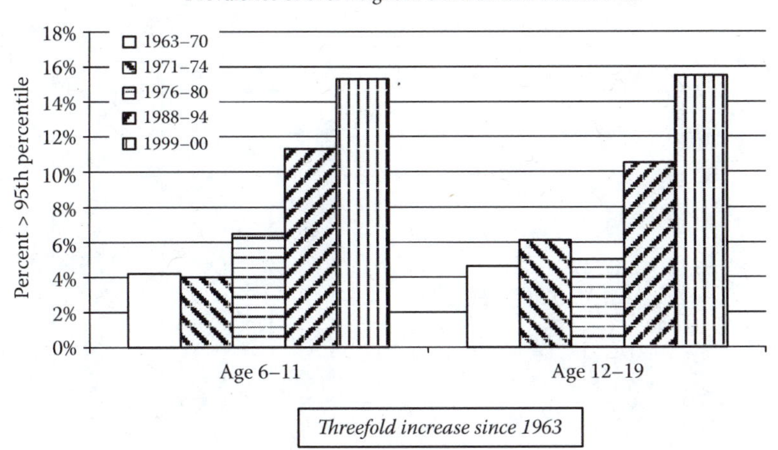

FIGURE 2.9 Prevalence of overweight in children aged 6 to 11 and adolescents aged 12 to 18 using data from the National Health and Nutrition Examination Surveys. (Redrawn from Ogden, C.L., et al., *JAMA* 295(13), 1549–55, 2006.)

of the distribution range were at higher risk, and that infants who grew more rapidly were also at an increased risk of overweight. These relationships held for infants born between 1927 and 1994, indicating the consistency of the pattern. These earlier growth patterns in girls are associated with an earlier age of menarche (Pierce and Leon 2005). An analysis of the development of overweight among children shows that not only have more children become overweight in the past three decades, but the overweight children have been getting even heavier (Jolliffe 2004). In an Australian birth cohort, overweight at age 5 years predicted earlier puberty and advanced puberty also predicts BMI of young adults at age 21. The effects of weight at age 5 are independent of the pubertal effect (Mamun et al. 2009). Using the 1958 British birth cohort, Li et al. (2009) found that weight gain in childhood, as well as in adulthood, was associated with a higher body weight (BMI) in their offspring.

METABOLIC SYNDROME

Waist circumference as a measure of central adiposity has not been as frequently collected as height and weight and there is, thus, less data. One thing is clear, however, and that is that the criteria, or cut-points, for waist circumference differ by gender and by ethnic group and several of these criteria were presented earlier in Table 2.3.

Central adiposity, as measured by the waist circumference, is the principal criterion now used to assess abdominal or visceral fatness. Although longitudinal data is limited, what there is suggests that it has increased, just as the BMI has increased. Using data from the NHANES conducted between 1988 and 1994 and the more recent survey from 1999–2000, Ford et al. (2003) found that the age-adjusted waist had increased in men from 96 cm to 98.9 cm and from 88.9 cm to 92.2 cm in women. These data suggested that the waist circumference distribution had shifted upward. Using age-specific rates of high-risk waist sizes, the authors estimated that there are about 35 million men and 58 million women who have high-risk waist circumference measurements.

The prevalence of the metabolic syndrome, using the ATP-III criteria described in Table 2.6, increases with age (Figure 2.10) and has been estimated at 23.7% of the adult population, or 47 million U.S. adults (Ford et al. 2002). The prevalence increases with age, rising from 6.7% in those aged

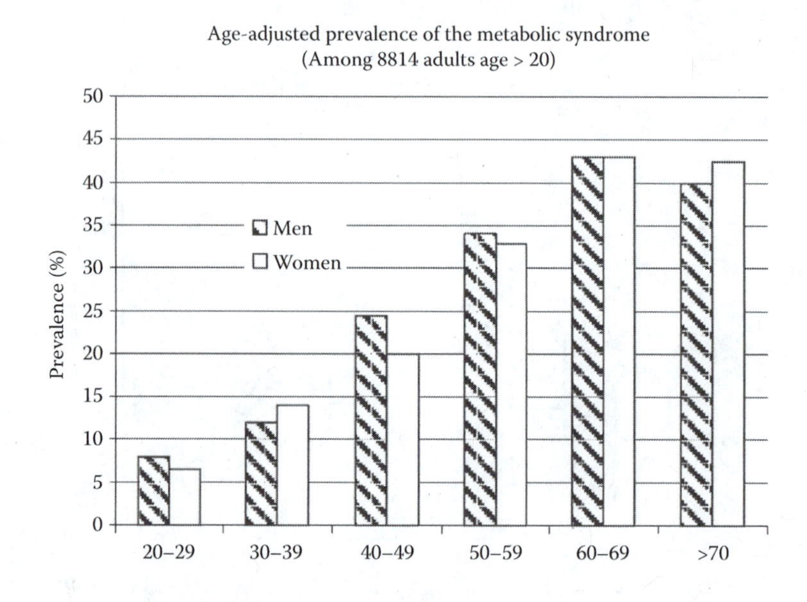

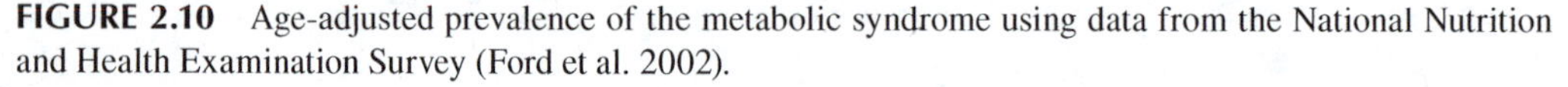

FIGURE 2.10 Age-adjusted prevalence of the metabolic syndrome using data from the National Nutrition and Health Examination Survey (Ford et al. 2002).

TABLE 2.10
Prevalence of the Metabolic Syndrome among Men and Women in Various Countries

Country	Men (%)	Women (%)
Australia (>24 years)	20	17
China (35–74 years)	10	13
Finland (42–60 years)	20	23
France (30–64 years)	10	8
India (>20 years)	8	18
Iran (>20 years)	26	42
Ireland (50–69 years)	22	21
Oman (>20 years)	20	23
Scotland (45–64 years)	28	—
Turkey (>31 years)	29	40
United States (>20 years)	25	29

Source: From Gu, D., et al., *Lancet*; 365, 1398–1405, 2005; Eckel, R.H., et al., *Lancet*, 365, 1415–1428, 2005; Ford, E.S., et al., *Diabetes Care*, 27, 2444–2449, 2004.

20–29 years to 43.5% in those aged 60–69 years, and 42% in people older than 70 years. There is an ethnic variation in this prevalence. The overall values are similar in men and women (24.0% versus 23.4%), but for African-American and Mexican-American women, the prevalence was 57% versus 31% for the men. The prevalence of the metabolic syndrome is increasing and is likely to lead to increases in the incidence of diabetes and cardiovascular disease (Ford et al. 2004). The metabolic syndrome is also a prevalent problem in other parts of the world (Table 2.10).

The metabolic syndrome is also a feature of overweight children. Because the set of measurements that are available differ from those in adults, different criteria are used in children. Caprio et al. have identified the prevalence of the metabolic syndrome in children to be 38.7% in the moderately overweight and 49.7% in the very overweight using the following criteria: A BMI > ninety-seventh percentile for age and gender, i.e., a *z*-score > 2; a triglyceride level > ninety-fifth percentile for age, gender, and ethnicity; an HDL-cholesterol < fifth percentile for age, gender, and ethnicity; a SBP and/or DBP > ninety-fifth percentile for age and gender; and impaired glucose tolerance (IGT) (Weiss et al. 2004).

CONCLUSION

One clear message from this discussion of body composition is that we now have good ways to measure body fat and most other body constituents. There is also agreement that the BMI is a useful criterion for assessing overweight as a surrogate for obesity in most, but not all, cases. It is also evident that the prevalence of obesity has increased markedly in the last quarter of the twentieth century in all parts of the world. Evidence from the beginning of the twenty-first century suggests that this may have begun to level off. Finally, there are significant differences in fat distribution and in the prevalence of obesity among ethnic groups, income levels, and parts of the world.

3 Genetic, Metabolic, and Social Origins of Obesity

KEY POINTS

- At least 17 genes have been associated with common forms of obesity, and 18 have been associated with type 2 diabetes.
- Positive energy balance is the essential ingredient required to store body fat and become overweight and obese.
- The concept of energy balance does not tell us all that is important: genetic factors, gender differences in fat distribution, or effects of age or medications.
- An epidemiological model of obesity describes the environmental factors such as maternal fatness, sleep time, viruses, toxins, and drugs as contributing mechanisms.
- Cost of food plays an important role in food choices.
- A homeostatic model for control of food intake and energy expenditure helps isolate the specific mechanisms that can be targeted for understanding and treating the problem.

INTRODUCTION

Differentiation of obesity into various subtypes was one of the important historical themes that began in the early twentiety century (Bray 2007b). There are case reports of individuals with massive obesity from the time of the Grecian god Dionysus onward. Some, like Daniel Lamber, sometimes called "The Great" because of his 739-pound weight, and Edward Bright, the miller from Billericay in England, have achieved long lasting fame because of pictures and etchings (Wadd 1816; Haslam 2009; Bray 2007). Some are in *Guinness World Records*. These reports provided little insight into the nature of obesity until the twentieth century, when we began to subdivide them into categories based on the factors that produced the obesity. This chapter will develop the theme of differentiation of obesity, from the reports in 1900 of individuals whose obesity resulted from an injury to their brain, through the discovery of leptin in 1994, and the massive obesity produced when leptin is deficient. It was the discovery of leptin that put obesity in the camp of "molecular diseases," rather than a "lack of willpower."

To put the genetic, physiological, and environmental factors into a conceptual framework, I will use the diagram in Figure 3.1. In the center is the energy balance model with food intake and energy expenditure as the two arms of the balance. When there is an excess on either side, there is a shift in energy balance and fat is stored or lost in the corresponding direction. Above this in the diagram are the genetic and physiological factors that influence the food intake and energy expenditure that will be described in this chapter. The growth of understanding about how food intake is regulated is another major theme of the twentieth century. Surrounding this metabolic balance in the circles of the diagram are the many environmental and societal factors, such as availability, cost, types of food, and social settings where we eat food that influence the amount eaten. This model will provide us with a basis for integrating the factors that affect obesity (Bray 2007a; WHO 2000).

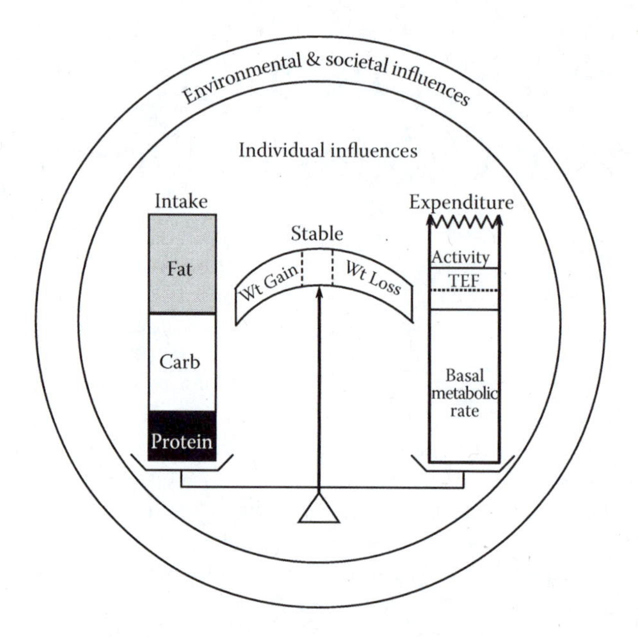

FIGURE 3.1 A model with the energy balance in the center showing energy intake and expenditure on opposite limbs surrounded by environmental and social determinants of how the energy balance system responds.

GENETIC FACTORS

Expansion of our knowledge about the physiological and molecular mechanisms regulating body weight and body fat (Schwartz 2006; Kershaw and Flier 2004) has been dramatic in the twentieth century, and particularly in the past quarter century (Bray 2007). One great step forward was the cloning of genes corresponding to five types of obesity in experimental animals that were due to defects in single genes—so-called monogenic syndromes of obesity—and the ensuing characterization of the human counterparts to these syndromes, including leptin deficiency and defects in the melanocortin-4 receptor system (Pérusse et al. 2005; Farooqi et al. 2008). Subsequent research has added a number of other genes with lesser effects to the list of genes modifying body weight (Willer et al. 2008). Extensive molecular and reverse genetic studies (mouse knockouts) have helped to identify critical pathways regulating body fat and food intake, and have validated or refuted the importance of previously identified pathways (Pérusse et al. 2005).

The epidemic of overweight is occurring on a genetic background that does not change as fast as the epidemic has been exploding in the twentieth century. It is nonetheless clear that genetic factors play an important role in its development. One of the earlier important demonstrations of this was from the work of Davenport on the offspring of families. For these studies, he used the body mass index as the criterion for examining the parental weights and the weights of their offspring. His data showed that fleshy parents, as he described them, had more fleshy children than pairings between less fleshy parents (Davenport 1924).

Genetic factors have been demonstrated subsequently in studies with twins (Verschuer 1927; Newman et al. 1937; Stunkard et al. 1990; Bouchard et al. 1990) and family studies (Davenport 1923; Stunkard et al. 1986). Most of these twin studies were conducted prior to the onset of the epidemic of obesity that began around 1980. To address the question of whether genetics are still strong, Wardle et al. (2008) carried out a study of 5092 twin pairs aged 8–11. There was 77% heritability for both BMI and waist circumference in this population—numbers that are similar to the earlier studies. This means that if one twin is fat there is a high likelihood that the other twin will be fat, in both adoption and twin studies. Studies evaluating the genome have shown that at least 17 genes are involved in obesity and 18 in diabetes (Pérusse et al. 2005; Willer et al. 2008).

Charles Benedict Davenport (1866–1944), in his 1923 monograph, clearly showed the relationship between the weight of parents and that of their offspring. Davenport was born in Stamford, CT, in 1866. Davenport's father, a founder and teacher in a private academy in Brooklyn, NY, was a key figure in his early development. His father taught his son at home until the age of 13 and was a demanding, and some say harsh, puritanical, and tyrannical, father. At 13, this mainly solitary youth entered the Polytechnic Institute of Brooklyn and was soon at the head of his class, despite his previous unorthodox schooling. After completion of his civil engineering degree in 1886, he entered Harvard College where he majored in zoology, receiving an AB degree in 1889 and a PhD in 1892. In 1899, Davenport left Harvard, where he was an instructor, to become an assistant professor at the University of Chicago, where he advanced to associate professor in 1901. He left the University of Chicago in 1904 following the establishment by the Carnegie Institution of the Cold Spring Harbor Station for Experimental Evolution. Shortly afterward, he established and directed the Eugenics Record Office at the same location (MacDowell 1946). He was elected to both the American Philosophical Society and the National Academy of Sciences. The rediscovery of Gregor Mendel's results in 1900 turned many scientists toward genetic studies directed at a variety of organisms (Mendel 1866; MacDowell 1946). As one Davenport biographer notes, "From 1907 Davenport's interest turned to human heredity and eugenics, a shift sparked at least partly by his wife" (McDowell 1946). Davenport published more than 400 communications. The great majority of these were without coauthor. Davenport became a "staunch advocate of an improved race of man . . . and urged great care in the selection of marriage partners, large families for those who had thus selected, a ban on racial mixing, and the excluding of undesirable immigrants from the United States" (McDowell 1946).

"Genes load the gun and the environment pulls the trigger" is one analogy for the role of genes in the obesity epidemic. Each year there is an increase in the number of genes identified that are involved in the development of obesity. From the time of the early twin and adoption studies more than 50 years ago (Verschuer 1927; Newman 1937; Pérusse et al. 2005), the focus has been on evaluating large groups of individuals for genetic defects related to the development of overweight (Farooqi et al. 2008; Willer et al. 2008). Obesity genes can be divided into two groups, the rare genes that produce excess body fat and a group of more common genes that underlie susceptibility to becoming overweight—the so-called "susceptibility" genes (Pérusse et al. 2005; Willer et al. 2008). The number of genetic factors has been given a recent boost by genome-wide association studies in which variants in populations with tens of thousands of people are examined (Willer et al. 2008). Using this genome-wide association strategy, at least 17 genes for common obesity and 18 genes for type 2 diabetes have been identified. Others will be identified in the future. These are summarized in Table 3.1.

Eight of these genes account for 0.84% of the variance in human body weight (FTO; MC4R; TMEM-18; NEGR-1; GNPDA-2; GABARA2; MTCH-2; KCTD-15; SH2B1), probably through actions in the central nervous system, which regulates food intake. The FTO gene accounts for half of this effect and is associated with increased energy intake in children (Cecil 2008). In the Women's Health Initiative Observational Study of 1517 diabetics and 2123 matched controls, polymorphisms in the FTO gene were associated with BMI and waist circumference in white women and Hispanic women, but not black or Asian/Pacific Islander women. Each copy of the allele was, on average, associated with a 0.45 kg/m^2 higher BMI (95% CI 0.16 to 0.74) and a 0.97 cm increase in waist circumference (95% CI 0.21 to 0.65) (Song et al. 2008). The FTO gene appears to primarily affect food intake (Cecil et al. 2008).

Genetic responses to the environment differ between individuals and affect the magnitude of the weight changes that we observe. Several genes have such potent effects that they produce obesity

TABLE 3.1
Some Genetic Loci Associated with Higher BMI Identified from Genome-Wide Association Studies

Gene & Chromosomal Location	Proposed Function	Additional Phenotypes	Where Expressed	Comments:
FTO (Fused toe 16q22.2)	Hypothalamic control of FI	Type 2 DM	Neuron	Adults & children
MC4R (Melanocortin-4 Receptor 18q11.2)	Hypothalamic signaling		Neurons	KO mice and human obese
PCSK1 (Neuroendocrine convertase 1)	Hypothalamic			
NEGR1 (1p31) (Neuronal growth regulator 1)			Neuronal growth	
TMEM18(2p25 closest gene) (Transmembrane protein 18)		Type 2 DM	Neuronal growth	
BDNF (11p13:locus with four genes) (Brain-derived neurotrophic factor)		Type 2 DM	Neuronal	BDNF knock-down hyperphagia
SH2B1(16p11.2 locus with 19–25 genes) (SH2-B Signaling Protein)	Energy homeostasis		Neuronal	SH2B1 KO mice obese and diabetic
MAF (c-MAF transcription factor 16q22-q23)				
NPC1 (endosomal/lysosomal Niemann-Pick C1 gene 18q11.2)				
KCTD15 (19q13.11)				
FAIM2 (12q13; locus contains BCD1N(N3D)) (FAS apoptotic inhibitory molecule 2)	Adipocyte apoptosis			
MTCH2 (11p11.2 ; locus with 14 genes) (proto-oncogene tyrosine-protein kinase ABL1)	Cellular apoptosis			
PTER (Phosphotriesterase-related gene 10p12)				
PRL (Prolactin gene)			Pituitary	
Gene desert (4p13) GNPDA2 is one of three genes nearby (glucosamine-6-phosphate isomerase)		Type 2 DM		
ETV5(3q27); locus with three genes (ERM)				
SEC16B, RASAL2 (1q25) (zipper transcription regulator 2)				

Source: Adapted from Hofker, M. and Wijmenga, C. *Nat. Gen.* 41, 139–140, 2009.

in almost any environment where food is available. Leptin deficiency, leptin receptor deficiency, and defects in the melanocortin-4 receptor are 3 of the most important (Farooqi et al. 2008). Most other genes that affect body weight and body fat vary under different environmental influences and produce only small effects. These small differences, however, account for much of the variability in the response to diet that we see.

A novel approach to the genetics of obesity came from a study of the fat organ in the fruit fly (Drosophila). In this gene expression study, the sonic hedgehog gene stood out. When this gene was

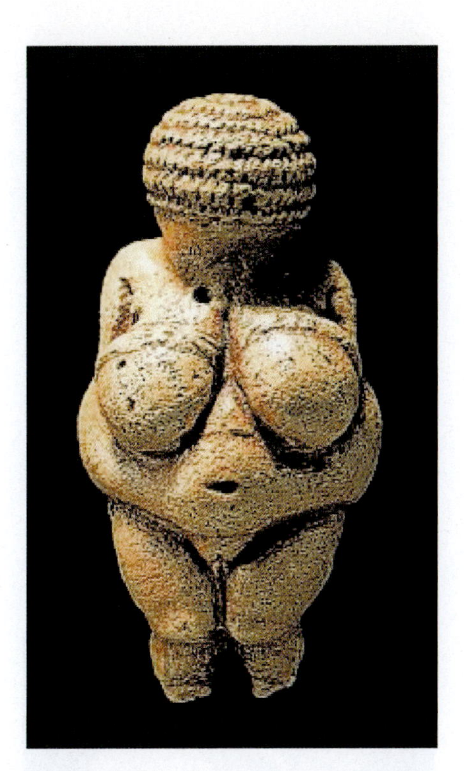

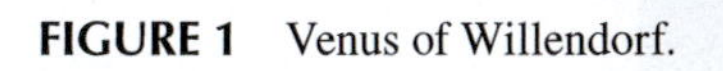

FIGURE 1 Venus of Willendorf.

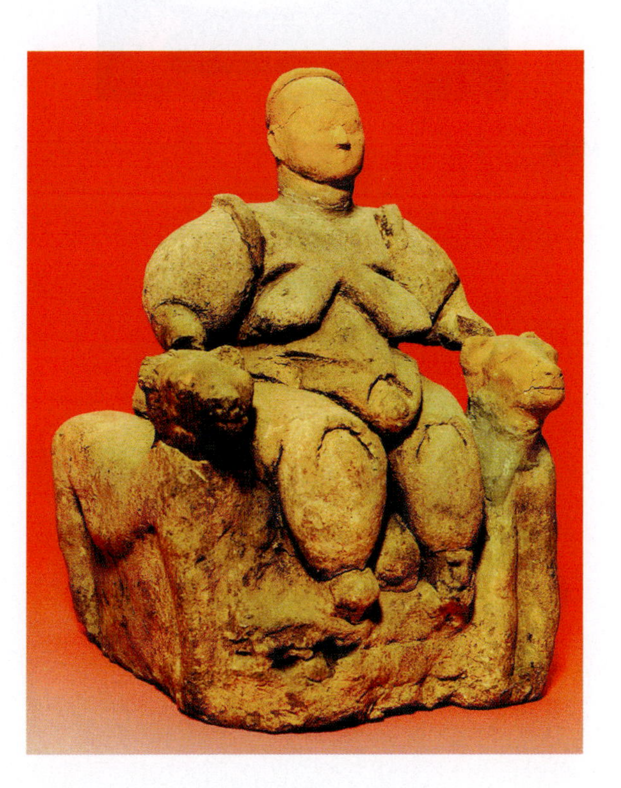

FIGURE 2 Baked clay goddess excavated from Çatalhöyük, Turkey.

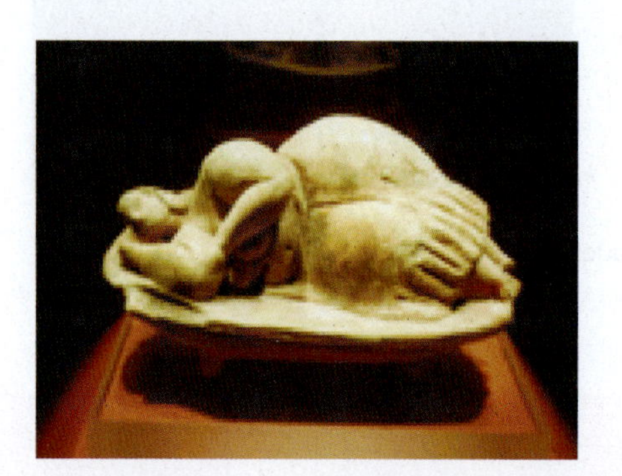

FIGURE 3 Venus of Malta.

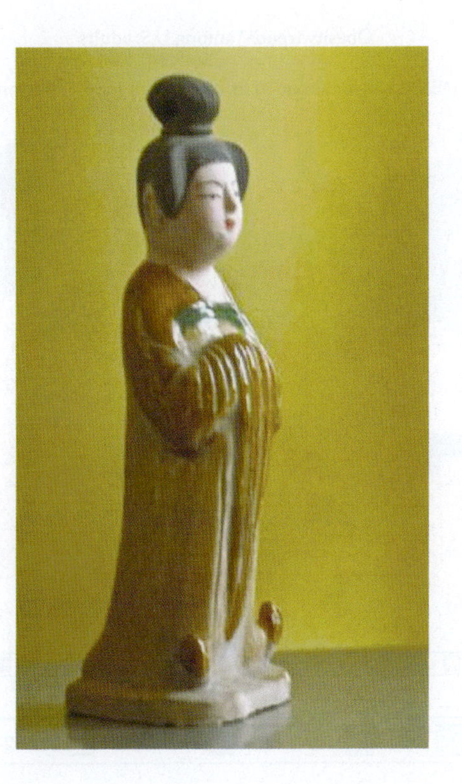

FIGURE 4 Tang dynasty woman.

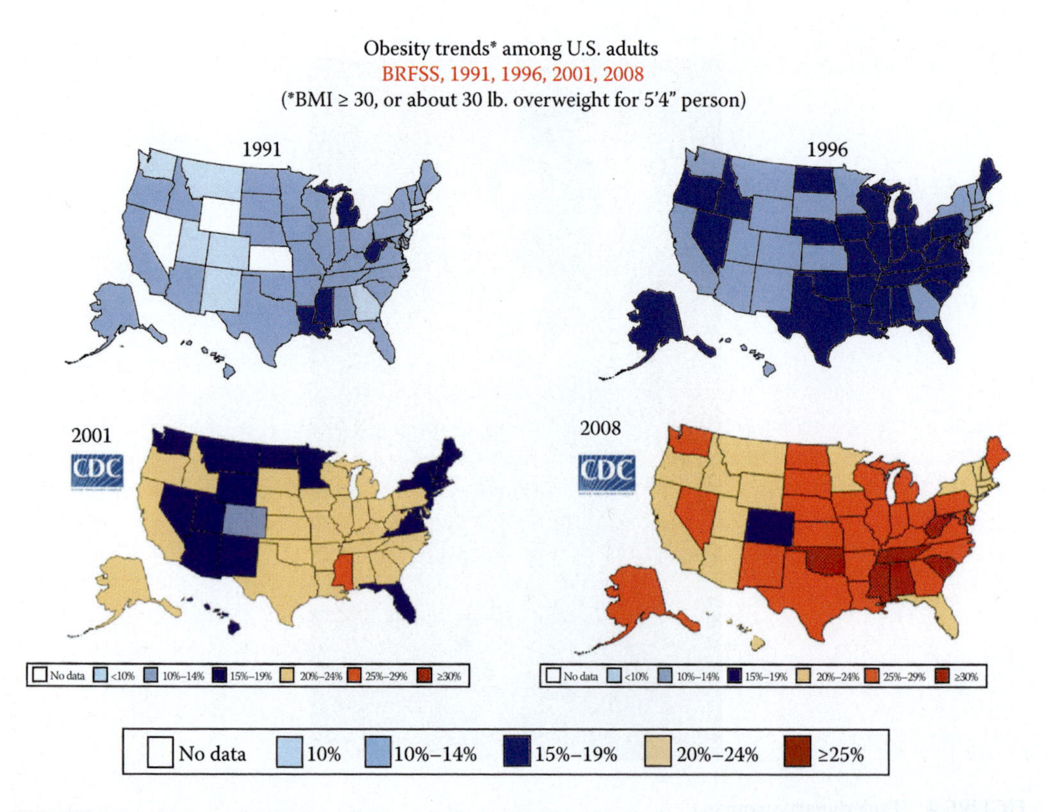

FIGURE 2.5 Changes in obesity between 1990 and 2010 by State in the United States using the Behavioral Risk Factor Surveillance Survey data from the Centers for Disease Control and Prevention.

over-expresed in mice they had almost no body fat, suggesting that this gene in adipose tissue may be a target for future treatment of obesity (Pospisilik et al. 2010).

EPIGENETIC AND INTRAUTERINE IMPRINTING

Over the past decade of the twentieth century, it became clear that infants who are small for their age are at higher risk for metabolic diseases later in life. This idea was originally proposed by Dr. David Barker and is often called the Barker Hypothesis (Barker et al. 1993, 2002). Several examples illustrate its role in human obesity. The first was the Dutch winter famine of 1944, in which the calories available to the residents of the city of Amsterdam were severely reduced by the Nazi occupation (Ravelli et al. 1999). During this famine, intrauterine exposure occurred during all parts of pregnancy. Intrauterine exposure during the first trimester increased the subsequent risk of overweight in the offspring (Ravelli 1998). This exposure also increased total cholesterol and triglycerides in women, but not men, around age 58 (Lumey et al. 2009).

Maternal diabetes, maternal smoking, and gestational weight gain are examples of fetal imprinting. In a study of infants born to Pima Indian women before and after the onset of diabetes, Dabelea et al. (1999) noted that the infants born after diabetes developed were heavier than those born to the same mother before diabetes developed (Fetita et al. 2006; Adams et al. 2005). This relationship is not entirely settled. In a systematic review, Whincup et al. (2008) found that among 28 populations, a 25% reduction in the risk of the pooled odds ratio of type 2 diabetes, adjusted for age and sex, was 0.75 (95% CI 0.70 to 0.81) per kg. They concluded that in most populations, birth weight is inversely related to type 2 diabetes risk, which is different from the conclusions reached with the Pima Indian study and the study of women who already have diabetes. The inverse relationship found by Whincup in their analysis would be more consistent with the observations of Barker and his colleagues, who observed an inverse relationship of birth weight with diabetes, that is, smaller babies are at higher risk of diabetes later in life (Barker et al. 1993).

The second example is the relation of body weight and smoking. In the offspring of diabetic mothers (Power et al. 2002) and the offspring of mothers who smoked during the intrauterine period (Power et al. 2002; Leary et al. 2006), the risk for overweight at age 3 was two times higher and predicted by smoking at first prenatal visit with an odds ratio of 2.16 (95% CI 1.05 to 4.47). Despite being smaller at birth, these infants more than caught up by age 3 (Fetita et al. 2006; Adams et al. 2005). Smoking during pregnancy increases the risk of overweight at entry to school from just under 10% to over 15% if smoking continued throughout pregnancy, and to nearly 15% if it was discontinued after the first trimester, indicating that most of the effect is in the early part of pregnancy (Toschke et al. 2003). Japanese and Swedish cohorts also show that maternal smoking increases childhood weight gain (Mizutani et al. 2007; Koupil and Toivanen 2008). There are clear racial differences in the response of children to maternal smoking in utero. In the Pregnancy Nutrition Surveillance System and the Pediatric Nutrition Surveillance System, including 155,411 low-income children born in the period 1995–2001, both the duration and quantity of smoking during pregnancy was positively associated with childhood obesity in a dose-response manner in non-Hispanic white children. Among Black children, only heavy smoking by the mother was associated with childhood obesity. Among Hispanics and Asian/Pacific Islanders, smoking during pregnancy was not associated with obesity in the offspring (Sharma et al. 2008).

A third example is the association of maternal weight and maternal weight gain to the birth weight and the risk of developing obesity in childhood. In the Mater-University Study of Pregnancy and Its Outcomes, maternal prepregnancy weight was significantly related to birth weight and to adiposity at age 14 (Lawlor et al. 2006). Similarly, in a retrospective analysis of the Collaborative Perinatal Project cohort with 10,226 infants, Wrotniak et al. (2008) found that the odds of overweight at age 7 increased 5% for every 1 kg of gestational weight gain (adjusted odds ratio 1.03 (95% CI 1.02 to 1.05)).

ENVIRONMENTAL AGENTS AND OBESITY: AN EPIDEMIOLOGIC APPROACH

During the twentieth century, many environmental factors were implicated in the risk for obesity. One way to view these factors is from an epidemiologic or environmental perspective. Food, medications, viruses, toxins, and sedentary lifestyle can each act on the host to produce increased fatness. But we need to remember that the response to each of these agents involves genetic components.

FOOD AS AN ENVIRONMENTAL AGENT FOR OBESITY

We obtain all of our energy from the foods we eat and the beverages we drink. Thus, without food and drink there could be no life, let alone excess stores of fat (Franco 2007) as shown in the Cuban famine of 1988–91. The cost and availability of food is an important determinant of food choices. In addition to cost and total quantity, food styles of eating and specific foods may be important in determining whether or not we become fat.

Costs of Food

Economic factors play an etiologic role in explaining the basis for the intake of a small number of "excess calories" over time that leads to overweight. What we consume is influenced by the price we have to pay for it. In the recent past, particularly since the beginning of the 1970s, the price of foods that are high in energy density (i.e., those that are rich in fat and sugar) have fallen relative to other items. The Consumer Price Index rose by 3.8% per year from 1980 to 2000 (Finkelstein et al. 2005), which outpaced by 3.4% the rise in food prices. In the period 1960 to 1980, when there was only a small increase in the prevalence of overweight, food prices rose at a rate of 5.5% per year—slightly faster than the Consumer Price Index, which grew at a rate of 5.3% per year. The relative prices of foods high in sugar and fat have decreased since the early 1980s compared with those of fruits and vegetables. For example (Finkelstein et al. 2005) between 1985 and 2000, the prices of fresh fruits and vegetables rose 118%, fish 77%, and dairy 56%, compared with the much smaller 46% rise for sugar and sweets, the 35% rise for oils, and the 20% rise for carbonated beverages. Is it any wonder that people with limited income eat more sugar- and fat-containing foods?

Human beings are price-sensitive when they buy food or any other item. The lower the cost of an item, the more likely we are to buy it and the more of it we are likely to buy. Thus, the cost of food is an important factor in the epidemic of obesity. During the period from 1960 to 1980, the price of food rose less than the cost of other components in the Consumer Price Index. Real wages also rose, providing additional money for consumption, some of which bought a wider variety of foods, some healthy such as fresh fruits and vegetables, fish, and dairy products, but others riddled with fat and sugar or high fructose corn syrup. This was a time when the rise in the prevalence of overweight was slow. However, between 1985 and 2000, the relative cost of fruits and vegetables increased much faster than the foods that contain more fat and sugar. This means that the food dollar buys relatively more food energy if we consume foods with more sugar and fat or more carbonated beverages. At the present time it costs between $0.30 and $1.50 per 1000 kcal for fats/oils, sugars, and grain, between $1.00 and $90.00 per 1000 kcal for meat, fish, and dairy products, and a similar amount for 1000 kcal of fruits or vegetables (Drewnowski and Darmon 2005). Is it any wonder that we eat a lot of good-tasting, high-energy-density foods that are inexpensive?

The food environment in which we live is determined more by the food processors and supermarkets than the farmers who grow the food or nutritionists who talk about them. The largest supermarket in the United States is Wal-Mart. The groceries sold by Wal-Mart account for about 1 in 5 dollars spent on groceries at supermarkets. Wal-Mart's food prices are, on average, 14% lower than other chains. Thus, Wal-Mart is a major player in the lower prices that people pay for food. Consumers can buy only what supermarkets offer to sell. In 2003, the 10 largest supermarkets had combined sales of $400 billion, with Wal-Mart having $130 billion of that. To the extent that they can provide lower-energy-density foods and smaller portion sizes at lower prices there may be a hope for moving the entire food industry toward a lower-weight America (Tollotson et al. 2005; Cutler et al. 2003; Lakdawalla and Philipson 2009).

Quantity of Food Eaten Is Enough to Produce the Obesity Epidemic

Eating more food energy over time than we need for our daily energy requirements produces extra body fat. In the current epidemic, the increase in body weight is, on average, 0.5 to 1 kg/year from the ages of 20 to 50 years (Norman 2003). You can calculate the amount of net energy storage required by an adult to produce 1 kg of added body weight, 75% of which is fat, by making a few assumptions. One kg of adipose tissue contains about 7,000 kcal (29.4 mJ) of energy. If the efficiency of energy storage were 50%, with the other 50% being used by the synthetic and storage processes, we would need to ingest 14,000 kcal (58.8 MJ) of food energy. Since there are 365 days in the year this would be an extra 20 kcal/day (40 kcal/day × 365 day/year = 14,600 kcal) (Hill and Peters 1998). For simplicity, we can round this to 50 kcal/day or the equivalent of 10 teaspoons of sugar. Other estimates of the amount of energy needed range from 100 kcal/day (Hill 2003) to 500 kcal/day (Swinburn 2009a, 2009b) for adults and 150 to 250 for children (Wang 2006).

Has the intake of energy increased? The energy intake (kcal/day) was relatively stable during the first 80 years of the twentieth century. During the past 20 years, however, there was a clear rise from about 2300 kcal/day to about 2600 kcal/day, or an increase of 300 kcal/day. This is more than enough to account for the 50 kcal/day net (100 kcal gross) required to produce the 1-kg weight gain each year (Putnam and Allshouse 1999). Table 3.2 shows several estimates of the increase in calories per day from the Centers for Disease Control and Prevention (CDC) and the Continuing Survey of Food Intake of Individuals (CSFII) by the USDA. The best analysis is that of Swinburn et al. (2009). They evaluated the relationship between food intake and energy expenditure using doubly labeled water. They showed that the rise in body weight could be entirely explained by the rise in energy intake between 1970 and 2000.

Portion Size

Portion sizes have dramatically increased in the past 40 years. Increased energy intake is associated with the larger portions of essentially all items examined (Nielsen and Popkin 2003). One consequence of larger portion sizes is that more food and more calories are consumed (Putnam and Allshouse 1999). The USDA estimates that between 1984 and 1994, daily calorie intake increased by 340 kcal/day or 14.7%. Refined grains provided 6.2% of this increase, fats and oils 3.4%, but fruits and vegetables only 1.4% and meats and dairy products only 0.3%. Calorically sweetened beverages that contain 10% high-fructose corn syrup (HFCS) are made from these grain products. These beverages are available in containers of 12, 20, or 32 ounces, which provide 150, 250, or 400 kcal if completely consumed. Many foods list the calories per serving on the NUTRITION FACTS label, but the package often contains more than one serving. Table 3.3 shows that in 1954, the burger served by Burger King weighed 2.8 oz and had 202 kcal. By 2004, the size had grown to

TABLE 3.2
CDC and USDA Estimated Increase in Caloric Intake for Men and Women between 1970 and 1995

Agency	Men	Women
CDC 2004	168 kcal/day	335 kcal/day
USDA CSFII	268 kcal/day	143 kcal/day

Source: CDC, *MMWR*, 53(04):80–82, 2004; USDA.

TABLE 3.3
Changes in Portion Sizes 1900–1954

Item	Year	oz/kcal	Year	oz/kcal
Burger King burger	1954	2.8/202	2004	4.3/310
McDonald fries	1955	2.4/210	2004	7/610
Hershey bar	1900	2/297	2004	7/1000
Coca-Cola	1916	6.5/79	2004	16/194
Movie popcorn	1950	3 cups/174	2004	21 cups/1700

Source: Newman C., *National Geographic* 206, 58, 2004.

4.3 oz and 310 kcal. In 1955, McDonald's served french fries weighing 2.4 oz and having 210 kcal. By 2004, this had increased to 7 oz and 610 kcal. Popcorn served at movie theaters has grown from 3 cups containing 174 kcal in 1950 to 21 cups with 1700 kcal in 2004 (Newman 2004).

Beverages are also a source of energy. Portion size influences what we eat in both controlled and naturalistic settings. Using a laboratory setting, both normal and overweight men and women were given different amounts of a good-tasting pasta entrée. They ate 30% more when offered the largest size than when offered half the amount (1000 g vs. 500 g) (Rolls et al. 2002). A similar finding was made when different-sized packages of potato chips were offered. Women ate 18% more and men 37% more when the package size was doubled (85 g vs. 170 g) (Rolls et al. 2004). The quantity of food eaten is also influenced by its proximity and the kind of container it is in. In a variety of experiments, Wansink et al. showed that when food is located close at hand, subjects tended to eat more than when the food was further away (Wansink et al. 2006) and eat more if it is in clear than opaque containers. Guidance for intake of beverages suggests intake of more water, tea, coffee, and low-fat dairy products with lesser consumption of beverages that contain primarily water and caloric sweeteners (Popkin et al. 2007). The importance of drinking water as an alternative to calorie-containing beverages is suggested by the inverse relationship between water intake, expressed per unit of food, and beverage intake and total energy intake. When the water intake was less than 20 g/gram of food and beverages, energy intake was 2,485 kcal/day. At the highest quartile of water intake, at or above 90 g/gram of food and beverage, energy intake had fallen to 1,791 kcal/day. Thus, drinking water may be one strategy for lowering overall energy intake (Stookey et al. 2007a). Replacing sweetened soft drinks with drinking water is associated with lower energy intake in adults (Stookey 2007b).

The size and shape of beverage containers influences portion sizes. Two articles from Wansink and van Ittersum showed that people poured less into tall glasses than into short, squat glasses of the same volume (Van Ittersum and Wansink 2007; Wansink and Van Ittersum 2007).

Energy Density

Energy density, the amount of energy in a given weight of food (kcal/g), interacts with portion size to affect how much we eat (Rolls 2009). Energy density of foods is increased by dehydrating them or by adding fat. Conversely, lower energy density is produced by adding water or removing fat. When energy density of meals was varied and all meals were provided for two days, the participants ate the same amount of food, but as a result got more energy when the foods were higher in energy density. In this experiment, they got about 30% less energy when the meals had low rather than high energy density (Bell et al. 1998; Stubbs et al. 1998).

When energy density and portion size were both varied, Rolls and her colleagues showed that they both influence the amount that is eaten. The meals with low energy density and small portion sizes provided the fewest calories (398 kcal vs. 620 kcal) (Kral et al. 2004). Energy density based on three-day food records from 682 children at ages 5 and 7 years was related to body fat at age 9. Energy density of the diet at age 7, but not age 5, predicted fat gain at age 9 (Johnson et al. 2008).

Styles of Eating

Breast feeding can be associated with later weight gain. For infants, breast milk is their first food and, for many infants, their sole food for several months. Three meta-analyses of observations found that the risk of obesity on entry to school was reduced by 15% to 25% with early breastfeeding compared to formula feeding (Rogers 2003; Harder et al. 2005; Gillman et al. 2007; Arenz et al. 2004). One hypothesis for this effect is the lower protein content of breast milk. In a controlled trial comparing over 1000 infants randomized to either lower or higher protein formulas, Koletzko et al. (2009) showed that after 2 years of follow-up, feeding the lower protein formula normalized early growth relative to a breast-fed reference group.

The composition of human breast milk may also play a role. The fats included in this nutritious food are obtained from the mother's fat stores. The composition of fat in human breast milk changed over the last 50 years of the twentieth century (Aihaud and Guesnet 2004). An analysis of samples taken over this time period showed that the quantity of the n-6 fatty acid linoleic acid has increased steadily. This fatty acid is common in fats from plants and probably reflects the increasing use of vegetable oils in Western diets. In contrast, the quantity of the essential n-3 α-linolenic acid has remained constant (Aihaud and Guesnet 2004). The way in which these fatty acids are metabolized differs, with the linoleic acid forming prostacyclin, which can act on receptors on the fat cell to modulate fat cell replication. It is conceivable that the changing fatty acid content of human breast milk may have modified the sensitivity to fats later in life.

Restaurants and Fast-Food Establishments

Eating meals away from home has increased significantly over the past 30 years. There are now more fast-food restaurants than churches in the United States (Tillotson 2005). The number of fast-food restaurants has risen since 1980 from 1 per 2000 people to 1 per 1000 Americans. Of the 206 meals per capita eaten out in 2002, fast-food restaurants served 74% of them. Other important figures are that Americans spent $100 billion on fast food in 2001, compared to $6 billion in 1970. An average of three orders of french-fried potatoes are ordered per person per week, and french-fried potatoes have become the most widely consumed vegetable. More than 100,000 new food products were introduced between 1990 and 1998. Eating outside the home has become easier over the past four decades as the number of restaurants has increased, and the percent of meals eaten outside the home reflects this. In 1962, less than 10% of meals were eaten outside the home. By 1992, this had risen to nearly 35%, where it has remained. However, in a telephone survey of BMI in relation to proximity to fast-food restaurants in Minnesota, Jeffrey et al. (2006) found that eating at a fast-food restaurant was associated with having children, with eating a high-fat diet, and with having a high body mass index, but not with the proximity to the restaurant.

Eating in a fast-food restaurant changes the foods consumed (Figure 3.2) (Paeratakul et al. 2003; Bowman et al. 2004), and increases the energy density of the diet (Prentice et al. 2003). Paeratakul et al. (2003) compared a day in which individuals ate at a fast-food restaurant with a day when they did not. On the day when food was eaten in the fast-food restaurant, less cereal, milk, and vegetables were consumed, but more soft drinks and french-fried potatoes were eaten. Similar findings were reported by Bowman et al. (2004), who reported, in addition, that on any given day, over 30% of the total sample group consumed fast food. In this national survey, several other features were also associated with eating at fast-food restaurants, including being male, having a higher household income, and residing in the South. Children who ate at fast-food restaurants consumed more energy, more fat and added sugars, and more sweetened beverages than children who did not eat at fast-food restaurants.

To test the effect of eating fast food in a controlled environment, Ebbeling et al. (2004) provided fast food in large amounts for a 1-hour lunch to normal-weight and overweight adolescents.

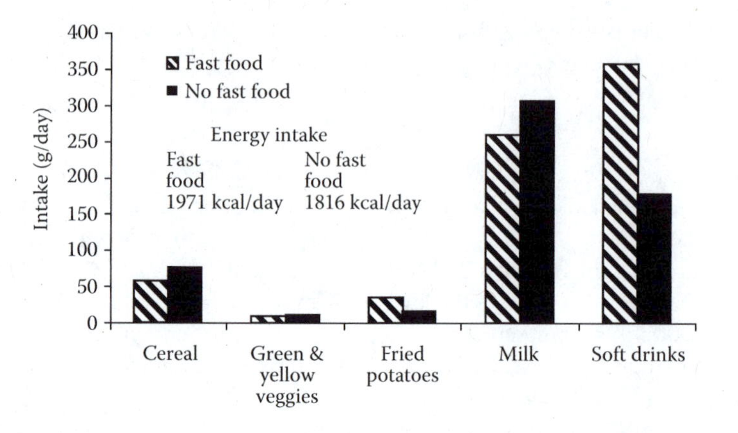

FIGURE 3.2 Effects of a day when a fast food meal was consumed, as compared to a day when no fast food was eaten. (Adapted from Paeratakul S. et al., *J. Am. Diet Assoc.* 103(10), 1332–1338.)

Overweight participants (weight > eighty-fifth percentile for height) ate 1860 kcal compared to 1458 kcal in the lean participants. The average intake for this lunch was over 60% of their estimated total daily energy requirements. During a second study, energy intake was significantly higher in the overweight subjects on the 2 days when the subjects ate fast food than on the 2 days when they did not (2703 kcal/day vs. 2295 kcal/day), a difference that was not observed in the lean adolescents. In a 15-year follow-up of the Coronary Artery Risk Development in Young Adults (CARDIA) study, Pereira et al. (2005) found that the frequency of consuming fast food at baseline was directly associated with weight gain in blacks and whites. Increases in the frequency of consuming fast food during the 15 years of follow-up were also associated with increased risk of weight gain. It thus seems clear that eating at fast-food restaurants increases the risk of ingesting more calories than are needed and becoming obese.

A decline in consumption of food at home is one consequence of eating out more often. To examine whether there was a relationship between frequency of family dinners and overweight status among 9- to 14-year-olds, Taveras et al. (2005) did a cross-sectional and longitudinal study of 14,431 children with 6647 boys and 7784 girls. They found that the frequency of eating family dinner was inversely associated with the prevalence of overweight in the cross-sectional study, but did not predict the degree of weight gain in the longitudinal study.

Breakfast

Eating breakfast is associated with eating more frequently, and with a lower body weight. As cereal intake increased from 0 to 3 times per week, there was a small, but significant, decrease in BMI (Barton et al. 2005). In the Physicians' Health Study, a longitudinal study of 17,881 men, eating more whole-grain and refined-grain breakfast cereals (Bazzano et al. 2005) was associated with less gain in body weight over 8 years after correcting for age, smoking, baseline BMI, alcohol intake, physical activity, hypertension, high cholesterol, and use of multivitamins. Compared to those who rarely or never consumed breakfast cereals, those who consumed ≥1 serving/day of breakfast cereal were 22% and 12% less likely to become overweight during follow-up periods of 8 and 13 years (relative risk 0.78 95% CI 0.67 to 0.91; 0.88 95% CI 0.76 to 1.00). The fiber content of cereal may influence cumulative calorie intake. In a small study with 32 healthy men and women, a breakfast high in insoluble fiber (26 g) reduced cumulative breakfast and lunch intake compared with a low fiber (1 g) cereal (Hamedani et al. 2009).

A study of 5823 white and 1965 African-American adolescents from the National Longitudinal Study of Adolescent Health also concluded that eating breakfast as an adolescent reduced the risk of obesity in young adulthood. In this study, only 64% had one or both parents present at breakfast.

Eating breakfast in adolescence increased the likelihood of eating breakfast as an adult and reduced the risk of obesity as a young adult (Merten et al. 2009).

Food Components

There have been a number of significant changes in the quantities of different foods eaten during the time the epidemic of overweight has developed, and they have no doubt changed the intake of other nutrients as well. From 1970 to 2000, per capita intake of fats and oils increased from 56 lb/person to 77 lb/person, sugars from 139 lb/person to 172 lb/person, fruits from 241 lb/person to 280 lb/person, vegetables from 337 lb/person to 445 lb/person, grains from 136 lb/person to 200 lb/person, and proteins from 588 lb/person to 621 lb/person. From an analysis of the changes in various food groups using the USDA guide (2006), it is clear that more food from all categories is being consumed, thus providing more energy to Americans with the resulting problem of overweight. Using data from the U.S. Department of Agriculture, Frazao and Allshouse (2003) reported that, whereas fruit and vegetable consumption increased 20% between 1970 and 2000, the consumption of calorie-sweetened beverages rose 70% and the consumption of cheese rose 162%.

Data from the National Health and Nutrition Examination Survey (NHANES) from 1999 to 2004 showed that those who ate more meat had a higher total daily energy intake. The upper fifth (quintile) had an intake of 700 kcal/day more than the lower 20% (quintile) (Wang et al. 2009). There was an association of both waist circumference and BMI.

Calorically Sweetened Soft Drinks

Sugar consumption has grown steadily for more than 400 years, and most dramatically since 1800 (Yudkin 1973). The high intake of sugar and the consumption of more refined and processed foods has heightened concern about their role in the epidemic of obesity. Cleave and Campbell argued this case and Yudkin picked up on it and focused on the potential role of sugar (sucrose) in the rising epidemic of heart disease after World War II.

One of the consequences of the lower farm prices in the 1970s was a drop in the price of corn, which reduced the price of corn starch that is converted to high-fructose corn syrup (Critser 2003). With the development of the isomerase technology to make fructose from glucose in the late 1960s, the manufacturers of soft drinks gradually switched from sugar to HFCS and we entered a new era (Bray et al. 2004). From the early 1970s through the mid-1990s, high-fructose corn syrup gradually

John Yudkin (1910–1995) is noted for his contributions to the role of sucrose in the epidemic of obesity. Yudkin was born in 1910 in London to Jewish parents who had fled the 1905 pogroms in Russia. His father died when he was 7 years old and his mother raised him and four other sons in very difficult circumstances. In 1933 he married Milly Himmelweit, who had fled from Nazi Germany. They were married for 60 years and had three sons. He received a PhD in 1938, but his interest in nutrition led him to enter medical school. In 1938, he undertook research into vitamin A and riboflavin at the Dunn Nutrition Laboratory. He examined the link between sugar and various degenerative illnesses. During World War II, he served as a military physician in West Africa and was busy with further studies. In 1945, he was appointed Professor of Physiology at the University of London. A bachelor's degree and master's degree in nutrition were established at University College. He advised the government of the young state of Israel on nutrition matters and was an energetic governor of the Hebrew University of Jerusalem. Since 1957, he showed that the consumption of sugar and refined sweeteners is closely associated with coronary heart disease. He became internationally famous with his book *Pure, White, and Deadly* in 1986 (published in 1972) (Wikipedia 2010).

replaced sugar in many manufactured products, and almost entirely replaced sugar in soft drinks manufactured in the United States. This was given a big boost when the major soft drink producers switched from sucrose to high fructose corn syrup in 1983. In addition to being cheap, high-fructose corn syrup is very sweet. We have argued that this sweetness in liquid form is one factor driving the consumption of increased calories that are needed to fuel the current epidemic of obesity. The increasing consumption of soft drinks and fruit drinks is shown in Figure 3.3. Data from the School Nutrition Dietary Assessment Study for 2004–2005 showed that sugar-sweetened beverages obtained at school contributed 29 kcal/day to middle school children and 46 kcal/day to high school children (Briefel et al. 2009). This study recommends removing sugar-sweetened beverages from school food stores and snack bars and reducing the frequency that French fries are provided.

Several meta-analyses on the effect of soft-drink consumption on changes in energy intake or changes in body weight have been published (Malik et al. 2006, 2010; Vartanian et al. 2007; Olsen and Heitman 2009; Forshee 2009). In a study by Malik et al., thirty publications (15 cross-sectional, 10 prospective, and 5 experimental) were selected. The large cross-sectional studies, in conjunction with those from well-powered prospective cohort studies with long periods of follow-up, showed a positive association between greater intakes of soft drinks and weight gain and obesity in both children and adults. Short-term feeding trials in adults also support the relation of soft drinks to positive energy balance and weight gain. The authors concluded that the weight of epidemiologic and experimental evidence indicates that consumption of soft drinks is associated with weight gain and obesity.

Another meta-analysis by Olsen and Heitmann (2009) included a total of 14 prospective and 5 experimental studies. The majority of the prospective studies found positive associations between intake of calorically sweetened beverages and obesity. Three experimental studies found positive effects of calorically sweetened beverages on body fat, but two did not. Eight prospective studies adjusted for energy intake and seven of them reported associations that were essentially similar before and after energy adjustment. They concluded that a high intake of calorically sweetened beverages is a determinant for obesity.

The most recent systematic review and meta-analysis by Malik et al. (2010) identified eight prospective cohort studies and five experimental studies that evaluated soft drink consumption and weight gain for qualitative review, and 10 prospective cohort studies evaluated intake of soft drinks and risk of cardiometabolic diseases (six for T2DM; three for MetSyn; and one for CHD) for inclusion in a random effects meta-analysis comparing soft drinks intake in the highest to lowest quantiles of intake. There was a clear and consistent positive association between consumption of soft drinks and weight gain, particularly in larger studies with longer durations of follow-up. These observations are supported by short-term feeding trials, which provide important insight into underlying biological mechanisms. In the meta-analysis including 294,617 participants and 10,010 cases of type 2 diabetes mellitus, 6236 cases of the metabolic syndrome, and 3105 cases of coronary heart disease in the highest quantile of soft drink intake had a 24% greater risk of cardiometabolic risk than those in the lowest quantile (relative risk 1.24 95% CI 1.12, 1.34). This increased to 30% when

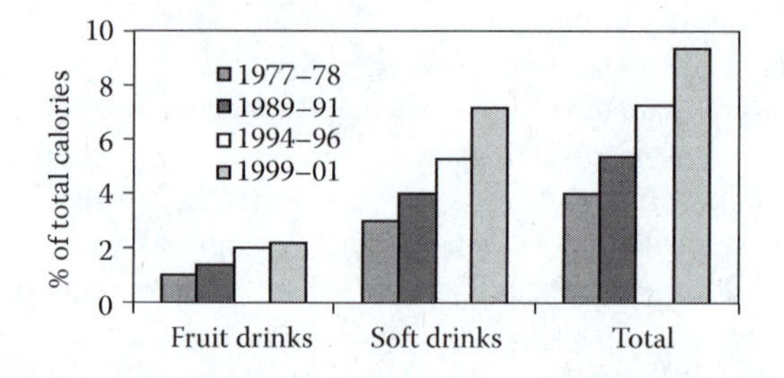

FIGURE 3.3 Intake of soft drinks and fruit drinks from 1977 to 2001 (Based on data from Nielsen S.J. and Popkin B.M., *JAMA* 289, 450–453, 2003).

studies that adjusted for mediating effects of energy intake and BMI were excluded from analysis (relative risk 1.30 (95% CI 1.20, 1.50)).

Several studies on the consumption of calorically sweetened beverages in relation to the epidemic of overweight have gotten significant attention (Bray et al. 2004). Ludwig et al. (2001) reported that the intake of soft drinks was a predictor of initial BMI in children in the Planet Health Study. It also predicted the increase in BMI during nearly 2 years of follow-up. Those with the highest soft drink consumption at baseline had the highest increase in BMI.

A few randomized, well-controlled intervention studies with fructose or sucrose have been published. Raben et al. (2003) showed that individuals consuming beverages sweetened with sugar for 10 weeks gained weight, whereas subjects drinking the same amount of beverages sweetened with aspartame lost weight. Equally important, drinking sugar-sweetened beverages was associated with a small, but significant, increase in blood pressure and an increase in inflammatory markers in the serum (Sorensen 2005). Women in the Nurses' Health Study (Shulze et al. 2004) also showed that changes in the consumption of soft drinks predicted changes in body weight over several years of follow-up. In children, a study focusing on reducing intake of "fizzy" drinks and replacing them with water showed slower weight gain than in the children not advised to reduce the intake of fizzy drinks (James et al. 2004).

In the Longitudinal Study of Child Development in Quebec (1998–2002) (Dubois et al. 2007), 6.9% of children who did not consume sugar-sweetened beverages between meals at 2.5 and 4.5 years of use were overweight at 2.5, 3.5, and 4.5 years, compared with 15.4% of children who did consume sugar-sweetened soft drinks four to six times or more per week between meals. The overall odds-ratio was more than doubled in multivariate analysis but was increased threefold in children from families with lower income.

As soft-drink consumption in the population has increased, the consumption of milk, a major source of calcium, has decreased. Milk, particularly low-fat milk, is a valuable source of calcium for bone growth during the time of maximal bone accretion. Intake of dairy products may be related to the development of overweight (Zemel et al. 2000). The level of calcium intake in population studies is inversely related to body weight (Davies et al. 2000; Pereira et al. 2002). However, a randomized clinical trial of calcium supplements found no effect (Yanovski et al. 2009).

Fructose consumption, either in beverages or food, may be detrimental (Figure 3.4). Fructose, unlike other sugars, increases serum uric acid levels. Nakagawa et al. (2006) propose that this happens when fructose is taken into the liver, where adenosine triphosphate (ATP) is used to phosphorylate

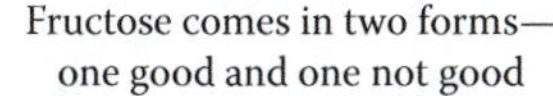

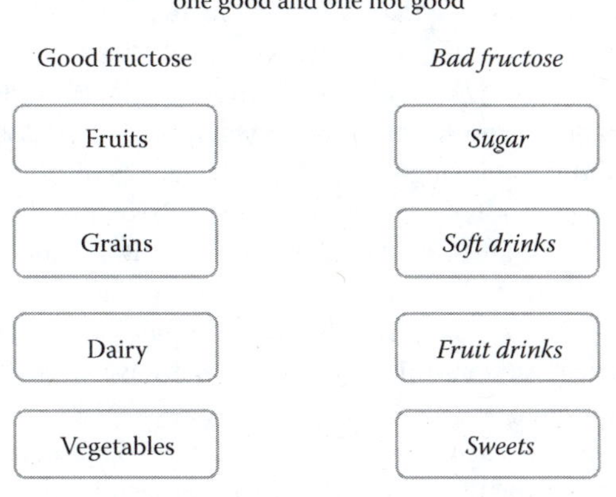

FIGURE 3.4 Fructose comes from two sources that can be classified as "good" and "bad" fructose, depending on the source. Good fructose is that obtained from fruits and vegetables. In contrast, bad fructose comes from the highly refined sources of sucrose and high-fructose corn syrup.

fructose to fructose-1-phosphate (Johnson et al. 2008). The adenosine-5′-diphosphate can be further broken down to adenosine-5′-monophosphate and to uric acid. Thus, the metabolism of fructose in the liver has as a by-product the production of uric acid. These authors propose that the high levels of uric acid could set the stage for advancing cardiovascular disease by reducing the availability of nitric oxide (NO), which is crucial for maintaining normal blood pressure and for maintaining normal function of the vessel walls (endothelium). If this hypothesis is borne out, it will provide another reason that nature preferred glucose over fructose as a substrate for metabolism during the evolutionary process (Nakagawa et al. 2006). In addition, soft-drink consumption has been linked to the development of cardiometabolic risk factors including diabetes, the metabolic syndrome, and coronary heart disease (Malik et al. 2010; Dhingra et al. 2007) and gout in men (Choi 2008).

Dietary Fat

Dietary fat may also play a role in the current obesity epidemic (Astrup et al. 2000; Bray and Popkin 1998; Bray et al. 2008). In epidemiologic studies, dietary fat intake is related to the fraction of the population that is overweight (Bray and Popkin 1998). In an 8-year follow-up of the Nurses' Health Study, Field and colleagues (2007) found a weak overall association of percent fat—and a stronger effect of animal fat, saturated fat, and trans fat—on fatness. In experimental animals, high-fat diets generally produce fat storage (Bray 2007a). In humans, the relationship of dietary fat to the development of overweight is controversial, but in a study of food intake records Bray et al. (2008) found a positive relationship between fat intake and calorie intake that, if continued without compensation in other sources of calories, would lead to obesity.

Foods combining fat and sugar may be a particular problem, since they are often very palatable and usually inexpensive (Drewnowski and Specter 2004). The Leeds Fat Study shows that people who were "high fat consumers" had an increased incidence of overweight (Blundell and MacDiarmid 1997). The high fat content of foods increases their "energy density," meaning that they have more available energy for each unit of food weight. From each gram of fat you get about 9 kilocalories of energy, whereas carbohydrate and protein yield only 4 kilocalories per gram. Thus, lowering the fat content of foods or raising the quantity of water in foods are ways of reducing the energy density. Providing an increased number of palatable foods with low energy density could be valuable in helping fight the epidemic of overweight. Alcohol is particularly problematic. When a high-fat snack is given with alcohol before lunch, subjects consumed just under 200 kcal (812 kJ) more at lunchtime than when there was no alcohol (Tremblay and St-Pierre 1996). Thus, alcohol may blunt decision-making about food and should be avoided during efforts to lose weight.

Gut Microbes

There are ten times as many bacteria in the GI tract as there are cells in the rest of the body—100 trillion bacteria versus 10 trillion cells in the body. There are 10 to 12 microorganisms per milliliter of GI colonic fluid with between 15,000 and 36,000 distinct species. These bacteria can be influenced by probiotics—nonpathogenic living microorganisms such as *Lactobacillus rhamnosus*—and prebiotics, which are indigestible oligosaccharides that act as fertilizers for colonic microbiota. Inulin and oligofructose are naturally occurring polymers of fructose that are digested in the colon to release fructose, which is not absorbed from that site and thus modulates intestinal bulk. The most common sources of probiotics are wheat, onions, bananas, garlic, and leeks. Americans consume 1 g–4 g of prebiotics per day, Europeans significantly more at 3 g–11 g per day. Combinations of prebiotics and protobiotics are controlled synbiotics and have been proposed as colonic foods with potential nutritional products.

The kinds of microbes in the gut may affect body weight. There are two groups of beneficial bacteria—Bacteroidetes and Firmicutes—in the gut, and lean individuals posses more of the bacteroidetes and the obese more of the Firmicutes (Ley et al. 2006). Both obese mice and obese humans have reduced numbers of Bacteriodetes and increased numbers of Firmicutes (Zhang et al. 2009). Mice that have gut bacteria are 40% heavier and have 47% higher gonadal fat pad weight than mice raised in a germ-free environment (Backhed et al. 2004). When bacteria from the distal gut were transplanted into germ-free mice, these mice had a 60% increase in body fat within 2 weeks, without a measurable increase in food intake or an obvious decrease in physical activity. A study in individuals with gastric bypass bariatric surgery showed that the bacterial colonization shifted toward the types of microbes seen in normal weight individuals and away from the obese (Zhang et al. 2009). Gut microbiota may also predict weight gain in children. The number of Bifidobacterial specials in fecal samples during infancy was higher in children remaining at a normal weight as compared to children becoming overweight (Kalliomaki et al. 2008).

A molecular basis for this effect may be through the toll-like receptor 5 (TLR5) in the gut mucosa, which is an innate component of the immune system in the intestine. Mice that lack this receptor develop hyperphagia, dyslipidemia, hypertension, and insulin resistance, which are characteristics of the metabolic syndrome (Vijay-Kumar et al. 2010).

Diet

The amount of energy intake relative to energy expenditure is the central reason for the development of overweight. Dietary factors can be influenced in a variety of ways and when the total energy intake is above what is needed for daily energy expenditure for an extended period of time, excess body fat is the result.

Overeating

Voluntary overeating, that is, consciously eating food in excess of that needed by the body can increase body weight in normal-weight men and women (Sims et al. 1973; Bouchard et al. 1990; Smith et al. 2000 p. 305). The use of this strategy to gain insight into the effects of excess caloric intake on human beings was pioneered by Ethan Sims and his colleagues at the University of Vermont. They produced a 25% increase in body weight in a group of prisoners in the Vermont State Prison who voluntarily overate. This procedure increased fat storage by increasing the size of existing fat cells (Salans 1968). It induced insulin resistance and impaired glucose uptake. Of interest, the subjects returned to their baseline weight when the overfeeding protocol was terminated.

This technique of voluntary overfeeding has subsequently been utilized in many different laboratories around the world (Levitsky et al. 2005; Tappy 2004; Teran-Garcia et al. 2004; Redden and Allison 2004; McDevitt et al. 2001; Schutz 2000). One of the most interesting is the study by Bouchard et al. (1990), who gave identical twins an extra 1000 kcal per day for 84 days under observed conditions. The pattern of weight gain is shown in Figure 3.5. The similarity of weight gain for each pair was closer than for weight gain between pairs of twins. This study shows two important things. First, there is a significant difference in weight gain between individuals and,

Ethan Allen Hitchcock Sims, MD (1916–2010) is noted for his pioneering studies with overfeeding as a strategy to unravel the effects of weight gain from chronic obesity. Sims was born in Newport, RI on April 22, 1916, the youngest of five children. His father was president of the Naval War College. Sims' interest in science began with the gift of a small 40-power microscope at age 7, followed by a much better microscope a few years later. He completed Harvard College in 1938 and received his MD from the Columbia University College of Physicians and Surgeons in 1942. His career in endocrinology began at Yale-New Haven Medical Center where he was a younger faculty member working in the laboratory of John P. Peters. In 1950, he moved to the University of Vermont, where he conducted an important series of experiments on the effects of voluntary weight gains of about 25% in healthy subjects who overate.

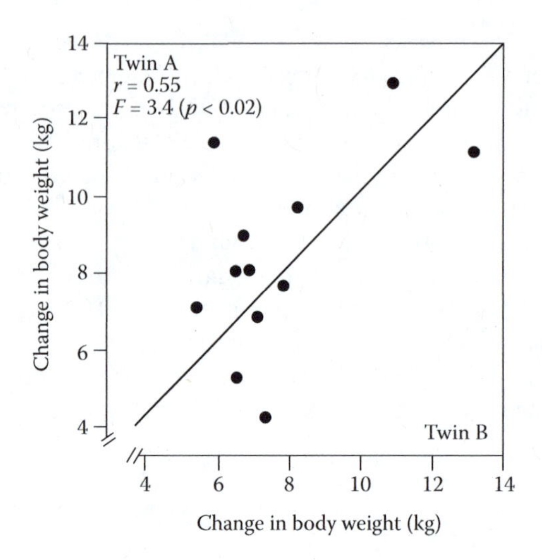

FIGURE 3.5 Effects of 84 days of overfeeding on 12 pairs of male identical twins. (Redrawn from Bouchard, C. et al., *N. Engl. J. Med.*, 322(21), 1477–1482, 1990.)

second, that genetic make-up influences weight gain and keeps the twins relatively close together. When these men stopped overeating, they lost most or all of the excess weight. The use of overeating protocols to study the consequences of food ingestion has shown the importance of genetic factors in the pattern of weight gain.

Overfeeding has also been practiced culturally among both women and men prior to marriage. Pasquet and Apfelbaum (1994) reported data on nine young men who participated in the traditional fattening ceremony called Guru Walla in northern Cameroon. These men overate during a 5-month period, gaining 19 kg in body weight and 11.8 kg of body fat. Before fattening, these men ate on average 3086 kcal per day (12.9 MJ per day) increasing to 6746 kcal per day (28 MJ per day). Over the 2.5 years following the overfeeding time the men returned to their pre-fattening body weight (Pasquet and Apfelbaum 1994).

A second form of overeating with clinical implications, I have called "progressive hyperphagia" (Bray 1976). A number of patients who become overweight in childhood have unrelenting weight gain. This can only mean that year by year their intake is exceeding their energy expenditure. Since it takes more energy as we get heavier this must mean that they are steadily increasing their intake of food. These individuals usually surpass 140 kg (300 lb) by age 30, for a weight gain of about 4.5 kg per year (10 lb per year). The recent death of a 13-year-old weighing 310 kg (680 lb) illustrates a nearly maximal rate of weight gain of 25 kg per year. These patients gain about the same amount of weight year after year. Because approximately 22 kcal per kg is required to maintain an extra kilogram of body weight in an obese individual, the energy requirements in these patients must increase year by year, with the weight gain being driven by excess energy intake.

Japanese sumo wrestlers are another example of conscious overeating. During their training, they eat large quantities of food twice a day for many years. While in training they have a very active training schedule and they have low visceral fat relative to total weight during training. When their active career ends, however, the wrestlers tend to remain overweight and have a high probability of developing diabetes mellitus (Li et al. 2005).

Carbohydrate Digestibility

The glycemic index is a way of describing the ease with which starches are digested in the intestine with the release of glucose, which can be readily absorbed. A high glycemic index food is one that is readily digested and produces a large and rapid rise in plasma glucose. A low glycemic index food, on the other hand, is more slowly digested and associated with a slower and lower rise in glucose. Comparative studies show that feeding high glycemic index foods suppresses food intake less than low glycemic index foods. The low glycemic index foods are the fruits and vegetables that tend to have more fiber. Potatoes, white rice, and white bread are high glycemic index foods. Legumes, whole wheat, etc. are low glycemic index foods.

In a review of six studies, Roberts documented that the consumption of higher glycemic index foods was associated with higher energy intake than when the foods had a lower glycemic index. This means that the higher fiber foods that release carbohydrate more slowly stimulate food intake less than the food where the glucose is rapidly released, as it is in the high glycemic index foods (Roberts).

Frequency of Eating: Grazers and Gorgers

For more than 40 years, there have been suggestions that eating fewer meals is more likely to lead to obesity than eating many meals (Bray 1976). One of the clear-cut effects of eating few meals is the increase in cholesterol (Bray 1972). Crawley et al. (1997) showed that among males, but not females, the number of meal-eating events per day was inversely related to the BMI. Males with a BMI of 20 to 25 ate just over six times per day, compared with less than six times for those with a BMI > 25 kg/m^2.

The frequency of eating in a controlled environment also affected the metabolic response to a test meal. In this trial, ten women with an average BMI of 37.1 participated in a counter-balanced crossover study. On one occasion, they ate four to six meals at regular times during the day for 14 days, and on the other occasion they ate three to nine meals at irregular times for another 14 days. Tests were done before and at the end of each period. During the time they ate meals at regular intervals, they had lower energy intake, lower total cholesterol, and higher TEF (Farshchi et al. 2005).

Low Levels of Physical Activity

Low levels of physical activity, as well as watching more television, predict higher body weight (Hancox et al. 2004). Recent studies suggest that individuals in American cities where they walk more tend to weigh less (Saelens et al. 2003). Low levels of physical activity also increase the risk of early mortality (Sui et al. 2007). Using normal-weight, physically active women as the comparison group, Hu et al. (2004) found that the relative risk of mortality increased 55%, from HR of 1.00 to HR of 1.55 (55%) in inactive lean women compared to active lean ones, to 92% (1.92) in active overweight women, and to 142% (2.42) in women who are overweight and physically inactive (Hu et al. 2004). It is, thus, better to be thin than fat and to be physically active than inactive.

Television has been one culprit blamed for the reduced levels of physical activity, particularly in children (Crespo et al. 2001; Dietz and Gortmaker 1985). Using data from the National Health Examination Survey, Dietz and Gortmaker (1985) provided some of the first evidence for this idea by using data from the National Longitudinal Study of Youth (Gortmaker et al. 1996), which showed a linear gradient from 11% to 12% overweight in children watching 0 to 2 hours per day to over 20% to 30% overweight children when watching more than 5 hours per day. A number of studies subsequently supported the proposition that, in both children and adults, those who watch more TV are more overweight. By one estimate, about 100 kcal of extra food energy is ingested for each hour of TV viewing.

Reducing sedentariness may have beneficial effects on body weight. In studies focusing on reducing sedentary activity, which mainly means decreasing TV viewing, there was a significant decrease in energy intake with increased activity (Epstein et al. 2005). Using the Early Childhood Longitudinal Study—kindergarten cohort—investigators found that between kindergarten and third grade, children watching more TV (odds ratio = 1.02) and eating fewer family meals together (odds ratio = 1.08) predicted a modest increase in weight (Gable et al. 2007).

Although television receives a good deal of blame, there is some evidence that the major increase in television viewing time occurred prior to the onset of the "epidemic" of overweight. Cutler et al.

(2003) found a 21% increase in television viewing between 1965 and 1975 (from 158 to 191 minutes per day), when color television became available at low prices. In contrast, between 1975 and 1995, when the epidemic of overweight was in full swing, the increase was only 11% (from 191 to 212 minutes per day). Although the use of television grew more slowly, other electronic devices, particularly computers and, more recently, the Internet, have grown faster. Television and other "screen" systems differ in that you can eat and watch television, but it is harder to do that when you need to respond to what is on the screen. The exposure to ten or more commercials per hour, most of which are for fast foods, soft drinks, and other energy-dense products associated with viewing television, may add an additional component to the epidemic of obesity (Finkelstein et al. 2005).

Sedentary Lifestyle

A sedentary lifestyle lowers energy expenditure and promotes weight gain in both animals and humans. Animals in zoos tend to be heavier than those in the wild. In an affluent society, energy-sparing devices in the workplace and at home reduce energy expenditure and may enhance the tendency to gain weight.

A number of additional observations illustrate the importance of decreased energy expenditure in the pathogenesis of weight gain. The highest frequency of overweight occurs in men in sedentary occupations. In contrast, a study of middle-aged men in the Netherlands found that the decline in energy expenditure accounted for almost all the weight gain (Kromhout 1983). According to the Surgeon General's Report on Physical Activity and Health, the percentage of adult Americans participating in physical activity decreases steadily with age, and reduced energy expenditure in adults and children predicts weight gain (HHS 1996). The number of automobiles is related to the degree of overweight in adults. Finally, the fatness of men in several affluent countries (The Seven Countries Study) was inversely related to levels of physical activity (Kromhout et al. 2001).

Has activity level declined? An estimate of energy expenditure over time was performed, utilizing a series of measurements in a relatively small (300 or so) group of people who were studied more than once with doubly-labeled water. This technique provides an estimate of total energy expenditure. Over a period of 25 years, there was no significant increase or decrease in the physical activity level (Westerterp and Speakman 2008).

Effect of Sleep Time and Environmental Light

Sleep time declines from an average of 14.2 ± 1.9 ($m \pm SD$) hours per day in infancy (11.0 ± 1.1 hours per day by 1 year of age) to 8.1 ± 0.8 hours per day at 16 years of age (Iglowinski et al. 2003). Sleep time declined across the cohorts from 1974 to 1993, due largely to later bedtime, but similar arising time. Five studies in children (Sekine et al. 2002; von Kries et al. 2002; Reilly et al. 2005; Agras et al. 2004; Al Mamun et al. 2007) found that there was a dose-dependent relationship between the amount of sleep and the body weight of children when they entered school. Von Kries et al. studied 6862 children of ages 5 to 6 years whose sleep times were reported in 1999–2000 by the parent. The follow-up was in 2001–2002 (von Kries et al. 2002). Overweight in this study was defined as a weight for height greater than the 97th percentile. Children with reported sleep times of less than 10 hours had a prevalence of overweight of 5.4% (95% CI 4.1 to 7.0), those who slept 10.5 to 11.0 hours per night had a prevalence of 2.8% (95% CI 2.3 to 3.3), and those who slept more than 11.5 hours had a prevalence of overweight of 2.1% (95% CI 1.5 to 2.9). Among the 8274 children from the Toyama Birth Cohort in Japan, Sekine et al. (2002) noted a graded increase in the risk of overweight at ages 6 to 7 years, defined as a BMI above 25 kg/m^2, as sleep time decreased. Children with reported sleep times of more than 10 hours at age 3 were the reference group with an odds ratio of 1.0, those with reported sleep times of 9 to 10 hours had an odds ratio of 1.49 (49% increase in risk of overweight), those with 8 to 9 hours had an odds ratio of 1.89 (89% increase), and those children who were reported to sleep less than 8 hours had an odds ratio for overweight of 2.87 (187%

increase). In an English study, Reilly (Reilly et al. 2005) found that the reported duration of sleep at age 3 years in 7758 children was related to their measured weight at age 7 years. Sleep assessed at 30 months of age predicted school-entry weight at age 7 years. The odds ratio comparing 10.5 hours with 12.5 hours or more was 1.45 (95% CI 1.10, 1.89). In an American study, Agras et al. (2004) found that sleep time at ages 3 to 4 years predicted body weight at age 9.5 years. Finally, Al Mamun et al. found that sleeping problems at ages 2 to 4 years were predictive of body weight at age 21 years (Al Mamun et al. 2007).

A dose-response relationship between the duration of sleep and body weight has been reported in adults too. Kripke et al. (2002) in a study of more than 1 million people ages 30 to 102 years found the same inverse relation between sleep time and body weight. Gangwisch et al. (2005), using the NHANES data, also found a relation between sleep duration and overweight that appeared to be "U" shaped. A similar "U" shaped relationship came from the Nurses Health Study (Patel and Hu 2006) where sleep times of <5 hours reported in 1986 was associated with a higher body weight of 69.5 kg versus 67.0 kg in those sleeping 7 hours and a rise to 68.3 kg in those getting more than 9 hours of sleep. With 16 years of follow-up, the same "U" shape was seen with those getting <5 hours of sleep gaining 9.6 kg versus 6.1 kg in those with 7 hours of sleep, but with more sleeping time the weight gain rose to 6.6 kg. When looking at the risk of obesity or a weight gain of more than 15 kg, only the short sleep time group in the Nurses Health Study showed a significant effect (Cox Proportional Hazard Ratio 1.15 and 1.28, respectively, for obesity and weight gain of 15 kg) (Patel et al. 2008).

These epidemiologic studies are buttressed by experimental studies that manipulate sleep time in the laboratory (Spiegel et al. 2004). First, reducing sleep time by sleep deprivation impairs glucose tolerance and increases insulin resistance. Reducing sleep time also lowers leptin levels and raises ghrelin levels, a setting that would favor weight gain.

Another setting in which lighting plays a role in the development of weight gain is "Seasonal Affective Depressive Syndrome," also called SADS. For some people, the shortening of the daylight hours with the onset of winter is associated with depression and weight gain. When the days begin to lengthen in the spring, this symptom complex is reversed. Current evidence suggests that it is related to changing activity of the serotonin system and can be treated with exposure to light or by manipulating brain levels of serotonin pharmacologically (Bray 2007b). In four longitudinal studies, depressive symptoms in childhood or adolescence were associated with a 1.9- to 3.5-fold increased risk of overweight later in life (Liem et al. 2008).

In a systematic review of epidemiological studies, Atlantis and Baker (2008) found a "weak" level of evidence supporting the hypothesis that obesity increases the incidence of depression. Studies from the United States tended to show a relation between obesity and depression, but other countries did not. Depressed patients often find benefit from weight loss (Dixon et al. 2003).

Medications That Produce Weight Gain

Several groups of drugs can produce weight gain and are shown in Table 3.4. The degree of weight gain is generally less than 10 kg and not sufficient to cause substantial overweight, but they can also increase the risk of future type 2 diabetes mellitus. Occasionally, patients treated with high-dose corticosteroid, with psychoactive drugs, or with valproate gain considerable weight.

Some phenothiazines and many of the "atypical" antipsychotics are prone to cause weight gain. This increase in weight is primarily fat and is associated with an increase in the respiratory quotient (RQ), a measure of the relative oxidation of carbohydrate and fat, suggesting that there is an increase in carbohydrate utilization that might stimulate food intake. Metabolic rate did not change (Graham et al. 1995). A multicenter trial compared changes in body weight among other outcomes during treatment of schizophrenia with antipsychotics. Olanzapine produced the most weight gain, 4.3 ± 0.4 kg (9.4 ± 0.9 lb) compared to smaller weight gains with the newer antipsychotics such as quietapine, 0.5 ± 0.45 kg (1.1 ± 0.9 lb), respiridone, 0.36 ± 0.45 kg (0.8 ± 0.9 lb), and ziprasidone,

TABLE 3.4
Drugs That Produce Weight Gain and Alternative Choices for Similar Problems

Category	Drugs That Cause Weight Gain	Possible Alternatives
Anti-psychotics	Thioridazine; Olanzepine; Quetiapine; Resperidone; Clozapine	Molindone; Haloperidol; Ziprasodone
Anti-depressants		
Tricyclics	Amitriptyline; Nortriptyline Imipramine	Protriptyline Bupropion;
Monoamine oxidase inhbitors	Mitrazapine	Nefazadone
Selective serotonin reuptake inhibitors	Paroxetine	Fluoxetine, Sertraline
Anti-convulsants	Valproate; Carbamazepine; Gabapentin	Topiramate; Lamotrigine; Zonisamide
Anti-diabetic drugs	Insulin Sulfonylureas Thiazolidinediones	Acarbose; Miglitol; Metformin; DPP-IV inhibitors
Anti-serotonin	Pizotifen	
Antihistamines	Cyproheptidine	Inhalers; Decongestants;
α-Adrenergic blockers	Propranolol	ACE inhibitors;
β-Adrenergic blockers	Terazosin	Calcium channel blockers
Steroid hormones	Contraceptives Glucocorticoids Progestational steroids	Barrier methods Non-steroidal anti-inflammatory agents

Source: © 2001 George A. Bray.

−0.74 ± 0.6 kg (−1.6 ± 1.1), compared to the older perphenazine, −1.8 ± 0.5 kg (−2.0 ± 1.1) (Lieberman et al. 2005).

Some antidepressants also can cause weight gain. The tricyclic antidepressant amitriptyline is a common culprit and may also increase the preference for carbohydrates. Lithium also has been implicated in weight gain. Two antiepileptic drugs, valproate and carbamazepine, which act on the *N*-methyl-D-aspartate (NMDA) (glutamate) receptor, cause weight gain in up to 50% of patients. Serotonin can inhibit food intake, and antagonists, such as cyproheptadine, are associated with weight gain.

Glucocorticoids cause fat accumulation on the neck and trunk, similar to that seen in patients with Cushing's syndrome. These changes occur mostly in patients taking more than 10 mg per day of prednisone or its equivalent. Megestrol acetate is a progestin used in women with breast cancer and in patients with acquired immunodeficiency syndrome (AIDS) to increase appetite and induce weight gain. The increased weight is fat.

Antidiabetic drugs are common causes of weight gain. Insulin probably produces weight gain by stimulating appetite with intermittent hypoglycemia as the most likely mechanism. Weight gain also occurs in patents treated with sulfonylureas, which enhance endogenous insulin release, and with glitazones, which act on the peroxisome proliferator-activated receptor-gamma (PPAR-γ) receptor to increase insulin sensitivity (Smith et al. 2005). In one clinical trial, 48 adult diabetics not treated with thiazolidinediones were randomized to receive either placebo or pioglitazone. Body weight decreased by 0.7 kg in the placebo group and increased by 3.6 kg in the pioglitazone group ($p < 0.0001$) with essentially all of the weight gain being subcutaneous fat (3.5 kg $p < 0001$). Using multislice, CT-scan measurements of visceral fat (VAT) showed no significant change in VAT during 12 weeks of treatment, 5.7 ± 2.2 to 5.5 ± 2.3 kg in the pioglitazone group ($p = 0.058$); 5.9 ± 1.9 to 5.8 ± 2.0 kg in the placebo group ($p = 0.075$). After 6 months, the visceral fat mass for both the placebo and pioglitazone-treated groups were not different from baseline or from each other. Stratifying the group into those who received sulfonylurea treatment and those who did not had no effect on the response to pioglitazone. Both pioglitazone and rosiglitazone cause significant increases in body fat, almost all of which is subcutaneous fat.

Some, but not all, beta-adrenergic antagonists can cause weight gain. In a comparison of metoprolol, a relatively pure beta-adrenergic antagonist and carvedilol, a beta-adrenergic antagonist with alpha-1 adrenergic antagonism, Messerli et al. (2007) found that during 5 months of treatment, those on metoprolol gained 1.19 kg, compared to only 0.17 kg with carvedilol. In the UKPDS study, atenolol produced a 3.4 kg weight gain compared to 1.6 kg with captopril (ACEI).

Toxins

Toxins from the environment are an additional factor that might influence body weight.

Smoking

Smoking increased from 1900 to 1970 and then declined during the last 30 years of the twentieth century. Smokers have a lower body mass index than nonsmokers and weight gain often occurs after stopping smoking with men gaining an average of 3.8 kg and women 2.8 kg (Williamson et al. 1991). In one analysis, men gained 4.4 kg and women 5.0 kg (Flegal et al. 1995) and it was calculated that this gain could account for about one-quarter to one-sixth of the increased prevalence of overweight. Several factors predict the weight gain, including younger age, lower socioeconomic status, heavier smoking, and genetic factors (Filizof et al. 2004). Economists have calculated that a 10% increase in the price of cigarettes could increase BMIs by 0.0251 kg/m^2 due to the decrease in smoking (Cutler et al. 2003). Snacks are the major component of food intake that rises when people stop smoking.

Organochlorines

In human beings, we know that many "toxic" chemicals are stored in body fat and that they are mobilized with weight loss. Backman first showed that organochlorines in the body decreased after bariatric surgery. The metabolic rate can be reduced by organochlorine molecules (Tremblay et al. 2004) and, conceivably, prolonged exposure to many chlorinated chemicals in our environment can affect metabolic pathways and energy metabolism. Thyroid hormone synthesis is decreased, plasma T3 and T4 are decreased, thyroid hormone clearance is increased, and skeletal muscle and mitochondrial oxidation are reduced.

In a review of possible relationships of environmental toxins and obesity Heindel states: "the current level of human exposure to these chemicals may have damaged many of the body's natural weight-control mechanisms" (Heindel 2003). "Examples of chemicals that have been tested for toxicity by standard tests that results in weight gain in the animals at lower doses than those that caused any obvious toxicity. These chemicals included: heavy metals, solvents, polychlorinated biphenols, organophosphates, phthalates, and bisphenol A" (Baillie-Hamilton 2002).

Monosodium Glutamate

Food additives are another class of chemicals that are widely distributed and may be involved in the current epidemic of overweight. In experimental animals, exposure during the neonatal period to monosodium glutamate (MSG), a common flavoring ingredient in food, produces fatness (Olney 1969).

Viruses as Environmental Agents

Several viruses produce weight gain in animals and it is possible that they also do so in human beings (Atkinson 2007). Injection of canine distemper virus, RAV-7 virus, Borna disease virus, scrapie virus, SMAM-1 virus, and 3 adenoviruses (types 5, 24, and 36) into the central nervous system produces fatness in mice. These observations were generally assumed to produce pathologic lesions and not to be relevant to humans. However, antibodies to adenovirus AM-36 appear in larger amounts in some overweight humans than in controls. The AM-36 viral syndrome can be replicated in the ferret, a nonhuman primate. The features of the syndrome are a modest increase in weight and a low cholesterol concentration in the circulation.

Behavioral, Psychological, and Social Factors

Psychological Factors

Psychological changes such as depression are widely recognized in obesity, but attempts to define a specific personality type that causes obesity have largely been unsuccessful.

Restrained Eating

A pattern of conscious limitation of food intake is called "restrained" eating. It is common in many, if not most, middle-age women of "normal weight." It also may account for the inverse relationship of body weight to social class; women of upper socioeconomic status often use restrained eating to maintain their weight. In a weight-loss clinic, higher restraint scores were associated with lower body weights (Konttinen et al. 2009). Weight loss was associated with a significant increase in restraint, indicating that higher levels of conscious control can maintain lower weight. Greater increases in restraint correlate with greater weight loss, but also with higher risk of "lapse" or loss of control and overeating. The ups and downs created by loss of restraint are followed by self-blame and then a period of recommitment that has been termed "The False Hope Syndrome" by Polivy and Herman (2002), because the cycle is likely to be repeated again and again.

Binge-Eating Disorder

Binge-eating disorder is a psychiatric illness characterized by uncontrolled episodes of eating, usually in the evening (Allison et al. 2005a). The patient may respond to treatment with drugs that modulate serotonin. Individuals with binge-eating disorder showed more objective bulimic and overeating episodes, were more concerned about their body shape and body weight, and were disinhibited on the three-factor eating inventory when compared to patients with the night-eating syndrome (Allison et al 2005b).

Night-Eating Syndrome

Night-eating syndrome involves the consumption of at least 25% of the day's energy between the evening meal and the next morning and finding oneself awakened at night to eat 3 or more times per week (Stunkard et al. 1955; Allison et al. 2006). The prevalence of this syndrome has ranged from a low of 1.5% in the general population (Lamerz et al. 2005) to a high of 12.6% in a psychiatric population (Lundgren et al. 2006). In an obesity clinic, the prevalence was 7.6 % and 9.0% (Striegel-Moore et al. 2006; Allison et al. 2006). In a study of monozygotic and dizygotic twins, the night-eating syndrome was found in 3.4% of the females and 4.3% of the males (Tholin et al. 2009). The heritability of 0.38 was lower than for obesity itself. In a comparison of overweight individuals (average BMI 36.1 kg/m^2) with the night-eating syndrome who ate on average 35.9% of their food after the evening meal and who awakened to eat an average of 1.5 times per night with comparably overweight individuals (BMI 38.7 kg/m^2) who did not have these features, Allison et al. (2006) showed that glucose and insulin were higher at night as expected from the eating pattern and ghrelin was lower. Plasma cortisol, melatonin, leptin, and prolactin did not differ, but there was a trend

Albert J. Stunkard (1922–present) described the night-eating syndrome and for his seminal contributions to the field of obesity over a period of 50 years, including work on the glucostatic theory of obesity, on the idea that there might be a characteristic behavior pattern behind obesity, on lifestyle treatment, and on inheritance of obesity. Stunkard was born in New York. He received his undergraduate education at Yale University, graduating in 1943. His MD was awarded by Columbia University in 1945. After serving in Japan in the late 1940s, he returned to train with Harold Wolff in New York. He became disillusioned with the psychoanalytic approach to human disease and turned to biological aspects of psychiatry. Stunkard has been a professor of psychiatry at the University of Pennsylvania School of Medicine much of his life. He served as chairman of the Department of Psychiatry there and for a short time at Stanford University. He founded the Center for Weight and Eating Disorders at the University of Pennsylvania. He has investigated both genetic and environmental influences on human obesity using adoptees, twins, differing social classes, and the Old Order Amish. He has been conducting a large-scale prospective longitudinal study of the growth and development of children at high risk of obesity. He also studies deviant eating patterns, having been the first to describe binge eating and having developed treatments for binge eating disorder. The night-eating syndrome was identified by Stunkard in 1955. He is the author of nearly 500 publications, mostly in the field of obesity and eating disorders and his research has been supported for 50 years by the National Institutes of Health. Dr. Stunkard has served as Past President of the American Association of Chairmen of Departments of Psychiatry, the Association for Research in Nervous and Mental Diseases, the American Psychosomatic Society, the Society of Behavioral Medicine, and the Academy of Behavioral Medicine Research and he serves on the editorial boards of seven journals in the fields of nutrition and behavioral medicine (Rossner 2009; Stunkard 1976).

for higher TSH. Patients with the night-eating syndrome were also more depressed (Allison et al. 2006). When sertraline, a serotonin reuptake inhibitor drug was tested in a randomized controlled trial of people who were "night-eaters," it produced weight loss and improvement in those with the night-eating syndrome (O'Reardon et al. 2006).

Eating at night is clinically important. In a study of weight gain over 3 years, 23 individuals who selected food between 11 PM and 5 AM while on a metabolic ward for three nights gained nearly 6 kg compared to about 0.5 kg in 69 subjects who did not eat at night (Gluck et al. 2009). Using a brain imaging technique called ADAM SPECT demonstrated an increased uptake of serotonin in the mid-brain and temporal areas.

Socioeconomic and Ethnic Factors

Social networks appear to modulate the risk of obesity. Christakis and Fowler (2007) examined the effects of social networks in participants in the Framingham Study, a densely interconnected social network of 12,067 people assessed repeatedly from 1971 to 2003. There were discernible clusters of obese persons that extended to three degrees of separation. The chances for an individual becoming obese increased by 57% (95% CI 6 to 123) if he or she had a friend who became obese in a given interval. Among pairs of adult siblings, if one sibling became obese, the chance that the other would become obese increased by 40% (95% CI 21 to 60). If one spouse became obese, the likelihood that the other spouse would become obese increased by 37% (95% CI 7 to 73). These effects were not seen among neighbors in the immediate geographic location. Persons of the same sex had relatively greater influence on each other than those of the opposite sex. From these data, we conclude that obesity appears to spread through social ties (Christakis and Fowler 2007).

Increased duration of living with a romantic partner was associated with obesity and obesity-related behaviors in the National Longitudinal Study of Adolescent Health. For women, living in a romantic relationship for more than one year was associated with increased odds of obesity; for men, this occurred between 1 and 1.99 years (Scharoun-Lee et al. 2009). Sexual abuse has been alleged as a factor in the development of obesity, but a review and meta-analysis of the literature could find no such relation (Paras et al. 2009).

Obesity, particularly in women, is more prevalent in those with less education. The inverse relationship of socioeconomic status (SES) and obesity is found in both adults and children. SES status and BMI are inversely related in most studies (Wang and Beydoun 2007; McLaren 2007). People of higher SES were more concerned with healthy weight-control practices, including exercise, and tended to eat less fat. The association of SES and weight is much stronger in Caucasian women than in African-American women. African-American women of all ages are more overweight than Caucasian women, but African-American men are less heavy than Caucasian men, and socioeconomic factors are much less evident in men. Among children and adolescents, the relationship between SES and obesity patterns is similar across race/ethnicity, but differs by gender during the transition to adulthood. Stronger associations with the persistence of obesity and enduring racial/ethnic disparities in obesity risk occur across socioeconomic groups suggesting that these social factors play a larger role in disparities earlier in life (Scharoun-Lee et al. 2009).

REGULATION OF BODY FAT: A HOMEOSTATIC MODEL OF ENERGY REGULATION

The genetic and environmental factors described above influence the energy balance by acting either on food intake or energy expenditure (see Figure 3.1). The basis for ideas about energy balance has its origin in the discovery of oxygen by Lavoisier in the 1780s (Chapter 1). The central theory and formulation of the law of conservation of energy, which is the basis of the energy balance concept, was published almost simultaneously by Helmholtz (1847) and by Mayer (1842). This theoretical construct was subsequently tested in both animals and man (Lust 1932). It was Atwater and Rosa and the metabolic chamber that they built at Wesleyan College that showed that the ideas of energy balance applied to human beings (Atwater and Rosa 1899). This important piece of equipment was put to masterful use by Francis Benedict over the next 20 years with seminal studies on starvation and nutrient needs. In the hundred years since the time of Atwater and Benedict, human nutrition research supported by the United States Department of Agriculture has expanded greatly and research centers—several of which have metabolic chambers that are the descendent of the one developed by Atwater and Rosa—are now located in Beltsville, Maryland, Boston, Houston, Grand Forks, North Dakota, Ames, Iowa, and San Francisco (Bray 2007b).

Francis Gano Benedict (1870–1957) is noted for his pioneering work with the respiration calorimeter developed by Atwater and Rosa and because of his studies on the effects of starvation on the human body. Benedict was born in Milwaukee and lived in both Florida and Boston during his youth. After a year at the Massachusetts College of Pharmacy, he received his AB and MA degrees from Harvard, and a PhD from Heidelberg in 1895. As fortune would have it, he began his academic career at Wesleyan University in 1895 as Atwater was completing his calorimeter. He began his work with Atwater and when Atwater died, Benedict was appointed director. Shortly after that, the nutrition laboratory was moved to Boston to be nearer clinical facilities. From 1897 to 1937, when he retired, more than 500 experiments were carried out that were presented in some 400 publications. His work on human starvation was conducted in 1915 and is a classic in the field (Maynard 1969).

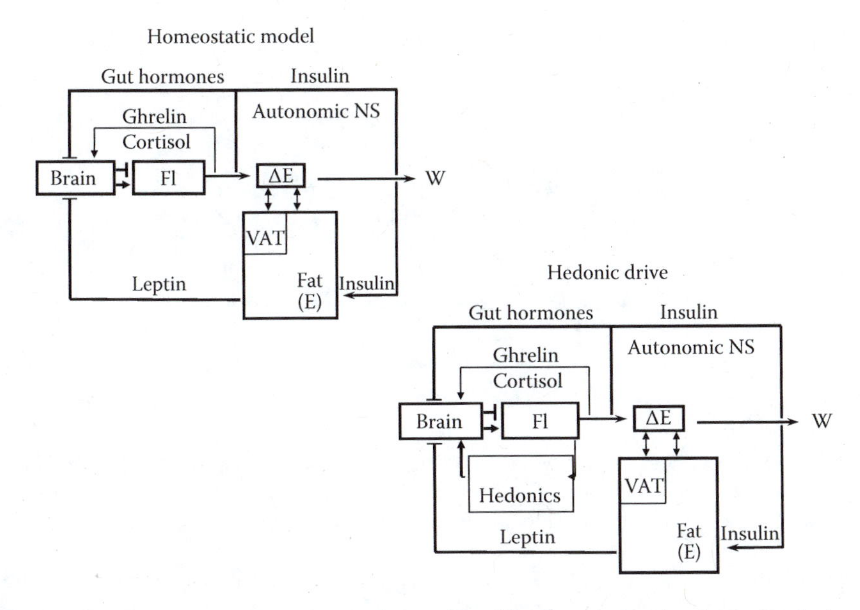

FIGURE 3.6 Two homeostatic models for regulation of food intake, one showing the feedback elements, and the other adding a hedonic component related to the taste and pleasure of food.

A homeostatic or feedback system between food intake and body energy (fat stores) is a useful way to view the problem of overweight (see Figure 3.6). Such a feedback system has four parts. The control center in the brain is analogous to the thermostat in a heating system. It receives information about the energy state of the animal or human being, transduces this information into neurochemical signals, and activates pathways that lead to or inhibit feeding and the search for food. The signals that the brain receives come from the environment through sense organs and from the body through neural, nutrient, or hormonal signals. The response the brain makes includes both the activation and inhibition of motor systems and the modulation of the autonomic nervous system and hormonal control system utilizing the orchestra of the endocrine glands. A systems approach has provided the basis for mathematical modeling of food intake, energy expenditure, and starvation (Hall 2006; Halgreen and Hall 2008; Thomas et al. 2009a, 2009b).

Outside of the brain is the so-called "controlled system," which for the purpose of this discussion includes the digestive track where food enters and is digested and absorbed, the metabolic systems in the liver, muscle, and kidneys that transform nutrients and metabolize them, and the adipose tissue, which both stores and releases fatty acids and acts as a secretory endocrine organ (Bray 2007a).

Digestion, Metabolism, and Fat Storage

The controlled system consists of the gastrointestinal track, liver, muscles, adipose tissue, the cardiovascular-pulmonary-renal system, and the supporting bone tissue. The ingestion, digestion, and absorption of food provide nutrients to the body and also provide signals from these nutrients to the vagus nerve, which relays the major neural control of GI function. Metabolism of food in the GI tract also releases hormones that can be secreted into the circulation or act on the vagus nerve. The nutrients that are absorbed can be metabolized to provide energy, or they can be stored as glycogen in the liver, as protein in muscle, or as fat in adipose tissue.

The largest part of the energy we expend each day is for "resting" metabolism and is consumed by the brain, liver, kidneys, heart, and intestinal track (Sparti et al. 1997a; Bosy-Westphal et al. 2009; Muller et al. 2002). This energy is involved in the metabolism of food, the transport of

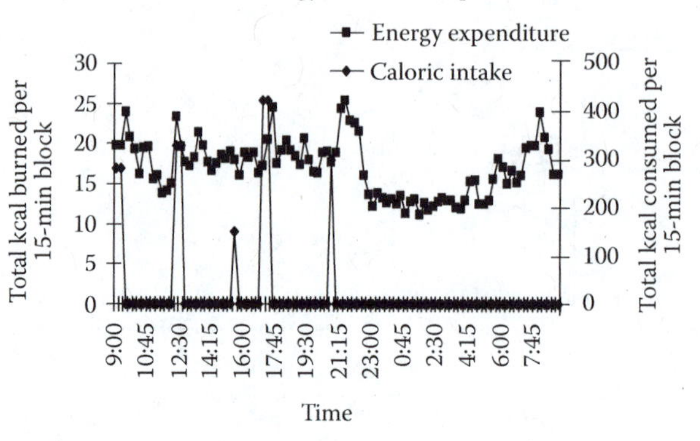

FIGURE 3.7 Twenty-four hour energy intake and energy expenditure of a healthy male living in a respiration calorimeter where all food and exercise were provided with an effort to maintain energy balance. (From Bray, G.A., *The Metabolic Syndrome and Obesity*, The Humana Press, Inc., Totowa, NJ, 2007.)

sodium, potassium, and other ions across cell membranes, repair of DNA, synthesis of protein, the beating of the heart, and functioning of the brain, liver, and kidneys. Resting energy expenditure, often called basal metabolic rate, is most strongly associated with fat-free body mass. The energy stores are controlled to within less than 1% error from year to year in most people, but declines slowly throughout adult life (Wang et al. 2005). Adults ingest between 750,000 and 1,000,000 calories during a 12-month period. A weight gain of 1 kg would represent storage of less than 7,500 to 10,000 calories or about 1% of this total and would produce a 1-kg weight gain. Estimates for the daily excess energy intake needed to produce the current epidemic has been estimated at between 100 kcal per day (Hill et al. 2003) and 500 kcal per day (Swinburn et al. 2009b).

Increased body fat results from a positive energy balance, which is regulated to varying degrees by an internal feedback system. Does this imply we are in energy balance each day? To examine this idea, we have attempted to produce "zero" energy balance, that is, to get subjects as close as possible over a 24-hour time interval to balancing energy intake and expenditure so that there was no difference. In our experiments, we can adjust either food intake or exercise to achieve balance. Meal intakes occur as spikes during the day, reflecting the periodic intake of energy (Figure 3.7). Energy expenditure continues throughout the day, but drops during sleep to about 80% of the daytime average. In our studies, an individual who spends 4 days in a row in the chamber gets no closer to energy balance than ±25 kcal (±105 kJ). Based on this and a number of other studies, we conclude that day-to-day energy balance is either positive or negative (Bray et al. 2008). We do not achieve meal-to-meal or day-to-day energy balance. Rather, if we are to avoid weight gain, we must achieve energy balance from week to week or month to month (Bray 2007a).

There is some evidence for regulation over a period of several days. The first study to support this idea was by Edholm et al. (1955). They measured food intake and energy expenditure in British military recruits. There was no correlation of energy intake and energy expenditure from day to day, but over a period of several days there was a correlation between the two. We have conducted a similar study with dietitians. They were enrolled in a study to see whether they could accurately record food intake over a 7-day interval when energy expenditure was being measured simultaneously by doubly-labeled water (Champagne et al. 2002; Bray et al. 2008). Their energy intake was not significantly lower than their energy expenditure during this period of time. However, there were striking day-to-day variations in energy intake (see Figure 3.8). Some individuals varied by more than 1000 kcal per day (4180 kJ per day), whereas others had much smaller variations. The coefficient of variation for the group was 24%, meaning that on a 2000 kcal average diet, the day-to-day difference could range from nearly 1500 to nearly 2500 kcal. When the day-to-day variations were examined, it became clear that there was a maximal relationship between intake and expenditure

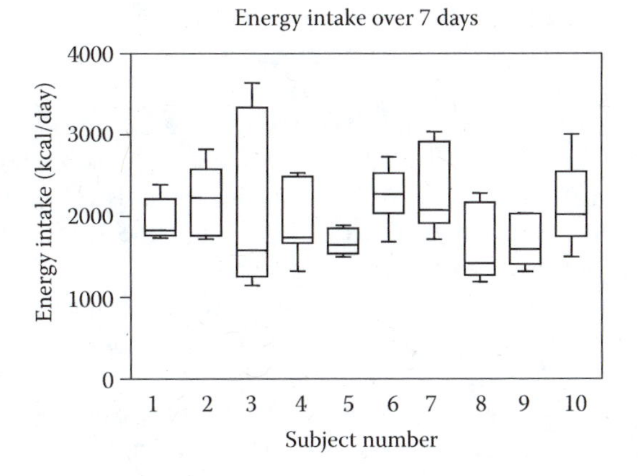

FIGURE 3.8 Day-to-day variation of food intake among 10 dietitians; the coefficient of variation is 24%. (Bray, G.A., et al., *Am. J. Clin. Nutr.* 88(6), 1504–1510, 2008.)

over an interval of 3 to 4 days, but not at days 1, 2, or 5 (Bray et al. 2008). This implied that there are feedback systems operating over periods of several days, and possibly longer, that are important in whether we can maintain energy balance over the long-term or whether the system is easily thrown off balance. Using baseline data from a study of calorie restriction, Racette et al. (2008) found that energy intake was higher on Saturday and lowest during the middle of the week.

If we are to maintain a stable body weight, the metabolic mix of carbohydrate, fat, and protein that is oxidized by the body must equal the amounts of these nutrients taken in as food. This concept has led to two broad hypotheses. The first is the nutrient balance hypothesis based on the work of Flatt who showed that experimental animals regulated food intake based on the shifts in carbohydrate balance from day to day (Flatt 1995). That is, maintaining energy balance requires that the mix of foods we eat be completely metabolized or oxidized. The capacity for storage of carbohydrate as glycogen is limited to about one day's supply of carbohydrate intake (about 1200 kcal or 300 g). The capacity to store protein is also limited, although not as much as for carbohydrates. Only the fat stores can readily expand to accommodate increasing levels of energy intake above those required for daily energy needs. Several studies now show that a high rate of carbohydrate oxidation, as measured by a high RQ, predicts future weight gain (Zurlo et al. 1990). One explanation for this is that when carbohydrate oxidation is higher, carbohydrate stores are depleted. To replace this carbohydrate, an individual must eat more carbohydrate or reduce the oxidation of carbohydrate by the body, since the body cannot convert fatty acids to glucose and the conversion of amino acids to carbohydrate mobilizes important body proteins (Flatt 1995; Sparti 1997b). Obese individuals who have lost weight do not increase fat oxidation in the presence of a high-fat diet as well as normal-weight individuals, and this may be one reason why they are so susceptible to regaining weight that has been lost (Raben et al. 1994).

A second hypothesis is the protein leverage hypothesis, based on a geometric model in which nutrient space is divided into two dimensions. One dimension is the protein intake, the other dimension is the sum of the carbohydrate and fat that is eaten. A protein target can be met by a number of different proportions of carbohydrate and fat (Simpson and Raubenheimer 2005). In this hypothesis, protein is prioritized over other nutrients. If that is the case, then the handling of fat and carbohydrate are adjusted to meet this goal. This hypothesis implies an important role for gluconeogenesis in the liver.

The final common pathway for retaining the energy from foods is through a mitochondrial chain of enzymes involved in oxidative phosphorylation. A growing number of studies have now shown that the genes controlling these enzymes are not expressed at normal levels in diabetic patients, in individuals with a family history of diabetes, or following ingestion of a high-fat diet (Patti and

Kahn 2004; Ukropcova et al. 2005). This defective expression of genes for oxidative phosphorylation may underlie the susceptibility of some individuals to becoming overweight when eating a high-fat diet that is so prevalent in Western societies.

Physical activity gradually declines with age. Thus, if we are to avoid becoming overweight as we age, we must gradually reduce our food intake or maintain a regular exercise program. A moderate level of exercise is beneficial in two ways. First, it reduces the risk of cardiovascular disease and type 2 diabetes and, second, it facilitates the oxidation of fat in the diet (Smith et al. 2000).

The concept of "energy wasting" or adaptive thermogenesis (or "luxuskonsumption," as it was once called), has a long and tortured history in obesity research (Schutz 2000; Wijers et al. 2009). Proteins that "uncouple" oxidation from phosphorylation in the mitochondrion are one mechanism that might underlie this kind of adaptive thermogenesis and keep us from storing extra calories. The uncoupling protein-1 (UCP1) found in brown fat has a well-established role in helping newborn infants and many smaller animals maintain body temperature. Increased expression and/or activation of this protein uncouples oxidation from phosphorylation by enhancing a leak of protons from the inner mitochondrial space, resulting in the conversion of energy to heat without storing the energy in adenosine 5′-monophosphate (ATP) molecules. If this occurred with overeating it could prevent us from gaining weight. If you eat more food energy than your body needs you could (theoretically) just "burn it off." As Hamlet said, "Tis a consummation devoutly to be wish'd."

The UCP1 molecule is important in human infants, but its importance in adults, due to the very low levels of brown fat (and hence UCP1 expression) in adult humans, has been questioned until recently (Nedergaard et al. 2007). This new evidence for active brown adipose tissue in adult humans comes from the use of sophisticated techniques combining glucose uptake in tissues (using the ^{18}fluoro-deoxy-glucose) measured by positron emission tomography (PET) and computed tomography (CT). Deposits of brown adipose tissue were demonstrated in the supraclavicular region, along the cervical vertebrae and along thoracic vertebrae. This activity can be blocked by propranolol, a beta-adrenergic-blocking drug, indicating that this glucose uptake is partly under control of the sympathetic nervous system. Higher temperatures eliminate the uptake and lower temperatures increase the uptake of labeled glucose. Whether the activity of this tissue can be enhanced by continued stimulation remains to be demonstrated. In one study, brown fat was found in 7.5% of women (76 of 1013 scans) and 3.1% of men (30 of 959 scans). The probability of finding brown fat was decreased in older people and with higher outdoor temperatures (Cypress et al. 2009). Uptake of glucose was increased 15-fold in the supraclavicular and paracervical fat by exposing five healthy subjects to the cold. Biopsies in three showed UCP1 (Virtanen et al. 2009).

The identification of two additional uncoupling proteins (UCP2 and UCP3) that are highly expressed in adult human tissues has attracted considerable interest. These two uncoupling proteins, in contrast, do not have the same effects as UCP1. That is, they do not seem to allow for heat dissipation by enhancing a mitochondrial proton leak. Rather, they appear to be involved in the transport of fatty acids into cells.

The Fat Cell

The discovery that fat is stored in "cells" and not as coagulated or congealed fat in the "lax tissues" of the body was a nineteenth-century discovery and followed the recognition of cell structure and the cell was the basic unit of biology in the 1830s (Schwann 1834, 1847). These fat cells are located in adipose tissue and serve two major functions. First, they are the cells that store and release fatty acids ingested in the food we eat or synthesized in the liver or fat cell. Second, fat cells are a major endocrine cell, secreting many important metabolic and hormonal molecules (Kershaw and Flier 2004).

Before fat cells can undertake these functions, however, they must be converted from precursor mesenchymal cells to mature fat cells. In vitro studies have shown a two-stage process—proliferation followed by differentiation. The development of a fat cell precursor that would become a fat cell when cultured outside the body was central to this work. Green and Meuth (1974) identified

Howard Green (1925–present) is noted for his contributions to developing a fat cell precursor that would differentiate into a mature fat cell in vitro. Green was born in Toronto, Ontario on September 10, 1925. He received his MD from the University of Toronto in 1947, and MS from Northwestern in 1950. He began his scientific work at the University of Chicago where he was an instructor from 1951 to 1953. He then moved to New York University where he rose to Chairman of the Department of Cell Biology. In 1970, he moved to the Massachusetts Institute of Technology in Cambridge, MA where he was chair of the Department of Cell Biology from 1970 to 1980. He then moved across the Charles River to the Harvard Medical School where he was chairman of the Department of Cellular and Molecular Physiology from 1980 to 1993 and since then he has been the George Higginson Professor in this department, continuing his work on the use of ketatinocytes in the regeneration of epidermis in severely burned patients. His laboratory is located in the Harvard Medical School Longwood Quadrangle, where the studies for the first life-saving use of this procedure were carried out.

the 3T3-L1 cell line that met these criteria, and it has been a major tool in understanding fat cell proliferation and differentiation. The proliferative phase is initiated by hormonal stimulation with insulin and glucocorticoids. After the cells begin to grow they enter a state of differentiation where they acquire the genetic state of mature fat cells that can store fatty acids, break down triglycerides, and make and release the many hormones that characterize the mature fat cell. Most of the fatty acids that are stored in human fat cells are derived from the diet, although these cells maintain the capacity for *de novo* synthesis of fatty acids (Hellerstein et al. 1993, p. 113).

The discovery of leptin catapulted the fat cell into the arena of endocrine cells (Zhang et al. 1994). The finding of a peptide released from fat cells that acts at a distance has refocused interest in the fat cell from primarily a cell that stores fatty acids to a cell with important endocrine and paracrine functions. In addition to leptin, the fat cell secretes a variety of peptides, including lipoprotein lipase, adipsin (complement D), complement C, adiponectin, tumor necrosis factor-α (TNF-a), interleukin-6 (IL-6), plasminogen activator inhibitor-1 (PAI-1), angiotensinogen, bradykinin, and resistin, in addition to other metabolites such as lactate, fatty acids, glycerol, and prostacyclin formed from arachidonic acid. This important endocrine tissue has thus greatly expanded its role. The endocrine products produced and secreted by the fat cell number close to 100 (Halberg, Wenstedt, and Scherer 2009).

Jeffrey Friedman, MD, PhD (1954–present) directed the laboratory that cloned leptin in 1994, a finding that changed the paradigm for viewing obesity. He was born in Orlando, Florida in 1954 but grew up in New York, graduating from Hewlett High School. Friedman graduated from Rensselaer Polytechnic Institute and received his MD from Albany Medical College of Union University in 1977. After completing two residencies at Albany Medical Center Hospital, he came to Rockefeller University as a postgraduate fellow and associate physician in 1980. In 1986, he received his PhD working in the lab of James E. Darnell Jr. In the same year he became an investigator at the Howard Hughes Medical Institute and in 1999 was appointed the Marilyn M. Simpson Professor. He has received a number of awards for his work in the discovery of leptin. He is an active basketball fan. Friedman is a member of the National Academy of Sciences and its Institute of Medicine. In 2009, he received the Shaw Prize in Life Science and Medicine and he has also received the Jessie Stevenson Kovalenko Medal, the sixth Danone International Prize for Nutrition, and the 2004 Passano Foundation Award.

Leptin has effects on many systems other than those controlling food intake (Dardeno and Sharon 2010). It is involved in the modulation of bone growth both peripherally and within the brain. It modulates growth of some cancers including breast. It influences endocrine function, including the onset of puberty and the function of the thyroid system.

In addition to its role as an endocrine cell, the fat cell is part of a tissue that has differing metabolic responses depending on its location. Orbital fat, fat in the heel (calcaneous fat pad), and bone marrow show little response to energy balance, in contrast to the changes in subcutaneous and visceral fat. Expansion of subcutaneous fat cells is one of the first responses to a positive energy balance. For this to happen, the fat cell must initiate a series of changes that will allow vessels to grow as it expands. Fibronectin, a structural element must be loosened or removed. Fat tissue from obese individuals is hypoxic (Pasarica et al. 2009; Halberg et al. 2009), a setting that stimulates a variety of messages including vascular endothelial factor (VEGF), collagen VI, hypoxia-inducible factor 1a, and macrophage chemotractant protein-1a that, among others, may facilitate the entry of inflammatory cells into adipose tissue. One hypothesis for the development of insulin resistance as fat cells enlarge is their resistance or "rigidity" resulting from these changes in the extracellular milieu.

Messages to the Brain from the Environment and from the Body

The brain receives a continuous stream of information from both the external and internal environments that plays a role in the control of feeding. The external information provided by sight, sound, and smell are all distance signals for identifying food. For many years, the contraction of the stomach was thought to be a major trigger for hunger and satiety—an old concept popularized by Cannon and Washburn (1912) and by Carlson (1912).

Taste and texture of foods are proximate signals generated when food enters the mouth. The classic tastes are sweet, sour, bitter, and salty as well as "umami," a fifth taste. In nature, most sweet foods also have vitamins and minerals, since they come from fruits. Sour and particularly bitter foods often contain unwanted and potentially hazardous chemical compounds. The extreme example of this is "bait-shyness" or taste aversion, the property that some items have

Walter Bradford Cannon (1871–1945) is noted for his seminal contributions to the function of the gastrointestinal track and for his concepts of homeostasis and the fight or flight modes of response to stress. Cannon was born in Prairie du Chien, a small town in Wisconsin on October 19, 1871. His mother died when he was ten. He received his early education in Milwaukee and St. Paul from where he went to Harvard College on a scholarship, graduating summa cum laude in 1896. He received his MD from Harvard Medical School in 1900 and joined the Department of Physiology as an instructor, only to be elevated to George Higginson Professor of Physiology in 1906, a position that he held until his retirement 36 years later in 1942. He was an internationally known physiologist and chairman of the Department of Physiology at Harvard Medical School for most of his professional life. His early work was focused on the gastrointestinal tract and his book entitled *The Mechanical Factors of Digestion* is a classic in its field (Cannon 1911). He was a skilled surgeon and used experimental animals frequently in his work. His devotion to animal welfare and to research led to his efforts throughout the pre-World War I period as an advocate of humane and proper care of experimental animals. His work on hunger, published in 1912, was followed 3 years later by one of his most popular books, *Bodily Changes in Pain, Hunger, Fear and Rage* (1915). His monograph *The Way of an Investigator* (1945) is a description of the life of a clinical investigator (Mayer 1965; Benison et al. 1987).

that produces a permanent rejection of future food with the same taste. This is a "hard-wired" response in the brain that overrides the usual feedback signals. There are several taste receptors that allow these tastes to be distinguished. Sweet tastants interact with a dimeric G-protein coupled receptor called T1R2 and T2R3. The G-protein in this case is the trimeric gustducin, which consists of a-gustducin and Gb3 and Gc13. The umami (monosocium glutamate taste) also has a dimeric receptor (T1R2 and T1R3 and possibly mGluR1 and mGluR4), which activate phosphatidylinositol 4,5-bisphosphate (PIP2), a second messenger. The salt taste appears to use vannilloid receptors (TRPV1 and TRPV1t). Sour taste involves PKD1L3 or PKD2L1 receptors. Finally, the bitter taste involves TAS2R50 and T2, which has 30 or so variants. Of interest is that the same receptors are also found in the intestine, suggesting that additional information on "tastes" is provided as foods are digested.

A taste for fats, specifically unsaturated fatty acids, may be a sixth taste. Receptors on the tongue can identify certain fatty acids. The discovery of taste and smell receptors for polyunsaturated fatty acids on the taste bud that involve a potassium rectifier channel offers an opening into modifying taste inputs into the food-intake system (Gilbertson et al. 2005). An important advance was showing that CD-36, a scavenger receptor that binds fatty acids, is one possible receptor for these fatty acids. These CD-36 receptors are located on the lingual papillae of the tongue. Mice that do not express the gene for the CD36 receptor do not prefer solutions enriched with long-chain fatty acids or a high-fat diet. These receptors are in close proximity to Ebner's glands, a source of lingual lipase, which cleaves triglycerides into fatty acids that can activate the CD36 receptor. When this receptor is activated, there is a rise in pancreatic secretions (Laugerette et al. 2005).

Several gastrointestinal peptides have been studied as potential regulators of food intake. Most of these peptides, including cholecystokinin, glucagon-like peptide-1, polypeptide YY3-36, oxyntomodulin, and neuromedin B (Howard et al. 2000; Beglinger and Degen 2006; Small and Bloom 2004), reduce food intake. Cholecystokinin (CCK) was the first peptide shown to reduce food intake in animals and humans alike (Bray and Greenway 1999).

Investigation of the growth hormone secretagogue receptor has led to the identification of ghrelin, a gastrointestinal hormone that stimulates food intake. Bowers found that secretion of growth hormone could be stimulated by oral administration of several small peptides with six to nine amino acids. The receptor for these peptides is called the growth hormone secretagogue receptor. The endogenous ligand for this peptide is ghrelin, which is produced in oxyntic cells of the gastric fundus. It has 28 amino acids with an n-octanoyl residue on the serine in the 3-position. It is encoded by a gene with the symbol GHRL (OMIM 506353, chromosome 3p26-p25), and is derived from a 117-amino-acid precursor. It stimulates food intake and reduces energy expenditure by acting on NPY/Agrp neurons that in turn inhibit anorexigenic neuromodulators that function through melanocortin and MC4R receptor. Ghrelin works in animals and human beings alike. The level is low in overweight people, suggesting that it may play a role in controlling appetite and weight gain (Cummings 2006; Abizaid et al. 2006; Theander-Carrillo 2006). Obestatin is a 23-amino-acid peptide derived from the carboxy-terminal end of the 117-amino-acid precursor of ghrelin. This peptide reduces food intake whether administered into the CNS or peripherally. It also reduces body weight gain, delays gastric emptying, and inhibits jejunal contractility. Its receptor is GPR-39, an orphan receptor with cyclic AMP as the second messenger (Zhang et al. 2005).

Glucagon-like peptide-1 is another important GI peptide for feeding that is produced in the L-cells of the intestine by processing preproglucagon into this or one of several other peptides (Figure 3.9). It has a relatively short half-life because it is cleaved by a ubiquitous dipeptidyl-dipeptidase. GLP-1 can reduce food intake when infused into normal and overweight human beings (Verdich et al. 2001). Two long-lasting derivatives of GLP-1, exenatide and liraglutide, reduce body weight when used to treat diabetics (Buse et al. Lancet 2009; Astrup et al. Lancet 2009).

Amylin is produced in the beta cell of the pancreas and is secreted along with insulin. In experimental studies, amylin reduces food intake by acting on the amylin (calcitonin-like gene product) receptor located in the hindbrain and hypothalamus (Barth et al. 2004). Pramlintide is a commercial

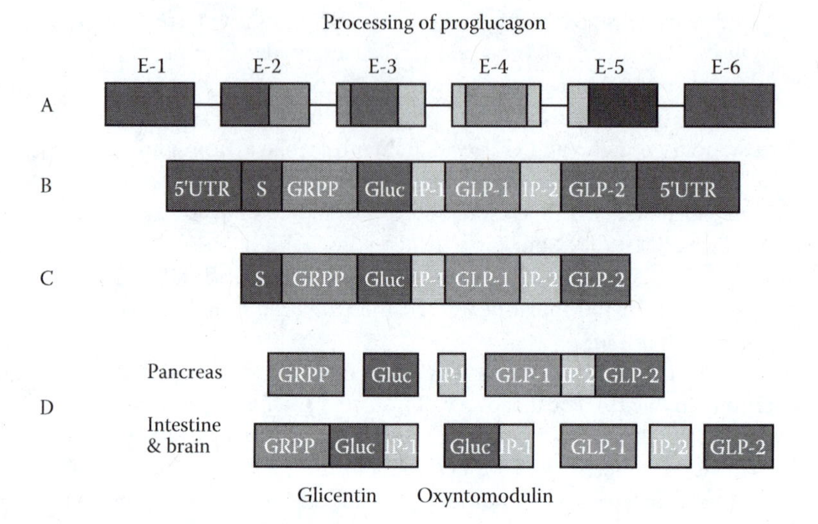

FIGURE 3.9 Structure of proglucagon and how it is processed in the intestine and pancreas to provide glucaton, glucagon-like-2 peptide, and oxyntomodulin.

analog of amylin that is currently used to treat diabetes. The combination of pramlintide with leptin produced augmented weight loss (Ravussin 2010). Pancreatic glucagon from the alpha-cells also reduces food intake in animals and humans, but most focus has been on the intestinal glucagon-like-peptide-1.

Nutrients may also be afferent signals to reduce food intake. A dip in the circulating level of glucose precedes the onset of eating in more than 50% of the meals in animals and human beings (Campfield and Smith 2003). This dip in glucose follows a small rise in insulin, and if the dip is blocked, food intake is delayed. The pattern recognized by this dip is independent of the level from which the drop in glucose begins (Campfield and Smith 2003).

The Brain and Food Intake

The brain undoubtedly plays a central role in whether or not obesity develops (Berthoud and Morrison 2008). Much emphasis has been placed on the neuroendocrine circuits involving the sensory system and gastrointestinal track feeding information to the brain that then activates efferent systems. The novel "right brain hypothesis," proposed by Alonso-Alonso and Pascual-Leone (Alonso-Alonso et al. 2007) describe unusual syndromes that disconnect the prefrontal lobes from the rest of the brain. Disconnection of the right prefrontal cortex (PFC) causes a passion for eating and a specific preference for fine food, the so-called "gourmand syndrome" (Table 3.5). In degenerative dementia, atrophy of the right PFC correlates with hyperphagia, whereas atrophy of the left PFC correlates with reduced appetite. The overeating of the Kleine-Levin syndrome is associated with hypoperfusion of the right frontal lobe as demonstrated by PET (Alonso-Alonso et al. 2007). Activation of areas in the PFC is also associated with people who are successful in maintaining weight loss. Hypoperfusion of the right frontal lobe using single photon emission computed tomography (SPECT) can be demonstrated in overeating conditions such as Kleine-Levin syndrome. In contrast, hyperactivity of the right PFC can lead to anorexia-like symptoms.

Imaging techniques have provided new insights into the role of the brain in regulating food intake and responding to stimuli that affect feeding. Areas activated by food intake include the orbitofrontal cortex, amygdale, parahippocampal gyrus, anterior fusiform gyrus, striatum, and cingulate gyrus (Pelchat et al. 2004). The technique for many of these studies involved measurement of blood oxygen level-dependent (BOLD) change during PET. It is of interest that drug and alcohol

TABLE 3.5
Areas of the Brain That Are Activated (+) or Inhibited (–) during Exposure to Food, in Response to Drugs or Alcohol, and to Leptin in a Weight-Reduced State

Area of the Brain	Activated by Food Cues	Activated by Alcohol/Drugs	Activated (+) or Inhibited (–) by Weight Loss	Activated (+) or Inhibited (–) by Leptin
Orbitofrontal cortex	+	+		
Amygdala	+	+	(–)	
Dorsolateral prefrontal	+	+		
Inferior parietal lobe				
Superior frontal gyrus				–
Middle frontal gyrus			–	+ and –
Inferior frontal gyrus			+	+ and –
Superior temporal gyrus				–
Middle temporal gyrus			+	+ and –
Middle occipital gyrus				–
Postcentral gyrus				+
Parahippocampal gyrus	+		+ and –	–
Anterior fusiform gyrus	+			
Precentral gyrus			–	
Supramarginal gyrus				
Insula	+	+		–
Striatum	+			
Anterior cingulate gyrus				

Source: Adapted from Pelchat, M.L., et al., *Neuroimage* 23(4), 1486–1493, 2004; Rosenbaum, M., et al., *J. Clin. Invest.* 118, 2583–2591, 2008.

also activate many of the same areas including the amygdale, anterior sicgulate gyrus, orbitofrontal cortex, insulin, hippocampus, caudate, and dorsolateral PFC (see Table 3.6). In the studies with leptin, individuals were studied before and after a 10% weight loss, and then after giving leptin to those who were 10% below their baseline weight. The effects of weight loss and leptin replacement are reflected in changes of activity in the hypothalamus, an area involved in integrating feeding information, and in brain areas involved in emotional responses such as the cingulated gyrus and Brodman area, and cognitive function such as the middle frontal gyrus. In the low-leptin state after weight loss, there is activity in the insula, cingulated gyrus, medial frontal gyrus, precuneus, middle occipital gyrus, superior frontal gyrus, and superior temporal gyrus (Rosenbaum et al. 2008).

The brain plays the central role as receiver, transducer, and transmitter of information from the peripheral organs (Berthoud and Morrison 2008). This control is accomplished through sensory organs and internal signals that are integrated through central neurotransmitters that in turn activate efferent neural, hormonal, and motor pathways. Diseases that affect this region, as well as the frontal leucotomies performed in the mid-1900s for psychosis, produce weight gain and overeating as common side effects.

Energy sensing in the brain may be a coordinated process that modulates feeding through the adenosine 5′monophosphate kinase (AMPK) system, which regulates the activity of two key enzymes, acetyl CoA carboboxylase and malonyl CoA carboxylase. Activation or inhibition of these enzymes by phosphorylation and dephosphorylation regulates the traffic of carbon atoms from glucose and fatty acids for oxidative processes in both the hypothalamus and liver, and possibly other key peripheral metabolic tissues (Xue and Kahn 2006; Levin et al. 2003; Bell et al. 1998).

TABLE 3.6
Weight Gain with Psychotropic Drugs

Drug Class/Type	Generic Name	Proprietary Names	Alternative Drugs That Are Weight Neutral or Weight Losing	
		Antidepressants		
Tricyclic antidepressants weight gain of 0.4 to 4.1 kg/mo; small number gain 15 to 20 kg in 2–6 months	anitriptyline	Elavil	bupropion	Wellbutrin*
		Vanatri		Wellbutrin SR*
	doxepin	Sinequan		Zypan*
	imipramine	Tofranil	nefazadone	Serzone†
	nortriptyline	Aventyl	*Black box warning for increased risk of seizure	
		Pamelor		
	tramipramine	Surmontil	† Blackbox warning for liver failure	
	metrazapine	Remeron		
Selective serotonin reuptake inhibitors (SSRI)	fluoxetine	Prozac		
	sertraline	Zoloft		
Initial weight loss followed by regain in 6 months in some patients		Sarafem		
	paroxetine	Paxil		
	fluvoxamine	Luvox		
Monoamine oxidase inhibitors (MAOIS). Weight gain less pronounced than tricyclics	phenelzine	Nardil		
	tranylcypromine	Parnate		
Lithium		Eskalith		
Gains of up to 10 kg occur in 11%–65% of patients		Eskalith SR		
		Lithobid		
Antipsychotics	haloperidol	Haldol	ziprasidone	Geodon
Weight gain very likely and variable	loxapine	Loxitane	quetiapine	Seroquel
	clozapine	Clozaril		
	risperidone	Risperdal		
	olanzapine	Zyprexa		

Source: Adapted from Pi-Sunyer, F.X. et al., *Obesity Management*, 3, 165–169, 2007.

Monoamine Receptors

Monoamines, such as norepinephrine, serotonin, dopamine, and histamine, as well as certain amino acids and neuropeptides, act through several receptors involved in the regulation of food intake. The serotonin system has been one of the most extensively studied of the monoamine pathways. Its receptors modulate both the quantity of food eaten and macronutrient selection. Stimulation of the serotonin receptors in the paraventricular nucleus reduces fat intake with little or no effect on the intake of protein or carbohydrate. This reduction in fat intake is probably mediated through 5-HT_{2C} receptors, since its effect is attenuated in mice that cannot express the 5-HT_{2C} receptor (Halford et al. 2005; Bray 2007; Bray and Greenway 1999).

Stimulation of α_1 noradrenergic receptors reduces food intake (Bray 2007; Bray and Greenway 1999), whereas stimulation of α_2 receptors increases food intake in experimental animals. A polymorphism in the α_{2a} adrenoceptor has been associated with a reduced metabolic rate in humans. Phenylpropanolamine is an α_1 agonist acting on this receptor that has a modest inhibitory effect on food intake (Wellman 2005). Some of the antagonists to the α_1 receptors that are used to treat hypertension produce weight gain, indicating that this receptor is also clinically active, but the weight gain is small. In contrast, the activation of β_2 receptors in the brain reduces food intake.

These receptors can be activated by agonist drugs (β-blockers), by releasing norepinephrine in the vicinity of these receptors, or by blocking the reuptake of norepinephrine.

Histamine receptors can modulate feeding (Masaki 2004). Stimulation of the H_1 receptor in the central nervous system reduces feeding. Experimentally, this has been utilized by modulating the H_3 autoreceptor, which controls histamine release. When the autoreceptor is stimulated, histamine secretion is reduced and food intake increases. Blockade of this H_3 autoreceptor decreases food intake. The histamine system is important in control of feeding because drugs that produce weight gain are modulators of histamine receptors.

Anticipation of hibernation or migration in animals is due to seasonally variable dopamine transmission in the suprachiasmatic nucleus, which drives the storage of food at the appropriate time of year. Loss-of-function mutations in the D2 receptor gene are associated with obesity in human beings, and dopamine antagonists can induce obesity in humans. One suggestion is that this is through modulation of nutrient partitioning, with obesity in man or fat storage in migratory and hibernating species as the results (Pijl 2003).

Peptide Receptors and Endocannabinoids

The opioid receptors were the first group of peptide receptors shown to modulate feeding. They also modulate fat intake (Barnes et al. 2006; Cowley et al. 1999). Both the mu- and kappa-opioid receptors can stimulate feeding. Stimulation of the mu-opioid receptors increases the intake of dietary fat in experimental animals.

Corticotrophin-releasing hormone (CRH) and the closely related urocortin reduce food intake and body weight in experimental animals. There are two different urocortin receptors, with food intake being modulated primarily by UR-2.

The discovery of leptin in 1994 opened a new window on the control of food intake and body weight (Bray 2007; Hida et al. 2005; Zhang 1994). This peptide is produced primarily in adipose tissue, but can also be produced in the placenta and stomach. As a placental hormone, it can be used as an indicator of trophoblastic activity in patients with trophoblastic tumors (hydatidiform moles or choriocarcinoma). Leptin is secreted into the circulation and acts on a number of tissues, with the brain being one of its most important targets. The response of leptin-deficient children to leptin indicates the critical role that this peptide plays in the control of energy balance.

Five variants of the leptin receptor have been identified. To act in the brain, leptin must be transported across the blood-brain barrier, or diffuse through the several areas that are permeable (Price 2010; Cowley et al. 1999). Once in the brain, leptin acts at several sites. Initial focus was on receptors in the arcuate nucleus near the base of the brain where it acts in a reciprocal fashion in the production and release of at least four peptides. It inhibits production of neuropeptide Y gene (NPY) and agouti-related peptide (AGRP) gene while enhancing the production of the pro-opiomelanocortin (POMC) gene, the precursor for α-melanocyte stimulating hormone (α-MSH) and cocaine- and amphetamine-related transcript (CART) (Schwartz Cowley 1999). NPY is one of the most potent stimulators of food intake. It produces these effects through interaction with either the Y-1 or the Y-5 receptor. Mice that do not make NPY have no disturbances (phenotype) in food intake or body weight.

Agouti-regulated peptide (AGRP) is the second peptide that is co-secreted with NPY into the paraventricular nucleus (PVN). This peptide antagonizes the inhibitory effect of α-MSH on food intake. Animals that overexpress AGRP overeat because the inhibitory effects of α-MSH are blocked. AGRP is a potent stimulator of fat intake as are the opioids. Using the AGRP deficient (knock-out) mouse, Barnes et al. (2010) showed that the stimulation of fat intake by opioids was blocked but total food intake was still stimulated. This implies that the stimulation of fat intake by mu-opioids involved release of agouti-related peptide.

The third peptide of interest in the arcuate nucleus is POMC, which is the precursor for several peptides, including α-MSH. There are five melanocortin receptors that mediate the effects on skin pigmentation (MCR-1), cortisol secretion from the adrenal gland (MCR-2), and in the brain that affect food intake (MCR-3 and MCR-4), and MCR-5, which is not a specific receptor. α-MSH acts on the melanocortin-3 and -4 receptors in the medial hypothalamus to reduce feeding. When these receptors are knocked out by genetic engineering, the mice become grossly overweight. In recent human studies, genetic defects in the melanocortin receptors are associated with hyperphagia and obesity. Many genetic alterations have been identified in the MCR-4 receptor, some of which are in the coding region of the gene and others in the regulatory components (Farooqi et al. 2003). Some of these genetic changes profoundly affect feeding, whereas others have little or no effect. A final peptide in the arcuate nucleus is CART. This peptide is co-localized with POMC, and like α-MSH, CART inhibits feeding.

Two other peptide systems with neurons located in the lateral hypothalamus of the brain have also been linked to the control of feeding. The first of these is melanin-concentrating hormone (MCH) (Ludwig et al. 2001). This peptide increases food intake when injected into the ventricular system of the brain. It is found almost exclusively in the lateral hypothalamus. Animals that overexpress this peptide gain weight and animals that cannot produce this peptide are lean. These observations suggest an important physiological function for MCH (Morens et al. 2005).

Orexin A, also called hypocretin, was identified in a search of G-protein-linked peptides that affect food intake. It increases food intake, but its effects are less robust than those described above. However, it does seem to play a role in sleep (Zheng et al. 2003).

Endocannabinoids acting through the cannabinoid receptor-1 are involved in modulating feeding (Pagotto et al. 2006; Richard et al. 2009). Tetrahydrocannbinol, isolated from the marijuana plant, stimulates food intake. Isolation of the cannabinoid receptor was followed by identification of two fatty acids, anandamide and 2-arachidonoylglycerol, which are endogenous ligands in the brain for this receptor. Infusion of anandamide or 2-arachidonoylglycerol into the brain stimulates food intake.

The cannabinoid-1 (CB-1) receptor is a preganglionic receptor, meaning that its activation inhibits synaptic transmission. Antagonists to this receptor have been shown to reduce food intake and lead to weight loss. There is also a peripheral ligand, oleylethanolamide, which inhibits food intake.

A recent addition to the list of peptides involved in feeding is the arginine-phenylalanine-amide group (called RFa). The first of these peptides was isolated from a mollusk and had only four amino acids. The structure of the RFa peptides is highly conserved, with nearly 80% homology between the frog, rat, cow, and humans (Dockray 2004). In mammals there are five genes and five receptors for these peptides. The 26- and 43-amino-acid members of the RFa peptide family stimulate feeding in mammals (Primeaux et al. 2008) and are the ligands for two orphan G-protein-coupled receptors located in the lateral hypothalamus and the ventromedial nucleus. This family of peptides has been involved in feeding from early phylogetic times including *Caenorhabdis elegans*. Their role in human beings is not yet established.

Nesfatin/nucleobindin 2 (NUCB2) is expressed hypothalamic and brainstem nuclei. Nesfatin/NUCB2 expression in the paraventricular nucleus was modulated by starvation and refeeding. Administration of nesfatin-1 into the ventricular system of the brain inhibited food intake for 6 hours in male Wistar rats in a dose-dependent manner. Nesfatin-1 and its mid-segment (M30) also act peripherally to inhibit food intake for 3 hours in male mice. It also inhibited food intake in leptin-resistant obese animals (ob/ob mice; db/db mice, and mice fed 45% fat diets). Intraperitoneal administration of nesfatin-1 (M30) increased expression of genes for proopiomelanocortin and cocaine- and amphetamine-related peptide in the nucleus of the solitary tract of mice. Intranasal administration of nesfatin-1 significantly inhibited food intake for 6 hours in male Wistar rats (Shimizu et al. 2009).

Neuropeptide W is the endogenous ligand for 2 G-protein coupled receptors, GPR7 and GPR8, that are expressed in the central nervous system. Administration of NPW into the ventricular system of rats increased food intake and stimulated prolactin release (Shimomura et al. 2003). Injection of the 23-amino-acid form of NPW into the paraventricular nucleus at doses ranging from 0.1 to 3 nmol increased feeding for up to 4 h, and doses ranging from 0.3 to 3 nmol increased feeding for up to 24 h. In contrast, only the 3-nmol dose of NPW increased feeding after administration into the lateral hypothalamus. NPW may thus have a modulatory role in feeding (Levine et al. 2005).

Neural and Hormonal Control of Metabolism

The motor system for acquisition of food and the endocrine and autonomic nervous systems provide the major efferent systems involved with acquiring food and regulating body fat stores. Among the endocrine controls are growth hormone, thyroid hormone, gonadal steroids (testosterone and estrogens), glucocorticoids, and insulin.

During growth, thyroid hormone and growth hormone work together to increase linear growth. At puberty, gonadal steroids enter the picture and lead to shifts in the relationship of body fat to lean body mass in boys and girls. A distinctive role for growth hormone has been suggested from studies with transgenic mice overexpressing growth hormone in the central nervous system. These mice are hyperphagic and obese, and show increased expression of neuropeptide Y and agouti-related protein as well as marked hyperinsulinemia and peripheral insulin resistance (Bohlooly-Y et al. 2005).

Testosterone increases lean mass relative to fat and reduces visceral fat. Estrogen has the opposite effect. Testosterone levels fall as human males grow older, and there is a corresponding increase in visceral and total body fat and a decrease in lean body mass in older men (Stanworth et al. 2008). This may be compounded by the decline in growth hormone that is also associated with an increase in fat relative to lean mass, particularly visceral fat (Bartke 2008).

Glucocorticoids may also be important in modulating fatness. One recent finding suggests that the activity of the enzyme 11-β-hydroxysteroid dehydrogenase type 1, which reversibly converts cortisone to cortisol, may be important in peripheral tissues in determining the quantity of visceral adipose tissue (Morton and Seckl 2008; Kannisto et al. 2004). Changes in the activity of this enzyme may also contribute to the risk of women of developing more visceral fat after menopause. A high level of this enzyme keeps the quantity of cortisol in visceral fat high and may provide a fertile ground for developing new fat cells.

The sympathetic nervous system is an important link between the brain and peripheral metabolism. It appears to be involved in the oscillation of fatty acids in visceral fat that accompanies the increased fat as dogs overeat a high-fat diet (Hucking et al. 2003). Using genetic homologous recombination (knock-out), mice lacking the β1, β2, and β3 receptors have been produced. These animals show normophagic obesity with cold intolerance. They have higher circulating levels of free fatty acids. Thus, sympathetic nervous system function is essential to prevent obesity and to resist cold (Himenex et al. 2002; Travernier et al. 2005).

In this chapter, I have tried to provide a snapshot of our understanding of the regulatory systems for factors involved in energy homeostasis that are etiologic in obesity. I have reviewed both epidemiologic and metabolic feed-back models in assembling this information. We have not reached the end of the story. However, it is clear that we have a much better glimpse into its operation—one that can provide us a better framework for thinking about both the etiology of obesity and its possible treatments.

4 Effects of Obesity on Health and Metabolism

KEY POINTS

- Overweight increases the risk of death.
- Underweight increases the risk of death.
- Detecting the levels of overweight that are clinically important requires either large epidemiological samples or smaller samples of subjects followed for an extended period of time.
- Early analysis of epidemiological studies has led to the conclusion that overweight is not a risk for early mortality, but this is an error.
- The metabolic syndrome, as a collection of signs and clinical findings, predicts heart disease and diabetes.
- The pathological basis for overweight is an increase in the size of fat cells.
- Increased numbers of fat cells may also contribute in some individuals.
- Large fat cells secrete a variety of peptides that can be pathogenetic for various conditions associated with overweight.
- Diseases associated with overweight can be divided into those that cause these effects through the enlarged fat cells and those that result from the increased mass of fat.
- The metabolic syndrome reflects the response to factors produced from fat cells.
- Weight loss reverses all of the associated risks.
- Only small amounts of weight loss are needed to significantly reduce the risk of developing diabetes in high-risk populations.
- Maintaining weight loss reduces the need for antihypertensive medication.
- Overweight increases hospitalization, use of the medical care system, and increases overall health care costs into old age.

INTRODUCTION

We start with the premise that we all want to have a healthy weight, and that no one wants to be labeled obese. One reason for this is self-image and another is that excessive weight is a harbinger of ill-health. In this chapter, I will develop the historical context for this understanding and then provide ideas about how fatness produces these problems. Overweight will refer to any individual whose body weight is above 25kg/m^2 (see Chapter 1). Some individuals who are overweight are not at risk from this weight—athletes and naturally muscular people. However, for most of the population, the rise in body weight with age is associated with increased fatness and the ill health it produces if the BMI exceeds 30 kg/m^2 (see Chapter 2).

HISTORICAL CONTEXT FOR THE RISKS OF OVERWEIGHT AS A DISEASE

More than 2500 years ago, a physician named Hippocrates, often called the "father" of medicine, recognized that people who were overweight had increased risk for sudden death. This theme was repeated throughout the eighteenth and nineteenth century, affirming that obesity is a disease. Quotes

Malcolm Flemyng (?–1764) clearly articulated the idea of obesity as a disease in 1760 in the second monograph on obesity (Flemyng 1760). The date of his birth is unknown, but was in the early eighteenth century. There is little information about Flemyng's early life. His medical studies were at Leyden where he was a contemporary of Haller and a student under the esteemed Hermann Boerhaave. He returned to Scotland and began the practice of medicine around 1725, but shortly afterward moved to Hull. In 1751, he moved to London with his three children when the life of a country practitioner had taken a toll on his health. He taught one course of physiology lessons in 1751–52, but then moved to Brigg in Lincolnshire. From his correspondence with Haller we know he was hopeful of teaching physiology at Oxford or Cambridge. Flemyng was both an experimenter and a clinician. His contribution relevant to us is "On Corpulency" read to the Royal Society in 1757 and published in 1760. It was translated into German by J.J. Plenk at Vienna in 1769 and reprinted in London as late as 1810. Flemyng continued to practice medicine in Lincolnshire until his death on March 7, 1764 (Bray 2007, p. 70).

from several are presented here as a prelude to the detailed documentation of these health risks and the benefits of weight loss that have been published during the twentieth century.

Dr. Malcolm Flemyng, an eighteenth century physician wrote one of the two earliest books on overweight in the English language. In it, he said this about the risks of obesity or, as he called it, corpulency:

> Corpulency, when in an extraordinary degree, may be reckoned a disease, as it in some measure obstructs the free exercise of the animal functions; and hath a tendency to shorten life, by paving the way to dangerous distempers. (Flemyng 1760)

The idea that excess fat obstructs the free and normal function of the body and tends to shorten life was articulated by William Wadd, Surgeon Extraordinary to King George IV, who said:

> Fat is, of all the humours or substances forming part of the human body, the most diffused; a certain proportion of it is indicative of health, and denotes being in good condition—nay, is even conducive to beauty; but when in excess—amounting to what may be termed OBESITY—it is not only in itself a disease, but may be the cause of many fatal effects, particularly in acute disorders (Wadd 1810).

At about the same time, Robert Thomas, quoted in D. Haslam (2007), noted "Corpulency, when it arrives at a certain height, becomes an absolute disease." Near the end of the nineteenth century, James Wood in "The Relation of Alimentation to Some Diseases" noted, "The accumulation of fat in the tissues, or obesity, is a pathological or diseased condition."

COSTS OF OBESITY

One consequence of obesity as a disease is its costs; obesity is an expensive disease. In 1998, the medical costs of obesity were estimated to be as high as $78.5 billion, with roughly half of the amount financed by Medicare and Medicaid (Thompson and Wolf 2001). Costs have continued to rise. The overall expenditure estimated in 2004 was $75 billion or 5.7% of the health care budget. For Medicare, it was 6.8% (17.7 billion), and for Medicaid 10.6% (21.3 billion) (Finkelstein et al. 2004). In a more recent analysis, Finkelstein et al. found that the increased prevalence of obesity is responsible for almost $40 billion of increased medical spending through 2006, including $7 billion in Medicare prescription drug costs. They estimated that the medical costs of obesity could rise to $147 billion per year by 2008 (Finkelstein et al. 2004, 2008, 2009; Trogdon 2008). If all of

TABLE 4.1
Health Costs Related to Obesity

Item	Cost in Billions
Food	$90 billion
Large size clothing	$30 billion
Weight loss programs	$20 billion
Out of pocket	$20 billion
Medicare/Medicaid	$60 billion
Commercial payers	$80 billion
Absenteeism	$30 billion
Presenteeism (low productivity)	$70 billion
Short-term disability	$30 billion
Other	$20 billion
Total	$450 billion

Source: Kinsey & Co. Reimbursement Presentation, personal communication, 2009.

the components of the costs related to obesity are included, one can reach a figure of nearly $500 billion (Table 4.1). In a review of articles from 1990 to 2009, Withrow and Alter (2010) found that obesity accounted for 0.2% to 2.8% of the country's health care expenditure, and that medical costs for obese individuals were about 30% higher than for people of normal weight.

Obesity increased disability costs (Sturm et al. 2004; Visscher et al. 2004; Alley and Chang 2007; Neovius 2008). Finnish men and women of ages 20 to 64 years experienced 0.63 years of disability at work, 0.36 years of coronary heart disease, and 1.68 years more use of long-term medication than their normal weight counterparts (Visscher et al. 2004).

Hospital costs and use of medication also increase with the degree of obesity (Trasande et al. 2009; Folmann et al. 2007). In a large health maintenance organization, mean annual costs were 25% higher in participants with a BMI between 30–35 kg/m^2 and 44% higher in those with a BMI greater than 35 kg/m^2 compared to individuals with a BMI between 20 and 25 kg/m^2 (Quesenberry et al. 1998). Costs for lifetime treatment of hypertension, hypercholesterolemia, type 2 diabetes, heart disease, and stroke in men and women with a BMI of 37.5 kg/m^2 were $10,000 higher than for men and women with a BMI of 22.5 kg/m^2, according to data from the National Center for Health Statistics and the Framingham Heart Study (Thompson et al. 1999). Sturm showed that the percentage of health care costs related to obesity for both men and women rose from 7% in 1985 to nearly 20% in 2000 for women and from 10% to 22% by 2000 in men (Sturm 2004). Lakdawalla found that obesity contributed significantly to disability between ages 20 and 50 (Lakdawalla 2004).

The expenditures by Medicare for health care from age 65 to age 83 (or death) were related to the body mass index in 1967–73, nearly 40 years earlier. There was a graded increase in total costs with each higher category of BMI from a normal BMI of 18.5 to 25 to overweight (BMI 25–30) and Grade I and II obesity (BMI 30–34.9 and BMI > 35) (see Figure 4.1) (Daviglus et al. 2004). A second examination of midlife weight status on mortality and hospitalization later in life from cardiovascular disease used the Chicago Heart Association Detection Project in Industry study (Yan et al. 2006). In this predominantly white cohort, risk of hospitalization and mortality was higher in all overweight people who survived to age 65 years and older than in those with normal weight who had a similar cardiovascular risk profile at ages 31–64. Obesity identified at the time of military conscription among 1,191,027 Swedish men evaluated between 1969 through 1995 increased the risk of future disability pensions (Neovius et al. 2008). Allison estimates that lifetime costs associated with grade I obesity were 4.3%.

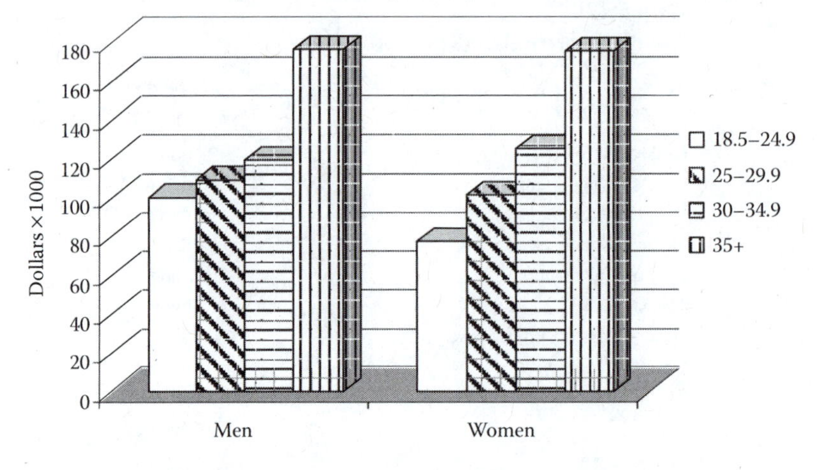

FIGURE 4.1 Relation of Medicare costs between ages 65 and 83 (or death) and the body mass index determined at age 45. (Adapted from Daviglus, M.L., et al., *JAMA*, 292(22), 2743–2749, 2004.)

In addition to the health care costs, there is increased use of medical services. Sturm, using the Healthcare for Communities Survey from 1998, found that annual medical expenditures were 36% higher in the grade I obesity (BMI > 30–35 kg/m^2) than for normal weight individuals (Sturm 2002). Finkelstein et al., using the Medical Expenditure Panel Survey, also found increased costs ranging from 26% for Medicare recipients to 39% for Medicaid recipients (Finkelstein et al. 2003). Both Quesenberry et al. and Thompson et al. have found that obese adults (BMI > 30 kg/m^2) have more physician visits and use more health-related resources such as medication, particularly diabetic medications, than normal weight individuals (Quesenberry et al. 1998; Thompson et al. 2001). This effect is evident in both adults and children. Obesity-associated hospitalizations, charges, and costs for children between 1999–2005 were obtained from a nationally representative sample of admissions to U.S. hospitals. In the interval from 1999 to 2005, hospitalizations for children nearly doubled when a diagnosis of obesity was present and this was reflected in an increase in costs from $125.9 million to 237.6 million (in 2005 dollars) between 2001 and 2005. Medicaid appears to bear a large burden of hospitalizations for conditions that occur along with obesity, while private payers pay a greater portion of hospitalization costs to treat obesity itself (Trasande et al. 2009).

Claims for employees at the Duke University Medical Center were evaluated and 11,728 individuals were followed up to 8 years. The number and cost of claims increased as the BMI increased with a 12-fold gradient between BMI 18.5 to 25 versus BMI > 40 kg/m^2. After adjusting for age, ethnicity, etc., the increase was reduced to 7.71-fold (Ostbye 2007). The main factors were injury to the limbs and back.

THE PATHOLOGY OF OBESITY

A number of bodily systems are affected by obesity. These are summarized in Table 4.2 (see also Figure 4.2). The remainder of this chapter will review these issues in more detail. These pathological changes can result from an increase in body weight itself or through the metabolic effect from the various adipokines secreted by enlarged fat cells.

BIG FAT CELLS

The etiology of obesity is an imbalance between the energy ingested in food and the energy expended. The excess energy is stored in fat cells that enlarge in size and/or increase in number. It

TABLE 4.2
Relative Risk of Health Problems Associated with Obesity in Developed Countries

Greatly Increased (Relative Risk > 3)	Moderately Increased (Relative Risk 2–3)	Slightly Increased (Relative Risk 1–2)
Diabetes	Coronary heart disease	Cancer (breast cancer in post-menopausal women, endometrial cancer, colon cancer)
Gallbladder disease	Osteoarthritis (knees)	Reproductive hormone abnormalities
Hypertension	Hyperuricemia and gout	Polycystic ovary syndrome
Dyslipidemia		Impaired fertility
Insulin resistance		Low back pain from obesity
Breathlessness		Increased anesthetic risk
Sleep apnea		Fetal defects from maternal obesity

Source: Adapted from World Health Organization, *Obesity: Preventing and Managing the Global Epidemic*. Report of a WHO Consultation on Obesity, Geneva, 1997.

is this hyperplasia and hypertrophy of these fat cells that is the pathologic lesion of the overweight patient. Enlarged fat cells produce the clinical problems associated with overweight either because of the weight or mass of the extra fat or because of the increased secretion of free fatty acids and numerous peptides from enlarged fat cells. Fat cells store and release fatty acids that flow to the liver and can modulate hepatic metabolism of insulin. Fat cells also secrete a variety of adipokines (adiponectin and visfatin) and cytokines (tumor necrosis factor-α and interleukin-6) that also flow to the liver and may provide part of the inflammatory environment that goes with being overweight. Finally, the secretion of leptin from fat cells provides a signal to the brain about the size of fat stores in the body. The fat cell, then, is an endocrine cell and adipose tissue is an endocrine organ. It is the hypertrophy and/or hyperplasia of this organ that is the pathologic lesion in overweight. One lesson of the late twentieth century was that "stress" as reflected in a rise in the activity of the hypothalamic pituitary adrenal axis was associated with increased visceral fat (Bjorntorp 2001).

Visceral Fat Cells and Central Adiposity

Visceral fat cells are very important units in the pathologic process that we call obesity. Visceral adipocytes are located strategically since they empty their products into the portal vein that flows initially through the liver. Thus, adipokines from visceral fat cells reach the liver in higher concentrations from these cells than from peripheral fat cells. Visceral fat cells also respond differentially to some drugs, particularly thiazolidinediones (glitazones) which increase subcutaneous fat without a significant change in visceral fat (Smith, De Jonge et al. 2005).

The recognition that central fat, and visceral fat in particular, is a health risk is a concept of the twentieth century. The insurance industry noted at the beginning of the twentieth century that

Professor Jean Vague (1911–2002) pioneered studies after World War II that identified an android or central type of adiposity as a risk for developing diabetes and heart disease. Jean Vague was born in 1911 and received his undergraduate education in Aix-en-Provence and his medical education at the University of Marseilles. Following an internship at the Hôtel Dieu Conception in Marseilles, he began his medical practice and research in endocrinology and rose through the ranks at the university to become professor in 1957. He served in the French army and was decorated with the Legion of Honor. Among many other distinctions, he is a member of the French Academy of Medicine (Bray 2007, p. 323; Haslam 2009, pp. 17–18; Jaffiol 2004).

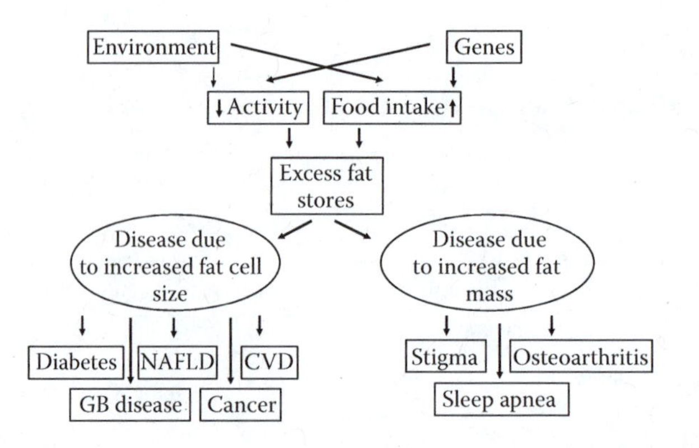

FIGURE 4.2 A model for the pathological changes associated with overweight, divided into those related to the metabolic changes associated with increased fat cell size and those related to the increased mass of fat.

obesity was a risk. In two short pieces in the transactions of the Actuarial Society of America published in 1901–1903 and 1904 (Actuarial Society of America 1901–1903; Weeks 1904), they noted that central fatness carried increased risk. It was nearly 50 years before the theme was taken up again by Jean Vague in France. Working after World War II, he recognized that women with "android obesity," that is obesity having a male pattern of distribution, had a higher risk for diabetes and cardiovascular risk than women with a lower body fat or gynoid distribution (Vague 1947, 1956). The method he used to make his measurements—the adipogenic index—was complex to use and it wasn't until the waist circumference and the ratio of the waist divided by the hip circumference came along that this important idea was readily recognized.

The accumulation of fat in visceral fat cells is modulated by a number of factors. Androgens and estrogen produced by the gonads and adrenals, as well as peripheral conversion of Δ^4-androstenedione to estrone in stromal cells in fat tissue are pivotal in regulating fat distribution and the estrogen levels of postmenopausal women. Male or android fat distribution and female or gynoid fat distribution develop during adolescence and can show further changes during adult life. The increasing accumulation of visceral fat in adult life is also related to gender, but the effects of cortisol, decreasing growth hormone, and decreasing testosterone levels are important in age-related fat deposition. Increased visceral fat enhances the degree of insulin resistance associated with overweight and hyperinsulinemia. Together, hyperinsulinemia and insulin resistance enhance the risk of the comorbidities described below.

Increased Fat Mass

Although fat cells were once thought to form primarily during growth, recent data suggest that adipocytes form throughout life (Spalding et al. 2008). The most marked expansion of the lineage occurs during the postnatal period. Most adipocytes descend from a pool of these proliferating progenitors that are already committed, either prenatally or early in postnatal life. These progenitors reside in the mural cell compartment of the adipose vasculature, but not in the vasculature of other tissues. Thus, the adipose vasculature appears to function as a progenitor niche and may provide signals for adipocyte development (Zeve et al. 2008).

In addition to the pathology produced by enlarged fat cells, additional pathology results from the extra mass of tissue and the effort that it requires for the overweight individual to move this extra mass. The consequences of these two mechanisms, increased fat cell size and increased fat mass, are diseases such as diabetes mellitus, gallbladder disease, osteoarthritis, heart disease, and some forms of cancer that are the hallmark of obesity as a disease (Bray 2004). The spectrum of medical, social, and psychological disabilities includes a range of medical and behavioral problems (Bray 2007).

Body fat also influences initiation of menstruation and the reproductive cycle. This important relationship was recognized by Rose Frisch (1978). She noted that menstruation occurred only after body fat in girls reached a threshold amount. If it subsequently fell to low levels, menstruation often stops (Frisch 1978).

THE PATHOPHYSIOLOGY OF CENTRAL AND TOTAL FAT

Risks Related to Enlarged Fat Cells and Central Adiposity

Excess Mortality

Data showing the relation of obesity to excess mortality have been published since the beginning of the twentieth century by the life insurance industry (Actuarial Society of America 1913). Concern for excess weight as a health problem attracted the attention of the life insurance industry because they pay money when people die. If excess weight carries increased risk of dying, they care. For people who were overweight, purchasing life insurance policies would be more expensive due to higher premiums. Beginning in 1913, the life insurance industry identified overweight as a risk for early mortality and then published tables of "ideal" or "desirable" weights—those weights associated with the lowest risks of mortality from overweight were in use until after 1980 when they were replaced by the Body Mass Index (BMI). The relationship that they found is shown in Figure 4.3.

The life insurance data were replicated in several other insurance studies during the twentieth century. One of the best known is the data from the Build and Blood Pressure Study of 1959. They showed the "J"-shaped relationship that has characterized almost all of the reports during the twentieth century. This data is shown in Figure 4.4.

Although the life insurance companies repeated their messages throughout the twentieth century, not everyone was convinced. There were several reasons for this. First, information developed from life insurance statistics did not represent the population as a whole—most insured people were men (90%) and most were white. To determine the truth of the assertion that "overweight is risking fate," a number of other epidemiological studies were started, many of which continue today.

A large study published in 2009 was a "déjà vu all over again" to use a saying from the great New York Yankees baseball player, Yogi Berra. This study pooled data from nearly 900,000 individuals (Whitlock et al. 2009). It showed, as did the earlier life insurance data, that the minimal mortality was at a BMI between 22.5 and 25 kg/m^2. It showed that increased body weight was

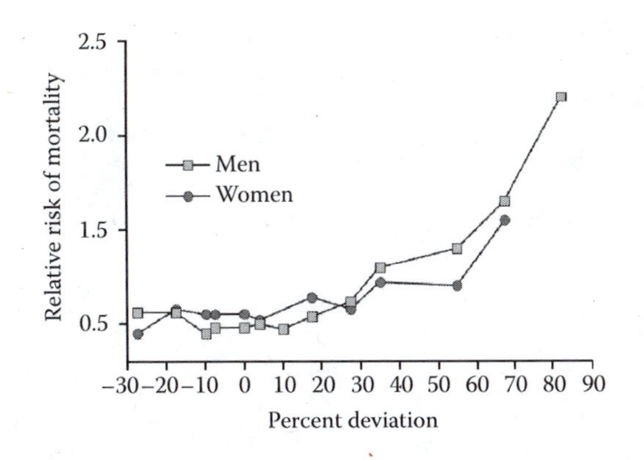

FIGURE 4.3 Relation of relative body weight to excess mortality. (Data from Actuarial Society of America and Association of Life Insurance Directors. *Medico-Actuarial Mortality Investigation*, Vol. 2, pp 5–9, 44–47. New York, 1913.)

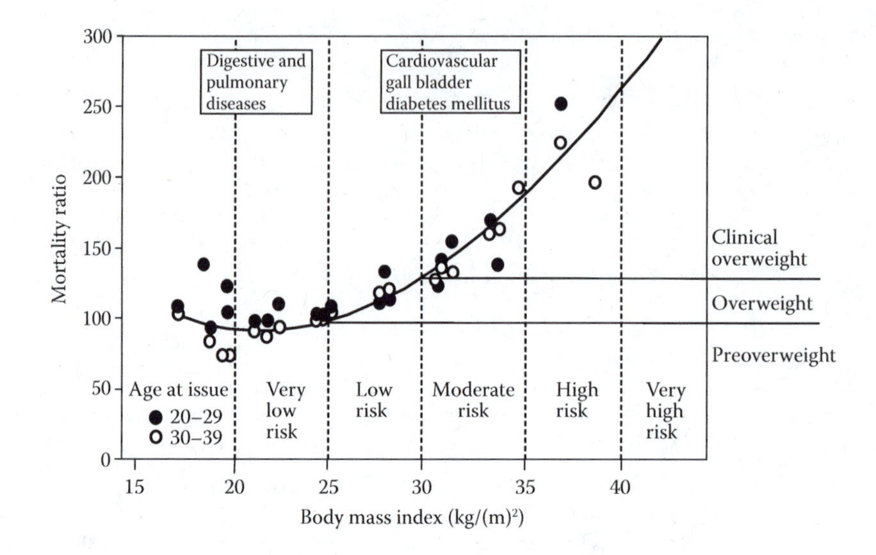

FIGURE 4.4 The body mass index has a curvilinear relationship to all-cause mortality.

associated with increased mortality and increased risk for diabetes, heart disease, gall bladder disease, and kidney disease. A strong relationship between body weight and mortality has been found consistently in most, although not all, studies for over 100 years (Sjostrom 1992). This is illustrated by the data obtained by pooling 57 studies with nearly 900,000 people. This curvilinear relationship is shown in Figure 4.4. For each 5-unit increase in BMI, there is a 20%–30% increase in mortality.

A number of other studies are entirely consistent with this set of findings as shown in Table 4.3. A decrease in life expectancy with increased fat mass and enlarged fat cells has been shown in many studies beginning with the life insurance data described earlier. One of the largest studies to examine the influence of ethnic differences used the Cancer Prevention Study II database, which enrolled more than 1 million people with nearly equal numbers of men and women. Among healthy people who never smoked, the nadir in BMI for longevity was between 23.5 and 24.9 in men and 22.0 and 23.4 in women. Among the heaviest individuals, relative risk of death increased by 2.58 for white men and 2.0 for white women. Black men and women had a lower relative risk with increasing body mass index. These authors concluded that over the range of BMI, there was an increased risk of death as BMI increased from all causes with cardiovascular disease (CVD) and cancer leading the list (Table 4.4).

TABLE 4.3
Change in Mortality Risk for Each Increase of Five BMI Units

Source of Mortality	Hazard Ratio	Percent Increase
Overall	1.29	30%
Cardiovascular	1.41	40%
Diabetic	2.16	120%
Renal	1.59	60%
Hepatic	1.82	80%
Neoplastic	1.10	10%

Source: Adapted from Prospective Studies Collaboration, *Lancet*, 373(9669), 1083–1096, 2009.

TABLE 4.4
Some of the Studies Relating BMI and Mortality since 1992

Author and Year	Population	No Participants	Follow-Up	BMI and Obesity		Comments
				25–30	>30	
Must 1992	Harvard Growth Study (M & F)	508		RR 1.8		Adolescent weight on adult mortality
Manson 1995	Nurses Health Study (F)	>110,000	16 years			
Calle 1999	Cancer Society I (M & F)	>1,000,000	14 years	RR 2.58 M	RR 2.00 F	Self-reported weight and height
Calle 2003		>900,000		5.2%	6.2%	Cancer deaths
Ni Mhurchu 2004	33 Asian cohorts	>300,000				Stroke—not death
Whiteman 2005	Cancer and Steroid Hormone Study (F)	>1300	14.6 years			
Flegal 2005	3 NHANES 1971–1974, 1976–1980, 1988–1994 (M & F)			No	Yes	
Pischon 2006	European Prospective Investigation on Cancer and Nutrition	>350,000	9.7 years	Yes	Yes	Waist and WHR and BMI
Jee 2006	Korean representative sample M & F	>1,200,000	12 years	Yes	Yes	
Mark 2005						
Calle 2005						
Price 2006	53 Family Practices in UK	>14,000	5.9 years	No	No	Subjects older than 75 years
Adams 2006	NIH-AARP (M & F)	>500,000	10 years	yes	Yes	Self-reported weight and height
McTigue 2006	Women's Health Initiative Observational Study	>90,000	7 years	Yes	Yes	
Freedman 2006	US Radiologic Technologists (M & F)	>80,000	14.7 years	Yes	Yes	
Gu 2006	Chinese M & F	>150,000	8–9 years	Yes	Yes	
Lawlor 2006	2 Scottish Towns (M & F)	>15,000	28 to 34 years	Yes	Yes	
Yan 2006	Chicago Heart Association Detection Project	>17,000	32	Yes	Yes	

(*continued*)

TABLE 4.4 (Continued)
Some of the Studies Relating BMI and Mortality since 1992

Author and Year	Population	No Participants	Follow-Up	BMI and Obesity		Comments
				25–30	>30	
Smith 2007	Chinese	>200,000	10 years	Yes	—	Inverse relation of BMI to death from esophageal carcinoma
Reeves 2007	Million Women Study	>1,200,000	5.4 to 7 years	Yes	Yes	
Simpson 2007	Melbourne Collaborative Cohort Study (M & F)	>40,000	11 years	Yes	Yes	Height, weight, and waist measured. BIA for fat
Moore 2008	Female Prospective Cohort	>50,000	10 years	Yes	Yes	Height and weight measured
Koster 2008	NIH-AARP	>225,000	9 years	Yes	Yes	BMI and smoking are independent predictors of mortality
Bjorge 2008	Norwegian Health Survey	>225,000	31.5 years			Adolescents
Matsuo 2008	Japanese	>90,000	10 years			
Zhou 2008	Chinese men	<200,000	10 years	Yes	NA	Stroke mortality BMI effect > 25
Whitlock 2009	57 pooled studies (M & F)	>890,000	Variable	Yes	Yes	Pooled data analysis

More than 2000 deaths occurred during the 14 years of follow-up in the Framingham Study. Using data from this study, Peeters et al. estimated that nonsmoking women who were overweight (BMI 25 to <30 kg/m^2) at age 40 lost 3.3 years and nonsmoking men lost 3.1 years compared to normal weight men and women (Peeters et al. 2003). Nonsmoking women with a BMI > 30 kg/m^2 lost 7.1 years and nonsmoking men lost 5.8 years compared to those with a BMI < 25 kg/m^2. Fontaine et al. (2003) using data from the Third Health and Nutrition Examination Survey found that the optimal BMI for longevity in whites was a BMI between 23 and 25, and in blacks was between 23 and 30 kg/m^2. Thirteen years of life were lost with a BMI > 45 kg/m^2 for white men and 8 years for white women. The effect on years of life lost in black women was considerably less, suggesting important ethnic differences in the health impact of overweight. Indeed, Olshansky et al. (2005) have concluded that there might be a decline in longevity in the United States related to the burgeoning epidemic of overweight.

The mortality associated with excess weight increases as the degree of overweight increases. One study estimated that between 280,000 and 325,000 deaths could be attributed to overweight annually in the United States (Allison, Fontaine et al. 1999). More than 80 percent of these deaths occur among people with a BMI > 30 kg/m^2. When the impact of a sedentary lifestyle is coupled with poor diet, the Centers for Disease Control and Prevention estimated that an extra 365,000 lives may be lost per year, putting these lifestyle issues just behind smoking as a leading cause of death in the United States (CDC 2005). A more recent estimate decreased the number of excess deaths to 112,000 (Flegal et al. 2005). Since all of these studies used the same data sources (NHANES I, II, and III), but with different assumptions, there remains uncertainty about the actual number of excess deaths. In a 10-year follow-up of the Breast Cancer Detection Demonstration Project cohort where height and weight were directly measured, Moore et al. (2008) showed that there was an increased risk of mortality across the range of overweight and obesity, regardless of disease and smoking history.

As the BMI increases, there is a curvilinear rise in excess mortality (Figure 4.4) (Bray 2003). In an analysis of BMI and mortality among 32,000 Japanese men and 61,916 Japanese women, the nadir for mortality occurred at a BMI of 23.4 kg/m^2 for men ages 40–59 and 25.3 kg/m^2 for men ages 60–79 and 21.6 kg/m^2 for women ages 40–59 and 23.4 kg/m^2 for women age 60–79 (Matsuo et al. 2008). This excess mortality rises more rapidly when the BMI is above 30 kg/m^2. A BMI over 40 kg/m^2 is associated with a further increase in overall risk and for the risk of sudden death.

The Women's Health Initiative Observational Study has provided 7 years of follow-up on all-cause mortality in relation to baseline BMI in 90,185 women. Compared to normal weight women, white women had no increase in the hazard ratio for all-cause deaths in the obese woman (BMI 25–29.9), but an increase to 1.18 for overweight class I (BMI 30–34.9), 1.49 for overweight class II (BMI 35–39.9), and 2.12 for overweight class III (BMI > 40 kg/m^2). Black women showed an increase in mortality at each increasing level of BMI (1.11 for overweight; 1.36 for obesity I; 2.00 for obesity II; 1.59 for obesity III—BMI > 40 kg/m^2). A similar graded increase was seen in coronary heart disease mortality and coronary heart disease incidence. Diabetes and hypertension were significant contributors to excessive mortality (McTigue et al. 2006).

Several studies published after 2005 again show the relationship between increasing body weight or body mass index and mortality (Freedman et al. 2006; van Dam et al. 2006; Price et al. 2006; Jee et al. 2006; Yan et al. 2006). Adams et al. (2006) did a 10-year follow-up of mortality using the NIH-AARP cohort of 527,265 men and women aged 50 to 71 years. In this group there were 61,317 deaths during follow-up. There was a "U"-shaped relation of BMI and mortality. Using a BMI of 23.5 to 24.9 kg/m^2 as an index BMI, there was increased mortality in the obese and in those with a BMI < 23.5 kg/m^2. Among women there was a small but significant increase in mortality with a BMI of 28.0 to 29.9 kg/m^2. In the Korean Study (Jee et al. 2006) 1.2 million people were included—about 11% of the adult Korean population. Men had an average age of 45 and women 49 years of age. Minimal mortality occurred at a BMI of 23.0 to 24.9 kg/m^2. There was increased mortality among nonsmokers with a BMI above 28. Cardiovascular deaths increased in men with a BMI between 25.0 and 26.4 kg/m^2 and for women between 16.5 and 27.9 kg/m^2. In this same population a low BMI (<18.5 kg/m^2) or a high BMI (≥35 kg/m^2) increased the risk of mortality 6 to 8 times compared to people with a normal BMI. Current smokers with a large waist circumference had a mortality risk about five times that of never smokers with a waist circumference in the second quintile (Koster et al. 2008).

There are at least three important reasons for the differences in estimates of excess mortality associated with overweight. The first is the way in which the comparison group is selected, the second is the size of the sample, and the third is the duration of follow-up. In the large population studies (Manson et al. 1995; Calle et al. 1999; Waaler and Lund 1983), the lowest mortality is associated with a BMI of 22–23 kg/m^2. As the BMI rises on either side of this lowest mortality, there is an increase in mortality. A re-examination of the original data from the Waaler trial showed that the relationship of BMI to the risk of mortality was not significantly affected by omitting socioeconomic status or educational level, except for type 2 diabetes mellitus, where the effect of BMI and height were substantially lower for both adults and adolescents (Koch 2010). When desirable body weights were obtained from life insurance tables, the normal body weight range was from a BMI of about 20 to 25 kg/m^2 for men and 19 to 24 kg/m^2 for women (Bray 1978). When the BMI was adopted by the NHLBI and WHO in 1998, they selected a lower limit of 18.5 for a BMI with the normal range of 18.5 to 25 kg/m^2. As seen in Figure 4.4, including this lower limit increased the number of people in the normal range. It also raises the overall mortality within the normal range because the risk of death rises when the BMI either falls below or rises above the minimal death rate, which is at a BMI of about 22–23 kg/m^2. When the relative risk of mortality for those with a BMI of 25–30 kg/m^2 is compared to the reference, it depends on what the reference number is as to the result you get. Within the range of BMIs from 18.5 kg/m^2 to 25 kg/m^2, there are more deaths in the short-term NCHS follow-up (Flegal et al. 2005) than among those with a BMI between 25 to 30 kg/m^2, suggesting, erroneously in my view, that it is better to be overweight than normal weight. If the comparison range were 20 to 25 kg/m^2, the relative difference within the 25–30 kg/m^2 category would be reduced. If the comparison were from 22 kg/m^2, the minimal death rate and the relative risk for a BMI of 25 to 30 kg/m^2 would be higher. Furthermore, if the study were of longer duration, we could be more confident of the death rates. Thus, the selection of BMI values becomes an important consideration in the conclusion that is reached (Flegal et al. 2005). Since few Americans or Europeans have BMI values below 20, including the range from 18.5 to 20 kg/m^2, this makes the slightly overweight group look better.

A second consideration in evaluating studies dealing with overweight and mortality is the duration of follow-up (Figure 4.5). Short-term follow-up tends to bias the results. As Sjostrom noted in his review of BMI and mortality (Sjostrom 1992), the BMI predicted increased mortality with large population groups followed for a short time or with smaller groups followed for a much longer time. The NCHS data samples range from 9,000 to 14,000 people and are thus, in epidemiological terms, relatively moderate compared to the Nurses' Health Study with more than 100,000, the Prospective Collaboration Studies with nearly 900,000 individuals (*Lancet* 2009), the American Cancer Society Follow-up Study with nearly 1 million (Calle et al. 1999; Stevens et al. 1998), The Norwegian Population Study with 2 million (Waaler and Lund 1983), and the Life Insurance Follow-up with 5 million (Lew et al. 1979). It may thus be unreasonable to conclude, as some have done, that there is no danger to being overweight with a BMI between 25 and 30 kg/m^2 as a recent NHANES study concluded, since this study is relatively small compared to those described above, and the subjects have not been followed for a long time period (Flegal et al. 2005).

A recent study from China shows a similar curvilinear relationship between BMI and mortality. Using a BMI of 24–24.9 kg/m^2 as the reference level, a higher or lower BMI in both men and women in this study of 154,736 Chinese showed an increase in the relative risk of mortality. The "U"-shaped relationship persisted even after excluding participants who were current or former smokers, heavy alcohol drinkers, or had chronic illness. This association was observed between BMI and mortality from cardiovascular disease, cancer, and other causes (Gu et al. 2006).

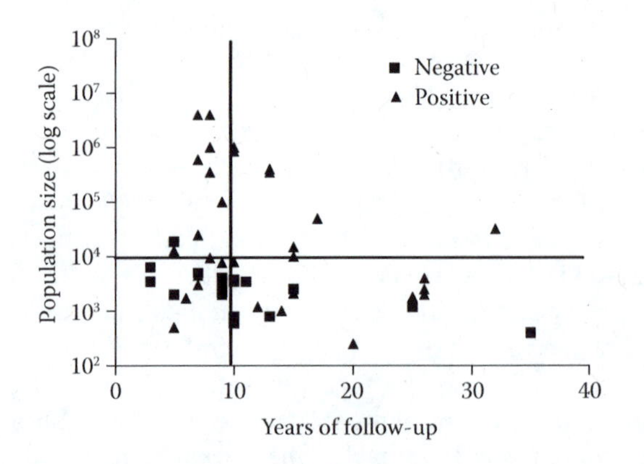

FIGURE 4.5 Relationship between size and duration of follow-up for cohort studies and whether they find a relationship between body mass index and mortality. (Adapted from Sjostrom, L.V., *Am. J. Clin. Nutr.*, 55(2 Suppl), 516S–523S.)

A recent assessment of "reverse causality" and confounding in the association of overweight and obesity with mortality examined data from two large studies—the Renfrew/Paisley Study and the Collaborative Study—showed that "among never-smokers and with the first 5 years of deaths removed, overweight was associated with an increase in all-cause mortality (relative risk ranging from 1.12 to 1.38) and obesity was associated with a doubling of risk in men in both cohorts (relative risk, 2.10 and 1.96, respectively) and a 60% increase in women (relative risk, 1.56) (Lawlor et al. 2006).

A long-term perspective on the effects of body weight on mortality can be obtained from data initially acquired in adolescence, although not all studies show this (Must 2003). Using the Harvard Longitudinal study, Must et al. (2003) found that overweight in adolescence was associated with increased risk of CVD and mortality in middle age. Another study by van Dam et al. using the Nurses' Health Study cohort found that a higher BMI at age 18 was associated with increased mortality later in life (van Dam et al. 2006). Similarly, a study of 227,000 Norwegian adolescents aged 14–19 found that overweight in adolescence predicted mortality in adult women. In a Norwegian study, adolescent obesity was related to increased mortality in middle age from several causes, including ischemic heart disease, colon cancer, and sudden death (Bjorge et al. 2008).

Preventing cardiovascular disease in diabetics is better accomplished by controlling blood pressure and lowering lipids than by lowering glucose (Ray et al. 2009). In older people aged more than 65 years, excess body weight is associated with impaired physical function, but not increased mortality (Lang et al. 2008).

Obesity increases the risk for many diseases that are described in more detail below.

Central Adiposity and the Metabolic Syndrome

Central adiposity is also a risk for mortality and is one of the components in the diagnosis of the metabolic syndrome. This concept was introduced from life insurance analyses near the beginning of the twentieth century (Actuarial Society of America 1901–1903; Weeks 1904), but it was Professor Jean Vague who championed this concept after World War II (Vague 1948, 1956). His initial prescient observation that central or android obesity compared to gynoid or peripheral obesity have been amply confirmed. In a prospective study from Muscatine, Iowa, the BMI was the strongest predictor in childhood of the risk of developing the metabolic syndrome in adulthood (Burns et al. 2009).

An example showing the impact of waist circumference on risk is the NIH-AARP study, which began in 1995 and has followed 154,776 men and 90,757 women aged 51–72 for 9 years. After adjustment for BMI and other covariates, a large waist circumference (fifth quintile vs. second) was associated with an approximately 25% increase in mortality in men (HR = 1.22 in men and HR = 1.28 in women). Compared to subjects with a combination of normal BMI and normal waist circumference, those in a normal-BMI group with a large waist circumference (men > 102 cm; women > 88 cm) had an approximately 20% higher mortality risk (HR = 1.23 for men and HR = 1.22 for women) (Koster et al. 2008).

In the European Prospective Investigation into Cancer and Nutrition (EPIC) study among 359,387 individuals in nine countries, the lowest risk of death was observed at a BMI of 25.3 kg/m^2 in men and 24.3 kg/m^2 in women. After controlling for BMI, both relative risk for mortality comparing first and fifth quintiles of waist circumference was 2.05 (95% CI 1.80 to 2.33) for men and 1.78 (95% CI 1.56 to 2.04) for women. For WHR, the relative risks were 1.68 for men and 1.51 for women. BMI remained significantly associated with risk of death in models that included either waist circumference or WHR (Pischon et al. 2008).

In the Aerobics Center Longitudinal Study follow-up, hypertension was the most potent risk factor for mortality and cardiovascular mortality, but central adiposity and hypertriglyceridemia remained associated with both all-cause and cardiovascular mortality. Risk for mortality increased incrementally as the number of components of the metabolic syndrome increased (Ho et al. 2008).

In the Canada Fitness Survey, waist circumference was positively associated with mortality whereas arm, thigh, and calf circumferences were significantly protective in men, and arm and thigh circumferences were protective in women (Mason et al. 2008).

A systematic review comparing the waist circumference, body mass index, and waist circumference to height ratio on the risk for diabetes and cardiovascular disease by Browning et al. (2010) found that both waist circumference and waist circumference divided by height were similar and slightly better than body mass index.

Diabetes Mellitus, Insulin Resistance, and the Metabolic Syndrome

Obesity is associated with a variety of diseases that are described in the sections below. Prime among these is diabetes, and it is the prevention of diabetes by weight reduction that has the greatest potential for being cost-effective (see Chapter 8). The overall increase in risk increases as BMI increases, as has been demonstrated repeatedly during the twentieth century (Bray 1976; Sjostrom et al. 2004) and the twenty-first century (Nguyen and Magno 2008).

Obesity is a strong predictor of type 2 diabetes mellitus in both genders and in all ethnic groups (Chan et al. 1994; Colditz et al. 1995). One estimate from the National Center for Health Statistics (NHANES III) reported that 78.5% of diabetics were overweight and 45.7% were obese (BMI > 30 kg/m^2). In the 1999–2002 survey, these numbers had risen slightly to 82.7% of diabetics being overweight and 54.8% being obese (2004). The prevalence varies, however, with the definition that is used, but the recent acceptance by most countries of a single set of criteria for the metabolic syndrome will facilitate comparisons (Alberti et al. 2009; Benetos et al. 2008).

The risk of type 2 diabetes mellitus increases with the degree and duration of obesity, and with a more central distribution of body fat (Figure 3.6). In a meta-analysis of ten publications, the pooled odds ratio for risk of diabetes was 2.14 (95% CI 1.70 to 2.71) (Freemantle et al. 2008). The relationship between increasing BMI and the risk of diabetes in the Nurses' Health Study is shown in Figure 4.6 (Chan et al. 1994; Colditz et al. 1995).

Weight gain also increases the risk of diabetes. The National Health and Nutrition Examination Survey showed an increase in diagnosed cases of diabetes as BMI categories increased in each of the national surveys from 1960–61 to 1999–2000 (Gregg et al. 2005). In the group with a BMI ≥ 30 kg/m^2, the prevalence increased from 2.9% in 1960–61 to 6.3% in 1976–80 and to 10.1% in the 1999–2000 survey. In contrast, hypertension and abnormal cholesterol values declined over the same time interval reflecting improved diagnostic and therapeutic intervention for cholesterol and blood pressure. For any given BMI, the risk of developing impaired glucose tolerance is higher with

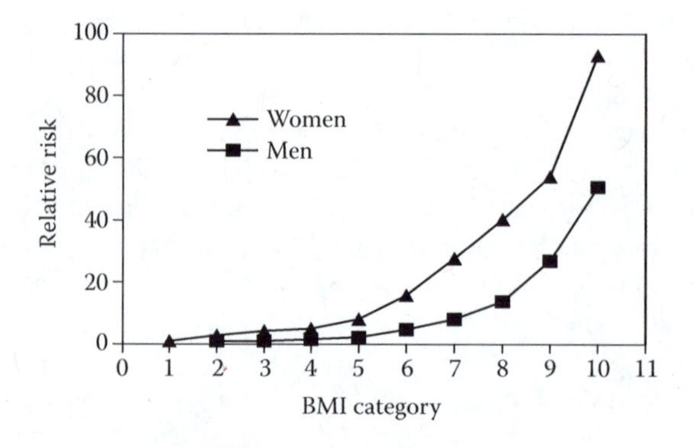

FIGURE 4.6 Relationship of body mass index and risk of diabetes in the Nurses' Health Study of Women and the Health Professionals Follow-up Study of Men. (Data from Chan, J.M., et al., *Diabetes Care*, 17(9), 961–969, 1994; Colditz, G.A., et al., *Ann. Intern. Med.*, 122(7), 481–486, 1995.)

greater weight gain since age 20 (Black et al. 2005). Obese men maintaining their weight since age 20 had a lower risk of IGT than nonobese men who became similarly obese by age 51.

Weight gain appears to precede the onset of diabetes. Among the Pima Indians, body weight steadily and slowly increased by 30 kg (from 60 kg to 90 kg) in the years preceding the diagnosis of diabetes (Knowler et al. 2002; Sjostrom et al. 1997). After the diagnosis of diabetes, body weight slightly decreased. In the Health Professionals Follow-up Study, relative risk of developing diabetes increased with weight gain, as well as with increased BMI. In long-term follow-up studies, the duration of overweight and the change in plasma glucose during an oral glucose tolerance test also were strongly related. When overweight was present for less than 10 years, plasma glucose was not increased. With longer durations, of up to 45 years, a nearly linear increase in plasma glucose occurred after an oral glucose tolerance test. Risk of diabetes is increased in hypertensive individuals treated with diuretics or beta-blocking drugs, and this risk was increased further in the overweight.

Weight loss or moderating weight gain reduces the risk of developing diabetes. In the Swedish Obese Subjects Study, Sjostrom et al. observed that diabetes was present in 13% to 16% of obese subjects at baseline (Sjostrom et al. 2004). Of those who underwent gastric bypass and subsequently lost weight, 69% who initially had diabetes went into remission, and only 0.5% of those who did not have diabetes at baseline developed it during the first 2 years of follow-up. In contrast, in the obese control group that lost no weight, the cure rate was low, with only 16% going into remission. This benefit has been demonstrated in a systematic review of bariatric surgery (Buchwald et al. 2009).

The incidence of new cases of diabetes was 7.8% in 2 years. The benefit of weight loss is also clearly shown in the Health Professionals Follow-up Study, in which relative risk of developing diabetes declined by nearly 50% with a weight loss of 5 to 11 kg. Type 2 diabetes was almost nonexistent with a weight loss of more than 20 kg or a BMI below 20 kg/m^2 (Colditz, Willett et al. 1995).

Both increased insulin secretion and insulin resistance result from overweight. The relationship of insulin secretion to BMI has already been noted. A greater BMI correlates with greater insulin secretion. Overweight develops in more than 50% of nonhuman primates as they age and gain weight (Hansen et al. 1999). Nearly half of these obese animals subsequently develop diabetes, which can be prevented by calorie restriction (Colman et al. 2009). The time course for the development of obesity in nonhuman primates, and in the Pima Indians, is spread over a number of years. After the animals gain weight, the next demonstrable effects are impaired glucose removal and increased insulin resistance as measured by impaired glucose clearance with a euglycemic hyperinsulinemic clamp. The hyperinsulinemia in turn increases hepatic VLDL triglyceride synthesis and secretion, increases plasminogen activator inhibitor-1 (PAI-1) synthesis, increases sympathetic nervous system activity, and increases renal sodium reabsorption.

Insulin resistance has a strong relationship to the metabolic syndrome, but there are no clinically easy ways to measure insulin resistance, except the Homeostatis Approach to Insulin Resistance (HOMA-IR). Thus, the National Cholesterol Education Program Adult Treatment Panel III has provided defining values for this syndrome without having to measure insulin resistance directly (see Chapter 1). When three of the five criteria, including waist circumference, blood pressure, plasma triglycerides, HDL-cholesterol, and fasting plasma glucose are abnormal, the patient is defined as having the metabolic syndrome (Alberti et al. 2009). A major feature of this syndrome is central adiposity, measured as a high waist circumference. The increased release of free fatty acids from visceral fat impairs insulin clearance by the liver and alters peripheral metabolism. The reduced production of adiponectin by the fat cell is another potential player in the development of insulin resistance. Using 16 cohorts, Ford et al. (2008) found that the metabolic syndrome, however identified, has a stronger association with diabetes than with coronary heart disease. A higher number of abnormal components were strongly related to incident diabetes, and limited evidence suggested that fasting glucose alone may be as good as the metabolic syndrome in predicting diabetes.

Liver and Gallbladder Disease

Nonalcoholic fatty liver disease, nonalcoholic steatohepatitis. Nonalcoholic fatty liver disease (NAFLD) is the term given to describe a constellation of liver abnormalities associated with overweight, including hepatomegaly, elevated liver enzymes, and abnormal liver histology that may progress to steatohepatitis, fibrosis, and finally cirrhosis. In a large sample ($n = 2287$) examined by proton magnetic resonance spectroscopy, almost one-third had hepatic steatosis that varied significantly by gender (42% in men, 24% in women) and ethnicity where the higher rate in Hispanics was strongly related to their higher body weight (Browning et al. 2004). NAFLD may reflect increased VLDL production associated with hyperinsulinemia. The accumulation of lipid in the liver suggests that the secretion of VLDL in response to hyperinsulinemia is inadequate to keep up with the high rate of triglyceride turnover. A retrospective analysis of liver biopsy specimens obtained from overweight and obese patients with abnormal liver biochemistries but without evidence of acquired, autoimmune, or genetic liver disease, demonstrated a 30% prevalence of septal fibrosis and a 10% prevalence of cirrhosis. Another study utilizing a cross-sectional analysis of liver biopsies suggests that in overweight patients, the prevalence of steatosis, steatohepatitis, and cirrhosis are approximately 75%, 20%, and 2%, respectively (Bellentani et al. 2000). The level with more marked insulin resistance as determined from the Homeostasis Assessment Model (HOMA) had a higher prevalence of severe steatosis (Angelico et al. 2005). Using ultrasound as a criterion for diagnosing increased liver fat, Hamaguchi et al. (2005) found that in a Japanese population there was a 10% incidence of new cases of nonalcoholic fatty liver disease after a mean follow-up of 414 days and that this was predicted by the metabolic syndrome. If increased fat in the liver is suspected, an ultrasound of the liver can provide a quantitative estimate that is much better than serum liver enzymes (AST, ALT). Although NAFLD is the most common cause of elevated serum alanine aminotransaminase (ALT) or aspartate aminotransferase (AST), up to 80% of the subjects with NAFLD have normal liver enzymes (Kotronen et al. 2009).

Gallbladder disease. Cholelithiasis is the primary hepatobiliary pathology associated with overweight (Ko 2002). The old clinical adage "fat, female, fertile, and forty" describes a number of epidemiologic factors often associated with the development of gallbladder disease. This is admirably demonstrated in the Nurses' Health Study (Stampfer et al. 1992). When the BMI was below 24 kg/m^2, the incidence of clinically symptomatic gallstones was approximately 250 per 100,000 person-years of follow-up. The incidence of gallstones gradually increases with increasing BMI to the level of 30 kg/m^2, and increases very steeply when BMI exceeds 30 kg/m^2.

Part of the explanation for the increased risk of gallstones is the increased cholesterol turnover related to total body fat (Caroli-Bosc et al. 1999). Cholesterol production is linearly related to body fat; approximately 20 mg of additional cholesterol is synthesized for each kilogram of extra body fat. Thus, a 10-kg increase in body fat leads to the daily synthesis of as much cholesterol as is contained in the yolk of one egg. The increased cholesterol is in turn excreted in the bile. High cholesterol concentrations relative to bile acids and phospholipids in bile increase the likelihood of precipitation of cholesterol gallstones in the gallbladder. Additional factors, such as nidation conditions, are also involved in whether gallstones do or do not form (Caroli-Bosc et al. 1999).

During weight loss, the likelihood of gallstones increases because the flux of cholesterol mobilized from fat is increased through the biliary system. Diets with moderate levels of fat that trigger gallbladder contraction and thus empty its cholesterol content may reduce this risk. Similarly, the use of bile acids, such as ursodeoxycholic acid, may be advisable if the risk of gallstone formation is thought to be increased.

Other gastrointestinal diseases. Overweight may also be a contributing factor in gastroesophageal reflux disease or GERD. A total of nine studies have examined the association of GERD with BMI (Hampel et al. 2005). In six of these studies, a statistically significant association between GERD and BMI was reported. Erosive esophagitis and esophageal adenocarinoma were more common.

The odds ratio for GERD was 1.43 in the overweight group (BMI 25–29.9 kg/m2) compared to the normal weight group and rose to 1.94 when the BMI was greater than 30 kg/m^2 (Utzschneider and Kahn 2006).

Hypertension

Blood pressure is often increased in overweight individuals (Rocchini 2004). In the Swedish Obese Subjects Study, hypertension was present at baseline in 44% to 51% of subjects. One estimate suggests that control of overweight would eliminate 48% of the hypertension in Whites and 28% in Blacks. For each decline of 1 mm Hg in diastolic blood pressure, the risk of myocardial infarction decreases an estimated 2% to 3%. A study where 1,145,758 Swedish men born between 1951 and 1976 were followed until 2006 observed a general increase among the obese in the magnitude of the association between blood pressure and subsequent CVD as BMI increased. Hypertension is just as serious among the obese as in lean individuals (Silventoinen et al. 2008). In the National Health and Nutrition Examination Survey (NHANES 1999–2004), the odds ratio for hypertension was 1.45 (95% CI 1.39–1.52) for every increase of five BMI units, and this effect was stronger in younger adults than in older ones (Chriinos et al. 2009).

Overweight and hypertension interact with cardiac function. Hypertension in normal-weight people produces concentric hypertrophy of the heart with thickening of the ventricular walls. In overweight individuals, eccentric dilatation occurs. Increased preload and stroke work are associated with hypertension. The combination of overweight and hypertension leads to thickening of the ventricular wall and larger cardiac volume, and thus to a greater likelihood of congestive heart failure.

Hypertension is strongly associated with type II diabetes, impaired glucose tolerance, hypertriglyceridemia, and hypercholesterolemia, as noted above in the discussion of the metabolic syndrome. Hyperinsulinemia in overweight and in hypertensive patients suggests insulin resistance and the metabolic syndrome. An analysis of the factors that predict blood pressure and changes in peripheral vascular resistance in response to body weight gain showed that a key determinant of the weight-induced increases in blood pressure was a disproportionate increase in cardiac output that could not be fully accounted for by the hemodynamic contribution of new tissue. This hemodynamic change may be attributable to a disproportionate increase in cardiac output related to an increase in sympathetic activity.

Hypertension is a major risk factor for stroke, which is the third leading cause of death and disability worldwide. This is true for both Western populations (Jood et al. 2004; Kurth et al. 2005) and Asians (Park et al. 2008). Among 154,736 Chinese men followed for an average of 8.3 years there were 7489 strokes, of which 3924 were fatal. Compared to a normal BMI of 18.5 to 24.9, the relative hazard of stroke increased to 1.43 (BMI 25–29.9), 1.72 (BMI ≥ 30). Both ischemic and hemorrhagic stroke incidence increased with BMI and so did stroke mortality (Bazzano et al. 2010).

The hypertension in obesity is related to altered sympathetic activity. During insulin infusion, overweight subjects have a much greater increase in the muscle sympathetic nerve firing rate than do normal-weight subjects, but the altered activity is associated with a lesser change in the vascular resistance of calf muscles (da Silva et al. 2009).

Kidney and Urological Disease

Overweight may also affect the kidneys. An obesity-related glomerulopathy characterized as focal segmental glomerulosclerosis has increased significantly from 0.2% of biopsies of pathological specimens between 1986 and 1990 to 2.0% in biopsies taken between 1996 and 2000 (Kambham et al. 2001). Kidney stones are also an increased risk of overweight patients (Taylor et al. 2005).

Body mass index is related to the risk of end-stage renal disease where dialysis is essential to maintain life. Waist-hip circumference ratio, but not BMI in this study, is also related to risk of CKD and mortality in the Atherosclerosis in Communities Study and the Cardiovascular Health Study

(Elsayed et al. 2008). In a study from the Kaiser Permanente Group of Northern California, Hsu et al. (2006) found that a higher BMI was a progressively greater risk factor for end-stage renal disease that persisted even after correcting for multiple potential confounding factors including baseline blood pressure or diabetes mellitus. Compared to normal weight individuals, those who were overweight (BMI 25–29.9 kg/m^2) had an 87% greater relative risk (RR = 1.87 (95% CI 1.64 to 2.14)). This risk increased to 3.51 (95% CI 3.05 to 4.18) with a BMI between 30 and 34.9 kg/m^2 and rose further to 7.07 (95% CI 5.37 to 9.31) when the BMI was above 40 kg/m^2. Similar data have been reported from the Framingham study (Foster et al. 2008) and from Japan (Yamagata et al. 2007). More recently, an increase in body weight, even in the normal weight range, is associated with an increased risk of chronic kidney disease (Ryo et al. 2008). Obesity is an important risk factor for urinary incontinence (Khong and Jackson 2008) that can be reversed by weight loss (Subak et al. 2009).

Heart Disease

Adults. Many studies show that as the body mass index increases there is an increased risk for heart disease (Kenchaiah et al. 2002). Data from the Nurses' Health Study indicate that the risk for U.S. women developing coronary artery disease is increased 3.3-fold with a BMI > 29 kg/m^2, compared with women with a BMI < 21 kg/m^2 (Flint et al. 2009). A BMI of 27 to <29 kg/m^2 increases the relative risk to 1.8. Weight gain also strongly affects this risk at any initial BMI (Meigs et al. 1997). That is, at all levels of initial BMI, weight gain was associated with a graded increase in risk of heart disease. This was particularly evident in the highest quintile in which weight gain was more than 20 kg. Similar effects are seen in men. Major risk of cardiovascular disease was increased 6% for each 1.1 kg/m^2 increase in BMI among 6452 British men (Emberson et al. 2005).

In spite of the data showing that body mass index is related to the risk of CHD, the data from Sjostrom et al. (2009) in the Swedish Obesity Study (SOS) failed to show that voluntary weight loss would reduce risk of fatal and nonfatal myocardial infarction. Two retrospective studies (Christou and Sampalis 2004; Adams 2007) showed that weight loss reduced the risk of death from MI, but the SOS study failed to find this relation in the prospective controlled trial with 2010 operated and 2037 control subjects. There were 104 cases of fatal and nonfatal MI in the surgery group and 113 in the control group [hazard ratio 0.90 (95% CI 0.69, 1.18)]. The cumulative incidence curves of the two groups were maximally separated in favor of surgery after 11 years, but converged thereafter and crossed each other after 18 years. When the groups were divided by median baseline fasting glucose (4.72 mM), those with the higher glucose had a lower incidence of fatal and nonfatal MI and had a favorable response to surgery (HR = 0.66 95% CI 0.47–0.92), but those with lower glucose did not, suggesting that a higher glucose and its potential for future diabetes may be an important component in the response to weight loss.

Both atrial fibrillation (Wang et al. 2004; Tsang et al. 2008) and congestive heart failure (Kenchaiah et al. 2002) have a higher risk in overweight subjects. During a mean 13.7 years of follow-up in the Framingham study, there was a 4% increase in the risk of new onset atrial fibrillation for each unit of BMI increase in men and women. In the Multi-Ethnic Study of Atherosclerosis (MESA), the risk of congestive heart failure in obesity was associated with elevated levels of inflammatory markers (interleukin-6 and C-reactive protein) and albuminuria (Bahrami et al. 2008).

In contrast to these studies reporting detrimental effects of increasing weight on cardiovascular endpoints, there is one paper that shows that overweight individuals survive better after coronary bypass surgery. Among 16,218 individuals who had a coronary artery bypass in the Providence Health System between 1997 and 2003, body size was not a significant factor for mortality but the authors note that the lowest mortality is found in the high-normal and overweight subgroups compared with the obese or underweight (Jin et al. 2005). In another study, obesity conferred an elevated risk of acute coronary syndrome in both healthy and less healthy subgroups (Jensen et al. 2008).

Dyslipidemia may be important in the relationship of BMI to increased risk of heart disease (Despres and Krauss 2002). A positive correlation between BMI and triglyceride has been demonstrated repeatedly. However, the inverse relationship between HDL cholesterol and BMI may be even more important because a low HDL cholesterol carries a greater relative risk than do elevated triglycerides. Central fat distribution is also important in lipid abnormalities. Waist circumference alone accounted for as much as or more of the variance in triglycerides and HDL cholesterol as either WHR or sagittal diameter, two other measures of central fat. A positive correlation for central fat and triglyceride and the inverse relationship for HDL cholesterol is evident for all measures (Franssen et al. 2008).

Dyslipidemia, however, is only part of the story. Inflammation is another part. Using C-reactive protein (CRP) as a marker of inflammatory status, Ridker and his colleagues have shown that the risk of myocardial infarction is predicted by CRP and by lipids. They operate independently and the worst risk is in individuals with high CRP and high LDL cholesterol and the best outcome is seen in those with low CRP and low LDL (Ridker et al. 2002).

Increased body weight is associated with a number of cardiovascular abnormalities. Cardiac weight increases with increasing body weight, consistent with increased cardiac work. Heart weight as a percentage of body weight, however, is lower than in a normal-weight control group. The increased cardiac work associated with overweight may produce cardiomyopathy and heart failure in the absence of diabetes, hypertension, or atherosclerosis (Kenchaiah et al. 2002). Weight loss decreases heart weight; this decrease was linearly related to the degree of weight loss in both men and women. An echocardiographic study of left ventricular midwall function showed that obese individuals compensated by using cardiac reserve, especially in the presence of hypertension. Interestingly, the heart rate was well within normal limits.

Central fat distribution is associated with small-dense low-density lipoproteins (LDL) (bad-LDL) as opposed to large fluffy LDL particles (good LDL) (Despres and Krauss 2002). For a similar level of cholesterol, the risk of coronary heart disease (CHD) is significantly higher in individuals with small dense LDL than with large fluffy LDL. Because each LDL particle has a single molecule of apo B protein, the concentration of apo B can be used to estimate the number of LDL particles. Despres et al. (2002) demonstrated that the level of apo B is a strong predictor of the risk for CHD. Based on a study of French Canadians, these researchers proposed that estimating apo B, the levels of fasting insulin, the concentration of triglyceride, the concentration of HDL cholesterol, and waist circumference could help identify individuals at high risk for the metabolic syndrome and coronary heart disease.

Central adiposity, as reflected in the waist circumference, is a strong predictor of the risk for cardiovascular disease. When increased central adiposity is added to other components of the metabolic syndrome, the prediction is even higher. Using the NHANES data, Janssen et al. (2004) showed that body mass predicted the risk of the metabolic syndrome in men, but when BMI is adjusted for waist circumference as a continuous variable, waist circumference accounts for essentially all of the risk for the metabolic syndrome. The importance of the waist circumference was also shown by Yusuf et al. (2005) in the INTERHEART study of myocardial infarction among 27,000 participants from 52 countries. The odds ratio of developing a myocardial infarction increased with each increasing quintile. The population attributable risks of myocardial infarction for increased waist-to-hip circumference ratio in the top 2 quintiles was 24.3% compared to only 7.7% for the top two quintiles of BMI, making waist circumference a somewhat more robust predictor. In a meta-analysis including 10 studies, indices of abdominal obesity were better discriminators of cardiovascular risk factors, including diabetes, hypertension, and dyslipidemia, than BMI, including waist to height ratio, waist-hip ratio, and waist circumference (Lee et al. 2008).

Children. Overweight children may be at higher risk for future cardiovascular disease. Longitudinal studies from the Bogulasa Heart Study, the Muscatine Study, the Harvard Growth Study, and the Boyd Orr cohort have all shed light on several dimensions of the problem (Clinton 2004). LDL cholesterol and triglycerides both increase in children above the 80th percentile (Freedman 2002). Blood pressure rises in children above the 90th percentile. Finally, carotid intima-medial thickness in children rises as the weight status rises (Freedman et al. 2004).

A long-term follow-up of children from Denmark has also shown important relationships between initial body weight and risk of heart disease in adult life.

Cancer

Certain forms of cancer are significantly increased in overweight individuals (see Table 4.5) (Brawer 2009; Calle et al. 2003). Males face increased risk for neoplasms of the colon, rectum, and prostate. In women, cancers of the reproductive system and gallbladder are more common. One explanation for the increased risk of endometrial cancer in overweight women is the increased production of estrogens by stromal cells in adipose tissue. This increased production is related to the degree of excess body fat that accounts for a major source of estrogen production in postmenopausal women. Breast cancer is not only related to total body fat, but also may have a more important relationship to central body fat (van Kruijsdijk et al. 2009). It may also help explain why breast cancer risk is increased at age 75 in women in the highest vs. the lowest quartile of the body mass index (Sweeney et al. 2004). The increased visceral fat measured by computed tomography shows an important relationship to the risk of breast cancer.

The Nurses' Health Study has added significant insight to the relation of body weight and breast cancer. Women who gained 25 kg or more after age 18 were at increased risk of breast cancer (RR 1.45 $p < 0.001$). Women who gained 10 kg or more after menopause were at increased risk for breast cancer compared to women whose weight remained stable (RR 1.18). Women who lost and maintained 10 kg or more and who did not use postmenopausal hormones were at lower risk than those who maintained weight (RR 0.43) (Eliassen et al. 2006). A pooling project with data from 13 cohort studies found a significant risk of renal cell carcinoma [RR BMI < 23 = 1; BMI 23 < 25 RR = 1.22 (1.02–1.46); BMI 25 < 27 RR = 1.39 (1.16–1.67); BMI 27 < 30 RR = 1.62 (1.35–1.93); BMI ≥ 30 RR = 1.84 (1.52–2.22)] (Mannistos and Smith-Warner 2006). Further support for the relation of obesity to cancer comes from Korean women where postmenopausal women showed overall increases (Song et al. 2008).

Endocrine Changes in the Overweight Patient

A variety of endocrine changes are associated with being overweight and they are summarized in Table 4.6 (Weaver 2008). The first ones I will discuss are the effects of increasing body weight on reproductive function and pregnancy. Polycystic ovary syndrome, which is one of these reproductive changes, is discussed in Chapter 4 as a clinical type of obesity. Even more than effects on pregnancy and reproductive function, overweight may be associated with insulin resistance. The diagnosis of

TABLE 4.5
Mortality from Cancer in American Men and Women

Men	Women
• Liver	• Uterus
• Pancreas	• Kidney
• Stomach/esophagus	• Cervix
• Colon/rectum	• Pancreas/esophagus
• Gallbladder	• Gallbladder
• Multiple myeloma	• Breast
• Kidney	• Non-Hodgkin's
• Non-Hodgkins	• Liver
• Prostate	• Ovary
	• Colon/rectum

Source: Calle, E.E., et al., *New Engl. J. Med.*, 348(17), 1625–1638, 2003.

TABLE 4.6
Endocrine Abnormalities Associated with Overweight

Endocrine Gland	Changes Noted
Hypothalamus	
Pituitary-adrenal axis	Normal 24-hour cortisol secretion
	Increased stress-induced ACTH
	Increased cortisol secretion
	Flat diurnal cortisol profile
	Increased cortisol clearance
	Reduced morning cortisol peak
	Impaired dexamethasone suppression
	Decreased cortisol binding protein
	Increased adrenal androgens production
Pituitary-growth hormone axis	Decreased FH secretion
	Increased GH binding protein
	Decreased IGF binding protein-1
	Decreased IGF binding protein-3
	Low or normal total insulin-like growth factor-1 (!GF-1)
	Decreased ghrelin secretion
Pituitary-thyroid axis	Increased thyrotropin
	Normal thyroid hormones
	Reduced TSH response to TRH
	Reduced prolactin response to TRH
Pituitary gonadal axis	Early menarche in obese girls
	Reduced sex-hormone binding globulin
Pancreatic-visceral fat	Increased insulin secretion
	Reduced hepatic insulin clearance
	Reduced aciponectin
	Insulin resistance

Cushing's disease is also discussed in more detail in Chapter 5. Hyperparathyroidism is associated with a clear increase in body weight.

Parathyroid hormone may also be related to metabolic syndrome. In a sample of 1017 obese Norwegian men (32%) and women (68%), parathyroid hormone, but not vitamin D (25-hydroxyvitamin D), was a predictor of metabolic syndrome by NCEP-ATPIII criteria (Hjelmesaeth et al. 2009).

Problems with pregnancy in the overweight woman. The changes in the reproductive system are among the most important endocrine effects of excess weight. Irregular menses and frequent anovular cycles are common, and the rate of fertility may be reduced (Grodstein et al. 1994). In the Nurses' Health Study, as BMI increased, the relative risk of infertility rose. Compared to the reference group that had a BMI of 20–21.9, the relative risk of infertility was 1.7 for a BMI 26–27.9 and 2.7 for a BMI above 30 kg/m^2 (Rich-Edwards et al. 1994). Some reports describe increased risks of toxemia during pregnancy. Hypertension and cesarean section may also be more frequent. Women with a BMI greater than 30 kg/m^2 have abnormalities in secretion of hypothalamic gonadotropin-releasing hormone (GnRH), pituitary-luteinizing hormone (LH), and follicle-stimulating hormone (FSH), which results in anovulation (Yen 1999). Increasing prepregnancy body weight produces a significant and weight-related increase in the likelihood of caesarean delivery. Preterm birth was higher in the smallest women, but heavier women had no increased risk of low birth weight in the infant. Weight gain of >18.6 kg (41 pounds) also increases the risk of Caesarean delivery. Low birth weight infants were less likely in heavier women and in those who gained more weight (Rosenberg et al. 2005). The risk of postpartum urinary tract infection also appears to be increased in overweight women based on an observational study of 60,167 women (Usha et al. 2005). Both smoking and obesity influence the risks of preeclampsia. Smoking protects against the risk of preeclampsia while increasing the risk of small-for-gestational-age infants. Obesity increases the risk of preeclampsia and overcomes this effect of smoking (Ness et al. 2008).

Increasing numbers of pregnancies are associated with future risk for developing the metabolic syndrome that is independent of prior obesity or weight gain related to pregnancy. The risk does vary, however, by whether the pregnancies were associated with gestational diabetes. The risk of metabolic syndrome is increased 33% (HR = 1.33 95% CI 0.93 to 1.90) with one pregnancy, and 143% (HR = 2.43 95% CI 1.53 to 3.86) with one pregnancy with gestational diabetes compared to nonparous women (Gunderson et al. 2009).

In a large retrospective study from Scotland, nulliparous women, more than multiparous women, had increased elective preterm delivery, neonatal death, and infant weights of less than 1000 g, with women above a BMI of 35 kg/m^2 having the largest effect (Smith et al. 2007). The Agency for Health Care Research and Quality, in a review of the literature, found that strong evidence supported an association between gestational weight gains and preterm birth, total birthweight, low birthweight, macrosomia, large-for-gestational-age and small-for-gestational-age infants (Viswanathan et al. 2008). A Danish national birth cohort with 60,892 term pregnancies also indicated that women may benefit from avoiding high and very high gestational weight gain (Nohr et al. 2008). A study from the Swedish Birth Registry of 186,087 women showed that 6.8% had postdate deliveries. Higher maternal weight during the first trimester was associated with longer gestation (Denison et al. 2008). In a large Missouri cohort of 459,913 singletons, obesity increased the risk for medically indicated but not spontaneous preterm birth in both singletons and twins (Salihu et al. 2008). Increasing BMI among 29,303 Chinese women increased the incidence of caesarean section, preeclampsia, gestational diabetes, preterm delivery, and large-for-gestational age as well as small-for-gestational age babies (Leung et al. 2008). Risk of preterm delivery decreased with increasing BMI and was highest among the underweight women. Overweight increased the risk of preeclampsia, but did not affect the risk of stillbirth in this study of Argentinian women (Hauger et al. 2008).

Obesity has also been shown to increase the risk of neural tube defects in a meta-analysis of 12 studies (Rasmussen et al. 2008). The relationship of overweight and obesity to congenital defects was explored in a meta-analysis and systematic review. Compared with mothers of recommended BMIs, obese mothers were at increased risks of neural tube defects (OR = 1.87 95% CI 1.62–2.15), spina bifida (OR = 2.24 95% CI 1.86–2.69), cardiovascular anomalies (OR = 1.30 95% CI 1.12–1.51), septal anomalies (OR = 1.20 95% CI 1.09–1.31), cleft palate (OR = 1.23 95% CI 1.03–1.47), cleft lip and palate (OR = 1.20 95% CI 1.03–1.40), anorectal atresia (OR = 1.48 95% CI 1.12–1.97), hydrocephaly (OR = 1.68 95% CI 1.19–2.36), and limb reduction anomalies (OR = 1.34 95% CI 1.03–1.73). The risk of gastroschisis among obese mothers was significantly reduced (OR = 0.17 95% CI 0.10–0.30). Women contemplating pregnancy should be made aware of these risks of maternal obesity and provided with help to maintain a lower weight prior to pregnancy and to maintain optimal weight gain during gestation (Stothard et al. 2009).

Pulmonary Disease

Pulmonary function. Alterations in pulmonary function have been described in overweight subjects, but subjects were free of other potential chronic pulmonary diseases in only a few studies. When underlying pulmonary disease was absent, only major degrees of increased body weight significantly affected pulmonary function. The chief effect is a decrease in residual lung volume associated with increased abdominal pressure on the diaphragm (Strohl et al. 2004).

Pneumonia. Community-acquired pneumonia may be an additional risk related to being overweight. In both the Health Professionals Follow-up Study and the Nurses' Health Study II, the risk

TABLE 4.7
Increasing Prevalence of Obesity and Asthma

	Year		
Prevalence	**1980**	**1991**	**2000**
Obesity	15%	23%	30%
Asthma	7.5%	10%	15%

of pneumonia was increased as the BMI increased (Baik et al. 2000). In addition significant weight gain in women after age 18 also increased the risk of pneumonia.

Asthma. Obesity increases the risk for asthma in both adults and children. As the prevalence of obesity has increased, so has the prevalence of asthma (Table 4.7) (Sin et al. 2008). In a meta-analysis of seven studies that included nearly 300,000 people followed for periods between 2 and 21 years, Beuther et al. (2006) found a significant increase in the odds ratio of developing asthma in the overweight with a BMI of 25–29.9 kg/m2 of 1.38 (95% CI 1.17–1.62) over 1 year and a further increase in the obese (BMI > 30 kg/m^2) to an odds ratio of 1.92 (95% CI 1.43–2.59). Males and females had similar risks. In a study of 46,435 African-American women, Coogan et al. (2009) found that the risk of asthma increased with the increasing BMI group. Compared to those with a BMI of 20–24.9, the overweight (BMI 25–29.9) had an odds ratio of 1.26; those with class I obesity (BMI 30–34.9) had an OR of 1.62, those with class II obesity (BMI 35–39.9) had an OR of 2.24, and those with class III obesity (BMI > 40 kg/m^2) had an OR of 2.85. In addition, these authors showed that a weight gain of >10 kg significantly increased the risk of developing asthma. Obesity is also related to risk of asthma in children. The *z*-score (deviation from median weight) at 6 months of age was significantly related to the risk of recurrent wheezing at 3 years of age (Taveras 2008).

The increase in asthma is mostly in the nonallergic group and can increase the likelihood of hospitalization in the Kaiser Health System (Peters 2006; Mosen 2008). The response of obese patients to asthmas medications, particularly glucocorticoids (steroids), is reduced (Sutherland 2009). The weight loss associated with bariatric surgery reduces the prevalence of asthma, and increased the 1-minute forced expiratory volume (FEV-1). One factor in the reduced response of more obese individuals may be the reduced production of MKP-1, the phosphatase for the MAPK kinase.

Dementia

Alzheimer's disease is the most common form of dementia. BMI and central adiposity may predict this problem, particularly in midlife. Publications over the past few years have shown that (a) central adiposity in middle age predicts dementia in old age; (b) waist circumference in old age may be a better predictor of dementia than BMI; (b) the relation between BMI and dementia is attenuated as people grow older; (d) lower BMI predicts dementia in elderly people; and (e) weight loss may precede a diagnosis of dementia by decades. Prevention of obesity may provide a means to prevent Alzheimer's disease (Luchsinger and Gustafson 2009).

Diseases Associated with Increased Fat Mass

In contrast to the relatively benign effects of excess weight on most components of respiratory function, overweight is often associated with sleep apnea, which can be severe and may require clinical care (Strohl et al. 2004; Coccagna et al. 2006). This is a condition for which weight loss can be beneficial. Obstructive sleep apnea (OSA) is considerably more common in men than women and, as a group, these people are significantly taller than individuals without sleep apnea. An increased snoring index and increased maximal nocturnal sound intensity are characteristic.

Nocturnal oxygen saturation is significantly reduced (Young et al. 2005). One interesting hypothesis is that the increased neck circumference and fat deposits in the pharyngeal area may lead to the obstructive sleep apnea of overweight. A study of obese diabetics using polysomnography as the criterion showed that over 86% had sleep apnea with a mean apnea-hypopnea index of 20.5 ± 16.8 events per hour. A total of 30.5% of the participants had moderate sleep apnea (15 ≤ AHI < 30), and 22.6% had the severe form (AHI ≥ 30). Waist circumference was significantly related to the presence of OSA and severe sleep apnea was most likely in individuals with a higher BMI (Foster et al. 2009).

Obstructive Sleep Apnea

Sleep apnea also benefits from weight loss. In twelve studies representing 342 patients that were identified for a meta-analysis, the pooled mean body mass index was reduced by 17.9 kg/m^2 (95% CI 16.5–19.3) from 55.3 kg/m^2 (95% CI 53.5–57.1) to 37.7 kg/m^2 (95% CI 36.6–38.9). The random-effects pooled baseline apnea hypopnea index of 54.7 events per hour (95% CI 49.0–60.3) was reduced by 38.2 events per hour (95% CI 31.9–44.4) to a final value of 15.8 events per hour, (95% CI 12.6–19.0). Although bariatric surgery significantly reduced the apnea hypopnea index, the mean apnea hypopnea index after surgical weight loss was still elevated and consistent with moderately severe OSA, suggesting that patients undergoing bariatric surgery should not expect a cure of OSA after surgical weight loss (Greenburg et al. 2009).

Asthma has been associated with overweight, and a systematic review has shown that in all 15 studies that were identified, weight loss improved at least one outcome of asthma (Uneli and Skybo 2008).

Diseases of the Bones, Joints, Muscles, Connective Tissue, and Skin

Osteoarthritis is significantly increased in overweight individuals. The osteoarthritis that develops in the knees and ankles may be directly related to the trauma associated with the degree of excess body weight (Felson et al. 1988). However, the increased osteoarthritis in other non-weight-bearing joints suggests that some components of the overweight syndrome alter cartilage and bone metabolism, independent of weight-bearing. Increased osteoarthritis accounts for a significant component of the cost of overweight. Increased body weight also produces disability from joint disease (Okoro et al. 2004). Using the Behavioral Risk Factor Surveillance System telephone survey data on individuals over 45 years of age, Okoro et al. found that Class III overweight (BMI > 40 kg/m^2) was associated with disability among individuals who reported arthritis as well as those who did not report arthritis. Even lighter individuals had increased likelihood of disability compared with those of normal weight respondents (Messier et al. 1998). BMI had a small effect on the need for and response to a unicompartmental knee arthroplasty (Naal et al. 2009).

Rheumatoid arthritis and body mass index have a paradoxical relationship. In a study of rheumatoid arthritis that accrued 123 deaths in 3460 patient years of observation, the BMI was found to be inversely related to mortality. The study was conducted between 1996 and 2000 and is thus relatively short-term with a small number of subjects and may thus not have a long enough follow-up (Escalante et al. 2005).

Several skin changes are associated with excess weight (Garcia Hidalgo 2002). Stretch marks, or striae, are common and reflect the pressures on the skin from expanding lobular deposits of fat. Acanthosis nigricans with deepening pigmentation in the folds of the neck, knuckles, and extensor surfaces occurs in many overweight individuals, but is not associated with increased risk of malignancy. Hirsutism in women may reflect the altered reproductive status in these individuals (Bray 2003).

Psychosocial Dysfunction

Psychosocial problems for children. Overweight is stigmatized (Puhl and Latner 2007; Williams et al. 2005; Strauss and Pollack 2003), that is, overweight individuals are exposed to the opprobrium from their fatness. This was recognized more than 40 years ago in a study of disabilities in children. Children were given six pictures of children of the same sex with different disabilities. One of the pictures was of an overweight child. They were asked to pick out the child that it would be easiest to play with until they had ranked all six pictures. In almost all settings—urban, rural, suburban, inner city, and affluent or poor—the children ranked the overweight child at the bottom or next to the bottom of the children they would like to play with. This occurred in both preschool as well as 11-year-old children. Latner and Stunkard returned in 2003 with the same technology to reexamine this question. They found that if anything, the stigma against the overweight child had worsened in the 40 years since the original studies by Richardson et al. (Richardson et al. 1961; Goodman et al. 1963; Latner and Stunkard 2003). Self-image is also negative for overweight children and their parents are often aware of this problem. Quality of life for children has been evaluated in several studies. In one report, children who were severely overweight had a quality of life similar to children diagnosed as having cancer, both of which were substantially lower than normal weight children (Schwimmer et al. 2003). This hospital-based study had a somewhat worse prognosis than a study cohort study based on a two-stage sampling design of primary school children in Australia (Williams et al. 2005). In this study, 4.3% were described as overweight and 20.2% as at risk for overweight. There were significant decreases in physical and social functioning for the overweight children when compared to the normal weight children, but not as severe as in the hospital-based population.

Stigma from overweight in adults. Stigma against obese adults occurs in education, employment, health care, and elsewhere (Puhl and Latner 2007). One group that used the Medical Outcomes Study Short-form Health Survey (SF-36) demonstrated that overweight people presenting for treatment at a weight management center had profound abnormalities in health-related quality of life (Fontaine and Barofsky 2001). Higher BMI values were associated with greater adverse effects. Overweight women appear to be at greater risk of psychological dysfunction, when compared to overweight men; this is potentially due to increased societal pressures on women to be thin (Carpenter et al. 2000). Intentional weight loss improves the quality of life (Fontaine et al. 2004). Severely overweight patients who lost an average of 43 kg through gastric bypass demonstrated improvements on all domains of the SF-36 to such an extent that their post-weight-loss scores were equal to or better than population norms (Choban et al. 1999).

Depression and psychological distress. An increasing body mass index may lead to psychological distress and future dementia (Whitman et al. 2005). Central adiposity has also been associated with the risk of a depressive mood (Lee et al. 2005). In a large study of 497 patients with BMI > 40 kg/m^2 who were preparing for bariatric surgery, the Beck Depression Inventory showed depression in 53% of the subjects with an average value of 17.7 (a score of 16 is depressed). Higher scores were found in young patients and those with poor self-image (Dixon et al. 2003). After weight loss, depression scores improved significantly averaging 7.8 one year after surgery and 9.6 four years after surgery. In a systematic review of epidemiological studies, Atlantis and Baker (2008) found that there was a weak level of evidence supporting the hypothesis that obesity increases the incidence of depression outcomes. Studies from the US tended to show this effect whereas those from other countries did not. A systematic review has shown that four of eight studies that met the criteria of the investigation had an increased risk of dementia (Gorospe and Davie 2007).

In a review of the literature, four cross-sectional studies showed an association between depressive symptoms and overweight in girls aged 8–15 years, with effect sizes including a correlation coefficient of 0.14 and a regression coefficient of 0.27. In four longitudinal studies, depressive symptoms in childhood or adolescence were associated with a 90% to 250% increased risk of subsequent overweight (HR = 1.90 to 3.50) (Liem et al. 2008). Using data from the 2005–2006 NHANES survey that contained 4979 individuals over 20 years of age, 509 of whom had diabetes and 4470 did not, Curtis et al. (2009) found that overweight (BMI 25–29.9 kg/m^2) and obese (BMI ≥ 30 kg/m^2) diabetic patients experience significantly higher rates of mild depression than the nondiabetic counterparts. Moderate depression was significantly higher across all BMI categories in diabetic than nondiabetic patients.

BENEFITS AND POTENTIAL RISKS OF WEIGHT LOSS

Weight loss improves many intermediate risk factors for disease states (1998; 2000; Douketis et al. 2005; Bray 2007a). Two simultaneous publications have clearly established that intentional weight loss lowers mortality. These papers have been termed the missing link because they completed the connection between improvement in risk factors with weight loss and reduced mortality with weight loss (Bray 2007). The first was the prospective matched control study called the Swedish Obese Subjects study (Sjostrom et al. 2007). They found that mortality was reduced by 39% after an average follow-up of 10 years. The second study by Adams et al. (2007) used driver's licenses to match controls to patients who had received a gastric by-pass to produce weight loss. In this study, the risk of death from cardiovascular disease was reduced 56%, diabetes 92%, and cancer 60%.

The risk of diabetes is also reduced by modest weight loss. The diabetes Prevention Program showed that after 3.2 years in an intensive lifestyle program with an initial weight loss of 7% of body weight that the conversion rate was reduced by 55% compared to the placebo-treated control group (Knowler et al. 2002; DPPOS 2008) after long-term follow-up for the DaQing Study (Li et al. 2008).

Weight loss is also beneficial in reducing the risk of diabetes, cancer, hypertension, cardiovascular disease, and sleep disorders but primarily in high-risk individuals. In the Framingham cohort, the effect of weight loss on blood pressure was examined in middle aged (30–49) and older (50–65) adults. After adjusting the confounding variables, they found that a 6.8% weight loss over 4 years was associated with a 21% to 29% decrease in risk of hypertension. After adjusting for cancer and cardiovascular risk, these percentages increased further with middle-aged individuals reducing their risk of hypertension by 28% and older adults reducing their risk of hypertension by 37%. Thus, a modest weight loss significantly reduced the risk of hypertension (Moore et al. 2005).

Hypertensive individuals who maintained their weight loss following a weight loss intervention were able to maintain lower blood pressure compared to the individuals who regained weight, where blood pressure returned to baseline levels (Stevens et al. 2001). In a meta-analysis of 25 studies with 4874 individuals, Neter et al. (2003) found that weight loss averaging 5.1 kg after diet and/or exercise programs reduced blood pressure by 4.44/3.47 mmHg. The studies with weight losses above 5 kg showed larger decreases in blood pressure than those with less weight loss.

Blood lipids and sleep disturbances also improve with weight loss (Peppard et al. 2000). Indeed, effective weight loss would be the first order of treatment for individuals with the metabolic syndrome, since it can reverse all of the components of this syndrome, including the insulin resistance. In a systematic review of long-term weight loss studies and their applicability to clinical practice, Douketis et al. (2005) found that dietary and lifestyle therapy provided <5 kg weight loss after 2–4 years, that pharmacological therapy could produce 5 to 10 kg weight loss over 1–2 years. Weight loss of ≥5% from baseline is not consistently associated with improvements in cardiovascular risk factors and these benefits appear primarily in the individuals with concomitant cardiovascular risk factors.

Weight loss also reduces the risk of cancer in women, but not men. In women, the number of first-time cancers after inclusion in the SOS prospective trial of bariatric surgery was lower in the surgery group ($n = 79$) than in the control group ($n = 130$; HR = 0.58 CI 0.44–0.77; $p = 0.0001$), whereas there was no effect of surgery in men (38 in the surgery group vs. 39 in the control group; HR = 0.97 CI 0.62–1.52; $p = 0.90$) (Sjöström et al. 2009).

Weight loss also benefits patients with osteoarthritis. In a cluster randomized trial comparing a standardized consultation focusing on weight loss and physical activity vs. usual care, patients assigned to the standardized consultation lost more weight and increased physical activity scores more than those in the usual care group (Ravaud 2009).

Weight loss, thiazolidinediones, metformin, and sulfonylureas all produce beneficial changes in inflammatory markers. We could not leave this discussion without noting the possibility that weight reduction may have detrimental effects. In a study of older men, bone mineral density declined with weight loss (Ensrud et al. 2005). In this study, the bone mineral density (BMD) at the hip increased 0.1% per year in men who gained weight over an average of 1.8 years of follow-up. In the men whose weight was stable, BMD declined 0.3% per year, and in men who lost weight the decline was 1.4% per year. The initial BMI, body composition, or intention to lose weight did not affect these changes. Among the men with a BMI $\geq$ 30 kg/m^2 who intentionally lost weight, there was a decrease in BMD of the hip.

In summary, this chapter has dealt with the costs and risks associated with being overweight. From the time that life insurance statistics became available there has been a growing body of information showing that overweight is risking fate. The effects are the result of enlarging fat cells and increased total fat mass each of which relates to one or more of the problems associated with being overweight. Diabetes, liver disease, high blood pressure, heart disease, and some forms of cancer are among the most important. There is also data arguing that weight loss is beneficial.

Part II

Treatment of Obesity

5 Prevention, Evaluation, and Introduction to Treatment

INTRODUCTION

Preventing further rise of body weight is a key public health challenge, and reducing the percentage of people who are obese an even greater one. More than 40 years ago the Fogarty International Center at the National Institutes of Health identified obesity as an important public health problem and organized one of their first two conferences around this topic (Bray 1976). In spite of this auspicious beginning, the problem has only gotten worse. We need to prevent obesity because doing so will prolong life and reduce the risk of developing diabetes, heart disease, and some forms of cancer. Obesity is a disease that can bankrupt the health care system, particularly in developing countries (Bray 1998).

How Can We Prevent the Current Epidemic?

Preventing the current epidemic of obesity and reducing its prevalence are major public health goals. Efforts to prevent overweight have been the subject of several recent reviews (Kumanyika and Daniels 2006; James 2008; Daniels et al. 2005; Swinburn et al. 2004; Koplan et al. 2005; Seidell et al. 2005; Jeffery and French 1999; Simkin-Silverman et al. 2003; Kuller et al. 2001). The most promising news comes from the National Center for Health Statistics, which suggests that the epidemic may have slowed or even reached a peak in the first decade of the twenty-first century (Flegal et al. 2010).

The first law of thermodynamics or the energy balance concept serves as the basis for both ancient and modern ways of treating obesity. If obesity results from an excess of energy intake over energy expenditure over some period of time, then to redress the problem we need to reverse this imbalance, either by eating less, exercising more, or a bit of both. This concept is shown in Figure 5.1, which also lists the general types of treatment that are available under one of two headings: cognitive and noncognitive. The cognitive treatments are so named because they require "thinking" on the part of the participant. The individual has to take the necessary steps to reduce their energy intake or increase their physical activity. No one can do it for them anymore than the horse that is led to water can be forced to drink. The other types of treatment do not require this same type of individual commitment. They include surgery and to some extent medications, although the patient does have to take the medication for it to work. One of the best examples of a truly noncognitive treatment is the use of fluoride added to water supplies in amounts that will reduce dental caries. The individual drinking water does not have to add fluoride, nor can they easily remove it. Surgery is like this. Once the bariatric operation (see Chapter 8) is done, the patient cannot undo it. Medications (see Chapter 7) also have some element of automatic response when the medication is taken.

The epidemic of overweight is occurring on a genetic background that has not changed significantly since the epidemic began 30 years ago. Nonetheless, it is clear that genetic factors play a critical role in the susceptibility to becoming obese in our modern toxic environment. One analogy is that "genes load the gun and the environment pulls the trigger." Modifying one or more

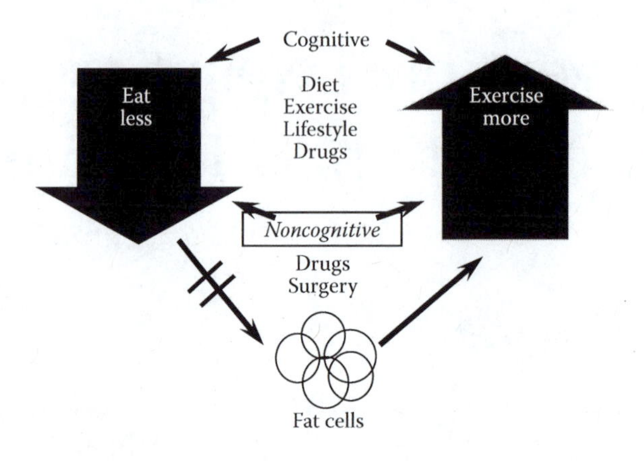

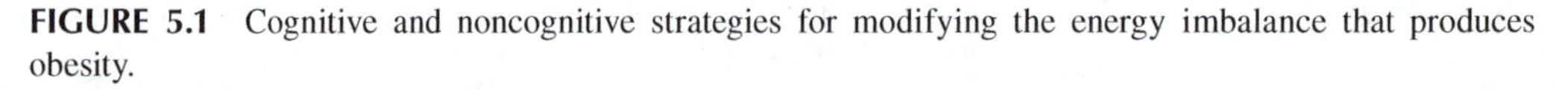

FIGURE 5.1 Cognitive and noncognitive strategies for modifying the energy imbalance that produces obesity.

environmental factors acting on our ancient genes must be the primary strategy if we are to prevent obesity. The belief that this can be done by the individual alone is to miss the argument of how environmental factors have acted on these ancient gene pools to produce the current epidemic, with major emphasis on the imprinting of the plastic brain of the growing child and adolescent and the low cost of tasty energy-dense foods.

The first law of thermodynamics and the idea of energy balance have lulled us into the uncomfortable place of believing that individuals through "will power," increased food choices, or more places to exercise can overcome the current epidemic of obesity. Cognitive approaches relying on individual commitment and resolve have been unsuccessful in stemming the epidemic so far and there is nothing to suggest that they will be more successful in the future.

It is what the first law of thermodynamics does not tell us about energy balance that is key to the strategies of prevention. In this context, it is the unconscious host systems on which environmental factors operate that produces the disease of obesity. If the vending machines that now provide kickbacks to schools contained beverages with no calories, either from sugar or high fructose corn syrup (HFCS), available calories would be reduced. The exposure of young children to the high levels of fructose found in either sucrose (table sugar) or HFCS may produce detrimental imprinting of the brain, making overweight more likely and more difficult to control (Bray et al. 2004).

PREVENTION OF OBESITY

At least four preventive strategies are available to deal with the epidemic: education, regulation, modification of the food supply, and changes in the cost of food energy. Education about good nutrition and healthy weight in the school curriculum would be beneficial in helping all children learn how to select appropriate foods and should be included in school curricula. Foods used in school breakfast and lunch programs should match these educational messages.

However, it is unwise to rely on educational strategies alone, since they have not, so far, prevented the epidemic of obesity. The program of knowing your BMI initially instituted on a state wide basis in Arkansas may have helped that state to reduce the upward trend in obesity. Regulation is a second strategy. Regulating an improved food label would be one good idea. Regulations on appropriate serving sizes and caloric value might be part of the information provided by restaurants on their menus. This is now required in New York City and will, hopefully, spread around the country.

Modification of some components of the food system is a third and very important strategy. Since the energy we eat comes from the food we eat, we need to modify this system to provide smaller portions and less energy density. One approach is to use differentiated food taxes to promote healthy diets. This is the approach New York State is trying with its tax on soft drinks introduced in 2007, and this approach has been encouraged by a group of prominent nutritional scientists (Brownell et al. 2009). This strategy has been argued both at the academic level (Smed et al. 2005; Smed and Denver 2005; WHO/FAO 2002), and at the policy level (FAO 2004). It may be that economic tools that will shift food choices using costs are the "fluoride" for treating the epidemic of overweight.

Some years ago, I proposed that the best strategy for prevention of obesity may be modeled after the use of fluoride for prevention of dental caries. The addition of fluoride to the water supply had a more profound effect on the incidence of dental cavities than brushing and flossing teeth. Brushing and flossing are like diet and exercise. They both require commitment on the part of the individual. Adding something like fluoride to the water supply doesn't require any commitment. Increasing the price of oil may be one such strategy. Between 1940 and 2005, Pollan pointed out that the number of calories from petroleum (oil) used to produce food energy has risen dramatically. In 1940, it was 0.4 cal of oil for each calorie of food energy. In 2005, it had risen over 20-fold with 10 calories of oil needed for each calorie of food. These calories come from the petroleum products used to make fertilizers, to transport food, to process and package it, and for pesticides and so on. If oil prices rise significantly, this will shift the use of oil for food production and distribution and our consumption patterns will change (Pollan 2008).

Strategies for Preventing Obesity Aimed at the Entire Population

Population-based messages aimed at the public concerning food and exercise are cognitive in nature requiring individual commitment (Kumanyika and Daniels 2006). If the individual follows the advice in the message, this strategy would be sufficient to overcome the epidemic of obesity. However, positive preventive messages are delivered in an environment in which there are many competing alternative messages urging consumption of this or that kind of food or eating at one or another of many different kinds of restaurants. The low-fat message of the 1990s is one example of a message that assumed obesity results from increased fat intake and that reducing fat intake would reverse it. Omitted from this was the realization that eating less fat did not necessarily mean eating fewer calories and thus redressing the energy imbalance. A test of the low-fat hypothesis as a public health message came from the Women's Health Initiative. Women were randomly assigned to normal or low-fat diets, but without calorie goals. The women assigned to the low-fat diet lost 2.2 kg at 1 year compared to 0.3 kg in the control group with normal fat intake, but after the low point, weight was regained, although those in the low-fat group remained on average 0.4 kg lighter after 7.5 years (Howard et al. 2005). Of particular interest is that the weight change over 7.5 years had a strong relation to the level of fat that the women actually ate. Those with the lowest quintile of fat intake remained over 2 kg lighter after 7 years than those in the highest fat intake group, indicating that dietary fat is one component of a diet for lowering body weight, but that it is not the whole story.

If one believed that the current epidemic of obesity were due to limited activity, then a campaign like "America on the Move," which enrolls individuals to use step counters as a way to increase their activity, should be an effective strategy (Hill and Peters 1998). The jury is still out on this strategy.

An alternative approach might be to reengineer the built environment to make it both easier to walk and make it more likely that individuals would do so rather than getting into their car (Sallis et al. 2009). The current housing model with clusters of houses off a main street where the automobile is essential for mobility will make this strategy a long-term one. A systematic review by Papas et al. (2007) identified 20 studies that examined the relation of obesity to the numbers of outlets for physical activity and food. Of these, 17 found a significant relationship between built environment (food outlets or access to physical activity) and risk of obesity. The number of recreational facilities and likelihood of overweight in adolescents were significantly related.

Food

Faith et al. (2007) reviewed research that used manipulations of the food environment to produce weight change. They concluded that ease of food access may influence food purchases, consumption, and possibly weight change, while restriction of food availability may accomplish the same goals although this requires further research. The food industry, for obvious reasons, favors the hypothesis that obesity results from reduced levels of physical activity and strongly supports providing more places for people to exercise and providing them with more healthy alternatives in food stores as a strategy to help overcome the obesity problem (Kumanyika and Daniels 2006; James and Cole 2008). However, "healthy" food items are likely to be more expensive than the ones already on the shelf, and since newer technologies and marketing are needed, it is unclear whether a price-sensitive public can be persuaded to buy them.

Strategies for improving access to healthful foods often focus on fruits and vegetables. A diet high in fruits, vegetables, and low-fat dairy products with a reduction in the level of fat- and sugar-containing products lowers blood pressure across the range of salt intake in individuals who were maintaining their body weight (Appel et al. 1997; Sacks et al. 2001). Access to fruits and vegetables through farmers' markets, subsidizing the availability of fresh fruits and vegetables to school children, lowering the cost of fruits and vegetables while increasing the price of high-fat or high-sugar foods in school or worksite cafeterias, and changing marketing strategies in other ways that increase fruit and vegetable consumption are some way to change food intake patterns (Kennedy et al. 2006; Buzby et al. 2003; www.ers.usda.gov/publications/efan03006; Glanz and Hoelscher 2004; Glanz and Yaroch 2004; French and Wechser 2004). Since we are all price-sensitive, these might move choices of food from the lower cost less healthy ones to more healthy choices. However, as Drewnowski has pointed out, the high-fat, high-sugar alternatives provide much more food energy for the money than the so-called "healthier options" (Drewnowski and Darmon 2005).

Another strategy toward this end is to limit availability of higher energy foods by making them more expensive. A review of the relationship of price for food items to their consumption in Europe by Smed et al. (2005) has shown that increasing the tax or reducing the subsidies on "unhealthy" items and reducing the tax on "healthy" items through the value-added tax system could shift consumption toward healthier foods (Smed and Denver 2005). The federally funded programs such as food stamps, school lunches, and meals on wheels could also be used toward this end. Pending the willingness of the public and the politicians to tackle some of the political implications of tax policy to combat the epidemic of obesity, this strategy is likely to remain unused (Brownell et al. 2009).

Increasing Physical Activity as a Focus for Prevention

An overall increase in physical activity would increase energy expenditure and is one strategy for prevention of obesity. One assumption of such a strategy is that activity may have decreased during the time that the epidemic of obesity developed.

How much has our daily activity level changed? To examine this question, Cutler et al. (2003) examined this problem in levels of activity in various tasks from 1965 to 1995, which covers the period before and to the peak of weight gain. These data are summarized in Table 5.1. They found that over the 30 years from 1965 to 1995, the major changes in activity have been a decrease in household work and an increase in recreation and communication. These are relatively small compared to the proportion of the daily routine that is spent in paid work and in personal needs and care. Another approach has used repeat measurements of total energy expenditure with doubly-labeled water. Total daily energy expenditure was measured twice in over 300 individuals, but did not show any decrease in physical activity level over the time when the epidemic of obesity was developing (Westerterp and Speakman 2008). Altering the "built environment" such as sidewalks and shopping centers is one way to increase daily activity (Sallis and Glanz 2009). Because there is a 30–40 year lag between initiation of changes in architectural land use and real changes in configuration of sidewalks, this is unlikely to impact this problem in the foreseeable future. We, thus, think food intake is a more viable strategy for rewarding.

TABLE 5.1
Changes in Level of Physical Activity for Various Categories of Activity from 1965 to 1995

Activity	1965	1975	1985	1995
Paid work	290	258	259	266
Household work	146	128	124	102
Child care	37	31	31	18
Obtaining goods and services	51	45	53	49
Personal needs and care	622	644	634	632
Education and training	12	16	18	23
Organizational activities	20	24	18	17
Entertainment/social	78	65	65	72
Recreation	27	37	43	47
Communication	158	191	95	212
TOTAL	1440	1440	1440	1440
Kcal/min/kg	1.69	1.57	1.62	1.53
E for 70 kg man	16.4	13.5	14.7	12.6
E for 60 kg woman	15.1	12.3	13.5	11.3

Source: Adapted from Cutler, D.M., et al., *J. Econ. Perspect.*, 17(3), 93–118, 2003.

Workplaces provide another location where prevention and intervention can occur. In a review of worksite nutrition and physical activity programs, Anderson et al. (2009) noted modest improvements in employee weight status at the 6 to 12-month follow-up where such programs exist. Based on nine randomized, controlled trials, there was a weight loss of 1.3 kg (2.8 pounds) (95% CI −4.6, −1.0) and a decrease of 0.5 BMI units (95% CI −0.8, −0.2) units based on six randomized controlled clinical trials. The findings were applicable to both male and female employees, across a range of worksite settings. Most of the studies combined informational and behavioral strategies to influence diet and physical activity; fewer studies modified the work environment (e.g., cafeteria, exercise facilities) to promote healthy choices. This is an area of potential future advance.

The nutrition-transition in China provides an interesting example of how the modern way of life makes preservation of physical activity so difficult (Zhai et al. 2009; Monda et al. 2008). As recently as 20 years ago, the bicycle was a major mode of transport for the Chinese, but no longer. The automobile and public transport systems are relegating the bicycle to museums. Whether understanding the need for people to move can provide a rescue strategy for weight gain is doubtful.

Use of Social Marketing

One element in trying to combat the epidemic is to focus on the needs of selected groups—so-called "social marketing." The idea is to provide focused messages targeted at specific subgroups. Another approach is to focus on specific food groups. The program by the National Cancer Institute to increase the consumption of fruits and vegetables through the "5 A Day for Better Health" program is an example of this idea. Although we would all agree that this is a desirable approach, its effectiveness in changing average fruit and vegetable intake has not been overwhelming (Stables et al. 2002).

"America on the Move" is another targeted program that encourages state by state involvement in public-private partnerships to improve eating and activity patterns of the public. Outcome results are awaited (www.americanonthemove.org).

Strategies Aimed at Children

There is a great deal of concern for the plight of obese children. The pioneering work of the psychoanalyst Dr. Hilde Bruch, a refugee from Nazi Germany working in the 1940s, did much to alert the public to this important issue.

Children of overweight parents are a high-risk group for development of overweight (Berkowitz et al. 2009). In a long term study, Berkowitz et al. followed 32 high-risk children whose maternal prepregnancy BMI was 30.4 kg/m^2 and compared them to 29 low-risk children whose maternal BMI was low at 19.6 kg/m^2. Four-year-old children consumed a test meal in which their eating behavior was assessed, including rate of caloric consumption, mouthfuls per minute, and requests for food. Parental prompts for the child to eat also were noted. Parental feeding prompts were not different between high-risk and low-risk children, but the rate of eating measured by mouthfuls of food per minute and total caloric intake per minute during the test meal predicted an increased risk of becoming overweight or obese at age 6. Thus, preschool years and the home environment are important in setting risks for future obesity.

Schools have also changed. They were once a place where children could be very active. With security issues and concerns about children walking home from school safely, there is less opportunity for physical exercise. Providing safe pedestrian walkways to school could increase physical activity for children more easily than changing the built environment for adults. In a review of school-based programs, Harris et al. (2009) examined 18 studies involving 18,141 children. They were primarily elementary school children and had programs that lasted from 6 months to 3 years. A meta-analysis showed that interventions involving physical activity did not improve BMI (Harris et al. 2009).

To provide more detail on prevention of childhood obesity, I have extracted data from a Cochrane Collaboration review of preventive strategies for children. The long-term studies described below lasted 52 weeks or more.

Long-Term Studies. One controlled trial that was deemed of good quality was conducted in the United States and randomized 26 children and their families to two conditions: 1) increasing fruit and vegetable intake and 2) decreasing fat and sugar intake (Epstein et al. 2001). The children were ages 6 to 11 years and at least one parent accompanied them. They received a comprehensive behavioral program. At the end of 12 months, the decrease in percentage of overweight was 1.10% in the fruit and vegetable group, and 2.40% in the group that decreased fat and sugar intake. These differences were not statistically significant, but are nonetheless tantalizing and suggest the need for applying this to high-risk groups like the children of overweight parents.

Hilde Bruch (1904–1984) is noted for her contributions to the study of childhood obesity and her book *The Importance of Overweight* published in 1957. Dr. Bruch grew up in a Jewish family with six siblings in Dulken, Germany. For practical reasons, she did not pursue mathematics or her interest in dress design, but graduated with a medical degree from the University of Freiburg in 1929. As the climate for tolerance deteriorated in Germany with the rise of Hitler, she immigrated to London, where she spent one year. Her initial work in pediatrics shifted into psychiatry as World War II began. In 1943, she became a professor of psychiatry at Columbia University, College of Physicians and Surgeons. Her early contribution showing that most childhood obesity was not due to Frohlich's syndrome or hypothalamic obesity was a landmark. As an older, single woman, she finally decided to leave New York and accepted a position at the Baylor College of Medicine in Houston, TX as professor of psychiatry. During these years she made significant contributions to understanding the psychiatric aspects of childhood obesity (Gallo 1994; Garfinkel 1986).

A second study of good quality was conducted by James et al. (2004) where 644 children were randomized by school class into 15 intervention and 14 control classes in 6 schools. The baseline prevalence of overweight was comparable. The intervention focused on decreasing consumption of carbonated beverages. The intervention was delivered in three one-hour sessions by trained personnel with the assistance of teachers. At 12 months, the change in BMI "z" scores was not significantly different between intervention and control classes (mean z score 0.7 (SD 0.2)). However, there was a reduction in the self-reported consumption of soft drinks.

A third trial was conducted in Thailand in randomized kindergarten children divided by class into an exercise group and a control group with five classes in each arm (Mo-Suwan 1998). The reduction in the prevalence of obesity tended toward significance ($p = 0.07$).

A U.S. trial including 549 children from six schools was stratified by percentage ethnicity (Dowda et al. 2005). The intervention, called SPARK (Sports, Play, and Active Recreation for Kids) was a physical education program with a self-management component. The results for boys showed that the control group had significantly lower BMIs at 6 and 12 months, but not at 18 months. In contrast, the girls in the control group had lower BMIs at each time point that reached statistical significance at 18 months.

The Pathways Study (Caballero 2003) is one of the largest studies for prevention of obesity in children. The participants included 1704 children from 41 American-Indian schools. Children were ages 8–11. Pathways was a school-based, multicomponent, multicenter intervention for reducing percentage of body fat. There were four components: 1) changing dietary intake; 2) increasing physical activity; 3) A classroom curriculum focused on healthy eating and lifestyle; and 4) a family-involvement program. At the end of the 3-year study, knowledge improved and fat intake at lunch decreased, but there were no changes in either body composition or activity level measured by motion sensor.

The Planet Health study is a high-quality randomized controlled trial (Gortmaker et al. 1999) conducted among 1295 ethnically diverse children in 10 U.S. schools in New England who were randomized by school. The children were ages 11–12 years and in the sixth to eighth grade. The program was a behavioral choice intervention and concentrated on the promotion of physical activity, modification of dietary intake, and reduction of sedentary behavior with an emphasis on reducing time watching television. At follow-up the percentage of obese girls in the intervention schools was reduced 53% compared with controls (OR = 0.47 95% CI 0.24 to 0.93). Each hour of reduction in television time predicted a 15% reduction in obesity (OR 0.85 95% CI 0.75 to 0.97) (see Figure 5.2). Among the boys, there was a decline in BMI in both groups, but no significant difference between them. Time spent viewing television was reduced among both boys and girls and fruit and vegetable consumption increased significantly. The authors concluded that the

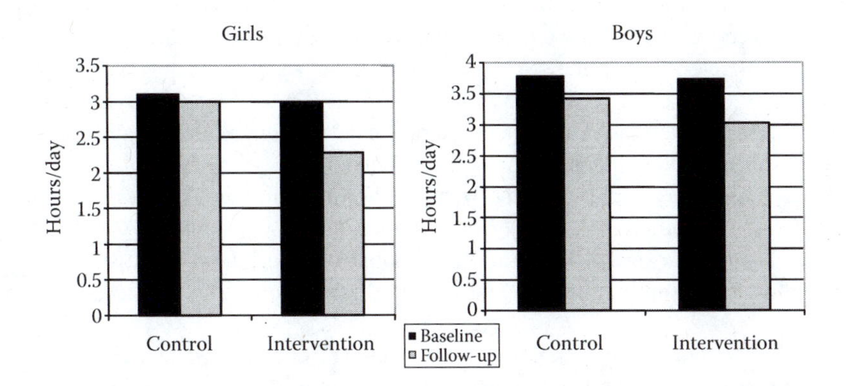

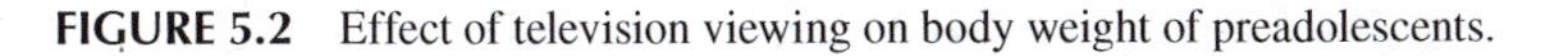
FIGURE 5.2 Effect of television viewing on body weight of preadolescents.

decline in television watching was a major factor in preventing obesity (Gortmaker Peterson et al. 1999).

In another clinical trial from Germany, Mueller et al. (2001) randomized a group of 414 children from six schools into control or intervention groups in the Kiel Obesity Prevention Study or KOPS. The key messages in the intervention group were to eat more fruits and vegetables each day, to reduce high fat foods, to keep active for at least 1 hour a day, and to decrease television viewing to less than 1 hour a day. At the end of 1 year there was no significant difference in change of BMI between the intervention and control groups.

In a program called Active Program Promoting Lifestyle in School, or APPLES, 634 children in 10 schools were randomized to intervention or control groups. The intervention included teacher training and resources, modification of school meals, support for physical education, and playgroup activities. At 1 year, there was no difference in the change in BMI between the children in the two groups, nor was there any difference in dieting behavior. However, children reported a higher consumption of vegetables. Although APPLES was successful in changing the ethos in the schools and the attitudes of the children, the trial was ineffective in changing weight status.

The program "VERB™—It's What You Do!" was developed by the U.S. Centers for Disease Control and Prevention and is another example of a social marketing strategy. It is designed to increase physical activity among ethnically diverse 9 to 13 year olds (Wong et al. 2004). The question of whether it is really possible to get long-term behavioral change in a society with a vibrant advertising industry providing opposing messages remains to be seen.

Mind, Exercise, Nutrition—Do it (MEND) is a British program held at a sports center, twice weekly, for 3 months that consists of behavior modification, physical activity, and nutrition education. In their pilot study, 11 obese children ages 7–11 years and their families were recruited and attended a mean of 78% (range 63%–88%) of the sessions. Waist circumference, cardiovascular fitness, and self-esteem were all significantly improved at 3 months and continued to improve at 6 months. BMI was significantly improved at 3 months but lost significance by 6 months. This program has now been expanded to many sites through the United Kingdom.

There is clearly some comfort in the fact that, in the state of Arkansas, measuring BMI in all school children and providing it to their parents was associated with a stabilizing of BMI over several years.

Strategies Aimed at Adults

A large number of trials have been conducted in adults and reviewed in detail by Kumanyika and Daniels (2006). The Pound of Prevention study (Jeffery and French 1999; Sherwood et al. 2000) is probably the largest and most general study for prevention of overweight reported to date. It demonstrated the feasibility of reaching a large number of people and producing some positive behavioral changes. However, as with many of the studies in children, the interventions were not successful in preventing weight gain relative to the control condition. The decrease of fat intake and increased physical activity were the strongest predictors of weight maintenance (Sherwood et al. 2000). Again, behavioral changes were positive and perhaps a higher intensity might have produced different results, but at the present time there is a reasonable argument to be made that money spent on behavioral efforts at changing behavior is unproductive.

The results of the 5-year trial from the Healthy Women Study is also worth noting (Simkin-Silverman et al. 2003; Kuller et al. 2001). Behavioral counseling at 6 months was effective in preventing a weight gain during the transition to menopause. The intervention program appears to have been well-received, judging from retention rates, but it seems to be labor- and cost-intensive to deliver.

Rural counties in the United States have higher rates of obesity, sedentary lifestyle, and associated chronic diseases than nonrural areas. To tackle this problem, Perri et al. worked with the U.S.D.A. Cooperative Extension Service. They recruited obese women from rural communities who had completed an initial 6-month weight-loss program at Cooperative Extension Service offices in six medically underserved rural counties in Florida ($n = 234$). The women were randomized to an extended care program or to an education control group. The extended-care programs entailed problem-solving counseling delivered in 26 biweekly sessions via telephone or face-to-face. Control group participants received 26 biweekly newsletters containing weight-control advice. The body weight at entry was 96.4 kg, and the women in the intervention group lost 10 kg during the 6-month intervention. One year after randomization, participants in the telephone and face-to-face extended-care programs regained less weight (mean [SE], 1.2 [0.7] kg, respectively) than those in the education control group (3.7 [0.7] kg; $p = .03$). The beneficial effects of extended-care counseling were mediated by greater adherence to behavioral weight-management strategies. Cost analyses indicated that telephone counseling was less expensive than face-to-face intervention, thus offering a strategy of working with the Cooperative Extension Service using behavioral weight strategies to modulate body weight (Perri et al. 2008).

INTRODUCTION TO TREATMENT

A great deal of effort has been expended on preventive strategies, but we still have a long way to go. When prevention fails, and an individual becomes obese, the focus shifts to treatment. From here on in this book, we will develop the procedures for evaluating and treating the overweight or obese individual, and describe the uses and limitations of the solutions that are available.

Evaluation of the Overweight Patient

The first step in deciding on treatment is to evaluate the individual and to decide whether they have an unhealthy weight, and, if so, what risk this carries for them. The basic components involved in the evaluation of the overweight patient are a medical examination and a laboratory assessment. This should include a record of the historical events associated with their weight problem, a physical examination for pertinent information and appropriate laboratory tests. We will use the criteria recommended by the U.S. Preventive Services Task Force, and also take into account the reports from the National Heart, Lung, and Blood Institute Report (1998) and the World Health Organization (2000). The importance of evaluating overweight individuals has increased as the epidemic of overweight has worsened and the number of potential patients needing treatment has increased.

Clinical History

Among the important features to identify are whether there are specific events that are associated with the increase in body weight. This would include the genetic and neuroendocrine conditions described below. Has there been a sudden increase in weight or has body weight been rising steadily over a long period of time? Weight gain is associated with an increased risk to health. Three categories of weight gain are identified: <5 kg (<11 lb); 5 to 10 kg (11 to 22 lb); and >10 kg (>22 lb). In addition to total weight gain, the rate of weight gain after age 20 needs to be considered when deciding the degree of risk for a given patient. The more rapidly they are gaining weight, the more concerned you should be.

Etiologic factors that cause obesity should be identified, if possible. If there are clear-cut factors, such as genetic syndromes, neuroendocrine diseases, drugs that produce weight gain, or cessation of smoking, they should be noted on the clinical evaluation form (Table 5.2). The presence of symptoms suggestive of sleep apnea such as snoring, plethoric face, or daytime somnolence should be noted along with abdominal symptoms that might suggest gall bladder disease.

Attempts to lose weight whether successful or unsuccessful should be identified for the insight it provides about what may have worked and what didn't. Assessing the level of physical activity is also important since a sedentary lifestyle increases the risk of early death. Individuals with no regular physical activity are at higher risk than individuals with modest levels of physical activity.

TABLE 5.2
Clinical Evaluation Form for Recording Vital Signs Related to Obesity

Clinical History
1. Are family members obese?
2. How fast are you gaining weight (lb/yr or kg/yr)?
3. Do you snore or fall asleep in the daytime?
4. Are you depressed?
5. Do you have pain when you eat food?
6. Are you treated for diabetes?
7. Are you treated for high blood pressure?
Vital Signs
Height
Weight
Calculate BMI or use table (kg/m^2)
Waist circumference (cm)
Laboratory Data for Diagnosis of Metaboic Syndrome
HDL-cholesterol
Triglycerides (fasting)
Fasting glucose
Blood pressure

Family History

It is important to determine whether the individual comes from a family where obesity is common—the usual setting—or whether they have become obese in a family where few people are overweight. It is well-known that children from families with overweight parents have a higher risk of obesity. This latter setting suggests a search for environmental factors that may be contributing to weight gain. Recent studies have shown that in children and adolescents with a BMI above 30 kg/m^2, alterations in the melanocortin-4 receptors occur in between 2.5% and 5.5% of these individuals. This genetic defect is among the most common that are associated with any chronic disease.

Physical Examination

Vital Signs Associated with Obesity

The first step in a clinical examination of an overweight patient (Bray 2008) is to determine their vital signs, which include weight and height, from which the body mass index can be calculated, and waist circumference as well as pulse and blood pressure. Measuring height and weight is the initial step in the clinical assessment because they are essential for determining the BMI, which is calculated as the body weight (kg) divided by the stature (height [m]) squared (wt/ht^2) and is shown in Table 5.2 (Bray 1978). BMI has a reasonable correlation with body fat, and is relatively unaffected by height (Gallagher et al. 2000). Table 5.2 provides a form to record the height, weight, BMI and other relevant clinical and laboratory data during this evaluation. This helps categorize the patient as preoverweight or overweight, with or without clinical complications.

BMI has a curvilinear relationship to risk (see Chapter 4). Several levels of risk can be identified based on cut-points that need to be interpreted in an ethnically sensitive manner. Different ethnic groups have different percentages of body fat for the same BMI (see Chapter 2) (Gallagher et al. 2000). Thus, the same BMI presumably carries a different level of risk in each of these populations. These differences need to be taken into consideration when making clinical judgments about the degree of risk for the individual patient. During treatment for weight loss, the body weight is more useful than the BMI, since the height will not change and the inclusion of the squared function of height makes it more difficult for physician and patient to evaluate.

Components of the Metabolic Syndrome

Waist circumference Waist circumference is a component of the metabolic syndrome and is the most practical measurement for determining central adiposity. Waist circumference is measured using a metal or nondistensible plastic tape placed around the abdomen at the level of the umbilicus or at the midpoint between the lower rib and the supra iliac crest or at the iliac crest, the most common locations. Although visceral fat can be measured more precisely with computed tomography (CT) or magnetic resonance imaging (MRI), these are expensive and clinical studies show that the waist circumference is essentially as good and much less difficult to obtain (Alberti 2009).

Measuring the change in waist circumference along with weight is a good strategy for following the clinical progress of weight loss. It is particularly valuable when patients become more physically active. Physical activity may slow loss of muscle mass and thus slow weight loss while fat continues to be mobilized. Waist circumference can help in making this distinction. The relationship of central fat to risk factors for health varies among populations as well as within them. Japanese Americans and Indians from South Asia have relatively more visceral fat and are thus at higher risk for a given BMI, particularly in diabetics or total body fat than are Caucasians.

Lipid abnormalities There are two lipids that contribute to the dyslipidemia of the metabolic syndrome, HDL-cholesterol and triglycerides. These have been referred to as the "atherogenic lipids." A low HDL-cholesterol, with different cut-points for men and women and high triglyceride number are the key elements. Another way to assess this risk is with what Depres calls the "dyslipidemic waist," which is the combination of a high triglyceride number and a large waist.

Glucose An elevated glucose and treated diabetes are also elements of the metabolic syndrome. The range for impaired fasting glucose is 100 mg/dL to 125 mg/dL. A value of 126 mg/dL or above, if confirmed, in a fasting individual who is not otherwise stressed is diagnostic of diabetes.

Blood pressure Careful measurement of blood pressure is important. Hypertension is amenable to improvement with diet (Appel et al. 1997) and hypertension or its treatment is an important criteria for the metabolic syndrome. Having the patient sit quietly for 5 minutes before measuring the blood pressure with a calibrated instrument will help reduce stress that can increase it.

Other Items for the Physical Examination

Acanthosis nigricans deserves a comment. This is a clinical condition with increased pigmentation in the folds of the neck, along the exterior surface of the distal extremities, and over the knuckles. It may signify increased insulin resistance or malignancy, and should be evaluated. If there are suggestions of sleep apnea—snoring, daytime somnolence—a sleep study may be indicated. If abdominal pain occurs after eating, a gall bladder study may be indicated. If symptoms of depression are present, the patient may need to be evaluated and possibly treated. If children are markedly obese, and there are suggestions of close ties in the family marriage, a genetic screen may be appropriate.

Laboratory evaluation. Laboratory tests in addition to those needed for the diagnosis of the metabolic syndrome are important for refining the clinical strategy and evaluating the risk associated with the BMI. The laboratory can measure lipids, glucose, and c-reactive protein (CRP) and help in the diagnosis of genetic and neuroendocrine disease. An increased fasting glucose, low HDL-cholesterol, or high triacylglycerol values are atherogenic components of the metabolic syndrome that have been defined earlier. Along with elevated blood pressure, it is possible to categorize the patient as having metabolic syndrome by one of several sets of criteria (see Table 5.3). In addition to the lipids that are determined as part of the assessment of the metabolic syndrome, a patient should have a measurement of their LDL-cholesterol, which is a key risk factor for coronary heart disease.

TABLE 5.3
Criteria for Metabolic Syndrome

	ATP-III Criteria	
Criterion	**Metric**	
Waist circumference	Use criteria specific for the population being evaluated	
Female	>35 inches*	>88 cm
Male	>40 inches*	>102 cm
HDL-cholesterol		
Female	<50 mg/dL**	
Male	<40 mg/dL**	
Triglycerides	>150 mg/dL&	
Glucose	100–125 mg/dL$	5.5–7.1 mmol/L*
Blood pressure	130/85#	130/85**

Source: Adapted from Alberti, K.G., et al., *Circulation*, 120(16), 1640–1645, 2009.
Note: Values for the United States from the NHLBI Report;
** or treatment for dyslipidemia; & or treatment of dyslipidemia; $ or treatment for diabetes; # or treatment for hypertension.

Also important is a measurement of highly-sensitive c-reactive protein (hs-CRP). It is now clear that risk for heart disease can be predicted from both the LDL-cholesterol and hs-CRP.

Genetic Factors in the Development of Obesity

Monogenic Causes of Excess Body Fat or Fat Distribution

The rare syndromes that produce obesity are listed in Table 5.4 (Farooqi et al. 2005). These include defects in the melanocortin-4 receptor, a deficiency in leptin or the leptin receptor, a defect in the processing of pro-opiomelanocortin, a defect in pro-convertase 1, a defect in TSH-beta, and a defect in peroxisome proferator-activated receptor-gamma (PPAR-γ). Although these defects are relatively rare, they have powerful effects on food intake and the deposition of body fat.

Mutations in the Melanocortin-4 Receptor

There are five different melanocortin receptors. The melanocortin 1-receptor is located on melanocytes and transmit signals for making pigment in response to α-melanocyte-stimulating hormone (α-MSH). The melanocortin 2-receptor is located in the adrenal gland and responds to adrenocorticotrophin (ACTH). Food intake and energy expenditure are modulated by α-MSH through the melanocortin 3-receptor and melanocortin 4-receptor that are located primarily in the brain. The melancortin receptor-5 is more widely distributed and doesn't have the specific effects of the other four.

Genetic engineering to eliminate the melanocortin-4 receptor (MC4R) in the mouse brain produces massive obesity. Numerous genetic defects in this receptor produce variable degrees of obesity, depending on their location. In surveys of large numbers of individuals, the prevalence of defects in this gene has been reported to range from 2.5% to over 5% (Farooqi 2003). The effect of defects in two different receptor locations on food intake in children is shown in Figure 5.3, which also includes data on food intake in normal children and in children lacking the leptin receptor. Leptin deficiency clearly has the biggest effect, but the difference between two children with defects in MC4R shows the variability of this receptor. Individuals with MC4R defects can be either sex. In contrast with leptin deficiency described below, individuals with the MC4R defects are generally normal height or tall, and are not as fat as those with leptin deficiency.

TABLE 5.4
Rare Genetic Syndromes That Produce Massive Weight Gain

Syndrome	Onset	Feature	Genetics
Leptin deficiency	Infant onset with hyperphagia	Delayed puberty; defects in T-cell # and function with recurrent infections; hyperinsulinemia	Frameshift mutation in OB gene
Leptin receptor deficiency	Infant onset with hyperphagia	Not as fat as leptin deficiency; poor linear growth; hypothalamic; hypothyroidism	Leptin receptor deficiency
POMC	Early onset with hyperphagia	Adrenal crisis in the newborn, pale skin, red hair	POMC mutations homozygous or compound
Melanocortin-4 receptor deficiency	Early childhood onset with hyperphagia	Increased lean body mass and body density with accelerated linear growth and hyperinsulinemia	MC4R mutations in many locations with variable penetrance
Prohormone convertase-1 (PC-1) deficiency	Early onset	Hypogonadotrophic hypogonadism; postprandial hypoglycemia; hypocortisolism; small intestine absorptive dysfunction	PC1 compound heterozygous mutation

Source: From Lustig, R.M., personal communication.

Mutations in the proopiomelanocortin gene

A defect in the production of proopiomelanocortin (POMC) results in loss or marked reduction in melanocyte-stimulating hormones (both α and β forms), adrenocorticotropin (ACTH), and β-endorphin, an opioid-like peptide. Because all of these peptides are deficient, individuals with POMC deficiency usually (but not always) have reddish hair because the melanocyte isn't being stimulated to make melanin, adrenal insufficiency because the adrenal gland is not being stimulated by ACTH, and hyperphagia and obesity because α-MSH is not produced to inhibit food intake (Krude et al. 1998). It is a rare form of obesity in children, and because of the adrenal insufficiency, many may die before they are recognized.

Mutations in the leptin gene

Leptin deficiency produces obesity in human beings and in the obese (ob/ob) mouse from which Friedman and colleagues (Zhang et al. 1994) identified leptin (Leibel 2008; Montague et al. 1997; Strobel et al. 1998; Ozata et al. 1999). Individuals with leptin deficiency are relatively rare. Leptin is a 167-amino-acid protein produced primarily in adipose tissue and the placenta, and possibly other tissues, that signals the brain about the size of adipose stores. Most, if not all, of the leptin-deficient individuals occur from consanguineous marriages. These very fat children are hypogonadal, but are not hypothermic. They lose weight when treated with leptin. The growth pattern for two children in one of these families is shown in Figure 5.4. Treatment of these children with leptin reduces food

FIGURE 5.3 Food intake in children with two different defects in the melanocortin-4 receptor and in leptin deficiency as compared to normal children. (Adapted from Farooqi, I.S., et al., *N. Engl. J. Med.*, 348(12), 1085–1095, 2003.)

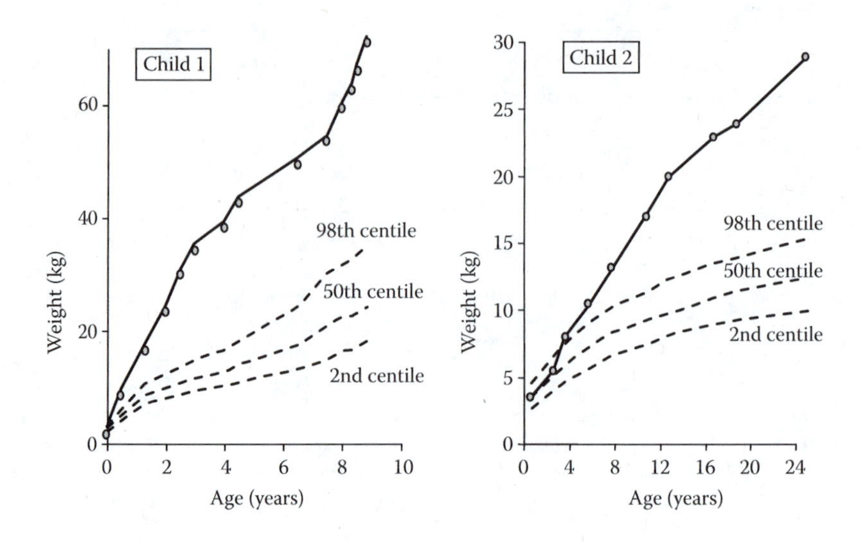

FIGURE 5.4 Growth pattern in two children lacking leptin.

intake and appetite, reduces fat mass and insulin, and rapidly increases thyrotropin (TSH), free thyroxine and triiodothyronine, and leads to pubertal development and improvement in function and number of CD4+ T cells (Farooqi et al. 2002). In thirteen heterozygotes from three families with the frameshift mutation in the leptin gene (deletion of a glycine residue at position 133 in leptin), leptin levels were significantly lower than in controls. In contrast to all other populations so far studied where leptin is positively correlated with body fat, there was no correlation in the heterozygotes of leptin with BMI. However, 76% of the heterozygotes had a BMI above 30 kg/m^2, compared to only 26% of the controls. Thus, the effects of leptin on body weight are gene-dose-dependent (Farooqu et al. 2001).

Leptin receptor defect

A defect in the leptin receptor has also been described (Clement et al. 1998; Farooqi et al. 2007). Among 300 hyperphagic subjects with severe early-onset obesity, nonsense or missense mutations of the leptin receptor were identified in eight (3%). Although obese and hyperphagic, neither of these phenotypes are as obese as seen in leptin-deficient individuals. The LepR-deficient subjects also showed delayed puberty due to hypogonadotrophic hypogonadism and alterations in immune function. Serum leptin levels were within the range predicted by the elevated fat mass in these subjects and clinical features were less severe than in those with congenital leptin deficiency. These individuals do not respond to leptin because they lack the leptin receptor.

Peroxisome proliferator-activated receptor-γ gene defect

The peroxisome proliferator-activated receptor-γ (PPAR-γ) is important in the control of fat cell differentiation (Ristow et al. 1998). Defects in the PPAR-γ receptor in humans have been reported to produce modest degrees of obesity that begin later in life. The activation of this receptor by thiazolidinediones, a class of antidiabetic drugs, is also a cause for an increase in body fat.

Proconvertase-1 gene defect

A defect in prohormone convertase-1 is a rare cause of obesity (Jackson et al. 1997; Snyder et al. 2004). In one family, a defect in this gene and a defect in a second gene were associated with overweight. Members of the family with only the PC-1 defect were not obese, suggesting that it was the interaction of two genes that lead to overweight.

Sim-1 (simple-minded) gene defect

The rare individuals with the Sim-1 syndrome and obesity are similar clinically to the Prader Willi syndrome. The main features include global developmental delay, hypotonia, obesity, hyperphagia, and eye/vision anomalies. In the five cases reported by Bonaglia et al. (2008), they could locate the defect in a 4.1 megabase section of chromosome 6q16.1q16.2. This syndrome thus differs from the Prader-Willi syndrome by its chromosomal location and relative rarity.

Syndrome Congenital Disorders

Several congenital forms of obesity exist that manifest themselves in childhood and may be more abundant than the single-gene defects (see Table 5.5).

Prader–Willi syndrome. The Prader–Willi syndrome (PWS) (Prader et al. 1956) is the commonest form of syndrome human obesity and results from an abnormality on chromosome 15 q 11-q13 that is usually transmitted paternally (Cassidy and Driscoll 2009). This chromosomal defect produces a "floppy" baby who usually has trouble sucking at birth. This poor feeding and poor weight

TABLE 5.5
Syndromic Obesity

Syndrome	Features of the Obesity	Key Clinical Features	Genetic Marker
Albright's hereditary osteodystrophy	Moderate obesity	Mental deficiency; short metatarsals and metacarpals; variable hypocalcemia and hyperphosphatemia	Mutations GNAS1 at 20q13,11, autosomal dominant
Fragile X syndrome	Early onset	Mental retardation; macroorchidism; macrocephaly; prominent jaw; high-pitched jocular speech	FMR1 gene
Bardet–Biedl	Obesity beginning as a toddler and short stature	Developmental delay; retinal dystrophy; abnormal kidneys; hypogonadism	Eight loci have been identified
Alstrom	Obesity develops in childhood	Neurodeafness; retinal degeneration; diabetes mellitus	ALMS1 at 2p13 autosomal recessive
Borjeson–Forssman–Lehmann	School age onset; moderate obesity	Hypotonia; developmental delay; hypogonadism and gynecomastia	X-linked with mutations PHF6 at Xq26-27
Killian/Teschler-Nicola (Pallister Killian Syndrome)	Postnatal obesity	Mental retardation; seizures; hypotonia	Tetrasomy 12p
Cohen syndrome	Truncal obesity beginning in mid-childhood	Hypotonia; prominent incisors; psychomotor retardation; retinochoroidal dystrophy and microcephaly	COH1 at 8q22-q23 as autosomal recessive
Carpenter syndrome	Late childhood onset obesity	Acrocephaly; syndactyly; polydactyly; mental retardation; hypogonadism	Autosomal recessive
Prader–Willi syndrome	Neonatal failure to thrive; early onset obesity	Voracious appetite; hypotonia; mental retardation; developmental delay	Paternally derives 15q11-q13 deletion or material UPD 15

Source: From Lustig, R.M., personal communication.

gain in infancy may require gavage feeding. The hyperphagia and subsequent overweight in these children begins between the ages of 2 and 6 and is associated with short stature and developmental delay with moderate mental retardation (Goldstone et al. 2008). There are characteristic facial features including narrow bifrontal diameter, almond-shaped palpebral fissures, downturned mouth, and small feet and hands with straight ulnar borders. Behavioral problems include temper tantrums, skin-picking, obsessive compulsive behaviors, and stubbornness. There may be eye problems with esotropia and myopia as well as thick viscous saliva and difficulties with articulating words. High pain threshold and altered temperature sensitivity can also be found.

There are several endocrine changes, including hypogonadism and growth hormone deficiency. Their hypothalamic-pituitary-gonadal system can be transiently activated with clomiphene, which modulates estrogen feedback to the hypothalamus (Bray et al. 1983). The levels of plasma ghrelin, a peptide that stimulates food intake, are very high in children with PWS (Cummings et al. 2002; Theodoro et al. 2006; Festen et al. 2006). Butobestatin produced from the ghrelin molecule is not elevated or correlated with insulin in children with PWS (Park et al. 2007).

Treatment of children with PWS is a major challenge for their parents and society. Use of growth hormone beginning in the early months has increased the height and reduced the degree of obesity in these children (Lindgren and Lindberg 2008). People with PWS do not respond well to appetite suppressant drugs. Vagotomy was tried with no success (Fonklesrud 1981). Bariatric surgical procedures have also been used (Schiemann et al. 2008).

The Bardet-Biedl syndrome. The Bardet-Biedl syndrome is a rare syndrome of congenital obesity (Grace et al. 2001). It has been labeled a ciliopathy that can be produced by a number of genes that affect the primary cilium (Marian 2009; Zaghloul and Katsanis 2009), producing the myriad of defects that characterize the syndrome. The Bardet-Biedl syndrome is named after the two physicians, Georges Bardet and Arthur Biedl, who independently described it in separate publications in the 1920s. It is a recessively inherited disorder that can be diagnosed when four of the six cardinal features are present. These six cardinal features are progressive tapetoretinal degeneration; distal limb abnormalities; overweight; renal involvement (O'Dea et al. 1996); hypogenitalism in men; and mental retardation.

More than a dozen different genes can produce this syndrome. The protein for the BBS-4 gene is involved as a subunit in ciliary machinery that recruits pericentrolar material 1 (PCM-1) to the satellites during cell division. Loss of this protein produces mislocation of the protein with cell death (Kim et al. 2004). It is allelic with the McKusick–Kaplan syndrome (MKKS). This latter syndrome is characterized by polydactyly, hydrometrocolpus, and heart problems, but without obesity.

Alstrom's syndrome. Alstrom's syndrome is another of the rare recessively inherited forms of obesity (Marshall et al. 2005). The syndrome consists of hyperphagia in childhood leading to obesity with BMI's that range from 20 to as high as 57. The obesity may moderate after puberty.

> Andrea Prader (1919–2001) headed the endocrinology laboratory where the syndrome that bears his name was identified in 1956. Prader was born in Zurich, Switzerland in 1919, just at the end of World War I. After graduating in 1938 from the Gymnasium in Zurich, he studied medicine at Lausanne and qualified in 1944. After graduating, he served in the army before becoming an assistant physician at the Children's Hospital in Zurich (Kinderspital). He trained with Emmett Holt at New York Hospital where his contacts with Lawson Wilkins at Johns Hopkins spurred his interest in endocrinology. Prader became chair of pediatrics in Zurich where he contributed to a number of endocrine problems, including growth and development of normal children, intersex-conditions, and defects of the steroid synthesis. He was involved in the discovery and delineation of lipid adrenal hyperplasia, hereditary fructose intolerance, and pseudo-vitamin-D deficiency. Prader described the syndrome that bears his name in 1956 with coauthors Alexis Labhart and Heinrich Willi. He died in Zurich in 2001 (Weidemann 1984).

Arthur Biedl (1869–1933) is known for the syndrome that he described. Biedl was born in Osztern, a part of Hungary, in 1869. He received his medical training in Vienna. He rose rapidly through the ranks from 1893 to 1899, when he was given the title of professor. In 1914, he became professor and chair of general and experimental pathology at the University in Prague. His interest in endocrinology dates from 1895, when he began his studies on the physiology of the adrenal glands. He published a short monograph on internal secretions entitled *Internal Secretion* in 1903, which was eventually expanded into the large two-volume work in 1910. With Aschner, he founded the journal Endokrinologie and in 1922 he published a monograph on the pituitary, the same year in which he presented his patients with mental deficiency, reduced metabolic rate, and a disturbance of digestion and polydactyly, (Medvei 1982).

These children typically have short, thick, wide feet and stubby fingers. There is no polydactyly. Hypogonadism is common in boys and hyperandrogenism in girls. Height is normal early, but final height may be low (Marshall et al. 2005).

Type 2 diabetes mellitus and retinal dystrophy begin in infancy. The typical child presents with severe light sensitivity and "wobbly" eyes and they are usually legally blind by age 12–16. Hearing is impaired, followed by slow, progressive, multiorgan failure including cardiac, pulmonary, urological, hepatic, and renal failure. There is a delay in developmental milestones, but mental retardation is rare. The fibrotic changes in all organs put this in the group of ciliopathies (Collin et al. 2002).

WAGR syndrome. WAGR is the acronym for this syndrome and comes from the names of its major components—Wilms tumor, aniridia, genitourinary anomalies, and mental retardation (Fischbach et al. 2005). The principal feature is cancer of the kidney called Wilms' tumors, which occur in about half the cases. The aniridia is a failure of the eyes to develop normally, leading to partial or complete absence of the irises and other ocular problems, including cataracts, nystagmus, and glaucoma. The genitourinary anomalies differ by sex. In males, they include hyopspadias, cryptorchidism, microphallus, and genital ambiguity. In females, there may be ovarian streaks, or malformations of the uterus or fallopian tubes. Mental retardation with cognitive impairment and developmental delay are common. The WAGR Syndrome is a rare genetic disorder caused by heterozygous gene deletions of variable size on chromosome 11p13. It is a sporadic defect arising de novo during ganetogenesis or embryogenesis. Over 100 genes can be involved in the region of deletion. Some of the clinical symptoms have been attributed to specific gene deletions. The WT1 deletion causes the kidney and genitourinary abnormalities; PAX6 the eye abnormalities; and BDNF, located at 11p14.1, the hyperphagia and obesity. A low level of brain-derived neurotrophic factor (BDNF) is seen in severe childhood obesity (Han et al. 2008). It is low in about 50% of cases.

Cohen syndrome. Cohen syndrome is an autosomal recessive disorder with variability in the clinical manifestations. It is characterized by developmental delay, visual problems, facial dysmorphisms, and intermittent neutropenia (Balikova et al. 2007). In a cohort of 10 patients affected by Cohen syndrome, ranging in age from 5 to 52 years, from nine Italian families, the authors found retinopathy and myopia in 9 of 10 patients, and truncal obesity in all patients older than 6 years (8/8). Mutations in COH1 were detected in DNA samples from all 15 patients. There were truncating mutations with only one being a missense change. Partial gene deletions were found in two families. Mutations in the VPS13B (COH1) gene underlie Cohen syndrome. In approximately 70% of the patients, mutations in the gene are identified on both alleles, while in about 30% only a mutation in a single allele or even no mutant allele is detected (Balikova et al. 2009). Copy number variations are common, so screening for copy number alterations of VPS13B should be an integral part of the diagnostic work-up of these patients.

Carpenter's syndrome. Carpenter's syndrome is a rare autosomal recessive disorder that belongs to a group of rare craniosynostosis syndromes (Carpenter 1901). Carpenter syndrome is the rarest, with only occasional patients seen (Hidestrand et al. 2009). There are three common features in all of these syndromes: craniosynostosis (skull base abnormalities with early fusion in different sutures), midface hypoplasia, and musculoskeletal abnormalities. Clinical features of Carpenter's syndrome include peculiar facies, asymmetry of the skull, polydactyly, brachymesophalangy, mild soft tissue syndactyly, obesity, hypogenitalism, congenital heart disease, and mental retardation. The brachycephaly is caused by early fusion in the coronal, sagittal, and lambdoidal sutures. Most of the affected patients have a surgical procedure between 3 to 9 months of age to open the cranial vault to make space for the brain to grow. The genetic basis for the syndrome appears to be alterations in RAB23 (Jenkins et al. 2007).

Albright's hereditary osteodystrophy. Albright's hereditary osteodystrophy (AHO) describes a constellation of physical features, including short adult stature, obesity, brachydactyly, and ectopic ossifications. Pseudopseudohypoparathyroidism is an older term for Albright's hereditary osteodystrophy. These individuals have normal end-organ responses to parathyroid hormone. The disease results from heterozygous deactivating mutations in the GNAS1 gene associated with a 50% reduction in bioactivity of the Gs alpha protein that it encodes. The GNAS1 gene is subject to tissue-specific genomic imprinting. Patients with mutations on their maternally derived allele are likely to have associated pseudohypoparathyroidism type Ia, whereas mutations on the paternal allele usually cause the Albright's hereditary osteodystrophy type (Wilson and Hall 2002).

Fragile X syndrome. The fragile X syndrome with permutation of between 55 and 200 CGG repeats in the fragile X mental retardation 1 gene (FMR1) leads to a broad spectrum of phenotypic involvement. Approximately 10% of the children in this group develop hyperphagia and lack of satiety at the end of meals. This often develops after 5 years of age and it typically leads to obesity. The major problems are a broad spectrum of intellectual impairments, although this is less common in the females. This fragile X syndrome is linked to about 30% of the cases of autism. Hyperactivity, anxiety, mood instability, hand-flapping, and hand biting occur in the majority of these children. The permutations can also cause primary ovarian insufficiency and a tremor ataxia syndrome.

The full mutation leads to methylation of the gene and subsequent block of transcription of FMR1. The level of the fragile X mental retardation protein (FMRP) is inversely correlated with the degree of clinical involvement, including IQ and the severity of the connective tissue involvement.

Börjeson–Forssman–Lehmann syndrome. The Börjeson–Forssman–Lehmann syndrome (BFLS) is a rare, X-linked, partially dominant condition with severe intellectual disability, epilepsy, short stature, obesity, microcephaly, coarse facial features, long ears, gynecomastia, tapering fingers, and shortened toes (Turner et al. 2004). The clinical history and physical findings in the affected males reveal that the phenotype is milder and more variable than previously described and evolves with age. Generally in the first year, the babies are floppy, with failure to thrive, big ears, and small external genitalia. As schoolboys, the picture is one of learning problems and moderate short stature with emerging truncal obesity and gynecomastia. Head circumferences are usually normal, but macrocephaly may be seen. Big ears and small genitalia remain. The toes are short and fingers tapered and malleable. In late adolescence and adult life, the classically described heavy facial appearance emerges. Some heterozygous females show milder clinical features such as tapering fingers and shortened toes. Of those with BFLS, 20% have significant learning problems and 95% have skewed X-inactivation. We conclude that this syndrome may be underdiagnosed in males in their early years and missed altogether in isolated heterozygous females. The mutations that cause this syndrome have been identified in the PHF6 gene (Mangelsdorf et al. 2009).

Neuroendocrine Causes of Overweight

Hypothalamic Causes of Overweight

The concept of "hypothalamic obesity" dates from the beginning of the twentieth century when two case reports of hypothalamic tumors producing obesity were published, one by Babinski (1900) and one by Frohlich (Frohlich 1901; Bruch 1939). This led to half a century of clinical and basic work

Joseph Francois Felix Babinski (1857–1932) published one of the first two cases of a child with a hypothalamic tumor and obesity, thus helping to separate obesity into causal mechanisms. Babinski was born in Paris of Polish parents. Under the influence of the famous Charcot, he became a neurologist and was appointed to the Hôpital de la Pitié in 1890, where he became a senior neurologist in 1914. He is best known for his description of the plantar reflex that bears his name. Babinski was a prolific writer, publishing in areas of physiology, neurosurgery, medical endocrinology, psychiatry, and medical editing. His first scientific contribution in 1882 concerned typhoid fever. His graduate thesis, published in 1885, was on multiple sclerosis. At age 30, he became chief assistant to Professor Charcot at Hôpital Salpetriere in Paris, and shortly after became Medecin aux Hôpitaux. He was an editor of the Revue Neurologique and a founder of the Societe de Neurologie de Paris (Talbot 1970).

identifying the ventromedial hypothalamus as a critical region whose damage produced obesity and formulating the hypothesis that hyperphagia produced by hypothalamic injury caused the obesity (Smith 1927; Hetherington and Ransom 1939; Brobeck et al. 1945). The past 50 years have seen two major refinements in the view of this syndrome. The first was the "neuroanatomic era" from 1945 to 1994. During this time, hyperphagia was shown to be sufficient, but not essential for the development of hypothalamic obesity (Han 1970; Frohman 1969), and that a disturbance of the autonomic nervous system was a key feature leading to many of the metabolic changes (Bray and York 1969; King 2006). The second was a "neurochemical era" that was initiated largely by the discovery of leptin in 1994 (Zhang et al. 1994), which provided a neurochemical basis for modulating food intake.

Hypothalamic obesity in humans may be caused by trauma, tumor, inflammatory disease (Bray and Gallagher 1975; Hochberg and Hochberg 2010), surgery in the posterior fossa, or increased intracranial pressure (Bray and Gallagher 1975). The symptoms usually present in one or more of three patterns: (1) headache, vomiting, and diminished vision due to increased intracranial pressure; (2) impaired endocrine function affecting the reproductive system with amenorrhea or impotence, diabetes insipidus, and thyroid or adrenal insufficiency; or (3) neurologic and physiologic derangements, including convulsions, coma, somnolence, and temperature dysregulation. Figure 5.5 shows the life history of a patient with hypothalamic obesity due to hypothalamic tuberculosis, diagnosed after death. The course lasted more than 3 years and, during the final year, there was a nearly 50-kg weight gain. In contrast to the Prader-Willi syndrome, where ghrelin is high, ghrelin levels in obese children and those with hypothalamic obesity due to craniopharyngioma are

Alfred Frohlich (1871–1953) is known for his description of a child with hypothalamic tumor and obesity. Frohlich was born in Vienna, where he received his MD degree in 1895. Following graduation, he joined the Department of Medicine under the direction of Dr. Nothnagel and worked in experimental pathology and in the neurology clinic. It was during his stay in Sherrington's Laboratory in Liverpool, England, that Frohlich met Harvey Cushing. Frohlich's first academic appointment with tenure was in the Department of Pharmacology and Toxicology in Vienna. He was subsequently appointed a full professor and served in that position from 1919–1939. He came to the United States in 1939, a victim of the German-Austrian Anschluss. He continued his pharmacologic studies as a member of the May Institute of Medical Research at the Jewish Hospital in Cincinnati, Ohio. Frohlich's work touched almost all areas of vertebrate and invertebrate pathology (Talbot 1970).

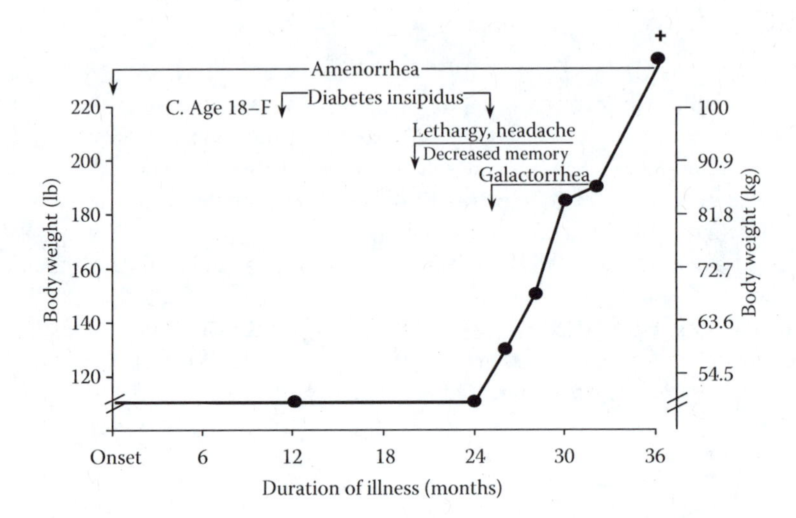

FIGURE 5.5 The natural history of a patient with hypothalamic injury and weight gain.

similar (1345 pg/ml vs. 1399 pg/ml) and significantly lower than in normal weight control children (Kanumakala et al. 2005; Daousi and MacFarlane 2005).

In human beings, the syndrome of hypothalamic obesity produces hyperphagia, hyperinsulinemia (Bray and Gallagher 1975) and reduced sympathetic activity (Roth et al. 2007; Coutant et al. 2003) and these disturbances have both been the target for therapeutic interventions. The appetite suppressants sibutramine (Danielsson et al. 2007) and amphetamine (Ismail et al. 2006) have only modest effects. The inhibition of food intake by cholecystokinin is not affected by hypothalamic lesions (Boosalis et al. 1992). The sympathomimetic combination of ephedrine and caffeine had modest effects (Greenway and Bray 2008). Surgical vagotomy aimed at reducing vagal overactivity was of limited effect (Smith et al. 1983) but gastric bypass produced larger weight losses (Schultes et al. 2009).

Rapid-Onset Obesity with Hypothalamic Dysfunction, Hypoventilation Autonomic Dysregulation, and Neural Tumor (ROHHADNET) Syndrome

A new syndrome with a variety of symptoms of hypothalamic origin has been described (Bougneres et al. 2008). The rapid onset of obesity before age 10 with a median age of 3 is characteristic of the syndrome. This was followed by symptoms of hypothalamic and autonomic dysregulation with a median onset of 3.6 years and the onset of alveolar hypoventilation slightly later at a median age of 6.2 years. High-resolution chromosome analysis, comparative genomic hybridization, and subtelomeric fluorescent in situ hybridization were negative in two patients (Ize-Ludlow et al. 2007). Increased serum sodium without diabetes insipidus was present in all six children in one review

TABLE 5.6
Use of the Body Mass Index (kg/m²) to Select Appropriate Treatments

Treatment	25–29.9	27–29.9	30–34.9	35–39.9	>40
Diet, exercise, lifestyle	+	+	+	+	+
Pharmacotherapy		With co-morbidities	+	+	+
Surgery				With co-morbidities	+

Harvey Williams Cushing (1869–1939) is known for his description of pituitary disease as a cause of obesity that became known as "Cushing's Disease," which appeared in the first American medical monograph and was central to the idea that obesity could be caused by identifiable conditions. Cushing came from a family with a long medical tradition (Loriaux). He could trace his ancestry back to the Massachusetts Bay Colony in 1638. Both his father and his grandfather were physicians in Cleveland, Ohio. Harvey Cushing was the youngest child in a family of ten. He received his collegiate education at Yale University, where he graduated in 1891. After Yale, he entered the Harvard Medical School, where he was a classmate of the famous diabetologist, Elliott Joslin, whose clinic in Boston still carries Joslin's name. Drawings from Harvey Cushing's notebooks in medical school (Fulton 1946; Thomson 1950) gave evidence of his skills as a minute and careful observer. Following one year of postgraduate education at the Massachusetts General Hospital in Boston, Massachusetts, Cushing began his work as an assistant surgical resident with the famous William Halsted (1852–1922) at the Johns Hopkins Hospital. Following two years of training at major European clinics, he returned to Johns Hopkins in 1901, where he remained until 1912, when he became professor of surgery at the newly opened Peter Bent Brigham Hospital in Boston, across the street from the Harvard Medical School.

Cushing's friendship with Sir William Osler during his years at Johns Hopkins made a significant imprint on the young Cushing's interest in the history of medicine. Cushing's collection of books, now residing in the Yale library, and his collection of works by and about the famous anatomist Vesalius, is evidence of his historical perspective. Cushing's bio-bibliography of Andreas Vesalius, published posthumously, is a classic in the field of historical bibliography (Cushing 1943).

In addition to his work on the syndrome that bears his name, Cushing, along with Sir Victor Horsley (1857–1916) in England, pioneered microsurgery. Cushing studied many neurosurgical diseases including acromegaly, meningiomas, gliomas, and intracranial physiology. He published 12 books. The first of these, on the pituitary gland, appeared in 1912 (Cushing 1912), the year in which Cushing moved from Johns Hopkins Hospital to become professor of surgery and surgeon-in-chief at the Peter Bent Brigham Hospital in Boston. His work in Boston was interrupted by World War I. The surgical unit at Base Hospital #5 in France was organized by Cushing and his wartime experiences were subsequently published in an account of this surgical unit (Cushing 1936). Cushing's most notable literary contribution, however, was his two-volume work entitled *The Life of Sir William Osler,* written between 1921 and 1924 (Cushing 1925). It earned him the Pulitzer Prize for biography in 1925. In 1932, at the age of 63, Cushing retired from the Harvard Medical School through an agreement Cushing made with Dr. Henry Christian, professor of medicine, upon his arrival in Boston in 1912. In spite of his long attachments to the Harvard Medical School, Cushing moved his book collection to Yale University, from which he had received his undergraduate degree, and bequeathed his library to Yale upon his death in 1938. The words used by Cushing in 1927 at the centenary of the birth of Lord Lister, the surgeon who introduced antisepsis into surgery, can equally be applied to Harvey Williams Cushing. He said:

> Rarely is it safe to prophesy any durability of recognition whatsoever the accomplishment. Fame that is contemporary, fame that for a time endures, and fame that actually accumulates, differ in quality as differ the flash of a meteor, the glow of a comet, and the permanence of a fixed star. Only when the contemplation of both the man and his achievement truly inspires and ennobles us will they remain indivisible to be praised by the people for time everlasting (Cushing 1928).

(Bougneres et al. 2008). TSH and thyroxine were abnormal in five of these children, and five of them had unilateral macroscopic adrenal ganglioneuromas. Abnormalities of growth hormone and adrenal steroids were also noted in some of the children.

Cushing's Syndrome

Central adiposity is one of the cardinal features of Cushing's syndrome (Beauregard et al. 2002). The differential diagnosis of overweight from Cushing's syndrome and pseudo-Cushing's syndrome is clinically important for therapeutic decisions. Pseudo-Cushing's is a name used for a variety of conditions that distort the dynamics of the hypothalamic–pituitary–adrenal axis and can confuse the interpretations of biochemical tests for Cushing's syndrome. It is a syndrome with "Cushingoid-like" features and can be caused by such things as depression, anxiety disorder, obsessive-compulsive disorder, poorly controlled diabetes mellitus, and alcoholism (Findling and Raff 2006; Arnaldi et al. 2003; Findling et al. 2005; Nieman 2002).

Polycystic Ovarian Syndrome

The polycystic ovarian syndrome was originally described in the first half of the twentieth century by Stein and Levinthal (1935) and bore their name for many years. It was characterized by polycystic ovaries and, thus, its name. The modern criteria for establishing the diagnosis of this syndrome come from a conference at NIH in 1990 and one in Rotterdam in 2003. The diagnosis can be made if two of the following three features are present, and other causes are eliminated. Those features are: 1) polycystic ovaries on ultrasound examination; 2) elevated testosterone; and 3) chronic anovulation manifested as prolonged menstrual periods—oligomenorrhea. Clinical studies show that 80%–90% of women with oligomenorrhea have PCOS. The syndrome has a prevalence in the population of 6%–8%.

Better understanding of the syndrome has come from studies of families where more than one woman has PCOS. In these families, the presence of hyperandrogenemia appears to be the central feature. In some women there is the additional presence of polycystic ovaries. Obesity appears in about half of the women and seems to exaggerate the appearance of the other features, including the insulin resistance, which is characteristic of the syndrome. The insulin resistance and the obesity make diabetes a common complication (Dunaif 2002).

The mechanism for the abnormalities seems to be an increase in the normal pulsatile release of luteinizing hormone (LH) from the pituitary due to the high androgens. LH is normally released in a pulsatile fashion responsive to the gonadotrophin releasing hormone (GnRH) released from the hypothalamus and is inhibited by estrogen from the ovary. The high androgen levels block this feedback of estrogen and allow the excessive secretion of LH. An animal model in nonhuman primates occurs when androgens are given to young female monkeys. One concept for the human condition is that there is early exposure to androgens by the mothers with subsequent impairment of the androgen-feedback system.

Insulin resistance is another characteristic feature of the polycystic ovarian syndrome. In the family study noted above, it occurred even when the individuals were not overweight, and it, too, probably reflects the influence of increased androgen on the responses in the insulin signaling system.

From the pathophysiology of the syndrome, effective treatment might result from inhibiting androgen production or action, or enhancing insulin sensitivity. Metformin, an insulin sensitizing drug, improves ovulation and increases the likelihood of pregnancy. A similar result of reduced insulin resistance is produced by blocking androgen production with spironolactone, flutamide, or buserelin (Gambineri 2006; Welt et al. 2006).

Growth Hormone Deficiency

Lean body mass is decreased and fat mass is increased in adults and children who are deficient in growth hormone, compared with those who have normal growth hormone secretion. However, the increase in fat does not produce clinically significant overweight. Growth hormone replacement reduces body fat and visceral fat (Franco 2009). Acromegaly produces the opposite effects with reduced body fat and particularly visceral fat. Treatment of acromegaly, which lowers growth hormone, increases body fat and visceral fat. The gradual decline in growth hormone with age may be one reason for the increase in visceral fat with age.

Hypothyroidism

Patients with hypothyroidism frequently gain weight because of a generalized slowing of metabolic activity. Some of this weight gain is fat. However, the weight gain is usually modest, and marked overweight is uncommon. Hypothyroidism is common, particularly in older women.

Hyperparathyroidism

Hyperparathyroidism is a disease with increased secretion of PTH that mobilizes calcium from bone, increases renal reabsorption of calcium, and indirectly increases intestinal calcium absorption by increasing production of 1,25 dihydroxyvitamin D2. In a meta-analysis of 13 studies, patients with hyperparathyroidism were 3.34 kg heavier than controls (95% CI 1.97 to 4.71). One explanation is that overweight may increase PTH and vitamin D, or vice versa (Bolland et al. 2005).

Risk-Benefit Assessment

Once the work-up for etiologic and complicating factors is complete, the risk associated with elevated BMI and increased waist circumference can be evaluated (Table 5.6). Several algorithms can be used for this purpose (Williamson et al. 1995; Yanovski et al. 1994; Stunkard 1955; Bray and Gallagher 1975).

I will use the algorithm in Figure 5.6 taken from the NHLBI monograph (NHLBI 1998). The BMI provides the first assessment of risk. Individuals with a BMI below 25 kg/m^2 are at very low

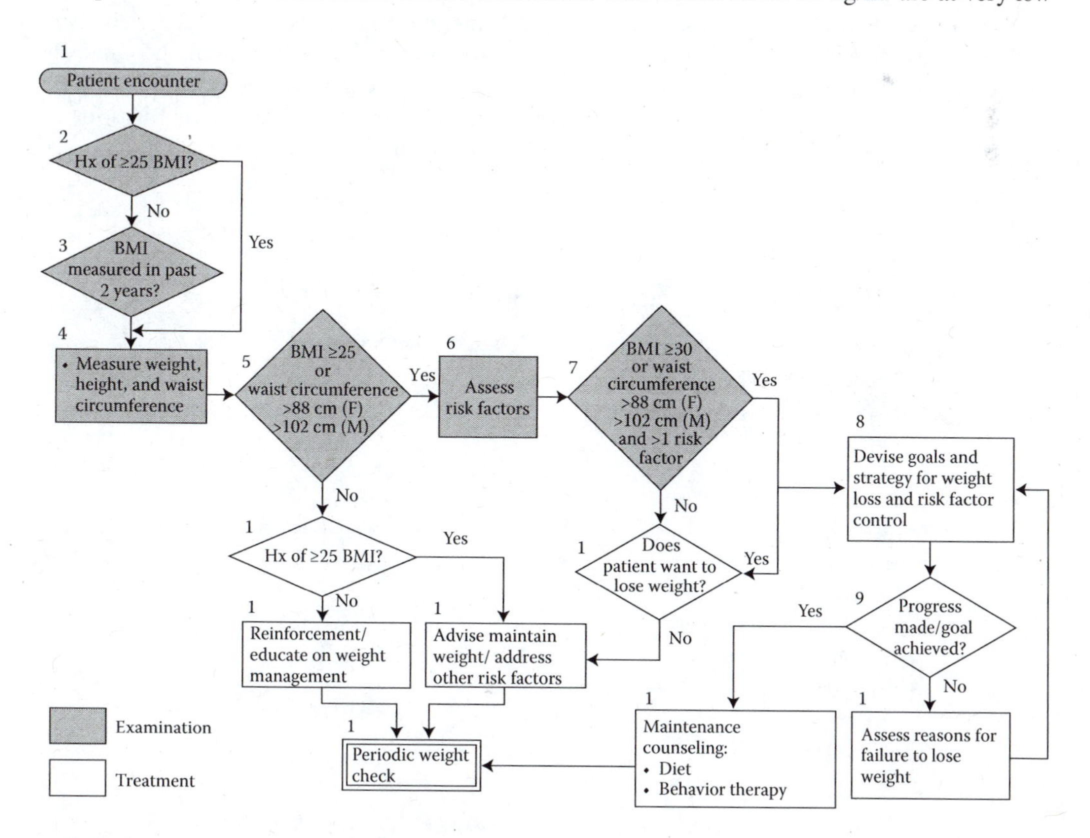

FIGURE 5.6 Treatment algorithm for the overweight patient (NHLBI).

risk but, nonetheless, nearly half of those in this category at ages 20 to 25 will become overweight by age 60 to 69. Thus, a large group of preoverweight individuals need preventive strategies. Risk rises with a BMI above 25 kg/m^2. The presence of the metabolic syndrome increases this risk. Thus, an attempt at a quantitative estimate of these complicating factors is important.

The body mass index is a useful guide to various types of treatment. This is shown in Table 5.7. Here the body mass index is divided into five-unit increases with a subdivision between 25 and 30 kg/m^2. For each five-unit increase in BMI, there is a 20%–30% increased risk of mortality and increased risks of 20% to 100% for such diseases as diabetes, hypertension, kidney disease, and cancer (Collaborative Prospective Studies 2009). The BMI thus provides a useful guide to assess initial risk when interpreted in an ethnically specific framework. A BMI above 23 is classified as obesity in many Asian countries, whereas the risk among African-Americans may only begin to rise when BMI exceeds 30 kg/m^2 (Calle et al. 1999).

Treatments for overweight can be risky. This is shown in Table 5.8, which summarizes a number of the untoward events associated with treatment of obesity. As can be seen, many treatments have been associated with unintended consequences. The use of thyroid hormone was associated with symptoms of hyperthyroidism. Dinitrophenol produced neuropathies, cataracts, and death. Amphetamine was addictive. Fenfluramine produced aortic value regurgitation and pulmonary hypertension. Rimonabant increased the risk of suicide. These unwanted side effects must temper enthusiasm for new treatments unless the risk of the new medication is very low. Because obesity is stigmatized, any treatment approved by the FDA will be used to achieve improved self-image (cosmetically desired weight loss) by people who suffer the stigma of being overweight. Thus, drugs to treat overweight must have very high safety profiles.

Cosmetic vs. Medical Weight Loss

There can be both medical and self-image (cosmetic) benefits to weight loss (Bray 2008). However, they do not necessarily occur together. For example, a 10% weight loss, which would be clinically significant for a 300 pound (145 kg) person, would only reduce body weight by 30 pounds to 270—a weight change that many people might not notice. At the other extreme, a 10% weight loss for an individual weighing 150 pounds would lower their weight to 135 pounds, which would have a very

TABLE 5.7
Clinical Features of Cushing's Syndrome

Feature	Percentage
Obesity/weight gain	95
Facial plethora/rounded face	90
Decreased libido	90
Thin skin	85
Decreased growth in children	70–80
Menstrual irregularity	80
Hypertension	75
Hirsutism	75
Depression/emotional lability	70
Easy bruising	65
Glucose intolerance	60
Weakness	60
Osteopenia/fracture	50
Nephrolithiasis	50

Source: Adapted from Newell-Price, J. et al., *Endocr. Rev.*, 19(5), 647–672, 1998.

TABLE 5.8
Unintended Consequences Associated with a Number of Treatments for Overweight

Year	Drug	Complication
1892	Thyroid	Hyperthyroidism
1932	Dintrophenol	Cataracts/neuropathy
1937	Amphetamine	Addiction
1968	Rainbow pills	Deaths—arrhythmias
1985	Gelatin diets	Cardiovascular deaths
1997	Phen/Fen	Valvulopathy
1998	PPA	Strokes
2003	Ma huang	Heart attacks/stroke
2007	Ecopipam	Suicidality from this dopamine receptor antagonist
2009	Rimonabant	Suicidality from this cannabinoid receptor-1A antagonist

Source: © 2005 George A. Bray

positive impact on self-image. We also know that cosmetically significant weight losses may not produce clinically significant effects. After liposuction that removed about 7% of body weight, there were no improvements in health-related risk factors. These distinctions are summarized in Table 5.9.

Patient Readiness

Before initiating any treatment, the patient must be ready to make changes that facilitate weight loss. A series of questions developed by Brownell in The Dieting Readiness Test can help make this assessment. When counseling patients who are ready to lose weight, accommodation of their individual needs as well as ethnic factors, age, and other differences is essential. The approach outlined above is not rigid and must be used to help guide clinical decision-making, and not serve as an alternative to considering individual factors and clinical judgment in developing a treatment plan. Because of increasing complications of overweight, more aggressive efforts at therapy should be directed at people in each of the successively higher risk classifications.

Doctor–Patient Expectations

The doctor or assistant who identified an elevated BMI or waist circumference in an overweight patient should take a moment to make sure the patient knows how to interpret the BMI and other components of the metabolic syndrome. If the patient knows their BMI, it means that the physician or assistant also knows the BMI. However, a recent survey showed that only 42% of overweight

TABLE 5.9
Clinically Effective and Cosmetically Effective Weight Loss

Type of Procedure	Weight Loss	Clinically Significant	Cosmetically Significant
Diet/Exercise	10% from 300 to 270 lb	Yes	No
	10% from 200 to 180 lb	Yes	Probably not
	10% from 150 to 135 lb	Yes	Yes
Liposuction	7% from 220 to 200 lb	No	Probably not
	7% from 160 to 149 lb	No	Yes
Surgery (Gastric Bypass)	40% loss from 264 to 165	Yes	Yes

patients seen for a routine medical check-up were told they needed to lose weight (MCR Paper Review 2009). We need to do better for our patients.

The realities of treatment for overweight often conflict with patients' expectations. When patients were asked to give the weights they wanted to achieve in a weight loss program, from their dream weight to a weight loss that would leave them dissatisfied, they provided a wide range of weight losses. These are listed in Column 2 of Table 5.10 (Foster 1997). Patients then participated in a weight loss program. The percentage achieving each goal is listed in the right-hand column. None of the patients achieved their dream weight, which was an average 38% below baseline. Nearly half failed to achieve even a weight loss outcome that at baseline would leave them disappointed. The patient's desired weight loss from the standpoint of their early self-image almost always exceeds the realistically achievable goals for weight loss. This mismatch between patient expectations and the realities of weight loss provides clinicians and their patients with an important challenge as they begin treatment. A weight loss goal of 5% to 15% can be achieved by most patients and is clinically reasonable.

Slowing and Cessation of Weight Loss during Treatment—Weight Plateau

One complaint about treatments for overweight is that they frequently fail, that is, they don't produce continuing weight loss or the desired level of weight loss. Since a plateau occurs with every treatment, patients need to anticipate this. Even when it is expected, a plateau is often viewed as a failure of the treatment and may lead the patient to terminate treatment if they are no longer losing weight. When treatment is stopped, weight is almost always regained. This is similar to what happens to patients with hypertension who are treated with drugs and who stop taking their antihypertensive drugs, and to patients with high cholesterol who stop taking their hypocholesterolemic drugs. In each case, blood pressure or cholesterol rises. Like the problem of excess body fat, these chronic diseases have not been cured, but rather palliated. When treatment is stopped, the risk factor recurs—and so does body fat.

One way of helping patients get a better feeling for their weight loss is to express the results as percentage of excess weight loss as opposed to percentage loss from baseline. Since a BMI of 25 kg/m^2 is a good goal, an individual with a BMI of 30 kg/m^2 who loses 10% of their body weight (3 kg/m^2) will have lost 60% of their excess weight (Bray et al. 2009).

Criteria for Successful Weight Loss

A weight loss of more than 5% from initial body weight is clinically significant for patients at high risk from obesity (Douketis 2005) and patients maintaining this can be called "conditionally successful." At this level one would expect improvement in the associated risk factors. If this does not occur with the 5% weight loss, then the treatment plan should be reevaluated. A weight loss of 5% to 10% is the outcome seen with most dietary, behavioral, and pharmacological treatments. Provided there are improvements in associated risk factors this would be "successful." A weight loss of more

TABLE 5.10
Patient Expectations for Weight Loss at the Beginning of a Weight Loss Study

Outcome	Weight (lb)	% Reduction
Initial	218	0
Dream	135	38
Happy	150	31
Acceptable	163	25
Disappointed	180	17

Source: Foster G.D., et al., *J. Consult. Clin. Psychol.*, 65(1), 79–85, 1997. With permission.

than 15% below initial body weight and maintenance of this weight loss is a very good result, even if the subject does not reach his or her "dream" weight.

Frequency of Treatment

The decision about duration and frequency of treatment is influenced by the effects of treatment on outcomes. My thinking about this was influenced by the results of the influential Diabetes Prevention Program (DPP 2002; DPPOS 2009). This trial showed that a weight loss averaging 7% reduced the development of diabetes by 58% over an average of 2.8 years. Other studies have shown similar results (Crandall 2009; Tuomilheto et al. 2001). At the end of the randomized trial, all participants in the DPP were offered a weight loss program of 16 sessions over 24 weeks (Venditti et al. 2008). Participants were then followed for conversion to diabetes. After 10 years, the conversion rate of the placebo group fell to just over 6% per year, a rate similar to the other groups. This would imply that short term programs of 6 months or less could have a major impact on some medically related problems associated with obesity. Since weight regain occurred over several years, a repeat treatment program might be available at 5-year intervals for those with a BMI below 30 and at 2 year intervals for those with BMI > 30 kg/m^2. This set of general recommendations for treatment are shown in Figure 5.7.

Types of Treatments

Figure 5.8 returns to the all-to-familiar energy balance concept that underlies both weight gain and weight loss. However, it adds a different dimension. The two potential treatment arms—energy intake and energy expenditure—can be affected by things we do through strategies over which we have control—our behavior—AND by things that happen in the environment, over which we have no direct control. I have labeled these "cognitive" and "noncognitive" strategies. Lifestyle, diet, and exercise are primary examples of cognitive strategies since they won't occur if the participant doesn't do them. As the old adage goes, "you can lead a horse to water, but you can't make it drink." We can design procedures for helping participants modify their lifestyle, give them advice on good diets and helpful hints on exercise, but they have to take responsibility for implementing them. Antiobesity drugs are a combination. The pharmacological effect occurs when the drug is taken. It

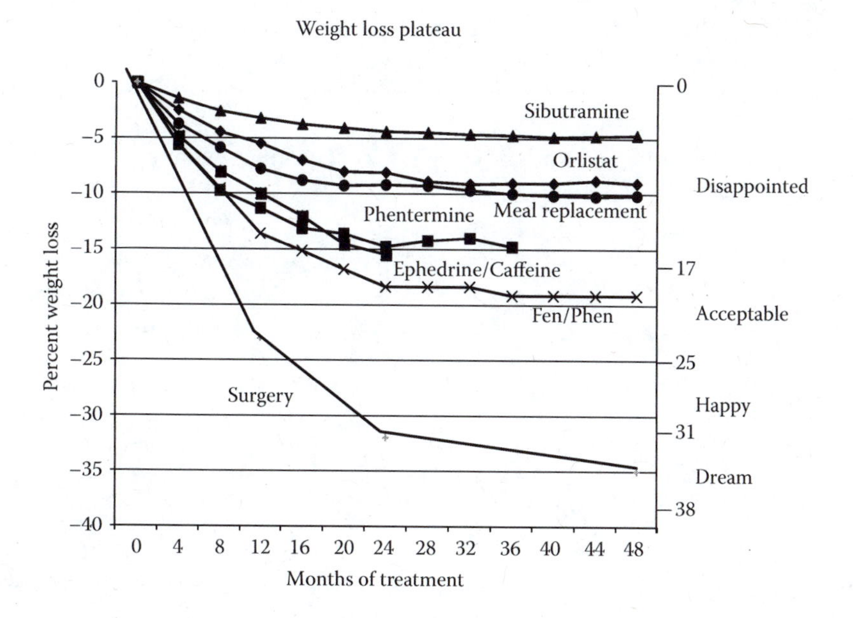

FIGURE 5.7 Slowing of weight loss with duration of treatment.

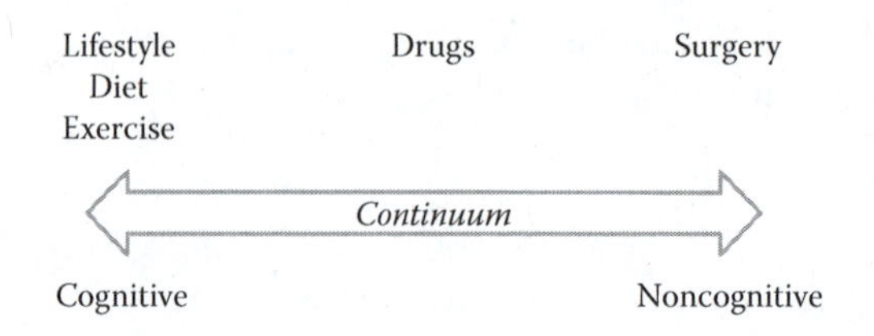

FIGURE 5.8 A continuum of treatment from cognitive to noncognitive.

is, however, the patient's responsibility to take the drug. I have thus labeled these as partly cognitive, partly noncognitive. Surgery is at the other end of the continuum. Once the surgery is done, the patient can't undo it, although they can eat around it.

Factors Affecting Weight Gain in Three Age Groups

Weight Gain during Pregnancy

Body weight gain and maternal weight, as well as smoking, are important features through which the mother can influence the future weight of her child. Recognizing the relationship between birthweight and maternal weight gain, the Institute of Medicine has issued new guidelines for weight gain during pregnancy (Rasmussen & Yaktine 2009; see Table 5.11). The higher the initial body weight of the mother, the smaller the recommended weight gain. Even more important would be to help women planning to get pregnant to reduce their body weight prior to conception. Gestational weight gain was associated with offspring BMI at all ages in a Danish birth cohort of 2485 individuals with long-term follow-up to age 42. Only half of the association was mediated through body weight and BMI up to 14, suggesting that weight gain during gestation may influence long-term susceptibility to an environment where genes load the gun and the environment pulls the trigger (Schack-Nielsen et al. 2010).

The importance of pregnancy for the future risk of obesity is highlighted in the estimation of risk of overweight at age 3 from information obtained at pregnancy or during the first year of life. Combining whether the maternal weight gain was normal or excessive with whether there was smoking during pregnancy, sleep duration in early infancy, and the duration of breastfeeding, Gillman et al. (2008) showed that infants of women with the best overall score had only a 6% risk of

TABLE 5.11
Recommendations for Total and Rate of Weight Gain During Pregnancy, by Prepregnancy BMI

Prepregnancy BMI	BMI (kg/m^2)	Total Weight Gain (Range) kg (lbs)	Rates of Weight Gain Second and Third Trimester Mean Range
Underweight	<18.5	28–40 lbs 12.7–18.5 kg	1 (1–1.3) lbs 0.45 (.36–.45) kg
Normal weight	18.5–24.9	25–35 lbs	1 (0.8–1.0) lbs 0.45 (.36–.45) kg
Overweight	25.0–29.9	1–25 lbs	0.6 (0.5–0.7) lbs .27 (.23–.32) kg
Obese (all classes)	≥30	11–20	0.5 (0.4–0.6) lbs .23 (.18–.27) kg

Source: Rasmussen, K.M. and Yaktine, A.L., eds., *Weight Gain during Pregnancy: Reexamining the Guidelines.* Washington, DC: The National Academies Press, 2009. With permission.

TABLE 5.12
Probability of Becoming an Overweight Child Based in Events in Utero and the First Year of Life

Variable	Lowest Risk	Highest Risk
Maternal smoking	No	Yes
Gestational weight gain	Inadequate	Excessive
Breastfeeding ≥ 12 months	Yes	No
Sleep duration > 12 hrs	Yes	No
Probability of weight at 6 months?	0.06	0.29
Percent risk	6%	29%

Source: Based on data from lecture by Parker, M., Gillman, M.W. Details available in Gillman M.W. et al., *Obesity* (Silver Spring) 16(7): 1651–1656.

having overweight children, compared to a 29% risk for infants of women in the highest risk group. This is summarized in Table 5.12.

Overweight Developing before Age 10

A number of factors are related to the risk of developing obesity later in life and can be the focus of preventive strategies, although many of them are not directly applicable. The data are presented in two tables. Table 5.13 shows data from a longitudinal study in England (Reilly et al. 2005). Also summarized are a group of metabolic changes that predict future obesity, but none of them is as valuable as the predictions that can be applied to the pregnant woman or the woman who is trying to get pregnant.

Prenatal factors Maternal smoking puts offspring at risk for obesity. Infants of mothers who smoked during pregnancy, whether for the first trimester only, or for the entire pregnancy, have infants who are at higher risk for increased body weight than infants from mothers who did not smoke during pregnancy (Toschke et al. 2005). Thus, advising women not to smoke during pregnancy has an important potential future impact on their infant.

Similarly, infants of mothers who have diabetes or who develop gestational diabetes are at greater risk of being macrosomic at birth and overweight in subsequent life (Landon et al. 2009). Treating

TABLE 5.13
Predictors of Weight Gain

Factors	Odds Ratio (95% CI)	
High parental BMI	10.44	(5.11, 23.12)
Birth weight (per 100 g)	1.05	(1.03, 10.7)
Weight gain in first year	10.6	(1.02, 1.10)
Catch-up growth	2.60	(1.09, 6.16)
SD for weight at 8 months	3.13	(1.43, 6.85)
SD for weight at 18 months	2.65	(1.25, 5.59)
Adiposity rebound	15.00	(5.32, 42.30)
>8 hours watching TV (3 year)	1.55	(1.13, 2.12)
Short sleep at 30 months (<10.5h)	1.45	(1.10, 1.89)

Source: Adapted from Reilly J.J., et al., *BMJ*, 330, 1357–1367, 2005.
Note: Obesity defined as BMI > 95th percentile; $N = 8234$ children age 7.

TABLE 5.14
Metabolic Predictors of Weight Gain

	Reference
Lower metabolic rate	Ravussin, E., S. Lillioja, W.C. Knowler, et al., *N. Engl. J. Med.*, 318, 467–472, 1988; Roberts S.B., J. Savage, W.A. Coward, B. Chew, A. Lucas., *N. Engl. J. Med.*, 318, 461–6, 1988; DeLany, J.P., *Am. J. Clin. Nutr.,* 84, 862–870, 2006.
Reduced nonexercise activity thermogenesis	Levine, J.A., N.L. Eberhardt, M.D. Jensen. *Science*, 283, 212–214, 1999.
Increase in carbohydrate oxidation	Zurlo, F., S. Lillioja, A. Esposito-Del Puente, et al., *Am. J. Physiol.*, 259, E650–E657, 1990; Seidell, J.C., D. C. Muller, J. D. Sorkin, R. Andres. *Int. J. Obes. Relat. Metab. Disord.*, 16, 667–674, 1992.
Increased insulin sensitivity	Swinburn, B.A., B.L. Nyomba, M.F. Saad, et al., *J. Clin. Invest.*, 88, 168–173, 1991; Travers, S.H., B.W. Jeffers, R.H. Eckel. *J. Clin. Endocrinol. Metab.*, 87, 3814–3818, 2002; Yost, T.J., D.R. Jensen, R.H. Eckel. *Obes. Res.,* 3, 583–587, 1995.
Low concentration of leptin	Filozof, C.M., C. Murua, M.P. Sanchez, et al. *Obes. Res.,* 8, 205–210, 2000.
Low cord blood leptin	Parker, M., S.L. Rifas-Shiman, M.B., Belfort, et al., *J Pediatr.*, 2010, epub ahead of print.
Reduced sympathetic nervous system activity	Spraul, M., E. Ravusesin, A.M. Fontvieille, R. Rising, D.E. Larson, E.A. Anderson. *J. Clin. Invest.*, 92:1730 –1735, 1993; Peterson, H.R., M. Rothschild, C.R. Weinberg, R.D. Fell, K.R. McLeish, M.A. Pfeifer. *N. Engl. J. Med.*, 318, 1077–1083, 1988.

the diabetes of the mother with gestational diabetes will reduce the risks of fetal overgrowth, but not the risks of stillbirth or perinatal death. Children who are born macrosomic showed twice as much overweight as nonmacrosomic children, and both macrosomia and maternal obesity were independent predictors of childhood weight status (Rijpert et al. 2009). There is also a factor related to weight gain that is transmitted from the mother to her infant through milk in the early weeks of life that enhances the risk of weight gain later. Maternal weight and maternal weight gain are important factors for both white women and African-American women. Thus, advising women to lower their body weight prior to pregnancy and to gain only the recommended amount of weight during the pregnancy are important.

Using clustered metabolic risk factors for the metabolic syndrome as the criterion, Ekelund et al. (2007) found that weight gain during infancy (0–6 months), but not during early childhood (ages 3–6), predicted clustered metabolic risk at age 17.

Breastfeeding Several recent cross-sectional studies have suggested that breastfeeding may reduce the prevalence of overweight in later life (Scholtens et al. 2008). In a large German study of more than 11,000 children, von Kries et al. (1999) showed that the duration of breastfeeding as the sole source of nutrition was inversely related to the incidence of overweight, defined as a weight above the 95th percentile, when children entered the first grade. In this study, the incidence was 4.8% in children with no breastfeeding, falling in a graded fashion to 0.8% in children who were solely fed from the breast for 12 months or more. A second large report (Gillman et al. 2001) also showed that breastfeeding reduced the incidence of overweight, but not obese adolescents. The third report with fewer subjects and more ethnic heterogeneity failed to show this effect (Hediger et al. 2001). However, the potential that breastfeeding can reduce the future risk of overweight is another reason to recommend breastfeeding for at least 6–12 months (Bergmann et al. 2003). In a study of breast-feeding by diabetic mothers, Rodekamp et al. (2005) concluded that it is the first week of life that has the most influence on subsequent changes in weight (Rodekamp et al. 2005); A randomized clinical trial in Belarus examined the effect of increasing breastfeeding for longer than 3 months on height, weight, adiposity, and blood pressure at age 6.5 years. A total of 17,406 healthy breastfed infants were included. The intervention increased breastfeeding duration but did not affect body weight, adiposity, or stature of blood pressure at 6.5 years of age (Kramer et al. 2007).

Childhood Overweight from Ages 3 to 10

Ages between 3 and 10 are high-risk years for developing obesity. At this age, as in the early ages, parental weight status is a strong predictor of which children will increase to overweight between ages 5 and 14 (Al Mamun et al. 2005; Danielzik 2004). Birthweight and weight gain over the first 6 months of life are positively associated with being overweight at age 5 and age 14 (Mamun et al. 2005). In infants and young children with overweight parents, an infant above the 85th percentile between ages 1 and 3 has a four-fold increased risk of adult overweight if either parent is overweight, compared with nonoverweight infants. If neither parent is overweight, this infantile overweight does not predict overweight in early adult life (Whitaker et al. 1997).

Adiposity rebound describes the inflection point between a declining BMI from birth to ages 5–7 and an increasing BMI that occurs after the low point (nadir) between ages 5 and 7 years of age. The earlier this rebound occurs, the greater the risk of overweight later in life. About half of the overweight grade school children remain overweight as adults. Moreover, the risk of overweight in adulthood was at least twice as great for overweight children as for nonoverweight children. The risk is 3 to 10 times higher if the child's weight is above the 95th percentile for their age. Parental overweight plays a strong role in this group as well. Nearly 75% of overweight children ages 3 to 10 remained overweight in early adulthood if they had one or more overweight parents, compared with 25% to 50% if neither parent were overweight. Overweight 3- to 10-year-olds with an overweight parent thus constitute an ideal group for intervention.

The weight gain over 2 years was predicted in 6–15-year-old children by their cardiorespiratory fitness. Both low initial fitness and a decline in fitness relative to their peers was associated with a significant risk of increasing BMI (McGavock et al. 2009).

When body weight progressively deviates from the upper limits of normal in childhood, adolescence, and adult life, I label it "progressive obesity" (Bray 1976). This is usually severe and lifelong, and is associated with an increase in the number of fat cells. These individuals are almost certainly the ones who have been characterized in case reports published by Wadd (1810) and many others in the nineteenth century and earlier.

A number of factors at age 2 predict weight status at ages 5–6 in 4289 German children (Toschke et al. 2005). Overall prevalence of overweight was 11%. High early weight gain accounted for 25% of the later obesity. Obese parents and high early weight gain accounted for a likelihood ratio of 3:6 with a corresponding positive predictive value of 40% and was found in 4% of the children.

Treatment Strategies by Age Group

Dividing treatment strategies by age group allows the physician and patient or family, when appropriate, to focus on the most important components related to their stage in life. The basic approaches to prevention and treatment are based on the patient's age.

Strategies for Age Group 1–10

Table 5.15 shows the strategies available for overweight and obese children. A variety of genetic factors can enhance body weight in this age group, which also contains a high percentage of pre-overweight individuals. Identifying individuals at highest risk for becoming overweight in adult life allows for a focus on preventive strategies. Among these strategies are the need to develop patterns of physical activity and good eating habits, including a lower fat intake and a lower energy-dense diet. Table 5.13 lists some predictors for developing overweight. Some of these are evident in children; others are not evident until adult life. For growing children, drugs for weight loss are generally inappropriate until the patient reaches adult height, and surgical intervention should only be

TABLE 5.15
Therapeutic Strategies Age 1–10

		Therapeutic Strategies		
Age	**Predictors of Overweight**	**Preoverweight at Risk**	**Preclinical Overweight**	**Clinical Overweight**
1–10	Positive family history Genetic defects (dysmorphic-PWS; Bardet-Biedl; Cohen) Hypothalamic injury Low metabolic rate Diabetic mother	• Family counseling • Reduce inactivity	• Family behavioral theraphy • Exercise • Low-fat Low-energy-dense diet	• Treat comorbidities • Exercise • Low-fat Low-energy-dense diet

considered after consultation with medical and surgical experts. Medications should be used to treat the comorbidities directly.

It is in this young age group that most of the genetic and congenital forms of obesity appear and the clinician should be aware of this possibility.

Strategies for Age Group 11–50

Table 5.16 outlines the available strategies for overweight adults. Since nearly two thirds of individuals move into the overweight categories in this age range, this age is quantitatively the most important. Preventive strategies should be used for patients with predictors of weight gain. These should include advice on lifestyle changes, including increased physical activity, which would benefit almost all adults, and good dietary practices, including a diet lower in saturated fat.

For patients in the overweight category, behavioral strategies should be added to these lifestyle strategies. This is particularly important for overweight adolescents, because good 10-year data show that intervention for this group can reduce the degree of overweight in adult life (NHLBI 1998; American Dietetic Association 2005; Snow et al. 2005). Data on the efficacy of behavior programs carried out in controlled settings show that weight losses average nearly 10% in trials lasting more than 16 weeks. The limitation is the likelihood of regaining weight once the behavior treatment

TABLE 5.16
Therapeutic Strategies Age 11–60

		Therapeutic Strategies		
Age	**Predictors of Overweight**	**Preoverweight at Risk**	**Preclinical Overweight**	**Clinical Overweight**
11–60	Positive family history of diabetes or obesity Endocrine disorders (PCO) Multiple pregnancies Marriage Smoking cessation Medication	• Reduce sedentary lifestyle • Low-fat low-energy-dense diet • Portion control	• Behavior therapy • Low-fat Low-energy-dense diet • Reduce sedentary lifestyle	• Treat comorbidities • Drug treatment for overweight • Reduce sedentary lifestyle • Low-fat Low-energy-dense diet • Behavior therapy • Surgery

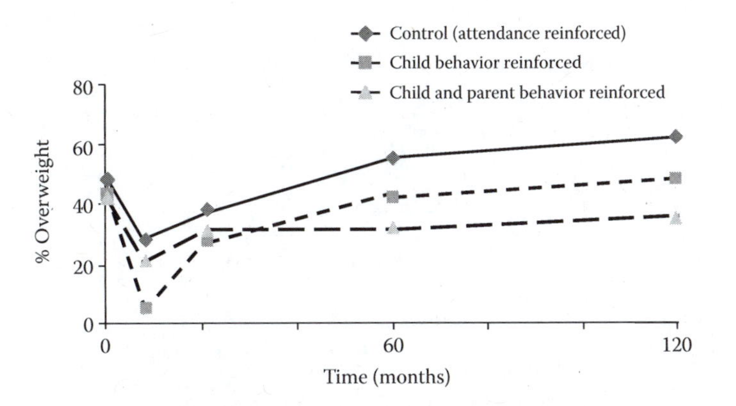

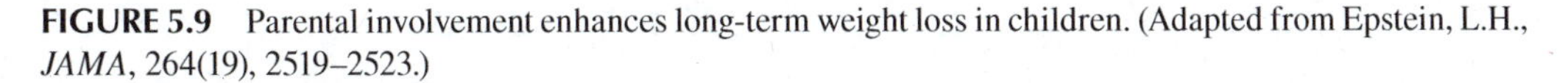

FIGURE 5.9 Parental involvement enhances long-term weight loss in children. (Adapted from Epstein, L.H., *JAMA*, 264(19), 2519–2523.)

ends, although, as shown in Figure 5.9, the long-term behavioral therapy in an early adolescent group did provide long-term weight loss (Epstein 1990).

Medication should be seriously considered for clinically overweight individuals in this group. Two strategies can be used. The first is to use drugs to treat each comorbidity, i.e., individually treating diabetes, hypertension, dyslipidemia, and sleep apnea. Current drugs include appetite suppressants (sibutramine, phentermine, diethylpropion, benzphetamine, and phendimetrazine), that act on the central nervous system and a pancreatic lipase inhibitor (orlistat). The availability of these agents differs from country to country, and any physician planning to use them should be familiar with the local regulations.

Overweight Developing in Adolescence and Adult Life

Adolescence Weight in adolescence becomes a progressively better predictor of adult weight status. In a 55-year follow-up of adolescents, the weight status in adolescence predicted later adverse health events (van Dam et al. 2006). Adolescents above the 95th percentile had a 5- to 20-fold greater likelihood of overweight in adulthood. In contrast with younger ages, parental overweight is less important, or has already had its effect. While 70% to 80% of overweight adolescents with an overweight parent were overweight as young adults, the numbers were only modestly lower (54% to 60%) for overweight adolescents without overweight parents. Despite the importance of childhood and adolescent weight status, however, it remains clear that most overweight individuals develop their problem in adult life.

Adult women Most overweight women gain their excess weight after puberty. This weight gain may be precipitated by a number of events, including pregnancy, oral contraceptive therapy, and menopause.

Pregnancy. Weight gain during pregnancy and the effect of pregnancy on subsequent weight gain are important events in the weight gain history of women (Crane et al. 2009; Olson 2008). A few women gain considerable weight during pregnancy, occasionally more than 50 kg. Not only is obesity in pregnancy detrimental to a woman's reproductive health and the outcomes of her pregnancy, it can also have a significant impact on the infant and risks for childhood obesity. Preventive strategies may be important during this period of a woman's life and during this interval when focus is on a "healthy baby" may be an optimal time to intervene (Birdsall et al. 2009).

Oral Contraceptives. Oral contraceptive use may initiate weight gain in some women, although this effect is diminished with the low-dose estrogen pills and are mainly seen with depot medorxyprogesterone. Obese adolescent girls who initiated the use of depot medoxyprogesterone gained

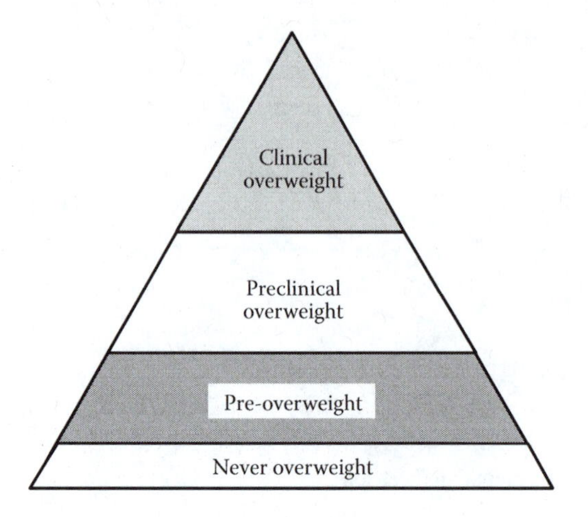

FIGURE 5.10 Weight loss pyramid showing the gradual transition from nonoverweight to clinically obese categories.

significantly more weight than obese girls starting oral contraceptive pills or girls not using birth control ($p < .001$ for both). After 18 months, mean weight gain was 9.4 kg for the girls receiving the depot preparation, 0.2 kg for the girls receiving oral contraceptives, and 3.1 kg for the control (Bonny et al. 2009).

Menopause. The changes in hormonal status at the time of menopause might anticipate changes in body fat and lean body mass. Most studies show only small changes in body weight, although visceral fat may increase. For example, Cagnacci et al. (2007), using bioelectric impedance to measure body fat, found that body weight increased in 87 perimenopausal women, decreased in 60 ovariectomized women, and did not increase significantly in 182 naturally postmenopausal women. When a small group of 8 healthy women were followed through menopause using magnetic resonance imaging to quantify total abdominal, subcutaneous, and visceral fat in both the premenopausal state and in the postmenopausal state, Franklin et al. (2009) found body weight and waist circumference did not change with menopause (pre- vs. postmenopause: body weight, 63.2 +/– 3.1 vs. 63.9 +/– 2.5 kg; waist circumference, 92.1 +/– 4.6 vs. 93.4 +/– 3.7 cm). Total abdominal fat, subcutaneous fat, and visceral fat, however, all significantly increased with menopause (pre- vs. postmenopause: total, 27,154 +/– 4268 vs. 34,717 +/– 3272 cm^3; subcutaneous, 19,981 +/– 3203 vs. 24,918 +/– 2521 cm^3; visceral, 7173 +/– 1611 vs 9798 +/– 1644 cm^3). Lean mass, fat mass, and physical activity, along with total cholesterol and triglyceride levels, did not change with menopause, whereas high-density lipoprotein and low-density lipoprotein both increased with menopause.

Adult men The transition from an active lifestyle during the teens and early 20s to a more sedentary lifestyle thereafter is associated with weight gain in many men. The rise in body weight continues through the adult years until the sixth decade. After ages 55 to 64, relative weight remains stable and then begins to decline. Evidence from the Framingham Study and studies of men in the armed services suggests that men have become progressively heavier for their height during this century. One group of concern is physically active men like football players and sumo wrestlers whose body weight doesn't decline and who are at high risk for metabolic syndrome (Buell et al. 2008) and early death (Croft et al. 2008).

Weight Stability and Weight Cycling

Weight cycling associated with dieting is popularly known as yo-yo dieting (National Task Force on the Prevention and Treatment of Obesity 1994). Weight cycling refers to the downs and ups in weight that often happen to people who diet, lose weight, stop dieting, and regain the weight they lost and

TABLE 5.17
Therapeutic Strategies for Ages over 61

		Therapeutic Strategies		
Age	Predictors of Overweight	Preoverweight at Risk	Preclinical Overweight	Clinical Overweight
11–60	Menopause Declining growth hormone Declining testosterone Smoking cessation Medication	Few individuals remain in this subgroup	• Behavior therapy • Low-fat Low-energy-dense diet • Reduce sedentary lifestyle	• Treat comorbidities • Drug treatment for overweight • Reduce sedentary lifestyle • Low-fat Low-energy-dense diet • Behavior therapy • Surgery

sometimes more. The possibility that loss and regain is more detrimental than staying heavy has been hotly debated. In an early review of the literature a group of experts concluded that most studies did not support any adverse effects on metabolism associated with weight cycling. This has been supported by a long-term follow-up in the Nurses' Health Study, where repeated intentional weight losses did not predict greater all-cause or cardiovascular mortality (Field et al. 2009).

Strategies for the Age Group over 51

Table 5-17 shows the proposed treatments for this age group. By age 51, most of the people who become overweight have done so. Thus, preventive strategies are less important and the focus is on treatment for those who are overweight. The basic treatments and treatment considerations are similar to those of the younger group. However, in this age group, the argument may be stronger for directly treating comorbidities and paying less attention to treating the obesity. For patients in this group who wish to lose weight, however, the considerations for patients between age 11 and 50 still apply. Surgery should only be considered for individuals who are severely overweight. This form of treatment requires skilled surgical intervention, and should only be carried out in a few places (see Chapter 8).

CRITERIA FOR EVALUATING OUTCOMES

Quality of Life

As the comparison of clinically significant and cosmetically significant weight loss makes clear, the quality of life is important for all overweight patients. This has effects in many areas. From the health care perspective, a reduction in comorbidities is a significant improvement. Remission of type 2 diabetes mellitus or hypertension can reduce costs of treating these conditions, as well as delay or prevent the development of complications. Weight loss can reduce the wear and tear on joints and slow the development of osteoarthritis. Sleep apnea usually resolves.

Psychosocial improvement is greatly important to patients. Studies of patients who achieved long-term weight loss from surgical intervention comment on the improved social and economic function of previously disabled overweight patients.

Loss of 5% or more of initial weight almost always translates into improved mobility, improvement in sleep disturbances, increased exercise tolerance, and heightened self-esteem. A focus on these, rather than cosmetic, outcomes is essential.

6 Lifestyle, Diet, and Exercise
Cognitive Solutions

KEY POINTS

Lifestyle

- Lifestyle became part of the treatment for obesity in the last quarter of the twentieth century and is now a cornerstone of treatment for obesity.
- It is based on the theory that obesity results from maladaptive behavior that can be improved by behavioral strategies.
- The extent of self-monitoring of behavior predicts weight loss.
- Set realistic goals and take small steps toward them.
- Behavioral contracting with rewards is a valuable strategy.
- A supporting family environment is helpful—a destructive one unhelpful.
- Learning positive thinking and assertiveness training is part of a lifestyle plan.
- Behavioral weight loss programs can produce weight losses of up to 10% over 6 months.
- The Internet may be useful for delivering a behavioral program and for helping with weight maintenance.
- Some of the best long-term results with behavioral strategies are in children.

Diet

- Current diets can be divided into those that reduce fat or carbohydrate selectively or that reduce overall intake of energy.
- Balanced deficit diets and the DASH Diet, a diet rich in fruits and vegetables and low fat dairy products, are recommended by the Dietary Guidelines.
- Adequate amounts of fluid intake are essential for life, and water, tea, coffee, and noncalorically sweetened beverages are preferred.
- Reduce intake of calorie-sweetened soft drinks and fruit drinks.
- Moderation and variety are valuable guidelines for a good diet.
- Low calorie diets produce significantly more weight loss than control diets, but the amount of fat, carbohydrate, and protein are not significant contributors to weight loss.
- Low carbohydrate diets can produce ketosis.
- Portion-controlled diets, also called meal replacements, can be useful in adhering to a lower calorie diet.
- Commercial weight loss programs can be helpful. Look for one where the diet has been tested.

Exercise

- The three main components of energy expenditure are
  - Resting metabolic rate
  - Energy consumed after eating a meal
  - Physical activity

  We only have conscious control over the last of these.

- Exercise alone is not very effective for inducing weight loss, but exercise is a very important component in maintaining a lower body weight. Exercise is valuable for preserving lean body mass.
- Fitness improves longevity, and you are better to be fit than unfit; and if obese, you are better to be fit and obese than obese and not fit.

INTRODUCTION TO COGNITIVE SOLUTIONS FOR WEIGHT LOSS

One central theme of this book is that obesity results from an increase in energy intake relative to energy expenditure that occurs over an extended period of time. A second theme is that this energy expenditure paradigm can be modified by a variety of environmental influences, including cultural settings, sleep time, epigenetic factors, and food availability. This concept is recapitulated in the figure below that shows the energy expenditure diagram in the center with the environmental influences around the outside (see Figure 6.1).

From this diagram, one approach to treatment of obesity is to eat less and another would be to exercise more. This is shown in Figure 6.2, along with the treatments that will be developed in the rest of this book. The three therapeutic approaches for treatment of obesity that are discussed in this chapter can be classified as cognitive therapies and are shown at the top of Figure 6.2. Cognitive pertains to the process of being aware, knowing, thinking, learning, and judging. Cognitive strategies require the individual to learn and practice skills, each of which involves learning skills that need to be practiced to put into play. They work when the individual adheres to the plan and the activities are followed. Adherence to behavior, dietary, and exercise programs is one of the keys to success with each of them. With high adherence, success is improved. When adherence wanes, success usually fades. The goal of this chapter is to develop each of the cognitive strategies and how they can be used effectively. As should be evident, all of these ideas have a historical past that will be part of this chapter as well.

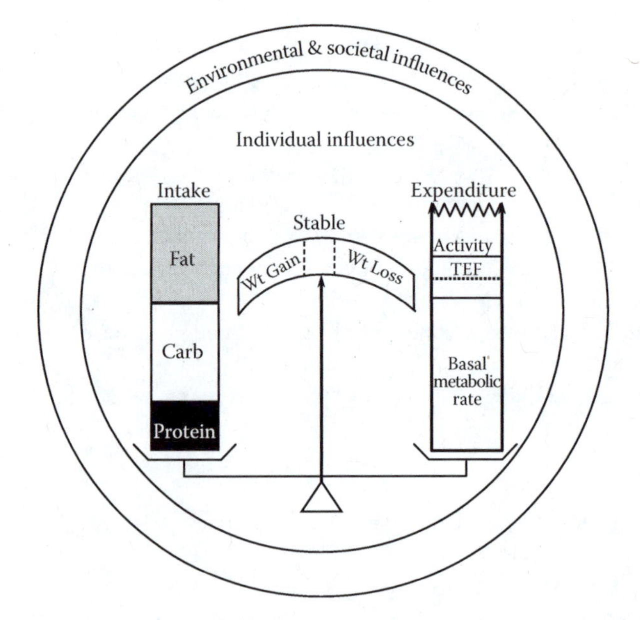

FIGURE 6.1 A model of obesity showing the energy balance concept as a scale in the center with the multiple environmental and social factors depicted in the circles surrounding the individual balance of energy intake and expenditure.

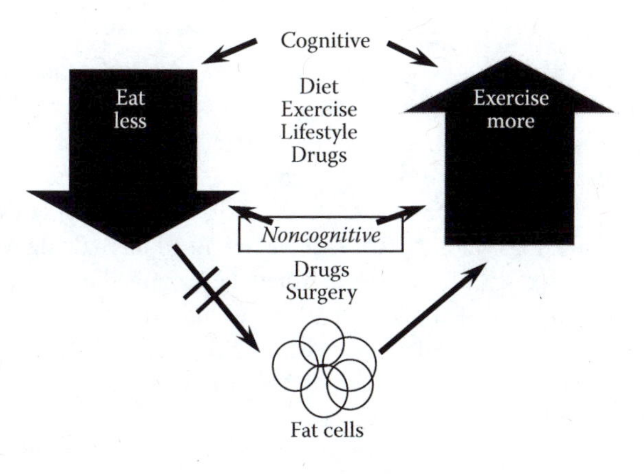

FIGURE 6.2 Eating less and spending more energy in physical activity can be influenced by both cognitive techniques that require important input from the individual and less cognitive strategies with surgery at one end.

LIFESTYLE CHANGE: A COGNITIVE SOLUTION

Historical Introduction to Lifestyle

Lifestyle strategies applied to obesity are a product of the twentieth century. They arose from two quite different research programs. The first was the psychoanalytic tradition that grew up from the teachings of Sigmund Freud. The second was the studies of the psychology of behavior epitomized in the work of Pavlov with conditioned reflexes and the work of Skinner with operant conditioning.

The psychoanalytic movement spearheaded by Sigmund Freud and his colleagues in the late nineteenth century (Freud 1913) provided several theories suggesting that obesity might result from "personality" disorders. As these theories have been tested, they have been found wanting as explanations for obesity (Stunkard and Mendelson 1967). That obesity had important social components, however, became clear from studies relating the prevalence of obesity to socioeconomic status (Moore et al. 1962). This study found that the prevalence of obesity is much higher in people from lower socioeconomic groups than in people from higher social and economic groups.

Behavior can be modified by two broad but different approaches. The first of these, known as conditioned behavior, uses the ability of animals and people to change their behavior in response to the association of external stimulus with unconditioned behavior patterns and arose from the work of Pavlov (1902, 1927). The classic example is the unconditioned salivary response in a dog when

Ivan Petrovich Pavlov (1849–1936) was the world famous physiologist who was awarded the Nobel Prize in 1904 with the citation "In recognition of his work on the physiology of digestion, in essential respects, he has transformed and enlarged our knowledge of this subject." Pavlov was born in the city of Ryazan, Russia, and received his early education in the theological seminary. His interest in science led him to St. Petersburg University, where he studied chemistry and physiology. He received his medical degree in 1883 from the Military Medical Academy. Postdoctoral research training in Leipzig with Ludwig and in Breslau with Heidenhain taught him techniques that would serve him well for his entire life. His chair in physiology, awarded in 1895, was the one he held until he retired in 1924. His most famous work is on the conditioned reflexes (Popper 1962; Mitchell 1966; Bray 2007).

Burrhus Frederic Skinner (1904–1990) is the father of "operant conditioning." Skinner was born in Susquehana, Pennsylvania, in 1904. His father was a lawyer, but Skinner was an independent soul. He attended Hamilton College in upstate New York and was an atheist in a school that required attendance in chapel. Although he tried his hand at writing, he didn't make the grade and, in 1928, he began his graduate studies at Harvard University where he received an MS in 1931 and a PhD in psychology in 1932. He remained there doing research until 1936 when he moved to the University of Minnesota, where he remained until he became chairman of psychology at the University of Indiana in 1945. He moved to Harvard in 1948 where he remained for the rest of his life. During his career, he guided many young men and women to become psychologists, and according to his biographer Boeree he may "perhaps be the most celebrated psychologist since Pavlov" (Ferster et al. 1962).

food is presented. When food is coupled with an unconditioned response such as the sound of a bell or a flashing light, animals and humans learn to respond to the flashing light or sound of a bell with salivation before presentation of the food. This conditioned salivary response will last for many trials when food is not presented, but will eventually be extinguished.

The second approach to modifying behavior is usually referred to as operant conditioning (Skinner 1988). It makes use of the behaviors that animals and humans perform spontaneously, and increases the likelihood of performing the desired ones by providing an appropriate reward. It is this latter approach that has been most widely used for changing behavior in lifestyle programs aimed at obesity.

The name of Richard B. Stuart is associated with the first application of behavioral techniques to the treatment of obesity. In his paper, Stuart (1967) outlines the four steps he used to achieve weight losses that averaged 17.1 kg (37.75 lb) or 19.1% of the initial weight of 89.2 kg (196.25 lb) in eight women. These four steps in self-control include:

1. An analysis of the response to be controlled along with its antecedents and consequences.
2. The identification of the behavior that facilitates eating the right amount of food.
3. The identification of the positive and negative reinforcers that control eating.
4. Using reinforcement to alter the probability of the prerelated response (1967). These are very similar to Ferster's ideas that I listed previously.

To carry out these steps, Stuart used several procedures (1967, 1972). Paper forms were used to allow his overweight subjects to record the time, nature, quantity, and circumstances for all eating events, related to both food and drink. Next, he kept a running record of fluctuations in body weight. He obtained a list of behavior patterns with a high likelihood of occurring in his patients such as reading, watching television, etc. Stuart also gathered information on the patients' fears that were most weight-related. These may be social, sexual, or health-related. During the first session, he introduced the behavioral curriculum in which he emphasized action as a means of attaining the desired goal. One piece of advice was to "eat slowly." Conscious interruption of eating, such as getting a glass of water during a meal, was another such example. The second step in the behavioral curriculum was to instruct the client or patient to remove food from all places in the house except the kitchen. Only one serving of food was to be prepared at a time. Complementing this was the third step, which focused on eating and how to make it a more circumscribed event. With none of his patients did Stuart consciously limit the intake of food.

Step 4 was introduced at the beginning of the second week. The patient was instructed to place a small amount of food in his mouth and then put the utensils down until the food was thoroughly chewed and swallowed. The patient was only trained to control eating under conditions of high arousal, such as when they were hungry. At step 5, the patient was instructed in substituting one

Richard Stuart (1933–present) was the first to apply the principles of behavioral therapy to a highly successful treatment program for obesity. Stuart was born in Newark, New Jersey, and received his undergraduate education at New York University. He then went on to Columbia University, where he received both a MS and DSW degree. He moved to the University of Michigan where he rose to become professor at the Center for Human Growth and Development and where he published his seminal paper in 1968 on behavioral therapy. He then moved to the State University of New York at Stony Brook and, finally, to the University of Utah. In addition to his initial paper, Stuart published "Slim Chance in a Fat World" in 1972 with Barbara Davis, which went through a second edition in 1978. He has contributed over 100 scholarly papers and books to the field. (Contemporary Authors Online, Gale, 2009. Reproduced in Biograph Research Center, Farmington Hills, MI.)

of their preferred activities for eating. The sixth and final step combines thinking about eating and then an aversive situation. It is interesting that Stuart, in his first paper, produced better results than almost any paper that has been published since (1967, 1972).

Elements of a behavior program. There are two basic assumptions underlying behavior therapy for overweight patients. The first is that obese individuals have learned maladaptive eating and exercise patterns that are contributing to weight gain and/or maintenance of their overweight state. The second is that these behaviors can be modified and that weight loss will result.

The lifestyle package that is currently used in most weight loss programs contains a number of components that are usually used together (Wing 2004; Wadden and Butryn 2005; Foster et al. 2005). These include self-monitoring (that is, keeping food diaries and activity records), control of the stimuli that activate eating, slowing down eating, goal-setting, behavioral contracting and reinforcement, nutrition education, meal planning, modification of physical activity, social support, cognitive restructuring, and problem-solving. The leading manual to help patients learn behavioral strategies is the LEARN Program for Weight Management 2000 by Kelly Brownell (Brownell 1991). Avenell et al. examined four clinical trials and found that adding behavioral therapy to diet increased the weight loss after 12 months by –7.67 kg (95% CI –11.97 to –3.36 kg).

Behavioral programs can be successful when administered individually as was done with the Diabetes Prevention Program, where weight loss averaged 7% below baseline by 6 months with only a slow gradual regain over the ensuing 3 years that leveled out after 5 years (Knowler et al. 2002; Wing et al. 2004; DPPOS 2009). Alternately, they can be done using groups, which is more economical since a single therapist can handle up to 15 or more participants. This is how the Look AHEAD (Action for Health in Diabetes) Trial of lifestyle for reduction of mortality and cardiovascular disease succeeded in producing an average weight loss of 8.4% in 1 year (Pi-Sunyer et al. 2007; Wadden et al. 2009). In an analysis of the 1-year data from the Look AHEAD weight loss trial, Wadden et al. (2009) showed a clear effect of adherence to the program on the amount of weight loss achieved. The more sessions people came to, the more weight they lost (see Figure 6.3). A meta-analysis of four trials comparing group and individual therapy by Avenell et al. found no difference in the weight loss between the two approaches after 12 months (1.59 kg [95% CI –1.81 to 5.00 kg]) (Avenell, Broom et al. 2004).

Self-Monitoring by Keeping Food Diaries and Activity Records

Self-monitoring is one of the key elements in a successful behavioral weight loss program. Participants are instructed in how to record everything they eat and the calories in the food as well as the situation where they are eating (Bray 2009). It is predictive of success during a weight loss program and is used daily during the first 4 to 6 months and then continued as needed (Wing and Phelan 2005). Self-monitoring also improves weight among patients in placebo groups in weight

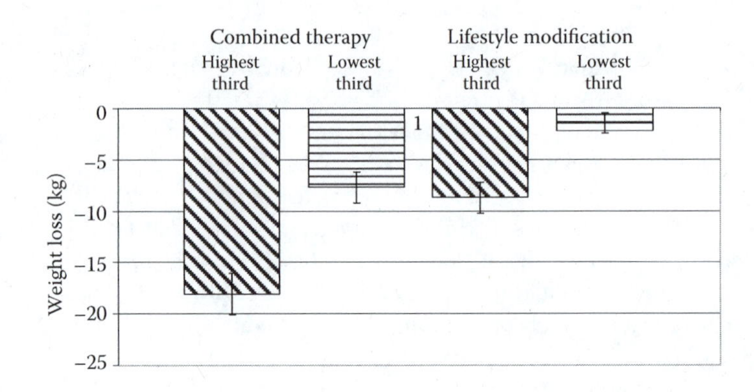

FIGURE 6.3 Effect of completing food intake records during 18 weeks on the weight loss after 1 year. (Redrawn from Wadden, T.A. et al., *N. Engl. J. Med.*, 353(20), 2111–2120, 2005.)

loss trials with drugs (Wadden et al. 2005; Berkowitz et al. 2003). In the trial with adolescents, those who were in the top third at self-monitoring and took the placebo lost 6.3% compared to only 1.2% for the lower third of the self-monitoring group. The value of self-monitoring was also shown in a study using sibutramine in adults (Wadden et al. 2005).

Stimulus Control: Gaining Control over the Environmental Factors That Activate Eating

Stimulus control is considered a key element in a behavioral program (Stuart 1967; Wing 2004; Bray 2009). Stimulus control focuses on eliminating or modifying the environmental factors that facilitate overeating. Part of this process is also to make the act of eating a focus of its own. Turning off the television set and putting down reading materials can allow the individual to concentrate on eating. Since food is a key issue in weight gain, participants are taught to buy more fresh fruits and vegetables, to prepare easy to eat lower calorie foods, and to place them prominently in the refrigerator or on the counter. The proximity of food and the kinds of containers that are used to serve it can influence how much is eaten. The elegant studies of Wansink and van Ittersum (2007) showed that when foods are close at hand, more is eaten, and that people pour out more fluid when they pour it into a short squat glass than when they pour it into a tall, thin glass. The message is: Buy and use tall thin glassware to reduce portion size from beverages.

Slowing Down the Rate of Eating

Since eating is central to ingesting food, slowing down eating may give physiological signals for fullness more time to come into play. A couple of ways of slowing down eating can be to concentrate on the tastes of the food—to savor what is being eaten. Other techniques might involve leaving the table during a meal to do something else if you are eating alone, or going to the bathroom, if eating away from home. Drinking water between bites can be another strategy to slow down eating and will increase the intake of noncaloric beverages (Bray 2009).

Setting Realistic Goals

Rome wasn't built in a day, and new ways of eating won't be learned overnight. It is important for both the patient and the therapist to set realistic goals, since expectations of the amount of weight that can be lost may be exaggerated (Foster et al. 1997). Small steps are better than trying to conquer the entire weight loss problem at once. It is also important to set concrete, achievable goals that the participant and the therapist agree on. A weight loss of 0.5 to 1 kg/week (1–2 lb/week) is a realistic goal (Wing and Phelan 2005). To achieve this goal, participants are encouraged to reduce energy intake by 1,000 kcal/day, which can be accomplished with diet instruction, provision of food, or the use of portion-controlled foods.

Behavioral Contracting and Reinforcement

Rewarding successful outcomes is important. Providing small tokens for success, such as gasoline purchase cards when gasoline prices are high or a small amount of money on a card for purchases at one of the local stores may have tangible effects. We all respond to positive encouragement, and this is particularly important when trying to lose weight.

Financial incentives can also serve to enhance weight loss. One randomized controlled trial lasting 16 weeks compared monthly weigh-ins, a lottery incentive program, and a deposit contract in 57 healthy but obese (BMI 30–40 kg/m^2) patients at the Veterans Administration (VA) Hospital who were predominantly male (94.7%). Weight loss in the control group (weigh-ins) was 1.77 kg (3.9 lb) compared to a significantly greater 6.36 kg (14.0 lb) in the deposit contract group and 5.95 kg (13.1 lb) in the lottery incentive group. The weight loss goal of 7.27 kg (16 lb) was met by 10.5% of the controls, 47.4% of the deposit contract group and 52.6% of the lottery group (Volpp et al. 2008). Weight regain occurred over the next 4 months of follow-up, but the treatment groups remained significantly lighter than the control group.

Diet and Structured Meals

Providing a defined meal structure, including portion-controlled foods and meal replacements, has helped individuals lose more weight than in the absence of such structure (Wing 2004). Use of portion-controlled diets is one of the strategies for providing this structured environment for eating. A lower fat diet is another approach that has been used.

Increasing Physical Activity

Increasing physical activity is another part of a successful behavioral program. It will be developed in detail later in this chapter.

Social Support

Enhancing social support may also be a means for improving long-term weight loss (McLean et al. 2003). Inclusion of family members or spouses is one of the best ways to accomplish this. There are both short-term and long-term benefits to programs that include strong family support. In a meta-analysis of four behavioral programs that included family members, Avenell et al. found that after 12 months, a family-based intervention had a weight loss of −2.96 kg (95% CI −5.31 to −0.60 kg) more than the control behavioral programs.

Cognitive Restructuring, Problem-Solving, Assertiveness Training, and Stress Reduction

We have internal conversations going all of the time. These can be negative or positive. For example, if you eat a piece of cake you can either blame yourself or you can decide to do some additional exercise to make up for the extra cake. Self-blame is negative self-talk. Cognitive restructuring is intended to increase positive self-talk, like exercising more to overcome the excess calories from the unintended cake. Problems dealing with food arise all the time. Learning how to handle restaurant situations, cocktail parties, and other social events is essential for success. Part of this is learning to control portion sizes of food and part is learning to say no and continuing to say no, even when food is being pushed on you. This is the task of assertiveness training. Finally, we need to reduce stress in our lives since stress for some people is a stimulus to eat. One approach is to think of a relaxing beach where you can take a deep breath and just relax. Whatever technique you use, stress reduction in this busy world is an important goal for a successful behavioral program.

Effectiveness of Lifestyle

Duration and Intensity Are Important

One of the major lessons of the past 30 years is that programs of greater length are more effective than shorter ones. In 1974, the average weight loss program lasted 8 weeks and had a weight loss of

3.8 kg. As treatment lengthened in the 1990s, the average weight loss increased to 8.5 kg after 21 weeks of treatment (Wing 2004). The efficacy of dietary counseling versus control therapy has been examined in a meta-analysis of 46 trials (Dansinger et al. 2007). A random-effects model showed a maximum net weight loss of 1.9 (95% CI −2.3 to −1.5) BMI units (approximately 6% weight loss over 12 months). There was a loss of about −0.1 BMI units per month for the 12 months of active treatment and a regain of about 0.02 to 0.03 BMI units per month during subsequent phases.

Benefits

Lifestyle programs have been effective in producing weight loss and improving the status of individuals with diabetes (Pi-Sunyer et al. 2007) and those at risk for diabetes (Knowler et al. 2002; Diabetes Prevention Program Research Group 2009; Venditti et al. 2008). In the diabetics assigned to the intervention group of the Look AHEAD trial, weight loss averaged 8.4% at the end of 1 year, and the participants required less insulin, had a reduction in blood pressure, and improved blood lipids. Among 357 pairs of participant-spouse pairs, there was a clear-cut ripple effect of weight loss. The spouses of those in the intervention group lost −2.2 ± 4.4 kg vs. −0.2 ± 3.3 kg in the spouses of pairs who were in the control group (Gorin et al. 2008).

A review of long-term effectiveness of lifestyle and behavioral weight loss interventions by Norris et al. (2004) found 22 studies that examined weight loss, with some studies lasting up to 5 years. Compared to weight loss among more than 500 diabetics receiving usual care, lifestyle strategies produced an added 1.7 kg of weight loss (95% CI 0.3–3.2 kg). If physical activity and behavioral strategies were combined with a very low calorie diet ($N = 117$ diabetics), weight loss was increased to 3.0 kg more than in the very low calorie diet comparison groups. With more intense physical activity added on top of lifestyle and dietary advice, added weight loss was 3.9 kg. The authors conclude that weight loss strategies involving behavior change, diet, and physical activity were associated with small between-group improvements in weight loss for diabetics.

Quality of life is also improved by weight loss. In the Look AHEAD trial (Williamson et al. 2009) health-related quality of life improved as indicated by less depression on the Beck Depression Inventory and by improved physical functioning as shown on the SF-36 physical function scales.

Digenio et al. compared five methods of delivering a lifestyle program to individuals who were also receiving sibutramine. A total of 376 obese (BMI 30–40 kg/m^2) participants from 12 obesity clinics were randomly assigned to one of five groups for 6 months using differing intensities of follow-up. At 6 months, weight loss was similar in the high-frequency face-to-face program compared to the high-frequency telephone counseling program (8.9% vs. 7.7%), and significantly greater than with low-frequency face-to-face counseling programs, high-frequency e-mail counseling, or self-help with no dietitian contact (Digenio et al. 2009).

In a review of randomized controlled trials involving behavioral weight control strategies (Tsai and Wadden 2009), brief counseling of patients alone by primary care physicians produced only 0.1 to 2.3 kg compared to 1.7 to 7.5 when the physician counseling was accompanied by pharmacotherapy or when the therapy was delivered by nonphysicians in collaboration with the primary care physician. This emphasizes the importance of the dietitian, behavioralist, and office staff in the effective management of body weight.

Internet-Based Programs

The Internet is all around us, and it would be surprising if it were not used as a strategy to deliver lifestyle change therapy to overweight individuals. The first use of computer-assisted therapy for weight loss programs was reported in 1985 (Burnett et al. 1985). Since 2000, use of the Internet has expanded rapidly (Tate et al. 2001; Harvey-Berino et al. 2002a; Tate et al. 2003; Harvey-Berino et al. 2002b; Womble et al. 2004; Harvey-Berino et al. 2004; Winett et al. 2005; Napolitano et al. 2003). It has been applied in commercial weight loss programs involving the internet (www.e-Diets .com) and in the clinical setting (Bennett et al. 2009).

The response to a commercial Internet Web site (www.e-Diets.com) has been compared in a randomized trial with a program that provided the LEARN manual in 47 women. The subjects had an initial visit and were then seen at 8, 16, 26, and 52 weeks to review progress. At 16 and 52 weeks, the weight loss of women assigned to the commercial program was smaller (−0.9% at 16 weeks and 1.1% at 52 weeks) than for the women using the weight loss manual (−3.6% at 16 weeks and −4.0% at 52 weeks). The significance of the data depended on the analysis used. The last observation carried forward provided a statistically significant advantage for the women using the weight loss manual, but the baseline-carried-forward analysis and the completers analyses did not, but the differences were small (Womble et al. 2004; Gold et al. 2004).

In a 12-week randomized controlled trial of a Web-based weight loss intervention among 101 primary care patients with obesity and hypertension, patients received four (two in-person and two telephonic) counseling sessions with a health coach. Weight loss at 3 months among intervention participants was 2.28 (±3.21 kg), relative to usual care (0.28 ± 1.87 kg). Retention was 84% and Web Site utilization and weight loss were greatest among those with a high frequency of Web site logins (quartile 4 vs. 1: −4.16 kg; 95% CI −1.47 to −6.84). This trial showed that a Web-based weight loss program can be delivered to primary care physicians via the Internet.

Smoking Cessation

Weight gain when trying to stop smoking is one of the deterrents to stopping, particularly among women (Parsons et al. 2009). In a review of the interventions, individualized interventions, very low calorie diets, and cognitive behavior therapy may be effective but do not reduce abstinence. In contrast, behavior interventions of general advice and exercise interventions are ineffective. Bupropion, fluoxetine, nicotine replacement therapy, and probably varenicline all reduced weight gain while being used, but are not maintained or there is insufficient information to provide clear-cut recommendations. Thus, current adjunctive measures to help people quit smoking need improvement.

Lifestyle Strategies for Children and Adolescents

Behavioral Treatment of Children and Adolescents

Some of the most effective studies of behavior therapy have been conducted in children. Epstein et al. (1990) made two important contributions to this area. First, they showed that when overweight children aged 10–12 were treated with members of the family (Figure 6.4), as opposed to

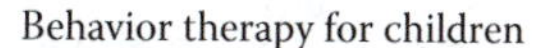

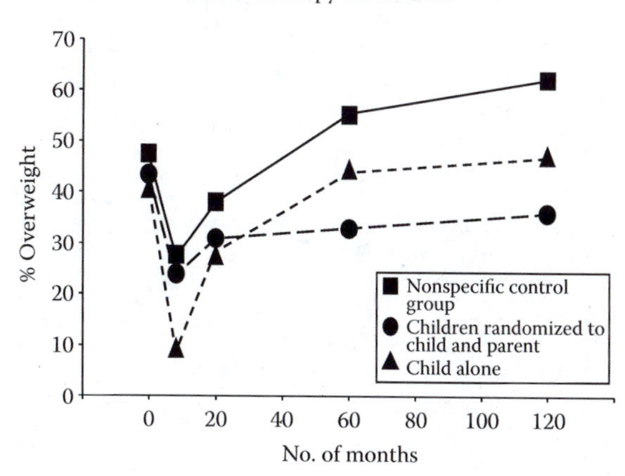

FIGURE 6.4 Comparison of weight over 10 years in overweight children who were treated alone or with one parent. (Redrawn from Epstein, L.H. et al., *JAMA*, 264(19), 2519–2523, 1990.)

individually, there was a weight loss that was largely retained over a 10-year period compared to when the children were treated without parents or when the parents were treated in separate sessions (Epstein et al. 1990).

In a second study, Epstein et al. showed that motivating adolescents to reduce inactivity (mainly decreasing television time) was more important than focusing on increasing activity. Not only did the adolescents gain less weight (or lose more), but there was a significant effect on reducing food intake. This is shown in Figure 6.5.

The Internet has also been utilized for weight loss and weight maintenance in adolescents and children. Baranowski et al. (2003) found that an 8-week Internet-based intervention for overweight eight-year-old African American girls did not yield significant weight changes in comparison to a control group. In contrast, a second study by Williamson and colleagues showed that in a program called Health Information Program for Teens (HIPTeens), weight increased 2.29 kg in the control group, but only 0.70 kg in the Internet-treatment group ($p < 0.05$). The body fat of the adolescent girls decreased by −1.12% in the behavioral group compared with a gain of 0.43% in the control group. Their parents also showed a greater decrease in body weight and body fat (Williamson et al. 2005).

An Internet lifestyle program for adolescent African-Americans compared to an Internet health education program produced small significant weight losses at 6 months (−1.12% vs. 0.43%), but by 2 years, there was no difference between the groups.

A 2-year multicomponent program enrolled 1349 students in grades 4 through 6 from 10 schools in a U.S. city in the Mid-Atlantic region with > or = 50% of students eligible for free or reduced-price meals. Schools were matched on school size and type of food service and randomly assigned to intervention or control. Students were assessed at baseline and again after 2 years. The School Nutrition Policy Initiative included the following components: school self-assessment, nutrition education, nutrition policy, social marketing, and parent outreach. The primary outcomes were the incidences of overweight and obesity after 2 years. The prevalence and remission of overweight and obesity, BMI *z* score, total energy and fat intake, fruit and vegetable consumption, body dissatisfaction, and hours of activity and inactivity were secondary outcomes. The intervention resulted in a 50% reduction in the incidence of overweight. Significantly fewer children in the intervention schools (7.5%) than in the control schools (14.9%) became overweight after 2 years. The prevalence of overweight was lower in the intervention schools. No differences were observed in the incidence or prevalence of obesity or in the remission of overweight or obesity at 2 years. Clearly, a multi-component school-based intervention can be effective in preventing the development of overweight

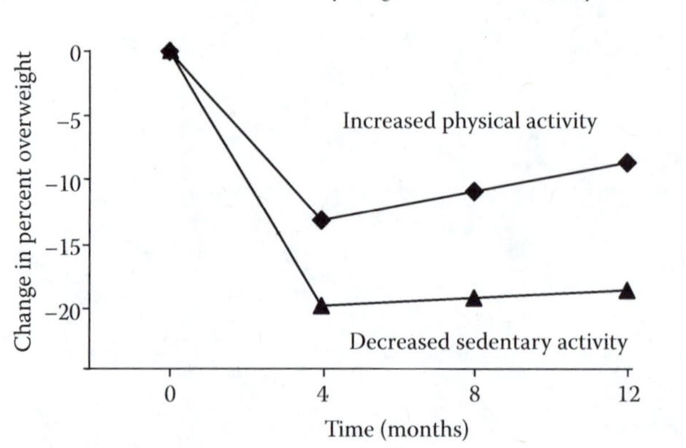

FIGURE 6.5 A comparison of advice to adolescents to be more physically active or to be less physically inactive.

among children in grades 4 through 6 in urban public schools with a high proportion of children eligible for free and reduced-priced school meals (Foster et al. 2008).

The Louisiana Health Study (LA Health) was a 30-month intervention in 17 schools located in seven of the parishes (counties) in Louisiana. It randomized schools by clusters with five assigned to the primary intervention, six schools to the primary plus a secondary prevention for those already overweight, and six schools to the control group. The children were enrolled in the fourth to sixth grades and followed with intervention through the sixth to eighth grade 2 years later. Those who didn't sign up got the educational materials, but weren't measured. The average number of students in each cluster was 290. Of those enrolled, 58.5% were female and 68.5% were African-American. Body fat averages were 12% in the males and 30% in the females using bioelectric impedance. The primary intervention focused on healthy eating, increasing activity to 60 minutes per day, reducing the vending machines in schools, and reducing television viewing to less than 2 hours per day. The nonoverweight individuals gained weight, but those who were overweight lost weight. Using digital photography to estimate food intake showed that the energy and fat intake were reduced. The Internet tools available to the participants during school time were used in 20% initially but fell to 13% over the course of the study. Physical activity also declined as the boys and girls grew older. Among white girls, the controls gained weight, but the intervention schools had less change. Among black girls, the weight gain was slowed over 30 months (Williamson et al. 2010). Other community-based programs may also be successful, but the magnitude and duration of the effects still leaves us with a challenge (Hoelscher et al. 2010; Chomitz et al. 2008; Sacher et al. 2010; Phillips et al. 2010).

DIET: A COGNITIVE SOLUTION

Historical Introduction to the Development of Diets

The modern diet has taken many centuries to develop (Cordain et al. 2005). During the period from 1500 to 1800 (see Chapter 1), diet therapy was largely used in the context of rebalancing the four humors—a concept that originated in Greco-Roman medicine. From the beginning of the nineteenth century, diet felt the influence of findings from experimental science such as those of Claude Bernard (1813–1878) and Justus Liebig (1803–1873). Claude Bernard discovered that the liver produced glucose. His ideas about glucose were used by some to promote diets with restriction of carbohydrates and were, in part, behind the diet that Dr. William Harvey gave to Mr. William Banting, who published the first popular diet book. The German school of nutrition led by Professor Liebig believed in the essential role of protein (McCollum 1957). In addition to these scientific concepts, much of the development depended on technical innovation, such as the growth and then decline of slavery in the West Indies, South America, and the United States, which was essential for the mass production of sugar (Mintz 1986). Progress depended on new techniques for processing of whole grains into refined wheat, corn, and rice; on the hydrogenization of liquid oils to produce saturated (solid) fats, which often contain trans fats and which in turn increase the risk of cardiovascular disease; and depended on the isomerization of glucose to produce high fructose corn syrup, which is used to sweeten most beverages and many other foods. With these industrial advances and national agricultural policies, consumption of a high-fat, high-sugar, high-salt diet—the Western Diet—was the outcome as cardiovascular disease, cancer, and obesity flourished when coupled with mechanization of many aspects of life.

The nineteenth century saw two important books on diet that continue to influence our thinking today. The first was the publication in French of *The Physiology of Taste* (*Physiologie du Gout*) by Anthelme Brillat-Savarin. This readable book has been through many editions and has been translated widely and beautifully illustrated by several artists.

The second was the publication in 1863 of the first "popular" diet book written by a layman. This book was titled *A Letter on Corpulence Addressed to the Public* and became wildly popular.

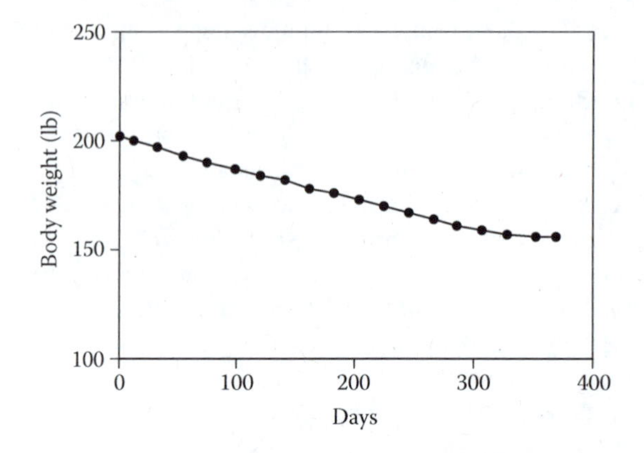

FIGURE 6.6 Weight loss curve for Mr. Banting during the first year on this diet during 1861–1862.

Mr. Banting published the first edition of his book at his own expense and gave it away to his friends in order to share his successful weight loss with them. Its popularity led almost immediately to a second printing. Subsequent printings continued until the early twentieth century. The terms "banting," "bantingism," or "to bant" became synonyms for dieting. Mr. Banting published his experience with dieting to bring the "miracle" of weight loss that he had experienced to the wider general audience.

Mr. Banting's diet consisted of the following:

Breakfast, 8 a.m.: 150 to 180 gm (5 to 6 oz) meat or broiled fish (not a fat variety of either); a small biscuit or 30 gm (1 oz) dry toast; a large cup of tea or coffee without cream, milk, or sugar.
Dinner, 1 p.m.: Meat or fish as at breakfast, or any kind of game or poultry, same amount; any vegetable except those that grow under ground, such as potatoes, parsnips, carrots, or beets; dry toast, 30 gm (1 oz); cooked fruit without sugar; good claret, 300 cc (10 oz). Madeira or sherry.
Tea, 5 p.m.: Cooked fruit, 60 to 90 gm (2 to 3 oz); one or two pieces of zwieback; tea, 270 cc (9 oz) without milk, cream, or sugar.
Supper, 8 p.m.: Meat or fish, as at dinner, 90 to 120 cc (3 to 4 oz); claret or sherry, water, 210 cc (7 oz).
Fluids were restricted to 1050 cc (35 oz) per day.

Following his diet over 1 year produced significant weight loss as is evident from his weight loss data (Figure 6.6).

Modern Diets

From these humble beginnings, diet books by professionals, self-styled professionals, and lay people have continued to appear, particularly as the concerns about obesity as a health and cosmetic problem have increased in the latter half of the twentieth century.

The dictionary defines diet as the "customary allowance of food and drink taken by any person from day to day, particularly one especially planned to meet specific requirements of the individual, and including or excluding certain items of food" (Dorland 2003). The foods and drink that comprise our diet must contain the nutrients that our bodies need to grow and function properly. You can be well-nourished and be either normal weight or overweight. Conversely, you can be poorly

William Banting (1797–1878) published the first "popular" diet book. The first edition of this small, 21-page pamphlet entitled *A Letter on Corpulence Addressed to the Public* was published privately by Mr. William Banting in 1863 (Banting 1863). The demand for this pamphlet was so great that a second and third edition were published within 1 year. In this pamphlet, Mr. Banting recounted his successful weight loss experience using a diet prescribed by his ear surgeon, Dr. William Harvey (Banting 1863), who was no relation to the William Harvey who discovered the circulation of the blood 200 years earlier. Why an "ear-surgeon," you might ask? Mr. Banting had become so heavy, weighing more than 200 pounds, that at his age of 60 he had begun to lose his hearing and his sense of balance, and was forced to come down stairs backward, lest he fall. He tried the diet recommended by Dr. Harvey and during the course of 1 year lost more than 50 pounds (23 kg). The immediate success of this pamphlet led to reprinting worldwide and a popularization of the term "Bantingism" as a reference to dieting.

nourished and be normal or overweight. That is, good nutrition and weight status are not directly related. Many different diets can satisfy our nutritional requirements.

Guidelines for a Good Diet

Two words, variety and moderation, are good general concepts to employ in selecting foods and beverages. Since each food has a different complement of nutrients, selecting a variety of foods from all food groups, particularly brightly colored foods that have many vitamins and minerals, is a good idea. Moderation, that is, controlling the amount of food we eat, is something we all need to do throughout our entire life. When this doesn't happen, overweight or malnutrition may be the result.

Much of the guidance for the public about foods is based on "food groups." There are several obvious ones including meats, milk, butter and cheese, fruits, vegetables, etc. In various forms, they have been used to guide the public in food selection for more than a half century. The Food Pyramid is one way to arrange food groups. This is shown in Table 6.1. The food groups are shown on the left side of this table and the serving size in the middle. On the right are the kinds of food that fall into

Carl Harko Hermann Johannes von Noorden (1858–1944) was a leading clinician and student of metabolism at the end of the nineteenth and beginning of the twentieth century. He came from an academic family with two great grandfathers who were physicians and a father who was a professor of history. He was born in Bonn, Germany and received his MD from the University of Leipzig in 1881. He was active in metabolic diseases in many German universities and the University of Vienna in Austria. His first academic appointment was in the Physiological Institute in Kiel and the Department of Internal Medicine at the University of Giessen. In 1889, he moved to Berlin where he was promoted to professor at age 34 in 1893. Next he moved to Frankfurt and then succeeded Nothnagel at the University of Vienna. He had a long interest in diet and in diabetes and he pioneered the use of the "weighed" diet. In 1900, the first volume of his *Encyclopedia of Metabolism and Nutrition* was published in 10 sections and translated into English in 1901. His *Handbook of Pathology of Metabolic Diseases* in 1906 was an equally monumental work. He continued his academic work for 77 years, only retiring in 1935 (Talbott 1970).

TABLE 6.1
Food Groups and MyPyramid Comparison of the USDA Food Guide and DASH Diet Eating Plans

Food Group	Servings	Comments
Grains	7 ounces (men)	Emphasize whole-grain bread, pasta, and brown rice.
		Be careful with white bread, white pasta, and white rice because refined grains are linked to higher risk of type 2 diabetes.
Vegetables	3 cups	Emphasize variety.
		Be careful about fried potatoes because these are the leading vegetable with more fat.
Fruits	2 cups	Emphasize variety with plenty of blue and red fruits.
		Moderation with bananas.
		Emphasize 100% fruit juices.
		Limit juices and punches made from concentrate, since "concentrate" is another name for sugar.
Meat and beans	6 ounces	Emphasize fish, poultry (skinless), beans, and nuts. Fish can be a good source of omega-3 fatty acids.
		Trim meats of fat and eat less red meat to reduce saturated fat intake.
Dairy products	3 cups	Emphasize skim milk and low fat yogurt. If you do not drink milk, take calcium and vitamin D supplements.
		Be careful with ice cream, butter, and cream.
Oils	6 teaspoons	Liquid vegetable oils without trans fats are preferred.
		Avoid products with trans fats because they are linked to high rates of heart disease.

Source: Adapted, with comments, from MyPyramid.gov.

this group. A comparison of MyPyramid with other population-based recommendations is provided in the JADA for May 2007 (Krebs-Smith et al. 2007).

The Dietary Guidelines Committee of 2010 recommended 2 diets for the general public. The first of these is the DASH Diet and the other is based on the USDA Food Guide and MyPyramid. The DASH Diet (Dietary Approaches to Stop Hypertension Diet) is derived from studies on dietary patterns that lower blood pressure (Appel et al. 1997; Sacks et al. 2001; Bray et al. 2004; Moore et al. 2003) and the USDA Food Guide from the MyPyramid Guide. The number of servings from each of the food groups and subgroups for the DASH and USDA Food Guide are shown in Table 6.2. Both recommend about 18% protein with significant amounts coming from vegetable sources. Fat intake is set at 27% in the DASH diet and 29% in the USDA Food Plan. Carbohydrate levels are 55% and 53%, respectively. Cholesterol intake at 136 mg/day is considerably lower than the 230 mg in the USDA Food Group. Potassium, calcium, and magnesium intakes are all higher in the DASH diet. Monounsaturated fat, saturated fat and fiber are similar—about 11%, 8%–9%, and 30%–31%.

Guidelines for Beverage Consumption

Guidelines have also appeared for beverages (Popkin et al. 2006) (Table 6.3). We need water as part of our daily diet, and we can meet all of our beverage needs with water alone (Popkin et al. 2010; Daniels and Popkin 2010). However, in addition to water, beverages may also contain many other nutrients, including vitamins and minerals that we find in fruit juices, but many beverages, particularly soft drinks, provide only water and calories. Reducing the intake of calorie-containing beverages would be good for all of us, and is particularly important when trying to lose weight. Table 6.3 provides guidance for the consumption of beverages from various categories. Water, black

TABLE 6.2
Comparison of the USDA Food Guide and DASH Diet Eating Plans

Food Groups and Subgroups	USDA Food Guide Amount	DASH Eating Plan Amount	Equivalent Amounts
Fruit group	2 cups = 4 servings	2–2.5 cups = 4–5 servings	½ cup equals ½ cup fresh, frozen, or canned fruit 1 medium fruit ¼ cup dried fruit USDA: ½ cup fruit juice DASH: ¼ cup fruit juice
Vegetable group	2.5 cups to 5 servings	2 to 2.5 cups/week	½ cup is equivalent to:
Dark green vegetables	3 cups/week		½ cup of cut-up raw or cooked vegetables
Orange vegetables	2 cups/week		
Legumes (dry beans)	3 cups/week		1 cup raw leafy vegetable
Starchy vegetables	3 cups/week		USDA: ½ cup vegetable juice
Other vegetables	6.5 cups/week		DASH: ¾ cup vegetable juice
Grain group	6 ounce-equivalents	7 to 8 ounce-equivalents or (7–8 servings)	1 ounce-equivalent =
Whole grains	3 ounce-equivalents		1 slice of bread
Other grains	3 ounce-equivalents		1 cup dry cereal ½ cup cooked rice, pasta, or cereal DASH: 1 oz dry cereal (½–1¼ cup depending on cereal type—check label)
Meat and beans group	5.5 ounce-equivalents	6 ounces or less of meat, poultry, or fish 4–5 servings per week of nuts, seeds, and dry beans	1 ounce-equivalent is: 1 ounce of cooked lean meat, poultry, or fish 1 egg USDA: ¼ cup cooked dry beans or tofu, 1 tbsp peanut butter, ½ oz nuts or seeds DASH: 1½ oz nuts, ½ oz seeds, ½ cup cooked dry beans
Milk group	3 cups	2 to 3 cups	1 cup equivalent = 1 cup of low-fat/fat-free milk or yogurt 1½ oz of low-fat or fat-free natural cheese 2 oz of low-fat or fat-free processed cheese
Oils	23 grams (6 tsp)	8 to 12 grams (2 to 3 tsp)	1 tsp equivalent = DASH: 1 tsp soft margarine 1 tbsp low fat mayo 2 tbsp light salad dressing 1 tsp vegetable oil
Discretionary calorie allowance	267 calories		1 tbsp equivalent = DASH: 1 tbsp jelly or jam
Example of distribution	18 grams	About 1 tsp (5 tbsp per week)	½ oz jelly beans
Solid fat Added sugars	8 tsp		8 oz lemonade

TABLE 6.3
Guidance for Beverage Intake

	Maximum Number of Servings per Day (*)	
Category	**Men**	**Women**
Total daily intake	13	9
Water	13	9
Coffee-unsweetened = 0 cal	4	4
Tea-unsweetened = 0 cal	8	8
Skim/low fat milk	2	2
Diet soft drinks or tea and coffee with artificial sweetener	4	4
100% fruit juice/whole milk or sports drinks	1	1
Soft drinks/juice drinks	1	1

*A serving is considered as 8 ounces (240 mL).

tea, and black coffee are preferred. Beverages prepared from whole fruit rather than concentrates, and skim or low-fat milk are also good choices. The beverages made from concentrate, another word for sugar, and soft drinks that have only water, caloric sweetener, and flavoring have the least nutritional value.

The relationship of drinking water to the quantity of food eaten has been examined in a retrospective analysis of a study of diet and obesity (Gardner et al. 2007). Absolute and relative increases in drinking water were associated with significant loss of body weight and fat over time (Stookey and Constant 2008). The caloric deficit attributable to replacing soft drinks with water was not overcome by compensatory increases in other food or beverages. Replacing all soft drinks with drinking water was associated with a predicted mean decrease in total energy of 200 kcal per day over 12 months (Stookey and Constant 2007).

Rate of Weight Loss with Dieting

The rate of weight loss is determined largely by the size of the caloric deficit, i.e., the difference between the number of calories required for daily activities, and what is consumed. The energy stored in fat cells can be viewed as a kind of bank account. A pound of fat tissue has approximately 3500 kcal of energy (7000 kcal/kg fat tissue), so that if an individual weighs 100 kg (220 lb) and has 40% body fat, the fat tissue represents 40 kg of weight and has 280,000 kcal of stored energy. If an individual eats 1600 kcal per day, 30% of which is fat, nearly 500 kcal of fat energy is received each day, or less than 0.5% of what is stored as body fat. If an individual eats 500 kcal less each day than the body needs to maintain its functions, the body will withdraw 500 kcal from body fat. Over 7 days, this will be 3500 kcal, or a pound (0.45 kg) of weight loss. To lose 50 pounds at this rate will take 50 days. This is why dieting takes so long to lose 50 lb of fat tissue, and why techniques for rapid weight loss are so popular. Such techniques usually rely on losses of water rather than fat. Figure 6.7 is a diagram showing the range of usual expected weight loss.

Total Energy Requirement

There are several key messages about calorie intake for patients and physicians alike. First, when caloric intake is reduced below that needed for daily energy expenditure, there is a predictable rate of weight loss. It is thus essential to adhere to the diet since adherence is the best predictor of success in losing weight (Sacks et al. 2009; Alhassan et al. 2008; Dansinger et al. 2006; Keys et al. 1950; Kinsell et al. 1964).

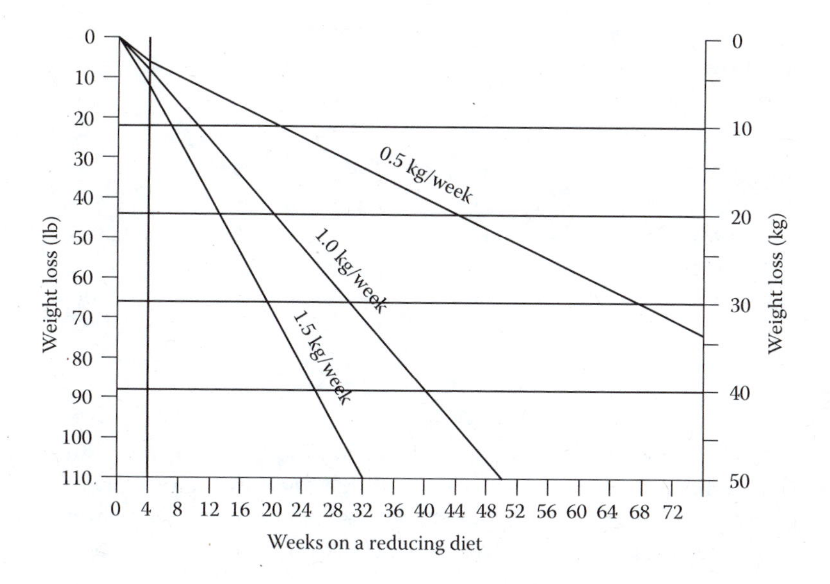

FIGURE 6.7 Anticipated rates of weight loss at 0.24 kg (0.5 lb) per week to 0.9 kg (2.0 lb) per week.

A second important fact to keep in mind is that men generally lose weight faster than women of similar height and weight on any given diet because men have more lean body mass and therefore higher energy expenditure. Similarly, older people have a lower metabolic expenditure than younger ones and as a rule lose weight more slowly since metabolic rates decline by approximately 2% per decade (about 100 kcal per decade) (Lin et al. 2003).

A third fact is that adherence to dietary programs is the essential component of success (Sacks et al. 2009; Al Hasan and Gardner 2008; Dansinger et al. 2006). In a small study where foods were labeled with nonradioactive carbon so that the amount eaten could be quantified, Lyon et al. (1995) found that the level of success was directly related to how well the subject adhered to the diet.

Finally, the breakdown of some protein is to be expected during weight loss. When weight increases from a positive energy balance, approximately 75% of the extra energy is stored as fat and the remaining 25% as lean tissue. If the lean tissue contains 20% protein, then 5% of the extra weight gain would be protein. Thus, it should be anticipated that during weight loss, at least 5% of weight loss will be protein. A desirable feature of any calorie-restricted diet, however, is that it results in the lowest possible loss of protein, recognizing that this will usually not be less than 5% of the weight that is lost.

Genetic factors are important in determining both weight gain and weight loss. Bouchard et al. reported a study in which 12 somewhat overweight identical male twins were put on a diet by reducing their food intake by an extra 1000 kcal per day, 6 days a week for 84 days or by exercising to produce a similar deficit (Bouchard et al. 1990). Five of the pairs dropped out, but among the 7 pairs that completed the trial, there was a strong relationship between the twins in the amount of weight that was lost, indicating that most of the difference in weight loss was due to the genetic factors, not environmental ones when subjects adhere to the diet.

Reducing Diets

Overview

The number of diets is enormous and grows each year as entrepreneurs and health care providers bring forth their latest ideas about how to reduce excess weight. Reducing energy intake below expenditure is essential for weight loss to occur, and all diets aim to do this in one way or another. Focusing strictly on reducing energy or calorie intake is one strategy. A second strategy is to reduce

TABLE 6.4
Types of Diets

Type of Diet	Calories kcal	Fat	Carbohydrate grams (%)	Protein
Typical American	2200	85 (35)	274 (50)	82 (15)
High fat, low carbohydrate	1400	94 (60)	35 (10)	105 (30)
Moderate fat	1450	40 (25)	218 (60)	54 (15)
Low and very low fat	1450	16–24 (10–15)	235–271 (65–75)	54–72 (15–20)

the intake of one of the more major nutrients, such as carbohydrate or fat, and a third is to manipulate the intake of protein. Diets can be defined by whether they are reduced in energy with a balanced reduction of foods, or whether they focus on reduction of one or other macronutrients in the food. Table 6.4 lists typical diets of each type (Freedman et al. 2001).

Types of Diets

Reduced energy diets

- Very low calorie diets with energy levels at or below 800 kcal per day. These are also called "protein sparing modified fasts" because they provide sufficient protein to reduce the loss of protein.
- Balanced energy deficit diets reduce all dietary components but have a total calorie intake above 800 kcal per day and usually above 1200 kcal per day for women and 1500 kcal per day for men.
- Portion-controlled diets using prepared meals, food bars, or portion-size liquid beverages to replace meals or as a key element of the meal.

Low carbohydrate diets

- Very low carbohydrate diets include those with a carbohydrate content that is less than 50 g per day, a level that will produce ketosis that can be measured by the presence of ketones in the urine.
- Low glycemic index diets that reduce intake of foods with readily digestible carbohydrate.
- The Mediterranean diet which lowers carbohydrate by replacing it with monounsaturated fats such as olive oil.

Low fat diets. These include:

- Very low fat diets with 10%–20% dietary fat.
- Moderate low fat diets with fat below 30%.

Fad diets. These are diets involving unusual combinations of foods or eating sequences. Many fad diets with various gimmicks have as one goal reducing dietary choices, which will reduce total intake by the mechanism of sensory-specific satiety, which was described in Chapter 3.

The compositions of various popular diets are presented in Figure 6.8. The gradations from higher to lower carbohydrate and fat are evident. Whether any of these combinations of macronutrients offer any special virtues for weight loss is discussed below after reviewing each of these dietary strategies in more detail.

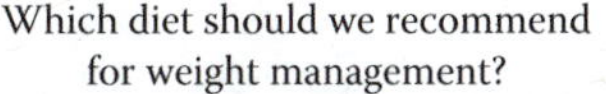

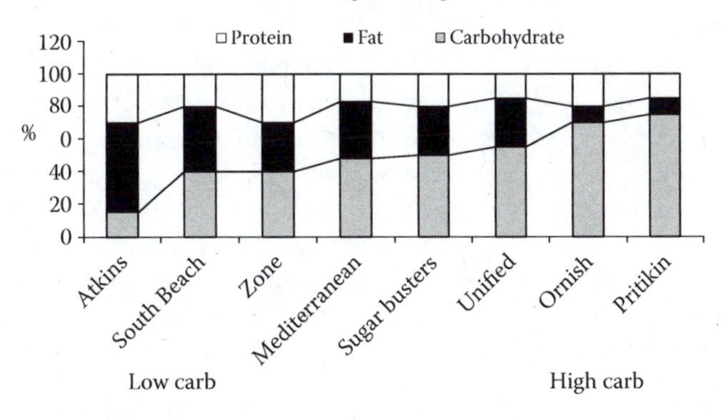

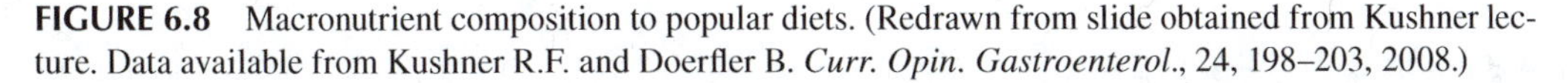

FIGURE 6.8 Macronutrient composition to popular diets. (Redrawn from slide obtained from Kushner lecture. Data available from Kushner R.F. and Doerfler B. *Curr. Opin. Gastroenterol.*, 24, 198–203, 2008.)

Starvation and semi-starvation. Total starvation has been used occasionally to treat obesity. The metabolic consequences of starvation were initially explored by Francis Benedict using the metabolic chambers designed by Atwater (Benedict 1915; Benedict et al. 1919) and, more recently, by several other authors (Fisler and Drenick 1987; Cahill 1976; Heilbron de Jonge 2006). Benedict found that human beings adapt to starvation by lowering energy expenditure and conserving protein and sodium and excreting water and potassium. At about the same time, the suggestion that calories could be dissipated by "burning them off," termed *luxuskonsumption*, was popularized by Gulick in the United States (Gulick 1922) and by Neumann in Germany (Neumann 1902), based on studies they conducted on themselves. This idea did not go unchallenged, however, and the debate about whether we can dissipate unneeded calories through changes in metabolism has been a recurring theme during the twentieth century (Wiley and Newburgh 1931). This concept is now termed "metabolic adaptation" to overfeeding.

A number of metabolic adaptations occur in fasting. Protein loss is rapid during the early phases of a very low calorie diet as the body's amino acids are used to produce glucose. As gluconeogenic mechanisms are brought into full activity, nitrogen loss falls. The brain adapts by oxidizing short chain fatty acids and sparing glucose. Glucose is also derived by salvaging the glycerol released when triglycerides are hydrolyzed to release fatty acids.

Very low calorie diets (VLCDs). Just before the beginning of the Great Depression in 1929, Evans (Evans 1926) showed that a VLCD had potential benefits for people needing to lose weight more quickly. Evans continued to publish on his VLCD as an approach to losing weight until the

> Francis Gano Benedict (1870–1957) is noted for his pioneering studies on human metabolism and for his classic studies on human starvation. Benedict was born in Milwaukee and lived in both Florida and Boston during his youth. After a year at the Massachusetts College of Pharmacy, he received his AB and MA degrees from Harvard and a PhD from Heidelberg in 1895. As fortune would have it, he began his academic career at Wesleyan University in 1895 as Atwater was completing his human calorimeter. He began his work with Atwater and when Atwater died, Benedict was appointed director. Shortly after that the Nutrition Laboratory was moved to Boston to be nearer clinical facilities. From 1897 to 1937, when he retired, Benedict did more than 500 experiments, which were carried out and published in some 400 publications. His work on human starvation was conducted in 1915 and is a classic in the field (Maynard 1969).

Frank Alexander Evans (1889–1956) was one of the first to introduce the idea of a "very low calorie diet" into clinical medicine. Evans was born in Pittsburgh in 1889. He graduated from Washington and Jefferson College in 1910 and attended Johns Hopkins Medical School where he received his MD in 1914. Following an internship at the Johns Hopkins Hospital, he received training in pathology at Presbyterian Hospital in New York City before returning to Johns Hopkins. Following service in World War I, he again returned to Johns Hopkins until 1922, when he joined Western Pennsylvania Hospital in Pittsburgh and rose from attending physician to physician-in-chief in 1931. In addition to his contributions to metabolism and low energy diets, Evans wrote a book on pernicious anemia, which had the unfortunate timing to appear in the same year that George Minot reported his Nobel-Prize-winning discovery that liver therapy prevented pernicious anemia, a discovery that did not appear in Evans's monograph (1926).

beginning of World War II, when this idea was lost sight of until fasting was reintroduced as a treatment for obesity by Bloom in 1959 (Bloom 1959).

Liquid formula diets, as a strategy to achieve a very low calorie diet, were initially popularized by the diet used at Rockefeller University in New York with the trade name Metrecal. Commercial use began gradually and then spread rapidly until 17 deaths occurred in patients using formula diets (Sours et al 1981). The use of gelatin in these diets provided an incomplete protein which was associated with fatalities from cardiac arrhythmias. Gelatin is a poor quality protein that is deficient in several essential amino acids. Although the 19th century Gelatin Commission in France had concluded that gelatin was an inadequate protein to support human life, this lesson had to be re-learned in the 1970's with fatal results (Magendie 1841; Carpenter 1994).

New liquid formula diets using high-quality protein replaced the gelatin-based diets, and sales reached another peak in the late 1980s, until the U.S. government raised concerns about the safety of these diets. Public interest in these diets faded rapidly and there was a loss of commercial profitability.

The theory behind the VLCD or protein-sparing modified fasting diet is that the lower the energy intake, the more energy would be withdrawn from fat stores and the faster weight and fat would be lost. Contrary to this theory, weight loss using a 400 kcal per day VLCD was not different than an 800 kcal per day diet, probably because the subjects adapted to the 400 kcal per day difference by modifying their energy expenditure during activity or during sleep (Blackburn and Bray 1985).

Although VLCDs, providing <800 kcal per day have been used since the 1970s to induce rapid weight loss, there is disagreement concerning their efficacy. In a review comparing VLCD and low calorie diets, Tsai and Wadden (2006) found six randomized trials that included a follow-up of at least 1 year after maximum weight loss. The VLCD diets induced significantly greater short-term weight losses (16.1 ± 1.6%) than the low calorie diets (9.7 ± 2.4%, $p = 0.0001$), but similar long-term losses (VLCD = 6.3 ± 3.2%; low calorie diets = 5.0 ± 4.0%, $p > 0.2$). Rates of discontinuation were similar with both dietary approaches. Benefits of the VLCD included reduction in blood pressure and improvement in hyperglycemia in diabetic patients. A fall in blood pressure is characteristic during the first week after starting a very low calorie diet, and may result in postural hypotension. Antihypertensive drugs, especially calcium channel blockers and diuretics, should usually be discontinued when a VLCD is begun. Most diabetics eating very low-calorie diets show marked improvement in hyperglycemia. Blood glucose concentrations fall within the first 1 to 2 weeks, and remain low as long as the VLCD is continued. Patients taking less than 50 units of insulin or an oral hypoglycemic drug will usually be able to discontinue therapy. Weight regain is often rapid when the diet is stopped. One clinical use for the very low calorie diet is in preparation for bariatric surgery. A 2- to 4-week period eating a VLCD can significantly reduce the size of the liver by mobilizing glycogen and, more importantly, lipid in the liver (Dixon et al. 2006). It can also reduce the size of the omentum, since the visceral adipose tissue stores are more responsive to a negative calorie balance than total body fat stores. A VLCD might also be considered for individuals with hepatic steatosis.

Balanced energy deficit diets. Planning a balanced low calorie diet requires the selection of a caloric intake and then selection of foods to meet this intake. It is desirable to eat foods with adequate amounts of protein, carbohydrate, and essential fatty acids. Thus, weight-reducing diets should eliminate alcohol, sugar-containing beverages, and most highly concentrated sweets, because they rarely contain adequate amounts of other nutrients besides energy. One concept is to buy and consume foods that are naturally nutrient-rich. This would mean eating more fruits, vegetables, whole grains, lower fat meats, fish, poultry, beans, and 100% fruit juices (not from concentrate) and yogurt, and eating less of the processed foods where the nutrients that are naturally present have been altered, removed, diluted, or otherwise changed (Drewnowski 2005).

Using a "diet score" concept to provide diets for weight loss and improving diet quality was the basis for the Oslo Diet and Exercise Study, which randomized 187 men to a 1-year trial comparing diet, exercise, and diet plus exercise against a control group. The diet score increased in both diet groups, but decreased in the exercise and control groups. Weight change was related to the change in diet score. In the diet groups, it was 5 to 7 kg compared to a 2-kg loss in the exercise group. Increased dietary score was also associated with improved systolic blood pressure, body size, blood lipids, glucose, insulin, and adiponectin, but was unrelated to cytokines (Jacobs et al. 2009).

In a meta-analysis of weight loss with "balanced deficit diets," Avenell et al. (2004) identified 12 studies that evaluated diet versus a control that lasted more than 12 months. At the end of 12 months, the difference between the control and treated groups was –5.31 kg (95% CI –5.86 to –4.77 kg). In another systematic review of studies having more than 100 subjects and a duration of more than 1 year without pharmacological intervention, Douketis et al. found 16 studies that met their criteria. After 2–3 years, weight loss was usually <5 kg below baseline (–3.5 ± 2.4 kg; range 0.9 to 10.0 kg) and after 4–7 years, where there was data, it was –3.6 kg ± 2.6 kg (Douketis 2005).

Portion-controlled diets and meal replacements. Portion-controlled diets are another strategy for achieving a balanced caloric deficit. This can be done most simply by the use of formula diet drinks based on powdered or liquid formula diets, nutrition bars, individually packaged frozen foods, cold-packed meals, or irradiated foods. Frozen low-calorie meals containing 250 to 350 kcal per package can be a convenient and nutritious way to do this. There are also portioned-controlled meals that can be stored at room temperature and cook in 90 seconds. With this strategy, it is easily possible to obtain a calorie-controlled intake of 1000 to 1500 kcal per day.

The Look AHEAD trial has nicely demonstrated the impact on weight loss of adherence to a portion-controlled meal replacement strategy (Figure 6.9). In the first year of this multicenter trial, the intervention group was prescribed a reduced calorie diet with meal replacements. The lowest quartile for use of meal replacements consumed an average of 117 meal replacements and lost 5.9%. This contrasted with the highest quartile using 608 meal replacements on average who lost 11.2% of their baseline weight (Wadden et al. 2009). In a university-based study, weight loss in the low calorie versus meal replacement groups was similar, but the nutritional adequacy was better in those using the fortified meal replacement products (Ashley et al. 2007).

In a meta-analysis of meal replacement studies, Heymsfield et al. (2003) showed more weight loss than with low calorie diets. Six randomized, controlled trials in adults that lasted at least 3 months in subjects with a BMI ≥ 25 kg/m^2 were evaluated. The prescribed calorie intake was the same for both low calorie and meal-replacement groups. Both groups lost weight, but the subjects prescribed the meal replacements lost more weight (7%–8% for meal replacement vs. 3%–7% for low calorie diets). Those completing the meal replacement programs lost 2.54 kg ($p < 0.01$) more at 3 months and 2.63 kg ($p < 0.01$) more after 1 year than the low calorie group. Cardiometabolic risk factors improved with weight loss in both groups. The rate of discontinuation was equivalent in the two groups at 3 months, but significantly less in the meal replacement group at 1 year. Thus, meal replacements offer an advance in the efforts to control calorie intake in a weight loss program.

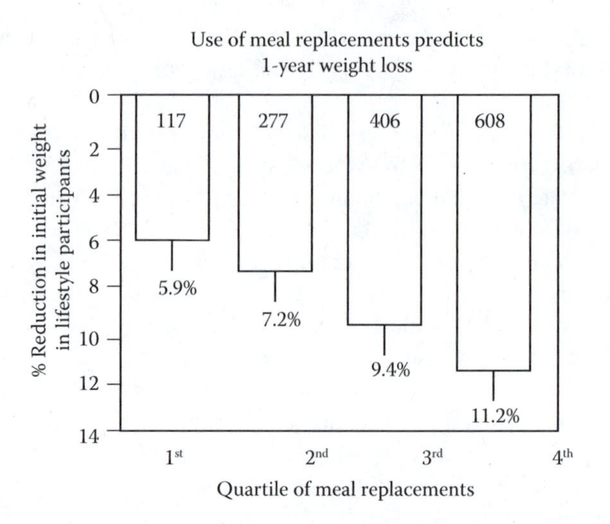

FIGURE 6.9 The effect of the number of meal replacements used in the Look AHEAD Clinical Trial on the weight loss in the intervention group. (Redrawn from Wadden, T.A. et al., *Obesity*, 17(4), 713–722, 2009.)

Low carbohydrate diets. These include:

- Low glycemic index diets
  The glycemic index is one way of expressing the rate at which glucose can be made available from foods. It is based on measurements of the rise in blood glucose in the test food compared to the rise after a 50-g portion of white bread (Ludwig 2002). Foods with a high glycemic index are those that are rapidly digested with a rapid rise in blood glucose. Low glycemic index foods usually come with fiber and are more slowly digested and thus produce a slower rise in blood glucose. Table 6.5 is a list of the glycemic index of some foods. The glycemic load refers to the quantity of carbohydrate in a food multiplied by the glycemic index of that food. Carrots, for example, have a high glycemic index because the carbohydrate they have is rapidly digested. However, they have a low glycemic load because there isn't much carbohydrate in carrots. In a review of six studies, investigators

TABLE 6.5
Glycemic Index and Load Values for Various Foods

Food	Glycemic Index	Glycemic Load
Instant rice	91	24.8
Baked potato	85	20.3
Corn flakes	84	21.0
White bread	70	21.0
Rye bread	65	19.5
Banana	53	13.3
Spaghetti	41	16.4
Apple	36	8.1
Lentil beans	29	5.7

Source: Adapted from Ludwig, D.S., *JAMA*, 287(18), 2414–2423, 2002.

documented that the consumption of foods with a high glycemic index was associated with higher energy intake than when the foods had a low glycemic index (Ludwig 2002).

The effects of low glycemic index diets on weight loss have been studied in a number of randomized clinical trials in adults (Thomas 2007). Thomas et al. identified six studies, including 202 participants that met their inclusion criteria (Bouche 2002; Ebbeling 2003; Ebbeling 2005; McMillan-Price 2006; Slabber 1994; Sloth 2004). Three of these studies compared low glycemic index diets with higher glycemic index diets, while the other three compared an ad-lib reduced glycemic load diet with a conventional energy-restricted reduced fat diet, or an energy-restricted low glycemic index diet with a normal energy-restricted diet. Interventions were relatively short, ranging from 5 weeks to 6 months. There was a small significant difference in body weight of 1.1 kg (95% CI −2.0 to −0.2) that favored the low glycemic index diets. The body mass decreased by 1.1 kg ($p < 0.05$) and fat mass by a similar amount compared to the change of weight in the control diet group. Both total and LDL cholesterol fell more with the low glycemic index diets (Thomas et al. 2007).

- Very low carbohydrate high protein diets
  Low carbohydrate high protein diets have been popular from the time of Banting nearly 150 years ago (1863). A number of well-done clinical trials examining the effects of low carbohydrate diets have been reported (Foster, Wyatt et al. 2003; Brehm et al. 2003; Samaha et al. 2003).
  In a meta-analysis of low-carbohydrate versus low fat diets, Nordmann et al. (2006) found significantly more weight loss at 6 months favoring the low carbohydrate diet (−3.3 kg 95% CI 5.3 to −1.4 kg) but that this benefit had been lost by 12 months (−1.0 kg 95% CI −3.5 to 1.5 kg). Changes in lipids varied between diets. The low carbohydrate diet produced a more favorable change in triglycerides and HDL-cholesterol, whereas the low fat diets were more favorable for changes in total cholesterol and LDL-cholesterol.
- Low carbohydrate moderate fat Mediterranean-type diets
  A clinical trial of a Mediterranean-style diet similar to the Mediterranean Step-1 diet of the American Heart Association (AHA) provided instruction in nutrition to reduce body weight by 10% by eating a 1300 kca/ld diet with 50%–60% carbohydrate, 15%–20% protein, and less than 30% fat (less than 10% saturated fat) with 10%–15% from monounsaturated fats and 5%–8% from polyunsaturated fat. Fiber was prescribed at 18 g per 1000 calories. Women were also given behavioral weight loss instruction on setting personal weight loss goals and self-monitoring with food diaries with regular behaviorally oriented sessions (Esposito et al. 2003). After 2 years in the trial, body weight had decreased 14 kg in the intervention group of 60 women but only 3 kg in the control group. Blood pressure, glucose, and insulin also improved more in the group eating the Mediterranean diet, as did adiponectin, IL-6, IL-18, and c-reactive protein. This moderate weight loss diet is clearly one of the most impressive longer-term follow-up studies. A modified Mediterranean style diet may also be beneficial for reducing hepatic steatosis in obese diabetics (Fraser et al. 2008).

High-protein diets. Dietary protein is essential for all aspects of growth and development, and it may play a role in modulating food intake and body weight regain after weight loss (Westerterp-Plantenga et al. 2009). The quantity of protein in the diet has been nearly constant for the past century since Atwater first estimated it to be about 15% of energy intake. Protein comes from both plant and animal sources. The percentage distribution of individual amino acids in animal proteins is closer to that of humans than it is to plant proteins, which are often low in one or another amino acid. For vegetarians it is thus desirable to get protein from a variety of plant sources, including beans, legumes, and nuts, to balance out the differences.

Several trials have tested the effects of varying protein levels in weight loss diets. One study compared 15% and 25% protein diets and a low fat diet. Weight loss over six months was greater with the higher protein diet (Skov et al. 1999). In a follow-up at 12 and 24 months, Due et al. (2004) found that the higher protein diet group had regained weight, but were still less heavy than the medium protein group and still 6 kg below their baseline weight, which was similar to the 5.5 kg weight loss in the control group. However, after 2 years of follow-up, there were only 5 of the original 23 in the medium protein group and 11 of the 23 in the high protein group. The body weights were the same and about 8–10 kg below their initial baseline. This is indeed a very impressive 2-year result for a lower fat diet, but does not suggest that one protein level is superior to the other.

In shorter-term trials, Hu (2005) found that higher-protein diets increase short-term weight loss and improve blood lipids, although long-term data are lacking. There was a significant relationship between increased protein intake and lower risk of hypertension and coronary heart disease in epidemiologic studies. Different sources of protein appear to have different effects on cardiovascular disease and there may be a potential benefit of partially replacing refined carbohydrates with protein sources low in saturated fat.

The interaction of dietary protein with exercise on body composition and weight loss was examined in a 4-month trial by Layman et al. (2005). A total of 48 women with a BMI > 26 kg/m^2 and a body weight < 160 kg were randomized to four groups. Two groups received 15% protein diets and the other two received 30% protein with energy levels of 7.1 MJ/d (1500 kcal/day). The two diet groups were divided into either a lifestyle activity group or a supervised exercise group that did supervised walking 5 days a week plus 2 days a week of resistance training. At the end of 4 months, the high protein group with or without exercise lost more body weight and body fat than the low protein group. Exercise preserved lean body mass and enhanced fat loss. In another pair of 3-month studies, however, there was no difference in weight loss with high protein compared to moderate protein diets, but there was no exercise program included, which may have been an important difference (Noakes et al. 2005; Luscombe-Marsh 2005, Noakes et al. 2005). Thus, the jury is still out on whether dietary protein influences weight loss.

Dietary fat, energy density, and low-fat diets. Many food items, particularly processed ones, have a considerable amount of fat and variable amounts of saturated fat. Substituting lower fat foods for high fat ones is a good strategy to reduce energy intake and lower intake of saturated fats. Table 6.6 shows the way in which reducing fats in the diet can also reduce energy intake. For example, cheese can contain up to 13% saturated fat, beef up to 11.7%, oils up to 4.9%, ice cream 4.7%, butter 4.6%, salad dressing 4.4%, poultry 3.6%, and sausage 3.2% (HH5 2005). In commercial foods, trans fats have been found in up to 40% of the fat in cakes, cookies, crackers, pies, and bread. In animal products, trans fats can be up to 20% or more of the fat. In some margarines, they were up to 17% but the presence of trans fat must now appear on the nutrition facts label and most margarines do not now have trans-fat in them. Fried potatoes can have 8%, potato chips, corn chips, and popcorn 5%, and household shortening 4% (2005).

- Low fat diets

  Low fat diets are one of the standard strategies to help patients lose weight. The rationale for these diets is that fat contains more than twice as much energy (calories) per gram (or pound) as either carbohydrate or protein. One concern about the recommendation of low fat diets is that the population has continued to gain weight and some have suggested that recommending a low fat intake may have played a detrimental role. A recent large randomized clinical trial of low fat versus control diets that included 48,835 women make this interpretation of the obesity epidemic unlikely. Howard et al. (2006) randomly assigned women from the Women's Health Initiative to low fat or control diets. The food records showed that the group assigned to the low fat diet reduced fat intake from 38.8% to an average of 29.8% compared to the 38.8% in the control group, which remained almost

TABLE 6.6
Comparison of Normal and Lower Fat Options

Food Item	Full Fat Option		Lower Fat Option	
	Saturated Fat (g)	Energy (kcal)	Saturated Fat (g)	Energy (kcal)
Cheese (1 oz)	6.0	114	1.2	49
Ground beef (3 oz cooked)	6.1	236	2.6	148
Milk (1 cup or 8 ounces)	4.6	146	1.5	102
Breads (medium croissant vs. medium bagel)	6.6	231	0.2	227
Frozen dessert (regular ice cream vs. low fat frozen yogurt (½ cup))	4.9	145	2.0	110
Table spreads (butter vs. soft margarine with zero trans fat)	2.4	34	0.7	25
Chicken (fried chicken leg with skin vs. roasted chicken breast no skin—3 ounces)	3.3	212	0.9	140
Fish (fresh fish vs. baked fish—3 ounces)	2.8	195	1.5	129

Source: HHS, *Dietary Guidelines for Americans*, U.S. Department of Health and Human Services, Washington, D.C., 2005.

constant at 38.1% at end of study. Weight loss was 2.2 kg at 1 year and 0.6 kg at an average of 7.5 years of follow-up. The reduction was similar across BMI groups, but there was a clear relationship between the decrease in percent fat and weight loss ($p < 0.001$ for trend) (Figure 6.10).

In contrast with the value of low fat diets for prevention of weight gain as discussed above is the issue of their role in weight loss. In the analysis by Bray and Popkin (1998), a 10% reduction

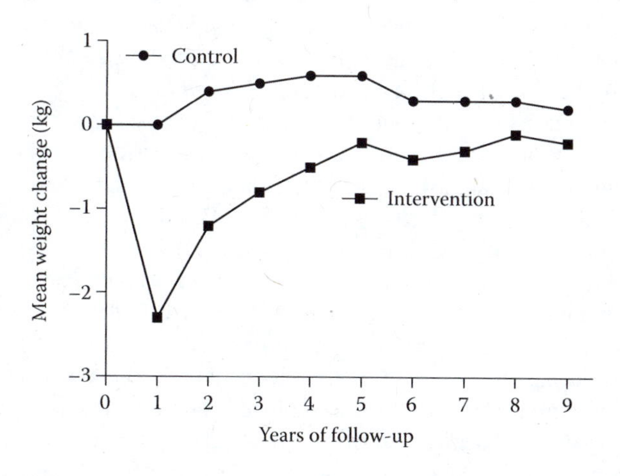

FIGURE 6.10 Effect of a low fat diet on weight loss in the Women's Health Initiative. (Redrawn from Howard, B.V. et al., *JAMA*, 295(1), 39–49, 2006.)

of dietary fat intake predicted an early fat loss of about 6 g per day or about 4 kg in 6 months. In a meta-analysis of weight loss studies, Astrup et al. (2000) found that over the first 6 months, low fat diets produced weight loss and that heavier individuals lost more weight.

Another shorter term trial compared a 35%–45% fat diet with more than 20% from monounsaturated fatty acids, a low fat (20%–30%) diet to a 35% fat control diet following an initial weight loss of ≥8%. All three groups regained weight, and no diet was better than another at preventing weight regain (Due et al. 2008).

A few randomized clinical trials of low fat diets have been conducted, and Pirozzo et al. (2003) conducted a meta-analysis of them. Five randomized controlled trials were included in this analysis. Both diet groups lost weight and the authors concluded that low fat diets produced significant weight loss, but not more so than the control diets against which they were compared. As shown in this study, weight regain occurs after the nadir of weight loss, whether the diet is low fat or low carbohydrate.

A low fat diet can be implemented in two ways (Bray 2009). First, the dietitian can provide the subject with specific menu plans that emphasize the use of reduced-fat foods. As a guideline, remember, that if a food "melts" in your mouth, it probably is high in fat.

Second, subjects can be instructed in counting fat grams (Bray 2009). Fat has 9.4 kcal/g. It is thus very easy to calculate the number of grams of fat a subject can eat for any given level of energy intake. Counting fat grams is an alternative to counting calories. Many experts recommend keeping calories from fat to below 30 percent of total calories. In practical terms, this means eating about 33 g of fat for each 1000 calories in the diet. For simplicity, I use 30 g of fat or less for each 1000 kcal. For a 1500 calorie diet, this would mean about 45 g per day or less of fat, which can be counted using the nutrition information labels on food packages.

Popular Diets

Overview

Many popular diets are on the bookshelf, and a new crop appears each year promising success where the others failed (Freedman et al. 2001; Dansinger et al. 2005). Among the current crop are *The Sonoma Diet,* which touts small portion sizes of sun-drenched California cuisine with red or white wine; *How the Rich Get Thin,* which stresses daily exercise, avoidance of processed foods, and a high intake of calcium and high quality protein; *Flavor Point Diet,* which has as its buzz-word monotony—that is, limiting your choices; *The Rice Diet Solution,* whose title tells the story; *The Supermarket Diet,* which steers you toward produce and away from processed foods; and the *QOD Diet* (QOD = every other day), which touts alternating 400 kcal on one day with a larger intake on the next. Based on the high intake of fructose, I have developed a strategy for weight loss that is published in my book, *The Low-Fructose Approach to Weight Loss.*

After ignoring the gimmicks, most popular diets can be grouped in very low-fat, moderate-fat, or high-fat categories. An analysis of these diets by Consumers Union has been adapted in Table 6.7 and included in this analysis are low carbohydrate diets, low fat diets, low glycemic index diets, along with computer diets, energy density, portion-controlled diets, and commercial groups. The Ornish diet (Ornish 1993) and the Pritikin diet (Pritikin 1991) (which is not included in the table) are two examples of very low-fat diets. Nutritional analysis has shown that the Ornish diet, if followed, provides only 13 g of fat (6%) (Freedman et al. 2001) (see Table 6.2). Carbohydrate intake in this dietary program is the highest of all the popular diets. Maintaining a very low fat diet can be difficult in a society with an abundance of high fat foods, but for those who do adhere to the diet, weight loss can be substantial. An additional benefit from this very low level of fat is the slowing or reversal of coronary artery disease. The Atkins diet is clearly the highest in fat, with the South Beach the second highest, the Ornish diet and the Volumetrics diet have the highest amount of fruits and vegetables.

TABLE 6.7
Nutritional Content of Several Popular Diets

Diet	Protein	Fat	Sat'd Fat	Carbohydrate	Fiber g/1000 kcal	F & V Daily Servings
Atkins	29%	60%	20%	11%	12	6
e-Diets	24%	23%	5%	53%	19	12
Jenny Craig	20%	18%	7%	62%	16	6
Ornish	16%	6%	1%	77%	31	17
Slim-Fast	21%	22%	6%	57%	21	12
South Beach	22%	39%	9%	38%	19	3
Volumetrics	22%	23%	7%	55%	20	14
Weight Watchers	20%	24%	7%	56%	20	11

Source: Adapted from *Consumer Reports*, June, 2005, 21.

Two examples of a moderate fat, low calorie diet are the *Sugar Busters!* diet (Steward 2002) and the Weight Watchers diet. Fat intakes with these diets are nearly the same, 44 g and 42 g per day, respectively (Freedman et al. 2001). Carbohydrate intakes are also similar, but the type of carbohydrate differs. The Sugar Busters! diet emphasizes the use of foods with a low glycemic index, that is, foods that have higher fiber contents and, thus, absorb glucose more slowly. *The Glucose Revolution* (Brand-Miller 2003) is another popular diet that uses foods with a low glycemic index as the basis for a higher-fiber, lower-calorie diet.

The third group of diets is the high fat, high protein diets. The most popular example in this category is the Atkins diet (Atkins 2002). Nutritional analysis of the Atkins diet has shown 75 g of fat in the induction diet, which increased to 114 g of fat during the maintenance diet (Freedman et al. 2001). Carbohydrate intake on the Atkins diet, if followed, is 13 g per day during induction, and this level increases to 95 g per day during maintenance. *The Carbohydrate Addict's Diet* (Heller 1993) has a similarly high level of fat but a somewhat less restrictive level of carbohydrate, at 87 g per day (Freedman et al. 2001). When carbohydrate intake is less than 50 g per day, ketosis uniformly develops. One concern with ketosis is the source of the cations needed to excrete the ketones. If the cations consist of calcium from the bone, this process may enhance the risk of bone loss.

Comparison of Diets

It should be clear by now that any diet that results in a decrease in calorie intake will achieve weight loss, but it is important to verify this by head-to-head comparisons. A number of trials lasting 1 to 2 years have been reported that have done just that (Dansinger et al. 2005; Gardner et al. 2007; Shai et al. 2008; Sacks et al. 2009; Brinkworth et al. 2009; Davis et al. 2009).

A 1-year head-to-head comparison of four popular diets in 168 men and women included the Atkins diet, the Ornish diet, Weight Watchers diet, and the Zone diet (Dansinger et al. 2005). Dansinger et al. found that each diet produced weight loss of about 5 kg. There was no significant difference between diets, but with each diet some patients lost significant amounts of weight. Adherence to the diet was the most important single criterion of success in this trial.

In another 1-year trial Gardner et al. (2007) compared the Atkins diet, the Zone diet, and the Ornish diet with the LEARN lifestyle manual in 260 premenopausal women. The Atkins diet produced more weight loss at 6 and 12 months compared to the other three, which were similar. There are at least two reasons for the differences between these trials. First, Gardner et al. (2007) had a more homogeneous population that included only premenopausal women. Second, the study by

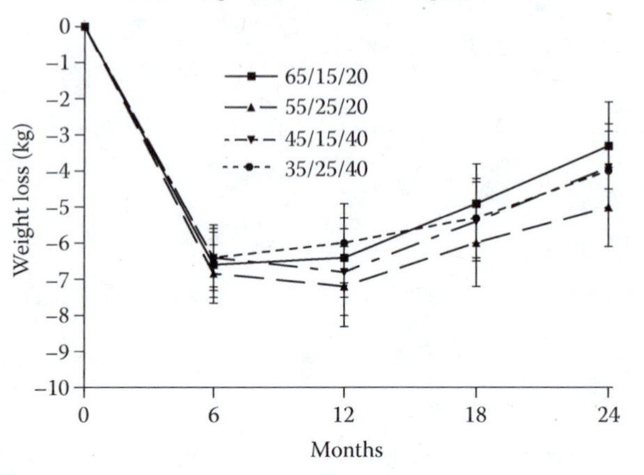

FIGURE 6.11 Weight loss in the POUNDS LOST trial over 2 years with diets that vary in their macronutrient composition. (Redrawn from Sacks, F.M. et al., *N. Engl. J. Med.*, 360(9), 859–873, 2009.)

Gardner et al. (2007) was larger and thus had more statistical power to detect differences. In a follow-up, Alhassan et al. (2008) showed that regardless of diet assignment, weight loss was greater for each diet among those who were most adherent to the diet.

In a third 1-year trial, providing an isocaloric low carbohydrate diet or a low fat diet for 12 months produced similar amounts of weight loss in 118 nondiabetic subjects, 59% of whom completed the trial and lost similar amounts of weight (14.5 ± 1.7 kg in the low carbohydrate group versus 11.5 ± 1.2 kg in the low fat group) (Brinkworth et al. 2009). Comparison of a low fat diet versus a high carbohydrate diet in 105 diabetic men and women, of whom 91 completed the trial, found a 3.4% weight loss in both groups (Davis et al. 2009).

In addition to these three 1-year trials, there are two trials lasting 2 years. The first of the 2-year studies compared three diets: a low fat diet; a Mediterranean-type diet; and a low carbohydrate diet

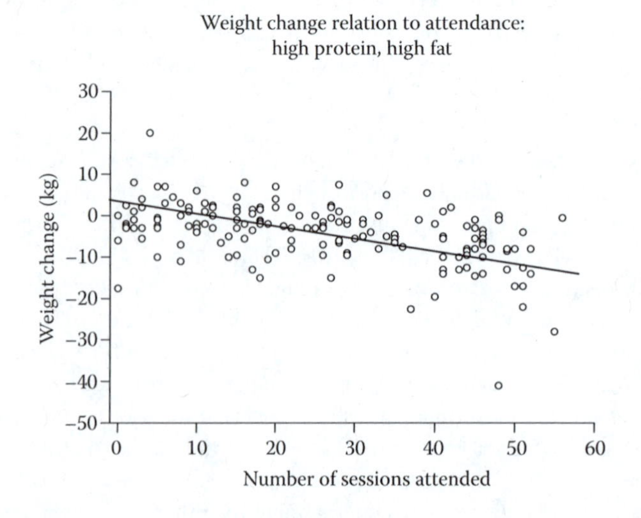

FIGURE 6.12 Effect of adherence to the intervention program on weight loss in the participants in the POUNDS LOST Trial. (Redrawn from Williamson, D.F. et al., *Int. J. Obes. Relat. Metab. Disord.*, 18, 561–569, 1994.)

like the Atkins diet in 322 subjects, 86% of whom were men (Shai et al. 2008). In the first 6 months, the group assigned the low carbohydrate group lost more weight, but surprisingly, in the next 6 months, the weight loss of the Mediterranean diet group accelerated to reach that of the low carbohydrate diet. The low fat diet group lost less weight, and all three groups had plateaued by 12 months in this two-year trial. The initial plateau followed by a subsequent weight loss after 6 months has not been reported in other trials, and it is unclear what was responsible for this effect.

The largest and most clear-cut of these head-to-head trials lasted 2 years and had 811 overweight and obese patients, which is more patients than the other three previous trials combined (Sacks et al. 2009). Participants were randomized to diets with a prescribed energy deficit of 750 kcal per day that had 20% or 40% fat, and 15% or 25% protein, giving a two by two factorial design. Maximal weight loss of 6.5 kg was achieved at 6 months and nearly 80% of this loss was retained at 2 years with an 80% follow-up rate (Figures 6.11 and 6.12). There was no difference between diets, but individuals who adhered better to each diet lost more weight (Sacks et al. 2009; Williamson et al. 2009).

Special Populations

Diabetics

Do weight loss diets work as well for diabetics as for nondiabetics? The Diabetes Prevention Program used an intensive lifestyle program in people with impaired glucose tolerance and the Look AHEAD trial examined an intensive lifestyle program in patients who already had diabetes. After 1 year, weight loss in the Diabetes Prevention Program was 7.5% and in the Look AHEAD trial it was 8.6%. The Look AHEAD trial had included meal replacements that may have accounted for their superior weight loss. It is clear, however, that diabetics can respond as well as those with impaired glucose tolerance but without diabetes. In both of these large studies, various ethnic groups (African-American, White, Hispanic, and Asian-Pacific) showed similar response to the lifestyle and dietary intervention. However, a paper from the Obesity Reduction Black Intervention Trial (ORBIT) raises questions about ethnic difference in the response (Stolley et al. 2009). In this trial with 213 black women aged 30–65, the intervention group lost 3 kg during 6 months and there was a weight gain of 0.2 kg in the control group (Figure 6.13).

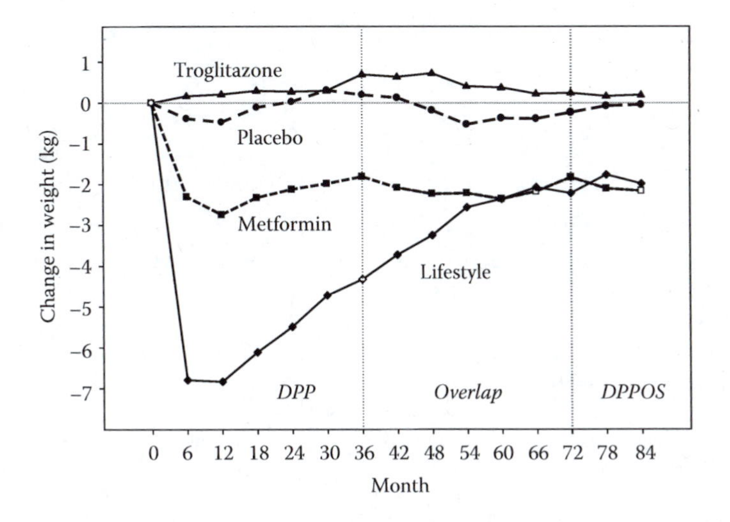

FIGURE 6.13 Weight loss over 8 years in the three randomized groups in the Diabetes Prevention Trial. (Redrawn from Venditti, E.M. et al., *Int. J. Obes.*, 32(10), 1537–1544, 2008.)

Hypertensives

Weight loss is an effective way to reduce blood pressure. The Dietary Approaches to Stop Hypertension trial (DASH) demonstrated that a diet high in fruits, vegetables, and nonfat dairy products with reduced fat and slightly higher protein reduced blood pressure significantly (Appel 1997; Sacks 2001). In a meta-analysis, Avenell et al. (2004) identified 12 studies, five in hypertensive groups, that evaluated diet versus a control that lasted more than 12 months. At the end of 12 months, the difference between control and treated groups was −5.31 kg (95% CI 5.86 to −4.77 kg), indicating that hypertensive and nonhypertensive patients responded to the diets with weight loss.

Commercial Weight Loss Programs

A number of commercial and self-help programs, including Overeaters Anonymous, Take Off Pounds Sensibly (TOPS), Weight Watchers, Jenny Craig, Herbalife, OPTIFAST, LA Health, and e-Diets are available to help the consumer. Tsai and Wadden (2005) have examined the effectiveness of a number of these programs. They included randomized trials that lasted at least 12 weeks and enrolled only adults, as well as case series that met their criteria and stated the number of enrollees and had an evaluation of 1 year or longer. Ten studies met their selection criteria.

There are three commercial weight loss programs shown in Table 6.8. The effects of the Weight Watchers program was evaluated in three randomized controlled trials. In one trial, lasting 2 years and including 423 subjects, the participants in the intervention group attended the Weight Watchers meetings and experienced a mean weight loss of 5.3% at 1 year and 3.2% at 2 years compared to 1.5% at 1 year and 0% weight loss for the control group that received the self-help intervention with two visits to a dietitian (Heshka et al. 2003). The Weight Watchers diet uses a balanced nutrient reduction to lower calories The Volumetrics diet (Rolls and Barnett 2000) emphasizes the need to eat less energy-dense foods. The theory is that filling the stomach with low-fat, high-fiber foods that have low energy density will reduce hunger and produce satiety. In a randomized clinical trial, 35 participants assigned to the commercial program (Jenny Craig) or control program for 1 year of treatment. At 6 months, weight loss in the commercial program was 7.2 (6.7) kg compared to 0.3 (3.9) kg weight loss in the control group ($p < 0.01$). At 1 year, weight loss was still 7.3 (10.4) kg for the commercial intervention group ($n = 32$) vs. a weight loss of 0.7 (5.6) kg for controls ($p < 0.01$) (Rock et al. 2007).

TABLE 6.8
Components of Three Commercial Very Low Calorie Diet Programs

Name	Group or Individual	Diet	Physical Activity	Staff
HMR (Health Management Resources)	Group sessions & weekly classes	Low-calorie or VLCD provided by meal replacement products	Walking and calorie charts	Physician & other health care providers
Medifast	Group classes included in Take Shape for Life	Low-calorie or VLCD provided by meal replacement products	May be included in Take Shape for Life	
OPTIFAST	Group classes and telephone support	Low-calorie diet provided through meal replacement products	Physical activity modules in lifestyle classes	Physician & other health care providers

Source: Adapted from Tsai, A.G. and T.A. Wadden, *Ann. Intern. Med.*, 142(1), 56–66, 2005.

Potential Problems with Diets

One concern with diets is the potential for loss of bone in excess of what would be expected from the lighter load on the bone matrix. One study comparing weight loss by calorie restriction in individuals with a BMI of >27 kg/m^2 with weight loss by exercise found that there were decreases in the bone mineral density of the total hip and the intertrochanter area (Villereal et al. 2006). A second clinical trial of 32 subjects aged 50 who were randomly assigned to a high or low protein diet using meat supplements of approximately 55 g per day for one group versus three g per day, exchanged isocalorically for carbohydrates, for the other group found that urinary calcium excretion was the same in both groups, but the high protein diet increased serum IGF-1 concentrations and decreased urinary N-telopeptides (Dawson-Hughes et al. 2004), suggesting that high protein diets can cause bone loss (Reddy et al. 2002).

Summary

My summary of dietary strategies is that any of them can work. If that is the case, then select the one you like best and adhere to it with religious fervor. All of the data shows that adherence is what makes any program work.

PHYSICAL ACTIVITY: A COGNITIVE SOLUTION

Introduction

Physical activity is the second largest component of energy expenditure. Changes in physical activity are particularly important in the pathogenesis of overweight and in its treatment. This is especially true for long-term maintenance of weight loss.

Components of Energy Expenditure

The components of energy expenditure are shown in Figure 6.14. They include energy needed for heat production, maintenance of body temperature, maintenance of ionic gradients across cells, and maintenance of resting cardiac and respiratory function and physical activity. Resting energy expenditure is the largest component of total energy expenditure and is measured in the early morning

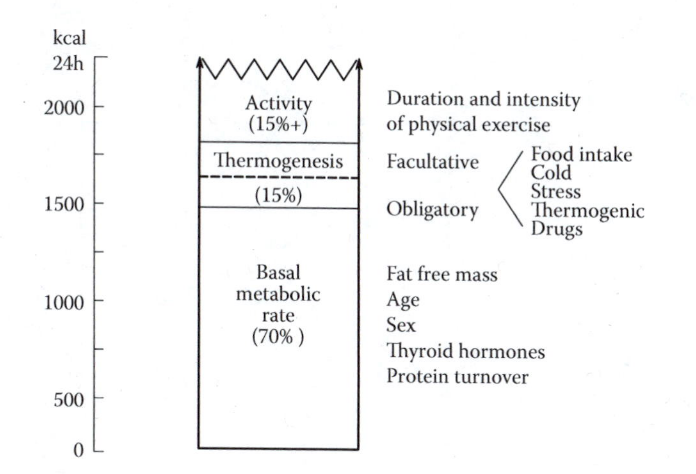

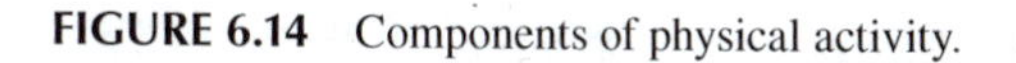
FIGURE 6.14 Components of physical activity.

when at rest. In a metabolic chamber, it is possible to identify the sleeping metabolic rate, which is about 15% lower than the resting energy expenditure. It is the component to which awakening energy expenditure is added to give the resting energy expenditure.

The second largest component of energy expenditure is physical activity, composed of both non-exercise activity thermogenesis and thermogenesis due to volitional activity of muscle groups. The smallest component, representing about 10% of the total, is the thermic effect of food. It is the rise in energy expenditure that follows a meal, a phenomenon first measured by Lavoisier more than 200 years ago. Physical activity energy expenditure (PAEE) can be calculated from the total energy expenditure and resting energy expenditure after correcting for the thermic effect of food (usually $0.9 \times$ TEE) (PAEE = $0.9 \times$ TEE − REE). The physical activity level is the ratio of total energy expenditure divided by the resting energy expenditure (TEE / REE) and is usually between 1.5 and 1.8.

Total Energy Expenditure

Total energy expenditure (TEE) can be measured in at least two different ways. The first is to house an individual in a calorimeter and measure their heat production or their intake of oxygen and release of carbon dioxide, from which their energy expenditure can be calculated. The first human calorimeter was developed in the mid-nineteenth century, but the widest application came from Atwater and Benedict at the beginning of the twentieth century and those who followed them (Atwater and Rosa, Benedict, Jecquier, Garrow, and Ravussin). They showed that human beings obeyed the laws of conservation of energy, just as other animals do. This important set of studies forms the basis for modern physiological thinking about energy balance and body weight.

Total daily energy expenditure can also be measured with a technique called doubly labeled water. During studies on distribution of oxygen among molecules in the body, Lifson et al. (1949) recognized that oxygen equilibrated with oxygen molecules in the body. Similarly, hydrogen equilibrated with the hydrogen in the body. By providing water labeled with stable isotopes of hydrogen and oxygen, they could measure the amount of oxygen, excreted either as carbon dioxide or water. They could thus trace the metabolism of the whole body by measuring hydrogen appearance in the

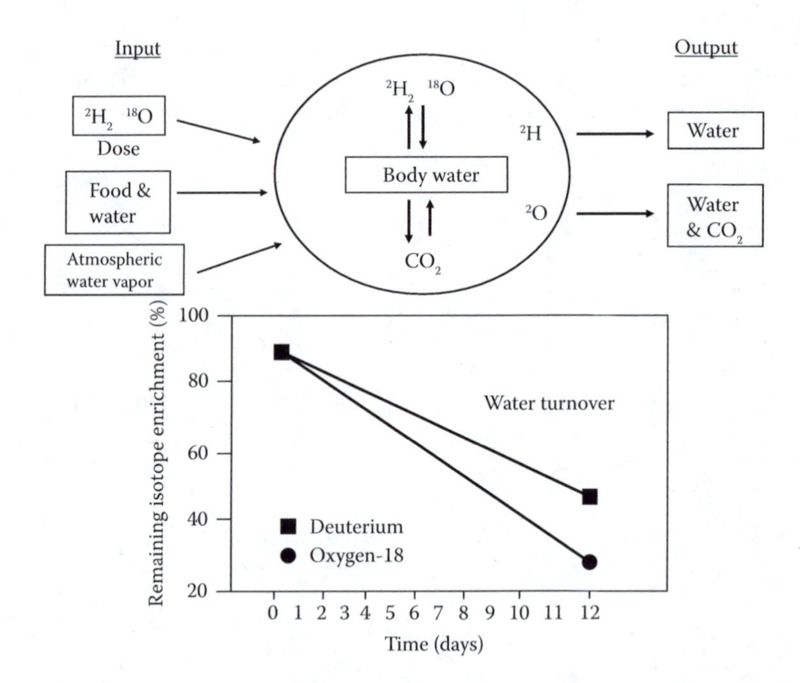

FIGURE 6.15 Model showing how doubly labeled water is used to measure energy expenditure.

urine as water, since hydrogen can only leave the body as water, whereas oxygen can leave as water or carbon dioxide. By measuring the differential rate of loss of these isotopes, they could estimate total carbon dioxide production and, thus, energy expenditure (Lifson et al. 1949). This technique was soon applied to human beings, and has since been used as a way of measuring total daily energy expenditure in children and adults during 7 to 14 day intervals of time. Figure 6.15 shows this process in a schematic form. The upper half shows the distribution of the two isotopes in the pool of hydrogen and oxygen, and the lower half shows the differential disappearance of the two isotopes (Schoeller et al. 1991; Westerterp and Speakman 2008).

Resting Energy Expenditure

Resting energy expenditure (REE) is the largest component of total energy expenditure and is measured in the early morning when at rest, usually with some device (mouth piece or hood) that is placed in the mouth or over the head while the individual is resting quietly in a low-light room. The REE is composed of both the sleeping resting energy expenditure, which is the low level of energy expenditure at night during times when there is no activity—usually between 2 a.m. and 5 a.m. (02:00 and 05:00) and the energy associated with arousal from sleep. The REE is related to lean body mass and surface area, is lower in women than men at the same body weight, age, and height due to the lower lean body mass in women. REE declines with age, and is altered by hormones such as thyroid hormone and growth hormone.

The resting, sleeping, and total energy expenditure and food intake for a single individual who spent 24 hours in a respiration chamber is shown in Figure 6.16. The REE is low at the beginning of the day and then rises with meals and activity and falls to sleeping energy expenditure during the night.

Thermic Effect of Food

The thermic effect of food (TEF) describes the increase in energy expenditure, measured as oxygen consumption that occurs after ingesting food (Figure 6.16). Lavoisier was the first to measure the rise in oxygen uptake following eating food more than 200 years ago (Lavoisier 1789). For a given energy load, protein produces the largest amount of heat, and carbohydrate and fat are similar. When a mixed meal is ingested, the thermic effect accounts for about 10% of the total energy value of the meal. There has been an ongoing argument as to whether overweight people have a reduced

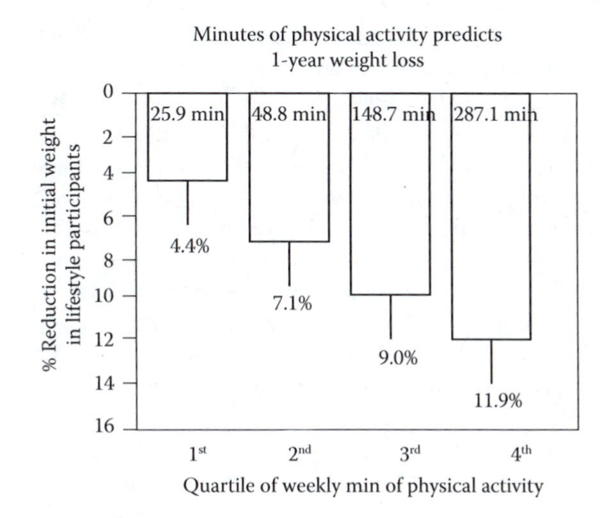

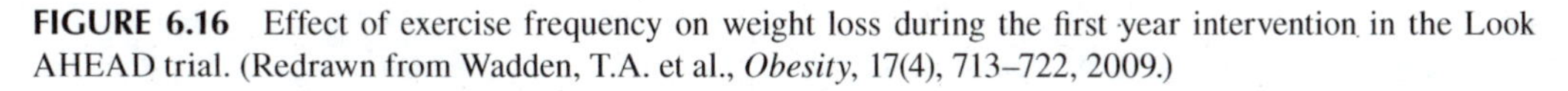
FIGURE 6.16 Effect of exercise frequency on weight loss during the first year intervention in the Look AHEAD trial. (Redrawn from Wadden, T.A. et al., *Obesity*, 17(4), 713–722, 2009.)

TEF. If the thermic response were reduced, this would provide a way to get up to 10% more energy to store after eating a meal. In a review on the TEF in obesity, it was noted that when similar methods were used, overweight people, particularly those who were more insulin resistant, had a lower thermic response to a meal (de Jonge & Bray 1997).

Energy Expenditure from Physical Activity

Energy expenditure associated with physical activity can be measured in a number of ways. The most accurate assessment is done by subtracting resting energy expenditure from total daily energy expenditure measured with doubly labeled water after correcting for the TEF. Assuming a 10% figure for the TEF physical activity energy expenditure (PAEE) equals 0.1 times TEE minus REE (PAEE = 0.1 × TEE − REE) (Westerterp 2009).

Accelerometers, particularly the triaxial models, provide useful information on the activity involved in energy expenditure (Bonomi et al. 2009). Pedometers worn on the waist provide a simple method for estimating the number of steps walked and, when used, increase the energy expenditure of individuals (Bravata et al. 2003). Measuring changes in heart rate above baseline is another technique for estimating energy expenditure. However, it is not effective for low levels of activity and must be calibrated for each individual.

Questionnaires of time spent in various activities, such as the Paffenbarger et al. questionnaire, the Modifiable Activity Questionnaire, and the Low Level Physical Activity Recall are widely used in epidemiological studies, but when compared with accelerometers have limited quantitative value.

Energy expenditure with physical activity is directly related to body weight. A key question is whether energy expenditure has declined over the past 30 years as the epidemic of obesity has developed and thus contributed to the obesity epidemic. Unfortunately, most measurements of energy expenditure are not very precise or easy to use and there is thus little reliable longitudinal data. To address this question, Westerterp and Speakman (2008) pooled data measuring total energy expenditure from doubly labeled water over the interval from 1980 to 2005. Their data showed no measurable change in the physical activity level (TEE/REE) over this interval in adults, suggesting that it is an increase of energy intake, not a decrease in energy expenditure that underlies the current epidemic of obesity. Swinburn et al. (2009) have reached a similar conclusion.

Physical Activity and Health

Physical activity appears to decline during adolescence and remain low in adults (Kimm et al. 2000; DeLany et al. 2004). In a longitudinal study of adolescent girls, the level of activity declined in both black and white girls each year during adolescence. By age 17, there was almost no spontaneous physical activity reported by the black girls and only slightly more by the white girls (Kimm et al. 2002). A similar decline was measured at ages 10 and 12 years in boys and girls in Baton Rouge, Louisiana, using doubly labeled water in boys and girls (DeLany and Bray 2004).

There is an important genetic component to the level of physical activity (Stubbe et al. 2005). In a study examining regular exercise among identical and fraternal twins that included both same and opposite sex pairs, environmental factors shared by children at age 13 accounted for 78%–84% of sports participation, whereas genetic differences provided almost no contribution. By age 17 to 18, the genetic influences represented 36% of the variance in the level of participation in sports and, by age 18 to 20, genetic factors accounted for almost all (85%) of the differences in participation in sports (Stubbe et al. 2005; Samaras et al. 1999).

Decreasing levels of physical activity are a predictor of weight gain in both men and women (Westerterp and Plasqui 2009). In this longitudinal study, 17 women and 23 men were followed for 11.4 years, from age 27 to 38 with measurements of doubly labeled water and REE. Body mass increased 1.5 kg/m^2 (from 22.8 to 24.3) and body fat increased. There was a small, but not significant, decrease in TEE and a small, but not significant rise in REE resulting in a significant decrease

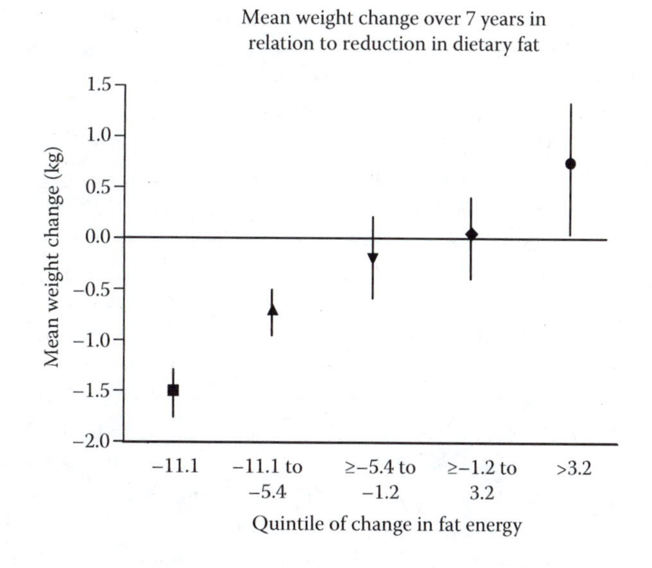

FIGURE 6.17 Dose response of reduced fat intake and 7-year weight change.

in physical activity level (TEE/REE). The increases in BMI and fat were related to initial physical activity level. Individuals with higher physical activity levels (PALs) at baseline gained more fat because their activity declined more than those with initially lower PALs. Improvements in cardiovascular fitness were more strongly associated with vigorous physical activity in black and white adolescents than in those with moderate physical activity (Gutin et al. 2005).

Television appears to be an important factor in the decreasing level of physical activity in children and adolescents (Manios et al. 2009; Crespo et al. 2001) and in adults (Swinburn and Shelly 2008). There is a graded increase in the BMI as the number of hours watching television increases (see Figure 6.17) (Crespo et al. 2001). A clinical trial comparing a school-based intervention aimed at reducing TV watching in one school with no intervention in another school found that the increase in BMI could be significantly slowed if TV viewing was reduced (Robinson 1999). The effect of TV viewing may be because children eat more while watching than by being less active (Jackson et al. 2009). Children who ate snacks in front of the television on a daily basis had higher BMIs than children who did so less frequently (Dubois et al. 2008). Reducing the behavior of eating while watching television is an important target for reducing potential weight gain.

Sedentary activity in adults is associated with increased mortality (Katzmarzyk et al. 2009). Data from 17,013 Canadians aged 18 to 90 years was used to examine mortality and daily sitting time. Over an average of 12.0 years, there were 1832 deaths (759 from cardiovascular disease (CVD) and 547 from cancer) during 204,732 person-years of follow-up. There was a progressively higher risk of mortality among those who sat less compared to those who sat more. The reference group consisted of those in the most active quintile. Among the five quintiles, the hazard ratios for death increased from 1.00, to 1.00, to 1.11, to 1.36, and to 1.54 in the least active group (p for trend < 0.0001). The risk of cardiovascular disease also increased with more sitting time (HR:1.00, 1.01, 1.22, 1.47, 1.54; p for trend < 0.0001) but no effect was seen on the risk of cancer. Similar results were obtained when the data were stratified by sex, age, smoking status, and body mass index. Age-adjusted all-cause mortality rates per 10,000 person-years of follow-up were 87, 86, 105, 130, and 161 (p for trend < 0.0001) in physically inactive participants and 75, 69, 76, 98, and 105 (p for trend $= 0.008$) in active participants across sitting time categories. These data demonstrate a dose-response association between sitting time and mortality from all causes and CVD, independent of leisure time physical activity.

The Nurses' Health Study has found that women who maintain vigorous physical activity have a smaller weight gain over 6 years of follow-up than those who do not (Field et al. 2001).

Spending more time in leisure activity can contribute to a lower body weight. Obese people stand on average 2.5 hours less in a day than normal weight people (Levine et al. 2008). In a comparison of community settings, one of which could be described as "high-walkability" versus "low-walkability" environments, Saelens et al. (2003) found that individuals living in the low-walkability neighborhoods had a higher mean BMI than people living in high-walkability neighborhoods. Both leisure-time physical activity and regular walking or cycling to work are associated with lower body weight and weight gain over 5 years in middle-aged men (Wagner et al. 2001). Church et al. reached a similar conclusion from a study that randomized 464 sedentary postmenopausal overweight or obese women (BMI 25–43) and SBP 120–159.9 to four groups: 1) No exercise; 2) 4 kcal/kg of exercise; 3) 8 kcal/kg of exercise; or 4) 12 kcal/kg of exercise. Over 90% returned for final evaluation (N = 427). There was a graded improvement in fitness levels across exercise levels, indicating that more is better in terms of training effect (Chuch et al. 2007). However, there was no effect on body weight.

Not everybody benefits from physical training. Improvements in physical conditioning in response to exercise have strong familial and genetic components. The HERITAGE study provided a 20-week program of physical training for 481 family members from two generations, including 95 fathers, 86 mothers, 141 sons, and 159 daughters in which the subjects' level of activity was observed. There were both nonresponders and high responders to the exercise training program (Rankinen and Bouchard 2008). Men had more improvement than women, and the children more than their parents. There was a strong intrafamily resemblance in their response to physical training, with some families showing considerable improvement in physical fitness after exercise (an increase of 500 mL/min in max V_{O2}) and others showing much less improvement (less than 300 mL/min, max V_{O2}).

Benefits of Exercise

Several studies have found a strong inverse relationship between habitual exercise and fitness and the risk of coronary disease and death (Sui et al. 2007; Fogelholm 2009). The value of exercise for reducing cardiovascular risk can be illustrated by the following observations. Data on fitness assessed by a maximal exercise test in 2603 men and women in Aerobics Center Longitudinal Cohort aged 60 years or older (mean age, 64.4 [SD, 4.8] years; 19.8% women) found 450 deaths during a mean follow-up of 12 years and 31,236 person-years of exposure. Death rates per 1000 person-years increased as BMI increased from 13.9 for BMI 18.5–24.9, to 13.3 for BMI 24–29.9, to 18.3 for BMI 30–34.9 to 31.8 for BMI ≥ 35 (adjusted for age, sex, and examination year) (p = .01 for trend). The mortality rate was 13.3 and 18.2 for normal and high waist circumference (≥88 cm in women; ≥102 cm in men) (p = .004); 13.7 and 14.6 for normal and high percent body fat (≥30% in women; ≥25% in men) (p = .51). Mortality rates declined with improving fitness from 32.6, to 16.6, to 12.8, to 12.3, and to 8.1 across quintiles of fitness ($p < .001$ for trend). In this study population, fitness was a significant predictor of lower mortality in older adults, independent of overall or abdominal adiposity (Sui et al. 2007).

Data from 33 eligible studies were evaluated for all-cause mortality among 102,980 participants with 6910 cases and CHD/CVD with 84,323 participants and 4485 cases. Pooled relative risks for all-cause mortality and CHD/CVD events per 1-MET higher level of maximal aerobic capacity (corresponding to 1-km/h higher running/jogging speed) were 0.87 (95% CI 0.84–0.90) and 0.85 (95% CI 0.82–0.88), respectively. Compared to participants with high cardiorespiratory fitness, those with low fitness had a relative risk for all-cause mortality of 1.70 (95% CI 1.51–1.92; p < .001) and for CHD/CVD events, a relative risk of 1.56 (95% CI 1.39–1.75; $p < .001$). Thus, better cardiorespiratory fitness was associated with a lower risk of all-cause mortality and CHD/CVD. Participants with the highest maximal aerobic capacity had substantially lower rates of all-cause mortality and CHD/CVD events compared with those with lower aerobic capacity (Kodama et al. 2009).

Exercise can improve glycemic control and insulin sensitivity, and may prevent the development of type 2 diabetes (Hu et al. 2006). Continued exercise programs cause a greater decrease in abdominal fat than lower body fat (Hunter et al. 2009) and help maintain it. This is important because subjects with abdominal obesity are at increased cardiovascular risk.

In a review of 36 papers published after 1990 that included adult participants with prospective follow-up, case-control or cross-sectional; data on cardiorespiratory fitness and/or physical activity; data on BMI (body mass index), waist circumference, or body composition; outcome data on all-cause mortality, cardiovascular disease mortality, cardiovascular disease incidence, type 2 diabetes, or cardiovascular and type 2 diabetes risk factors. Fogelholm et al. (2009) observed that having a high BMI, even with high physical activity, had a greater risk for the incidence of type 2 diabetes and the prevalence of cardiovascular and diabetes risk factors than a normal BMI with low physical activity. The data also indicate that the risk for all-cause and cardiovascular mortality was higher in individuals with normal BMI and poor fitness than in those with high BMI and good aerobic fitness (Fogelholm 2009).

Higher cardiorespiratory fitness, as measured by maximal oxygen uptake, reduces the risk of mortality. Women who were overweight or obese and unfit having a low cardiorespiratory fitness were at more than twice the risk of death as women who were of normal weight and fitness (Lyerly et al. 2009). Exercise can also have beneficial effects on serum lipoprotein concentrations, body composition, aerobic capacity, and hemostatic factors associated with thrombosis. Long-term aerobic exercise regimens have, in most studies, had a beneficial effect upon the systemic blood pressure.

Calorie restriction and exercise to produce weight loss have different effects on muscle mass. A group of 34 men and women aged 50–60 with a BMI between 23.5 to 29.9 kg/m^2 were assigned to calorie restriction or exercise to produce weight loss. After 12 months, body weight had decreased by 10.7% in the calorie-restricted group and 9.5% in the exercise group. Lean mass also decreased 3.5% vs. 2.2%, but exercise prevented the decline in thigh muscle and knee flexion strength observed in the calorie-restricted group. Maximal oxygen uptake declined in the calorie-restricted group by 6.8%, but increased in the exercise group by 28.3%. These data provide evidence that muscle mass and absolute physical work capacity decreases after 12 months of calorie restriction, but not in response to weight loss induced by exercise (Weiss et al. 2007). In older women, resistance training preserves fat-free mass without impacting changes in protein metabolism after weight loss (Campbell et al. 2009).

For men and women with knee pain, a home-based, self-managed program of simple knee-strengthening exercises over a 2-year period significantly reduced knee pain and improved knee function in overweight and obese people with knee pain. A moderate sustained weight loss is achievable with dietary intervention, but has less effect on knee pain than the exercises (Jenkinson et al. 2009).

Risks of Exercise

Exercise is not without its intrinsic risks. It has been associated with an increased risk of musculoskeletal injuries, cardiac arrhythmia, acute myocardial infarction, and bronchospasm.

Treatment of Overweight Using Exercise

Exercise has been evaluated as a single treatment for obesity. It has also been combined with diet, and has been used to help maintain weight loss. Table 6.9 summarizes good studies relating to exercise and weight loss. Ostman et al. (2004) performed a Medline search for studies related to physical exercise and overweight, and identified six randomized control trials from among 186 articles that dealt with overweight with physical activity as a treatment, that had treatment interval of 12 months (with one exception), and a drop-out rate of <40%. This table has been adapted with addition of two newer trials, one of 16-months duration and one of 8-months duration.

TABLE 6.9
Clinical Trials of Exercise in Overweight Individuals

Author	Inclusion Criteria	Intervention Groups	Duration	# Patients/ # Follow-up	Weight Fat	Comments
Wood 1988 (27)	Men 120%–160% overweight	1. Diet to give 1 kg/week weight loss; Fat reduced by 30% 2. Individual instruction to get 1 kg/week wt loss; Training at 60%–80% max physical capacity 40–50 mins, 3–4 times/week	1 year	1. 51/42 2. 52/47 3. 52/42	Weight 1. −7.2 kg 2. −4.0 kg 3. +0.6 kg Fat 1. −5.9 kg 2. −4.2 kg 3. −0.3 kg	TG and HDL-chol also improved; Diet and physical activity yield same reduction in weight and fat at same negative calorie balance
Wing 1988 (28)	Women: 30–60 yr with Type 2 diabetes; >20% above ideal weight	1. Diet (−1000 kcal/day + 3 miles 3 times/ week 2. Free diet + training (+ 3 miles, 4 times/ week) 3. Diet + stretching	12 months	1. 12 2. 15 3. 13	1. −7.9 kg 2. −7.9 kg 3. −3.8 kg	Hemoglobin A1C reduced and medications reduced in groups 1 and 2
Wood 1991 (29)	Men and women: 25–49 years; Overweight 120%–160%	1. Diet (moderate reduction of energy, fat, cholesterol) 2. Diet (as above) + physical activity (60%–80% of max) 25–45 mins, 3 times/ week	Top of Form Bottom of Form	1. 87/71 2. 90/81 3. 87/79	Men: 1. −5.1kg 2. −8.7 kg 3. +1.7 kg Women: 1. −4.2 kg 2. −5.5 kg 3. +1.3 kg	BP decreased in groups 1 and 2. Cholesterol decreased (women) (both groups 1 & 2) HDL-chol increased in group 2 (both men & women) TG decreased in men in group 2

(continued)

Exercise as Treatment for Obesity

The two best trials, in terms of design and execution, are those by Wood et al. (1988, 1991). In men, diet alone produced more weight loss than exercise alone, but when combined, diet and exercise were better than diet alone. In women, there were no significant additive effects of exercise to that of diet (−4.2 kg vs. −5.5 kg).

Several studies have evaluated the effect of exercise alone in inducing weight loss (Slentz et al. 2004; Wood et al. 1988; Irwin et al. 2003; Donnelly et al. 2003) (Ross et al. 2000; Ross et al. 2004;

TABLE 6.9 (Continued)
Clinical Trials of Exercise in Overweight Individuals

Author	Inclusion Criteria	Intervention Groups	Duration	# Patients/ # Follow-up	Weight Fat	Comments
Wood 1991 (29)	Men and women: 25–49 years; Overweight 120%–160%	1. Diet (moderate reduction of energy, fat, cholesterol) 2. Diet (as above) + physical activity (60%–80% of max) 25–45 mins, 3 times/ week	Top of Form Bottom of Form	1. 87/71 2. 90/81 3. 87/79	Men: 1. –5.1kg 2. –8.7 kg 3. +1.7 kg Women: 1. –4.2 kg 2. –5.5 kg 3. +1.3 kg	BP decreased in groups 1 and 2. Cholesterol decreased (women) (both groups 1 & 2) HDL-chol increased in group 2 (both men & women) TG decreased in men in group 2
Svendsen 1994 (30)	Women: 49–58 yr; BMI 25–42 kg/m²	1. Diet (4.2 MJ/d = 1000 kcal/day) 2. Diet (as above) + physical activity (submax aerotics and body building) 3. Controls	12 weeks with 6 month follow-up	1. 51/47 2. 49/47 3. 21/16	12 weeks: 1. –6.6 kg 2. –10.9kg 3. 0.0 kg 6 months: 1. –8.0 kg 2. –8.0 kg 3. 0.0 kg	TG decreased HDL-chol increased. No effect from physical activity
Pritchard 1997 (31)	Men: Overweight Mean BMI = 29 kg/m²	1. Diet: Reduction of 500 kcal/day with low fat 2. 65%–75% of max physical capacity 45 min, 3–7 times/week 3. Controls	12 mo	66/60	1. –6.3 kg 2. –2.6 kg 3. +0.9 kg	Diet self-controlled

(continued)

Lee et al. 2005). Weight losses were, in general, quite small (approximately 0.1 kg per week), except in military recruits where it rose to 1.8 kg per week (Lee et al. 1994), and the exercise program was more rigorous and supervised.

When the amount of energy expenditure resulting from exercise matches the reduction of energy intake, the weight losses for both men (Ross et al. 2000) and women are similar (Ross et al. 2004). In a 3-month trial, Ross et al. (2000) randomized 52 men to one of four treatments—diet-induced weight loss, exercise-induced weight loss, exercise without weight loss, and a control group. Cardiovascular fitness improved in the exercise groups relative to control. Weight loss was 1.3 kg more in the exercise group than the diet group ($p = 0.03$). Subcutaneous and visceral fat decreased in both groups of men who lost weight. A similar study was conducted in 54 women (Ross Janssen et

TABLE 6.9 (Continued)
Clinical Trials of Exercise in Overweight Individuals

Author	Inclusion Criteria	Intervention Groups	Duration	# Patients/ # Follow-up	Weight Fat	Comments
Irwin 2003 (32)	Overweight nonsmoking postmenopausal women age 50 to 75 years with a BMI > 25 kg/m^2 or BMI 24–25 and body fat > 33% by DXA who were sedentary at baseline (<60 min/week of moderate—vigorous activity) and maximal oxygen uptake of <25 mL/kg/min	1. Exercise consisted of at least 45 min of moderate intensity exercise 5 days/week for 12 months (months 1–3 they attended three sessions/week; months 4–12 they attended 1 session/week) 2. Weekly stretching sessions of 45 min for 12 months	12 mo	1. 87/84 2. 86/86	1. Exercise 3 months: B.W. – 0.5 kg. 12 months: B.W. – 1.3 kg Fat – 1.4 kg VAT – 8.5 cm^2 Top of Form 3 months: BW. 0.0 kg 12 months: BW. 0.1 kg Fat – 0.1 kg VAT 0.1 cm^2 Bottom of Form	Advised to maintain usual diet. Weight loss related to degree of exercise
Donnelly 2003 (33)	Overweight men and women age 17 to 36 with a BMI of 25.0 to 34.9 kg/m^2	1. Exercise targeted at 400 kcal/day 5 days a week with walking on a treadmill at 55%–70% of maximal oxygen uptake 2. Control group had same testing but no exercise program	16 months of verified exercise	1. 87/41 2. 44/33	16 months: Group 1: MEN: Weight – 5.2 kg Fat – 4.9 kg VAT -22.4 cm^2 WOMEN Weight + 0.4 kg Fat –0.2 kg VAT – 3.2 cm^2 Group 2: MEN: Weight – 0.5 kg Fat – 0.7 kg VAT – 6.3 cm^2 WOMEN: Weight + 2.9 kg Fat + 2.0 kg VAT + 3.1 cm^2	Exercise produced weight loss in men and prevented weight gain in women

(continued)

TABLE 6.9 (Continued)
Clinical Trials of Exercise in Overweight Individuals

Author	Inclusion Criteria	Intervention Groups	Duration	# Patients/ # Follow-up	Weight Fat	Comments
Slentz 2004 (2)	Men and women age 40 to 60 years and BMI 25 to 35 kg/m^2 and mild to moderate lipid abnormalities	Top of Form Top of Form Top of Form Top of Form Bottom of Form Bottom of Form Bottom of Form Bottom of Form	9 month Exercise was observed; This was not a weight loss study and diet was provided to maintain body weight	1. 44/17 2. 52/24 3. 42/14 4. 44/7	1. High/ Vigorous Intensity: Weight – 3.5 kg Fat – 4.9 kg Waist – 3.4 cm 2. Low/ Vigorous Intensity: Weight – 1.1 kg Fat – 2.6 kg Waist – 1.4 cm Low Moderate Intensity: Weight – 1.3 kg Fat – 2.0 kg Waist – 1.1 cm Control: Weight – 1.1 kg Fat – 0.5 kg Waist – 0.8 cm	

Source: Some data from Ostman M., et al. *Physical Exercise. Treating and Preventing Obesity*, Wiley-VCH Verlag, Weinheim, Germany, 142–143, 2004.

al. 2004). The diet and exercise weight loss groups lost 6.5% and abdominal and visceral fat losses were similar with both types of weight loss in women.

To examine further the effects of exercise on body composition, Lee et al. (2005) conducted a subsequent study in lean and obese men with and without diabetes. Reductions in total and subcutaneous fat were similar, but the loss of visceral fat was greater in the obese and diabetic groups compared to the lean men. It is thus clear that exercise can induce weight loss and modify body composition.

For many people it is difficult to lose weight with exercise alone, probably because of low adherence to the exercise program. However, even with limited weight loss, exercise may have a benefit on body fat and its distribution. In a 12-week study of diet-induced versus exercise-induced weight loss (of approximately 7.5 kg) on body composition and insulin sensitivity in 52 obese men (Lee et al. 1994). There was a greater reduction in total body fat in the exercise-induced weight loss group and similar reductions in abdominal adiposity, visceral fat, and insulin resistance in the two treatment groups. In the treatment group assigned to exercise without weight loss who increased caloric intake to match energy expenditure, abdominal and visceral fat were decreased, but to a lesser degree than in the other treatment groups.

Exercise also has beneficial effects on body composition. In a study in postmenopausal women, subjects were randomized to moderate-intensity exercise (most commonly brisk walking, on average three hours per week) versus a stretching program (control group) for 12 months. Women in the exercise group lost more weight, and had greater decreases in body fat, intra-abdominal fat, and subcutaneous fat (Irwin et al. 2003).

For a given amount of exercise, men appear to lose more weight than women. In a study of 74 sedentary, overweight, or moderately obese young men and women randomly assigned to exercise at an energy equivalent of 2000 calories per week, compared to a control group for 16 months, significant decreases in weight, BMI, and fat mass were seen in the men (5.2 ± 4.7 kg, 1.6 ± 1.4 kg/m^2, and 4.9 ± 4.4 kg, respectively) (Donnelly et al. 2003). In contrast, women assigned to exercise maintained their baseline weight, BMI, and fat mass, while increases in all three outcome variables occurred in women in the control group.

Exercise can be particularly beneficial for the elderly. In a 6-month trial in 136 men and women who were 60–80 years old, combined aerobic and resistance exercise improved insulin resistance and physical functioning more than aerobic exercise alone with resistance being least effective compared to the control group with no exercise (Davidson et al. 2009).

Exercise Combined with Diet

Exercise programs added to diets with moderate to severe caloric restriction often have little additional effect on weight loss. Whether lean body mass is spared by exercise during caloric restriction is controversial. In one study, 6 of 12 obese families eating a diet of approximately 800 kcal per day were randomly assigned to exercise for one hour, four days per week at 50% to 60% of their maximum aerobic capacity, or no exercise. Both groups lost 12 to 13 kg, and there was no difference between them in the loss of body weight, body fat, or lean body mass. One clear-cut example of where increasing levels of physical activity measured in minutes of walking per week was related to weight loss was during the first year of the Look AHEAD trial (Wadden et al. 2009). This is shown in Figure 6.17, where increasing amounts of time spent in activity were associated with progressively greater weight loss.

Suggestions for Physical Activity

Increasing the level of physical activity would be beneficial to all ages and for all groups. A consensus statement has outlined the types of exercise programs that are recommended. Any exercise program should be designed to fit into the health and physical conditions of the subject. Existing medical conditions, age, and preferences for types of exercise should all be considered in the decisions.

Subjects who are about to begin an exercise program, even those whose only exercise will be walking, should be advised of the possibility of musculoskeletal stresses and strains and joint injury. For those who are able, walking 150 to 210 minutes per week (30 min per day, 5 to 7 days per week) would be beneficial.

The role of exercise stress testing before beginning an exercise program has been controversial because of the frequency of false-positive tests. A joint 2002 American College of Cardiology/American Heart Association task force did not recommend routine exercise testing in this setting. However, it did give a class IIa recommendation (weight of evidence supports usefulness) to exercise testing in asymptomatic persons with diabetes mellitus who plan to start vigorous exercise and a lesser recommendation in patients with multiple risk factors for coronary heart disease (Gibbons et al. 2002).

Physical activity should be performed for 30 to 60 minutes, five to seven days a week. This will increase energy expenditure by 1000 to 2000 calories per week, or slightly more than 100 calories per day. The amount of energy expended depends upon the duration and intensity of the exercise, and the subject's initial weight. As an example, a 120-pound person walking three miles per hour expends slightly less than 2 calories per minute more than standing still. At 160 pounds, the difference is 2.4 calories per minute, and at 200 pounds it is 3 calories per minute. Thus, a 30-minute walk at three miles per hour for a person weighing 200 pounds would dissipate an extra 90 calories as compared with 60 calories for a person weighing 120 pounds.

A dose-response relationship has been demonstrated in overweight adult women between the amount of exercise and long-term weight loss (Jakicic et al. 1999; Slentz et al. 2004; Schoeller 1991). Jakicic et al. (1999) showed that after losing weight, 200 minutes of exercise maintained the lost weight over 18 months, but that 150 and 100 minutes of activity per week did not.

Finding appropriate places to exercise can facilitate any program of exercise. Health clubs may be helpful, but for most people walking is the most appropriate form of exercise. In one study of obese women, the combination of diet plus advice to increase physical activity by incorporating short periods of activity into daily schedules (e.g., walking instead of driving short distances, taking stairs instead of elevators) was as effective for inducing weight loss as diet plus structured aerobic activity (aerobics classes) (Andersen et al. 1999).

COGNITIVE STRATEGIES TO MAINTAIN WEIGHT LOSS

Lifestyle

One of the most difficult problems for individuals who lose weight is to maintain that weight loss. Important clues come from randomized clinical trials and from the National Weight Control Registry, which studies individuals who have lost weight on their own and maintained it for more than a year.

Randomized Trials

Both the intensity and duration of follow-up are key factors in maintaining weight loss. Using a maintenance program based on self-regulation theory, Wing et al. tested the efficacy of delivering the program face to face as compared to the Internet. A group of 314 people who had lost a mean of 19.3 kg (42.5 lb) of body weight in the previous 2 years were randomly assigned to one of three groups: a control group, which received quarterly newsletters (105 participants), a group that received face-to-face intervention (105 participants), and a group that received Internet-based intervention (104 participants). The two intervention groups had the same program but by different means. The emphasis was on daily self-weighing and self-regulation. Over the following 18 months, the weight regain was less in the face-to-face group (2.5 ± 6.7 kg) than the Internet group (4.7 ± 8.6 kg) or the control group (4.9 ± 6.5 kg). That is, those who adopted the self-weighing and other maintenance strategies were more successful in maintaining their weight loss. More than 70% of the control group regained 2.3 kg or more over the 18-month period (72.4%) compared with only 45.7% of the face-to-face group, and 54.8% of the Internet group (Wing et al. 2006). In a further analysis of those who maintained weight loss, Phelan et al. (2009) found that the factors that identified those who maintained weight loss included more physical activity, more conscious restraint, and environmental variables such as the presence of equipment for physical activity, less high fat foods, and fewer televisions in the home (Wing et al. 2008). This suggests that "environmental engineering" of the home can provide important strategies for helping to maintain weight loss.

To investigate the intensity of intervention on maintenance of weight loss, Svetkey et al. (2008) compared monthly personal contact against unlimited access to an interactive technology-based intervention or a self-directed control intervention in a randomized trial with subjects who had lost at least 4 kg during a 6-month weight loss program. The majority of subjects who initially lost weight maintained it below their baseline level. Monthly brief personal contact provided modest benefit. The interactive technology-based intervention provided early improvement in maintenance of weight loss, but the benefit waned and by 30 months the three groups had regained almost the same amount of weight.

One of the key strategies for self-monitoring is weighing yourself regularly (self-weighing) (Linde and Jeffrey 2005; Wing et al. 2007; Bray 2009). In one paper that combined two prevention trials (Linde and Jeffrey 2005), self-weighing at baseline was associated with lower fat intake. Those who lost weight increased the frequency of self-weighing over time regardless of treatment group, whereas those who gained weight reduced the frequency of self-weighing over time. In the STOP Regain trial, increased daily self-weighing was associated with reduced risk of regaining 2.3 kg or more (Wing et al. 2006).

National Weight Control Registry

The National Weight Control Registry is following a group of more than 4000 individuals who have lost at least 13.6 kg (30 pounds) and kept it off for at least 1 year. Several elements emerge as important among the successful people. Self-monitoring is one of the techniques that is most frequently used by successful people in this group (Wing and Phelan 2005). As with self-monitoring, increasing physical activity was also a key element reported by successful members of the National Weight Control Registry (Wing and Phelan 2005). Among the individuals who lost an average of 33 kg and maintained it for an average of 5.7 years, women in the Registry reported expending 2545 kcal per week and men 3293 kcal per week. This would be equivalent to about 1 hour a day of moderate-intensity activity such as brisk walking (Wing and Phelan 2005). Weighing oneself more frequently was associated with lower BMI. At 1 year of follow-up, weight gain (4.0 kg) was significantly greater for those whose frequency of self-weighing had decreased, compared to those whose self-weighing had increased (1.1 kg) or remained the same (1.8 kg). This registry has also been used to compare long-term weight loss among its volunteers with patients who have undergone bariatric surgical operations for obesity (Bond et al. 2009). In this case-control study, 105 surgical patients were matched with two nonsurgical participants (n = 210) on gender, entry, weight, maximum weight loss, and weight-maintenance duration and compared prospectively for 1 year. The authors concluded that despite marked behavioral differences between the two groups, there were no significant differences in weight regain.

Internet for Maintaining Weight Loss

The Internet has been used as a strategy to maintain weight loss and prevent weight regain. In the Study TO Prevent Regain (STOP), Tate and her colleagues have investigated five cohorts enrolled between 2000 and 2005 with the goal of preventing a more than 2.4 kg (5 lb) regain. A total of 314 adults who had lost more than 10% of their body weight in the previous 2 years were enrolled. They were on average 51 years old, had a BMI of 28.6 kg/m^2, and a weight loss of 20 kg (44 pounds). They were divided into three groups. The control group received only a newsletter, one intervention group received their program via the Internet and chat room with a leader, and the other intervention group had face-to-face group meetings for 4 weeks and then monthly. Lesson content was identical and they were to exercise 60 minutes per day and weigh themselves daily. Weight gains were classified into three categories: <3 pounds, 3–4 pounds, and >5 pounds. The latter group received active intervention with the use of pedometers, calorie books, scales, and menu plans. Both intervention groups did better than the control group in maintaining their weight loss, but there was no difference whether the maintenance techniques were delivered via Internet or in person. Weighing frequently was related to success.

Two studies by Harvey-Berino and her group have examined the value of the Internet in maintaining weight loss produced by direct patient contact (Harvey-Berino et al. 2002). In the first study, 122 participants were treated with an intensive behavioral program for 6 months and then joined the group to which they had been randomly assigned. One group was an Internet support group, the second was an in-person support group, and the third was a minimal in-person support program. The randomized part of the trial began at the end of the 6 months of in-person treatment and continued for the ensuing 12 months. Attrition was 18% at 6 months and 24% over the entire 18 months. In this study, Internet support did not appear to be as effective (–5.7 kg at 18 months) as either the frequent in-person support or minimal in-person support (–10.4 kg at 18 months for both groups). In a subsequent study, the group assigned to the Internet support group did just as well as those with continued face-to-face contact (Harvey-Berino et al. 2004). In a third trial from this group, the initial 6-month treatment for which 255 individuals enrolled was conducted over interactive television.

The mean weight loss for those completing 6 months was –7.8 kg or about 8.9%. The subjects were then randomized to an Internet support group, minimal in-person support, frequent in-person support, or minimal in-person support. At the end of 18 months, there was no significant difference between maintenance of weight loss between the three conditions (–8.2% for the Internet support, –5.6% for the frequent in-person support, and –6.0% for the minimal in-person group), suggesting that Internet strategies, when appropriately used, can be as helpful with weight maintenance as the more expensive in-person meetings. In this study, attendance at treatment meetings and chat room sessions, as well as frequency of self-monitoring, were related to successful maintenance.

Review of Randomized Clinical Trials

A review of 42 randomized clinical trials aimed at maintaining weight loss including the Internet, use of very low calorie diets, use of drugs, behavioral strategies, physical activity, and alternative strategies, showed that treatment with orlistat or sibutramine combined with dietary modification, caffeine or protein supplementation, consuming a diet lower in fat, adherence to physical activity routes, prolonged contact with participants, problem-solving therapy, and the alternative treatment of acupressure were efficacious in reducing weight regain after weight loss treatment (Turk et al. 2009).

The False Hope Syndrome: A Key to Overcoming Failure

One of the key elements of human nature is that "If at first you don't succeed, try-try again." This concept applies admirably to the search for new ways to lose weight and maintain it that happens on an almost annual basis. Polivy and Herman (2002) have labeled this cycle of failure and renewed effort as a "false hope syndrome." They posit a number of reasons why self-change attempts fail. First, expectations often exceed what is feasible. Second, people often predict that they will change more quickly and more easily than is possible. Third, people overestimate their abilities in many domains and are unaware that they are inaccurate, and finally, people often believe that making a change will improve their lives more than can reasonably be expected. Dieters go through a number of explanations for their failure. The failure was because something outside of them caused a relapse, and if they only tried harder to control their environment they could succeed. The plateau that occurs with all weight loss efforts can be viewed by the dieter as the result of not trying hard enough—maybe next time they could try harder and succeed. If a particular diet didn't work, it is the diet's fault. For the counselor, the option is to try another diet, which is why there is a ready market for new diets. Polivy and Herman see disadvantages to cycling through the false hope syndrome. The weight regain produces negative feelings and frustrations for the dieter. Obsessions with food may also be a consequence of this cycling through failure. At present some people overcome these barriers and succeed as the national Weight Loss Registry attests. Our goal as behavioralists is to increase these numbers.

Maintenance Strategies in Children and Adolescents

Helping children and adolescents maintain weight loss is just as important as in adults. Wilfley et al. (2007) reported a randomized clinical trial comparing a control group with a behavioral skills maintenance group or a social facilitation maintenance treatment. Of 204 children aged 7–12 who were 20%–100% overweight and entered the weight loss component with one parent, 150 were randomized to one of the three groups.

Summary. Lifestyle techniques based on behavioral theory are relatively newcomers to the treatment of obesity, but have proven their value. The recent emphasis on strategies for maintenance will dovetail well with my conclusions that adherence is the key element for any lifestyle program. Dedication with a variety of religious fervor will make any lifestyle program more effective.

Diet

People who are successful in maintaining weight loss used a variety of dietary strategies including reduction of fat intake, use of fat- and sugar-modified foods, reduced consumption of sugar-sweetened beverages, and increased consumption of artificially sweetened beverages (Phelan and Lang 2009).

Lower fat diets may also be an important strategy for maintaining weight loss as suggested from the National Weight Control Registry (Wing and Phelan 2005). This is also shown in the Women's Health Initiative. Women were randomized to control and lower fat diets, which produced an initial weight loss and a difference after 7.5 years of 1.8 kg. Subgroup analysis showed that women who lowered their fat intake more were more successful in maintaining their weight loss and had a reduced incidence of diabetes ($p = -0.04$). This dose-response relationship of decreasing fat intake to weight differential over 7.5 years is shown in Figure 6.17. Weight loss was also associated with greater consumption of fruits and vegetables. Thus, low fat diets can produce modest and prolonged benefit.

High protein diets may also enhance weight maintenance (Westerterp et al. 2004). Following weight loss with a very low calorie diet (VLCD) for 4 weeks, 148 male and female subjects with a baseline BMI of 29.5 kg/m^2 were stratified by age, BMI, body weight response to a restrained eating questionnaire, and REE and randomized to a control condition or a supplement of 48.2 g per day of additional protein. Both groups received regular visits and counseling by the dietitian at the University clinic. At the end of 3 months, the group receiving the protein supplement to bring protein to 18% had a 50% lower body weight regain than the unsupplemented group, whose protein intake was about 15%. The protein supplemented group had increased satiety and a lower increase in triglycerides and leptin. REE, RQ, and TEE were similar between the two groups.

Physical Activity

Exercise is an important factor in maintaining weight loss after weight reduction (Slentz et al. 2004; Donnelly et al. 2003; Jakicic et al. 2003; Wadden et al. 1997). One example is an 8-week study of diet plus exercise in which the subjects were followed up for 18 months. Weight loss with diet or diet plus exercise was not significantly different. However, during the subsequent follow-up period, the subjects who maintained their activity levels regained less weight than those who became sedentary again.

The National Weight Control Registry provides another example. The sample in this registry is defined by a 10% weight loss that is maintained and documented for 1 year before entering the registry. This group has on average lost 33 kg and maintained the loss for more than 5 years. The individuals in the registry report high levels of physical activity amounting to an hour or more per day that help them maintain their lower weight (Wing and Phelan 2005).

Exercise consistently stands out as an important factor in maintaining weight loss after any weight reduction (Jakicic and Marcus 2008; Avenell and Brown 2004; Turk and Yank 2009; Donnelly and Blair 2009; Mekary and Feskanich 2009).

The American College of Sports Medicine concluded that evidence supports moderate-intensity physical activity between 150 and 250 minutes per week as an effective strategy to prevent weight gain, but will provide only modest weight loss. Greater amounts of physical activity (>250 minutes per week) have been associated with clinically significant weight loss. Moderate-intensity physical activity between 150 and 250 minutes per week (−1) will improve weight loss in studies that use moderate diet restriction but not severe diet restriction. Cross-sectional and prospective studies indicate that after weight loss, weight maintenance is improved with physical activity continued at >250 minutes per week. However, no evidence from well-designed randomized controlled trials exists to judge the effectiveness of physical activity for prevention of weight regain after weight loss. Resistance training does not enhance weight loss but may increase fat-free mass and increase loss of fat mass and is associated with reductions in health risk. Existing evidence indicates that endurance physical activity or resistance training without weight loss improves health risk. There is inadequate evidence to determine whether physical activity prevents or attenuates detrimental changes in chronic disease risk during weight gain.

Using self-report, an increase of 30 minutes per day of total discretionary activity between 1991 and 1997 was associated with less weight regain in 4558 premenopausal women aged 26–45 years who had lost >5% of their body weight in the two previous years. Between 1991 and 1997, 80% of women regained >30% of their previous intentional weight loss. An increase of 30 minutes per day in total discretionary activity between 1991 and 1997 was associated with less weight regain (–1.36 kg, 95% CI −1.61 to −1.12), particularly among overweight women (BMI ≥ 25) (–2.45 kg, –3.12 to –1.78). Increased jogging or running was associated with less weight regain (–3.26 kg; −4.41 to –2.10) than increased brisk walking (–1.69 kg; −2.15 to −1.22) or other activities (–1.26 kg; −1.65 to −0.87). Compared to women who remained sedentary, women who were active were less likely to regain >30% of the lost weight if they maintained 30+ minutes per day of discretionary physical activity (OR = 0.69, 0.53 to 0.89) or increased to this activity level (OR = 0.48, 0.39 to 0.60). Conversely, risk of weight regain was elevated in women who decreased their activity. Increased physical activity, particularly high intensity activities, is associated with better maintenance of weight loss (Mekary and Franksich 2009).

It is clear from this discussion that being more physically active is an important component of weight management. The data suggests that physical activity is particularly important in maintaining a lower weight once weight is lost than as a primary strategy for weight loss.

7 Medications for Obesity

KEY POINTS

- Only a few drugs are available to treat obesity.
- Drugs significantly increase weight loss compared to placebo in most trials.
- Weight loss with medications usually reaches its nadir after 20 and 28 weeks of treatment.
- Patients can expect a weight loss of 6%–10% below baseline, provided they adhere to the weight loss program and take medications regularly.
- Sibutramine and orlistat are the only drugs that have been approved by the FDA for long-term use.
- All medications have side effects that need to be considered.
- The FDA has placed a "black box" warning on the label for sibutramine because of risks of cardiovascular problems.
- Sibutramine can raise blood pressure and heart rate, which may require its discontinuation.
- For orlistat the principal sided effects are gastrointestinal resulting from undigested fat in the lower bowel.
- Phase 3 trials have been completed for lorcaserin, a serotonin agonist, and for two combination drugs (bupropion/naltrexone and topiramate/phentermine).
- Other medications are in early clinical trials.
- Orlistat at a dose of 60 mg three times a day (half the prescription dose), is the only over-the-counter medication that is currently available.
- The herbal products that are available in health food stores usually have little data on effectiveness or safety.

BRIEF HISTORY OF THE DRUG TREATMENT FOR OBESITY

Tenth Century

One of the most fascinating stories from the history of drug treatment for obesity is the use of "theriac" to treat King Sancho the Fat. Theriac is an ancient remedy containing up to 64 or more ingredients. The leading ones are opium, myrrh, saffron, ginger, cinnamon, and castor. It originated in Grecian times with Mitridates VI and came into Roman hands when he was defeated. For Sancho, theriac had a dramatic success—Sancho lost weight and got his kingdom back.

Sancho was King of León in Spain in the tenth century. He was nicknamed "Sancho the Fat" because of his size (Hopkins and Lehmann 1995). His reign, which began in 958 AD, was cut short because his fatness became an impediment to his rule, and his noblemen deposed him. The physicians in León were unsuccessful in helping Sancho lose weight. Not wanting him to lose his throne, his strong-willed mother sought the help of a brilliant and learned Jewish physician named Hisdai ibn Shaprut, who was a physician to the Caliph in the southern Spanish city of Cordoba. In a day when "house calls" were still in fashion, Shaprut traveled several hundred miles from Cordoba to Pamplona to evaluate Sancho. Shaprut agreed to take Sancho as a patient, but advised him that it would be a long treatment requiring him to move to Cordoba. The medicine prescribed by Shaprut was "Theriaca," a mixture that probably contained opiates and that was often taken with wine and oils. Over time Sancho gradually lost weight. When he returned to León as a lean man, he was restored to his throne. Thus, a happy ending to a successful treatment of obesity over 1000 years ago.

Sixteenth Century

I now skip to the sixteenth century, which was one of discovery. Christopher Columbus had just discovered the New World in 1492 and brought tobacco, tomatoes, and many other products back to Europe. Tobacco became a treatment for obesity and we know today that the nicotine it provides both reduces food intake and stimulates energy expenditure, which reduces body weight. Daily doses of vinegar were also used as a treatment for obesity—a theme that has resurfaced time and again between AD 1500 and 1900. However, obesity was not common in the sixteenth century, and diet and exercise remained the principal rules for good health.

Seventeenth Century

Obesity had become enough of a concern that descriptions of its treatment appeared in medical texts in the seventeenth century. Below are five separate vignettes for treating "obesitas or corpulency," as it was called, that were published in a widely used textbook by Theophile Bonet (Bonetus), a leading physician of the time. They give a flavor of the strategies that were used by physicians to treat "Obesitas or corpulency." To quote Bonet:

> I. Chiapinius Vitellius, Camp Master-General, a middle aged man, grew so fat, that he was forced to sustain his belly by a swathe, which came about his neck: And observing that he was every day more unfit for the Wars than other, he voluntarily abstained from Wine, and continued to drink vinegar as long as he lived; upon which his Belly fell, and his Skin hung loose, with which he could wrap himself as with a Doublet. It was observed that he lost 87 pounds of weight. [Note: Vinegar and cleansing, or cathartic agents have a long history for treating obesity].
>
> II. Lest any great mischief should follow, we must try to subtract by medicine, what a spare diet will not; because it has been observed, that a looseness either natural, or procured by Art, does not a little good. But this must be done by degrees and slowly, since it is not safe to disturb so much matter violently, lest it should come all at once. Therefore the best way of Purging is by Pills, of Rheubarb, *Aloes* each 2 drachms [1drachm = 1/8 ounce or 60 grains], Agarick 1 drachm, Cinnamon, yellow Sanders, each half a drachm. Make them up with Syrup of Cicory. They must be taken in this manner; First, 1 Scruple* must be given an hour and a half before Meal; then two or three days afterwards, take half a drachm or two scruples before Meal. Thus purging must be often repeated at short intervals, till you think all the cacochymie is removed. *[scruple—a unit of apothecary weight equal to about 1.3 grams, or 20 grains]
>
> III. A certain Goldsmith, who was extreme fat, so that he was ready to be choaked, took the following Powder in his Meat, and so he was cured; Take of Tartar two ounces, Cinnamon three ounces, Ginger one ounce, Sugar four ounces. Make a Powder.
>
> IV. *Horstius* found the things following to take down fat Men; especially onions, Garlick, Cresses, Leeks, Seed of Rue, and especially Vinegar of Squills: Let them purge well: Let them Sweat, and purge by Urine: Let them use violent exercise before they eat: Let them induce hunger, want of Sleep and Thirst: Let them Sweat in a Stove and continue in the Sun. Let them abstain from Drink between Dinner and Supper: for to drink between Meals makes Men fat.
>
> V. I knew a Nobleman so fat, that he could scarce sit on Horse-back, but he was asleep; and he could scarce stir a foot. But now he is able to walk, and his body is come to it self, only by chewing of Tobacco Leaves, as he affirmed to me. For it is good for Phlegmatick and cold Bodies.
>
> VI. Let *Lingua Avis*, or Ash-Keyes be taken constantly about one drachm in Wine. According to *Pliny* it cures Hydropical persons, and makes fat people lean (Bonetus T. 1700, p. 390).

Eighteenth Century

The eighteenth century witnessed publication of the first two English books dealing exclusively with obesity. In each book, the author proposed a new way of treating obesity based on his theory of how it developed. The first book was by Thomas Short published in 1727 (Short 1727). From Short's perspective, treatment of obesity required restoring the natural balance and removing the secondary causes. If possible, one should pick a place to live where the air is not too moist or too soggy and one should not reside in flat, wet countries or in the city or the woodlands. He thought that exercise was important and that the diet should be "moderate spare and of the more detergent kind" (Short 1727).

The second eighteenth-century book was by Malcolm Flemyng, a graduate of the medical school in Edinburgh (Flemyng 1760). His approach to the treatment of obesity was based on the results of a patient that he presented to the Royal Society in London in 1757 and subsequently published in 1760. Flemyng's theory was that sweat, urine, and feces all contained "oil" and that the treatment for obesity was to increase the loss of "oil" by each of these three routes. Thus, laxatives, diuretics, and sweating were his principal approach to the treatment of obesity. To quote his approach:

> Now we are so happy as to be in possession of a diuretic medicine, which has that quality increases the quantity of urine and renders the animal oil more mixable with the watery vehicle of the blood, that otherwise it would be (a diuretic which) in a singular degree; and is withal so safe, as that it may be taken in large quantities every day for years together, without remarkably impairing the general health: that medicine is soap (Flemyng 1760).

Flemyng believed that soap could both prevent and cure corpulency.

Nineteenth Century

The nineteenth century saw the isolation of many different natural products and the beginning of their chemical identification. For obesity, the recognition that the thyroid gland in the neck produced a hormone that prevented myxedema was important because it stimulated the search for and isolation of "thyroid extract," which was first used to treat obesity in 1893. When its pure components, thyroxine and triiodthyroinine were isolated, they too were used to treat obesity.

The following summary of nineteenth- and early twentieth-century treatments for obesity is taken from a textbook by Sajous (7th edition 1914):

> Hyoscine hydrobromate 1/100 grain t.i.d. (three times a day) assists the reducing process by increasing the propulsive activity of the arterioles and causing them to drive an excess of blood into the fat-laden areas. Carlsbad, Homburg, and Marienbad waters owe their virtues mainly to the alkaline and purgative salts they contain, especially sodium sulphate. As a beverage alkaline Vichy water is advantageous to enhance the osmotic properties of the blood and facilitate the elimination of wastes (Sajous 1914).

Shortly after the discovery of endocrine glands in the nineteenth century, extracts were prepared and used for the treatment of obesity as early as the 1890s (Sajous). As Sajous says,

> The fact that thyroid preparations in sufficient doses promote the rapid combustion of fats has caused them to be used extensively in this disorder . . . In large doses (thyroid gland) . . . imposes hyperoxidation upon all cells . . . we behold gradual emaciation beginning with the adipose tissues, which are the first to succumb. Hence the use of thyroid preparations in obesity. Briefly, in all cases of obesity in which thyroid gland is rationally indicated, the feature to determine is whether directly or indirectly hypothyroidia underlies the adiposis (Sajous 1914).

Sajous also describes the use of testicular extracts:

> Testicular preparations, including spermine, have been recommended in a host of disorders, particularly . . . obesity . . . but others again have failed to obtain any favorable results (Sajous 1914).

Twentieth Century

In the twentieth century, the principal story is the introduction, development, and use of drugs derived from the aniline dye industry, which produced the dyes for colors in fabrics. The basis for the advances were the "Lock and Key" concept of Paul Erhlich (1854–1915) who, in the late nineteenth century, developed salvarsan, an arsenical for the treatment of syphilis based on this concept.

Amphetamine and dinitrophenol are two derivatives of the aniline dye group that have effects on body weight. Amphetamine was first synthesized by Edeleano in 1887, but it was not until 1927 that Alleges described its psychopharmacologic effects. Its two major effects are an increase in alertness, and a decrease in food intake (Leake 1958). Amphetamines produce weight loss by reducing food intake (Harris et al. 1947). The first clinical trials with amphetamine were conducted in the 1930s (Lesses and Myerson 1938), but after World War II, amphetamine became a street drug that was widely abused and its use was restricted. It no longer has a place in the treatment of obesity.

Dinitrophenol is another member of this group. It is a chemical used in the munitions industry during World War II (1914–1918). A number of cases of acute poisoning were reported associated with high fever, profuse sweating, nausea, vomiting and diarrhea, and often death. With subacute exposure, however, weight loss was one of the effects. Maurice Tainter at Stanford University was intrigued by this finding (Colman 2007). He conducted some initial studies in animals and noted the narrow margin between the therapeutic and toxic doses (Colman 2007). His first clinical trial in nine obese subjects lasted 10 weeks and produced a weight loss of about 20 pounds with a dose of 3–5 mg/kg body weight and there were no reports of acute toxicity. When this was published in 1933, the word spread quickly and it was estimated that over 100,000 Americans had taken the drug within the first 1–2 years. Gradually, the reports of significant side effects such as cataracts mounted. By one estimate, 25,000 people lost their sight using dinitrophenol. Neuropathy and deaths soon appeared. Notwithstanding, the drug was marketed as Compound 281 and was widely sold. It was during this time that the U.S. Food and Drug Administration (FDA) was increasing its capacity to deal with drugs like this, and eventually dintrophenol was removed from the market, only to make sporadic appearances since (Colman 2007).

Paul Ehrlich (1854–1915) was the one who crystalized the concept of the magic bullet for treating disease. He was born in Strehlen, a small town in Silesia, now part of the Czech Republic. After completing his basic education at Breslau, he moved to Strasbourg, where he received his medical education. His initial interest in aniline dyes formed the basis for his work in histology. He was forced to give up his work for a year-and-a-half after contracting tuberculosis in 1886. In 1896, he was appointed director of the newly opened Serum Institute at Steglitz, Germany. From there, he moved in 1899 to become director of the Royal Institute for Experimental Therapy in Frankfurt am Main, a position he held until his death in 1915. In addition to his early work on the application of aniline dyes as stains to the study of tissues, he also contributed pioneering studies to immunology, for which he won the Nobel Prize in 1908. His legacy is famously associated with his work on chemotherapeutics. His concept of the "magic bullet" as a concept for a drug targeted for a specific disease is an important part of his legacy (Stevenson 1953; Garrison 1914).

MECHANISMS THAT MODULATE FOOD INTAKE AND ENERGY EXPENDITURE: THE BASIS FOR PHARMACOLOGICAL INTERVENTIONS

The remainder of the chapter will be divided into five parts. The first is a description of the drugs that have already been developed, approved by the FDA, and are now on the market for treatment of obesity and related conditions. This will be followed by a description of drugs that are in advanced stages of clinical development, where they are nearly ready for review by the FDA. The third section will discuss drugs in earlier stages of evaluation. The fourth section will discuss the herbal and mineral preparations that some people use for obesity. The final section will examine why it has been difficult to develop drugs to treat obesity. In contrast with the treatment of hypertension and diabetes, where there are several different drugs with differing types of action that can be used, the armamentarium for the treatment of obesity is relatively sparse with only two drugs approved for long-term use by the FDA and four others for short-term use that come from only three biological mechanisms.

In Chapter 2, I developed a feedback model for regulation of body weight. This regulatory system has afferent signals from the gastrointestinal track and adipose tissue and possibly other organs that are transmitted to the brain by nerves or through the circulation. Molecules from the gastrointestinal (GI) track include ghrelin, which stimulates feeding and contrasts with the inhibitory effects on feeding of the other GI peptides, including glucagon-like peptide-1, peptide YY3-36, oxyntomodulin, and cholecystokinin. Drugs that mimic or block these pathways are areas of active research for new drugs. Blockade of intestinal nutrient digestion has been the strategy for orlistat, one of the FDA-approved drugs and for another drug, cetilistat, which is being tested. The pancreas produces amylin, glucagon, and insulin, all of which modulate feeding. Pramlintide, a commercially available version of amylin, reduces body weight in human beings and is under investigation in combination with other drugs.

Food intake often follows a vagally mediated rise in insulin which produces a 12%–15% drop in blood glucose (Campfield and Smith 2003). Modulation of this regulatory system may be worth pursing. Neurotransmitters in the CNS involved in feeding include gamma-aminobutyric acid, the monoamines, norepinephrine, serotonin, dopamine, and histamine, and the fatty acid derivatives anadamide and arachidonyl 2-glycerol that act on cannabinoid CB-1 receptors. Neuropeptides, which increase food intake, include neuropeptide Y (NPY) acting through one of its five receptors (Y-1, Y-2, Y-4, Y-5, Y-6), dynorphin, β-endorphin, agouti-related peptide, melanin concentrating hormone (MCH) orexin A and B. Another group of neuropeptides reduce food intake including α-melanocyte stimulating hormone (α-MSH), which is produced from proopiomelancortin, cocaine-amphetamine-related transcript (CART), urocortin, nesfatin-1, obestatin, and peptides of 26 or 42 amino acids ending with arginine-phenyalanine-amide (RFa). Some of these mechanisms may provide the base for new drugs.

DRUGS APPROVED BY THE FOOD AND DRUG ADMINISTRATION FOR THE TREATMENT OF OBESITY

When Do We Decide to Use the Currently Available Drugs?

The option of using drugs to help weight loss should only be done after lifestyle, diet, and exercise have been started. There are currently only two medications approved by the FDA for long-term use in the treatment of obesity, and four other drugs approved for short-term use. First, I will deal with the two drugs approved for long-term use and then those approved for short-term use. Following that I will describe a pragmatic clinical trial in which the currently available drugs were used by primary care physicians to obtain significant weight loss for their patients.

Currently Available Drugs

Table 7.1 lists the drugs approved by the FDA for treatment of obesity. For individuals desiring more detail or additional guidance in the use of medications to treat overweight, information can be found

TABLE 7.1
Drugs Approved by the U.S. Food and Drug Administration That Produce Weight Loss

Generic Name	Trade Names	Status	Usual Dose	Comments
	Drugs Approved by the FDA for Long-Term Treatment of Overweight Patients			
Orlistat	Xenical		120 mg, tid, with meals	May have GI side effects; daily vitamin pill in the evening; may interact with cyclosporine
Sibutramine	Meridia; Reductil		5–15 mg/day	Raises blood pressure slightly Do not use with monoamine oxidase inhibitors, selective serotonin reuptake inhibitors, sumatriptan, dihydroergotamine, meperidine, methadone, pentazocine, fentanyl, lithium, tryptophan
	Drugs Approved by the FDA for Short-Term Treatment of Overweight Patients			
Benzphetamine	Didrex	DEA-III	25–50 mg, qd-tid	All sympathomimetic drugs are similar Do not use with monoamine oxidase inhibitors, guanethidine, alcohol, sibutramine, tricyclic antidepressants
Diethylpropion	Tenuate, Tepanil, Tenuate dospan	DEA-II	25 mg, bid 75 mg in a.m.	
Phendimetrazine	Bontril, Plegine Plegine-XR Prelu-2 X-Trozine	DEA-III	35 mg bid-tid 105 mg in a.m.	
Phentermine	Adipex-P Fastin Phentercot Ionamin	DEA-II	15–37.5 mg 15–30 mg in AM	

Source: Trade names from http://www.drugs.com/, accessed July 2009.
Benzphetamine: Didrex
Diethylpropion: Tenuate Dospan; Tepanil Ten-Tab
Phendimetrazine: Adipost; Bontril PDM; Bontril Slow-Release; Melfiat; Obezine; Phendiet; Phendiet-105; Plegine; Prelu-2; PT 105
Phentermine: Adipex-P; Fastin; Ionamin; Obenix; Phentercot; Phentride; Pro-Fast; Termine; Zantryl
Orlistat: Xenical
Sibutramine: Meridia (U.S.); Reductil (Other countries). Sibutramine was withdrawn from the market in the United States, Canada, Australia and European Union Countries in 2010, but remains on the market in Argentina, Indonesia, Singapore, Azerbaijan, Israel, Brazil, Jamaica, Syria, Cambodia, Kazakhstan, Taiwan, Chile, Korea, Trinidad, Tobago, China, Kuwait, Turkmenistan, Colombia, Kyrgystan, United Arab Emirates, Costa Rica, Lebanon, Venezuela, Dominican Republic, Malaysia, Vietnam, Ecuador, Mexico, Egypt, Nambia, El Savador, New Zealand, Georgia, Nicaragua, Guatemala, Pakistan, Honduras, Panama, Philippines, India and Russia.

in a variety of sources (National Heart and Blood Institute et al. 2000; Yanovski and Yanovski 2002; Bray and Greenway 1999; Snow et al. 2005; Padwal et al. 2005; Vettor et al. 2005; Padwal et al. 2004; Haddock et al. 2002; Li et al. 2005; Kim et al. 2003; Colman 2005; Lloret-Linares et al. 2008).

The quantity of drugs used for treatment of obesity has gone up and down. Using information from patient visits to office-based physicians, Stafford and Radley (2003) evaluated national trends in use of drugs to treat obesity between 1991 and 2002. Following relatively stable use in the early 1990s, the number of prescriptions increased substantially in 1996 (10.6 million), and in 1997, 9.4 million compared to 1.4 million to 2.4 million drug-use occurrences between 1991 and 1994. This coincided with the widespread use of the combination of two active drugs, phentermine and fenfluramine. Then, following the removal of fenfluramine and dexfenfluramine from the worldwide market in 1997, a sharp drop occurred in drug use for obesity, with 3.7 million uses in 1998 and 2.8 million in 2002. As of 2002, phentermine, the only generic medication, was the most commonly used antiobesity medication, with an annualized rate of about 1.2 million uses per year, followed by orlistat (0.6 million), and sibutramine (0.4 million). In spite of the rising prevalence of obesity, relatively few of those who might benefit from weight control pharmacotherapy were actually prescribed such medications by their physician. Between 1996 and 1998, for example (prior to the availability of orlistat (Xenical®) and just following the availability of sibutramine (Meridia®), prescription weight loss pills were used by only 3.1% of obese men (i.e., BMI ≥ 30 kg/m^2) and 10.2% of obese women (Khan et al. 2001). Using national insurance claims data from 2002, it was estimated that fewer than 2.4% of adults clinically eligible for these medications used them, even when they were covered by their employer's health insurance (Encinosa et al. 2005).

Orlistat

Orlistat was approved by the FDA in 1999. It is an inhibitor of intestinal lipase and pancreatic lipase by binding to the active center of the enzyme and reduces digestion of some of the dietary fat we eat. The drug increases fecal fat loss up to 30% in a dose-dependent manner when the diet contains 30% fat. It also increases the loss of some of the fat-soluble vitamins. Orlistat has little effect in subjects eating a low fat diet. Orlistat reduces plasma triglycerides, remnant lipoprotein cholesterol, and free fatty acids in the early postprandial period following a mixed meal with 70 g fat (Tan and Tso 2002).

Clinical studies on orlistat are summarized in Table 7.2 and Figure 7.1. Figure 7.1 shows the 2-year weight loss in pooled data from several clinical studies that compared both the 120 mg three times a day that is available in prescription form and the 60 mg three times a day that is available over the counter. It shows a maximal weight loss at 6 to 12 months and then a modest regain over the next 12 to 18 months. There is a clear separation between each active dose and placebo.

The data in Table 7.2 show some characteristics of each study group and the weight loss achieved by the drug-treated and placebo-treated patients at 12 or 18 months. Attrition, or loss to follow-up, was a problem with all of the studies. I have presented the placebo and drug effects separately because the patient will receive the "placebo benefit" in addition to the "drug benefit" provided they take the drug. The widely used "placebo-subtracted" values cover up the important overall effects that the patient may experience.

In the trials of obese patients, the weight losses ranged between 7.3 kg and 10.6 kg (16.1 lb to 23 lb), except one study where the weight loss was only 3.29 kg. There is no obvious explanation for the small weight loss in this study. Weight losses were also more modest among the hypertensive and dyslipidemic patients (Table 7.2).

Maintenance of weight loss in patients treated with orlistat was demonstrated in two studies summarized in Table 7.2. In the 3-year study by Richelsen et al. (2007), patients received a very low energy diet for 8 weeks, and those who lost a minimum of 5% of their body weight were randomized to lifestyle or lifestyle plus orlistat. Weight loss continued to decline for 3 months and remained below randomization levels at 12 months in the orlistat group, but had risen above randomization level by 6 months in the lifestyle controls. At the end of 3 years, those on orlistat were still 2.4 kg lighter than the controls.

Initial weight loss is a useful criterion for longer term success. Using pooled data from several 2-year trials, Rissanen et al. (2003) found that a weight loss of >5% at 3 months predicted weight loss > 5% and improvement in major cardiovascular risk factors after 2 years of treatment with orlistat (Toplak et al. 2006).

Several meta-analyses of orlistat have been published that have pooled both nondiabetic and diabetic patients whose weight losses, as shown in Table 7.2, were different (Haddock et al. 2002; Li et al. 2005; Avenell et al. 2004; Rucker et al. 2008). In the meta-analysis of Li et al. (2005), the overall mean difference after 12 months of therapy in 22 studies was –2.70 kg (95% CI –3.79 to –1.61 kg). Since the patient will receive both the placebo and the drug effect, both the drug and placebo group data are useful. For orlistat, the mean weight loss is 7.3 kg after 1 year, compared to

TABLE 7.2
Randomized Clinical Trials Comparing Orlistat and Placebo

Author	Mean Age	Weight (kg)	Number Orlistat/ Placebo	Percent Attrition Orl/Plac	Weight Loss Orlistat	Weight Loss Placebo	Study Design and Comments
Trials in Obese Patients							
Davidson 1999	44	101	657 / 223	42% / 41%	8.76 (9.48)	5.81 (10.00)	1-year wt loss + 1-year maintenance; orlistat 120 mg tid; 600–700 kcal/day deficit diet
Finer 2000	41	98	110 / 108	34% / 39%	3.29 (6.05)	1.31 (6.05)	1-year wt loss trial; orlistat 120 mg tid; 600–800 kcal/day deficit diet
Hauptman 2000	42	101	210 / 213 / 212 120mg / 60mg/ Placebo	28% / 28% / 42%	7.94 / 7.08 (8.26)	4.14 (8.15)	1 year + 1-year maintenance; orlistat 120 mg tid or 60 mg tid; 1000 MJ/day deficit + food diary + exercise + video education
Krempf 2003	41	97	346 / 350	35% / 43%	7.3 (9.3)	4.4 (9.35)	18-month trial; orlistat 120 mg tid; 20% energy reduced diet; food diary
Rossner 2000	44	98	242 / 239 / 237	26% / 35%	9.4 / 8.5 (6.4)	6.4 (6.7)	1-year wt loss + 1 year maintenance; orlistat 120 mg tid; 600 kcal/day energy deficit
Sjostrom 1998	45	100	343 / 340	17% / 20%	10.3 (16.61)	6.1 (16.61)	1-year + rerandomized for the second year of maintenance; orlistat 120 mg tid
Torgerson (XENDOS) 2004	43	111	1640 / 1637	48% / 66%	10.6 (24.3)	6.2 (24.30)	4-year parallel arm—1 year wt loss used; orlistat 120 mg tid; 21% had impaired glucose tolerance

				Trials in Diabetic Patients			
Berne 2005	59	96	111 / 109	14% / 14%	5.0	1.8	1-year trial; orlistat 120 mg tid; type 2 DM receiving oral hypoglycemics; 2.5MJ/day deficit diet; exercise; educational counseling
Hollander 1998	55	100	162 / 159	15% / 27%	6.2 (6.51)	4.3 (7.18)	1-year trial; orlistat 120 mg tid; type 2 DM; 500 kcal/day deficit diet
Kelley 2002	58	102	274 / 276	50% / 54%	3.89 (4.48)	1.27 (4.59)	1-year trial; diabetics on insulin; orlistat 120 mg tid; diet counseling
Miles 2002	52	102	250 / 254	35% / 44%	4.7 (6.74)	1.8 (4.78)	1-year trial; orlistat 120 mg tid; 2.5–3.3 MJ/day deficit diet; exercise
Lindgarde 2000	54	96	190 / 186	16% / 12%	5.6 SE (0.7)	4.3 SE (0.7)	1-year trial; orlistat 120 mg tid; 2.5–3.8 MJ/day deficit diet
Hanefeld 2002	56	98	383		5.3 SE (0.4)	3.4 SE (0.4)	1-year trial; orlistat 120 mg tid; 2.5 MJ/day deficit diet
				Trials in Hypertensive or Dyslipidemic Patients			
Bakris 2002	53	101	278 / 276	42% / 61%	5.4 (6.4)	2.7 (6.4)	1-year trial; orlistat 120 mg tid; 600 kcal/day deficit diet; education
Broom 2002	46	101	259 / 263	30% / 40%	5.8 (8.5)	2.3 (6.4)	1-year trial; orlistat 120 mg tid; 2.5–3.8 MJ/day deficit diet; food diary
Derosa 2005	52	95	27 / 23	7% / 0%	8.60 (5.00)	7.60 (3.36)	1-year trial; orlistat 120 mg tid; 600 kcal/day deficit diet
Swinburn 2005	52	105	170 / 169	22% / 19%	4.7 (7.7)	0.9 (4.2)	1-year trial; orlistat 120 mg tid; diet and exercise counseling; ≥1 CVD risk factor
				Trials to Assess Maintenance of Weight Loss			
Hill 1999	46	90	181 / 173 / 187 / 188 30 / 60 / 120 mg/ Placebo	30% / 23% / 25% / 27%	2.62 / 3.84/ 4.91	4.40	1-year trial; orlistat 30 mg tid; 60 mg tid; 120 mg tid
Richelsen 2007	47	111	153 / 156		9.4	7.2	3-year trial; orlistat 120 mg tid; 8 week VLCD

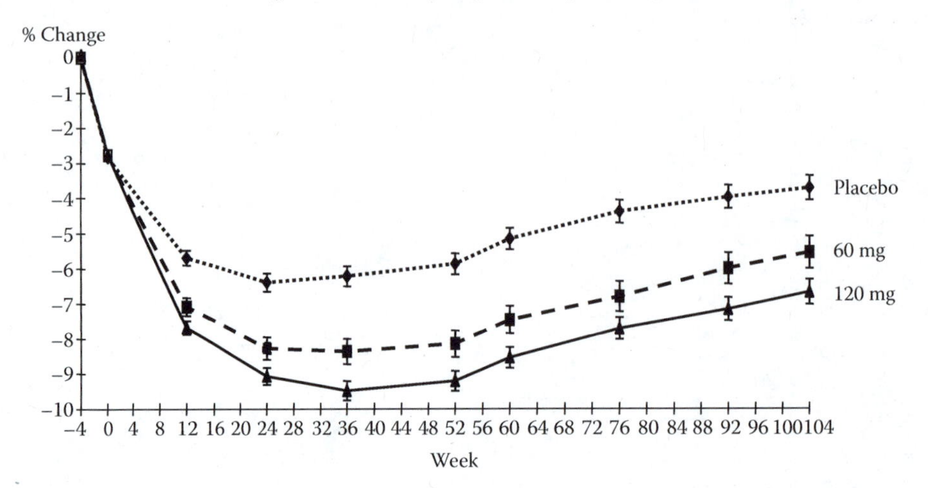

FIGURE 7.1 Two-year weight loss with orlistat 60 or 120 mg three time a day. (Drawn from data obtained in conversation with J. Hauptman. Details available in Hauptman, J., *Endocrine*, 13(2), 201–206, 2000.)

5.0 kg in the placebo group (Greenway and Bray 2010). In another meta-analysis of orlistat, including eight studies lasting 1 year or more, the overall effect of orlistat on weight loss at 12 months was 3.01 kg (95% CI −3.48 to −2.54 kg). After 24 months, the overall effect of orlistat on weight loss was 3.26 kg (95% CI −4.15 to −2.37 kg).

Another way to look at response to orlistat is the number of patients who achieve a 5% weight loss or a 10% weight loss compared to placebo. In the meta-analysis of 11 trials by Padwal et al. (2004), 52% of the patients treated with sibutramine lost more than 5% compared with 31% in the placebo group. At the 10% weight loss level in 10 trials, 25% of the orlistat-treated patients achieved this goal compared to 13% in the placebo group.

Treatment with orlistat is associated with improvement in cardiometabolic risk factors and a number of these are summarized in Table 7.3, adapted from the meta-analysis of Li et al. (2004).

TABLE 7.3
Effects of Orlistat on Waist Circumference, Blood Pressure, and Metabolic Variables

Outcome	Number of Studies	Number in Population	Weighted Mean Difference	95% Confidence Interval
BMI (kg/m^2)	3	1276	−1.05	−1.40 to −0.71
Waist circumference (cm)	9	4631	−2.06	−2.86 to −1.26
Systolic BP (mmHg)	13	6965	−1.52	−2.19 to −0.86
Diastolic BP (mmHg)	12	8322	−1.38	−2.03 to −0.74
LDL-cholesterol (mmol/l)	13	5206	−0.26	−0.30 to −0.22
HDL-cholesterol (mmol/l)	11	4152	−0.03	−0.04 to −0.02
Triglycerides (mmol/l)	11	4456	−0.03	−0.12 to 0.07
Fasting glucose in diabetics (mmol/l)	5	1678	−1.03	−1.49 to −0.57
Hemoglobin A1C in diabetics (%)*	5	1678	−0.38	−0.59 to −0.18
GI adverse events*	14	8938	0.24	0.20 to 0.29
Fecal incontinence*	4	1636	0.06	0.05 to 0.08
Discontinuation due to GI symptoms*	12	5994	0.02	0.01 to 0.03

* Risk difference—all other values are weighted mean differences.

Using the pooled data shows significant overall effects favoring orlistat after 1 year of treatment for the change in cholesterol (–0.34 mmol/L [95% CI –.41 to –.027] [$N = 7$ studies]), the change in LDL-cholesterol (–0.29 mmol/L [95% CI –.34 to –0.24] [$N = 7$ studies]), the change in HbA1c (–0.17% [95% CI –0.24 to –0.10] [$N = 3$ studies]) (Broom et al. 2002; Hollander et al. 1998; Lindgarde 2000), the change in SBP (–2.02 mmHg [95% CI –2.87 to –1.17] [$N = 7$ studies]), and the change in DBP (–1.64 mmHg [95% CI –2.20 to –1.09] [$N = 7$ studies]). In contrast, the change in HDL-cholesterol favored placebo (–0.03 mmol/L [95% CI –0.05 to –0.01] [$N = 6$ studies]), and the change in triglycerides was not statistically significant (0.03 mmol/L [95% CI –0.04 to 0.10] [$N = 6$ studies]). Another systematic review identified 28 studies comparing orlistat and placebo (Hutton and Fergusson 2004). The weight loss was 3.86 kg favoring orlistat in low risk patients, 2.50 kg favoring orlistat in diabetic patients, and 2.04 kg favoring orlistat in high risk patients.

Orlistat is also effective in diabetics. The diabetic patients in Table 7.2 were older and their weight loss is less, ranging from 3.9 kg to 6.2 kg (8.6 lb to 13.6 lb), which is something often reported in trials with diabetic patients. In a Swedish study of 220 diabetic patients treated with either metformin or metformin and a sulfonylurea for 52 weeks, weight loss was 5.0% in the orlistat group and 1.8% in the placebo-group with corresponding 4.8-cm and 2.8-cm reductions in waist circumference. Hemoglobin A1c decreased by 1.1% in the orlistat group and by 0.2% in the control group. HDL-C was slightly reduced (–0.01) in the orlistat group vs. a small rise (0.07 mmol/l) in the control group ($p = 0.0085$). Triglycerides declined slightly but not significantly in both groups (0.12 mmol/l in the orlistat and 0.04 mmol/l in the control group NS). The decline in fasting glucose was greater in the orlistat group (1.9 mmol/l vs. 0.3 mmol/l $p < 0.0001$). Insulin sensitivity, as assessed by the HOMA-IR model, improved (Lloret-Linares et al. 2008). In a meta-analysis focused on the use of orlistat in diabetics, Norris et al. (2004) reported a weighted mean difference in weight loss that favored orlistat of –2.6 kg (95% CI –3.2 to –2.1) after 52 to 57 weeks of treatment.

Three studies have examined whether weight loss with orlistat prevents diabetes (Heymsfield et al. 2000, Richelsen et al. 2007), and this has been reviewed in a meta-analysis (Gillies et al. 2007). In one study, data on 675 subjects were pooled from each of three 2-year studies with orlistat (Heymsfield et al. 2000). Fewer patients taking orlistat converted from a normal to an impaired glucose tolerance (6.6% for orlistat-group vs. 10.8% in the placebo-treated group), and none of the orlistat-treated patients who originally had normal glucose tolerance developed diabetes, compared with 1.2% in the placebo-treated group. Of those who initially had normal glucose tolerance, 7.6% in the placebo group, but only 3% in the orlistat-treated group, developed diabetes.

In a 3-year study on the prevention of diabetes, Richelsen et al. (2007) reported a reduction from 10.9% to 5.2% ($p = 0.041$) in the conversion rate to diabetes. In a large 4-year double-blind, randomized, placebo-controlled trial with over 3300 overweight patients, orlistat reduced the conversion to diabetes by 37% (HR = 0.63; 95% CI 0.46 to 0.86) among the 21% who had impaired glucose tolerance (Torgerson, Hauptman et al. 2004).

Clinical use of orlistat and other weight loss drugs has been evaluated in 714 French general medical practices that provided information on 6801 patients (Vray et al. 2005). Only 40% were treated with orlistat and followed for an average of 11 months with a maximum of 23 months. Between 64% and 77% stopped taking orlistat, primarily because of cost. The average weight loss was 5% after 3 months and 9% after 12 months in those who continued treatment.

Adolescents have also been treated with orlistat. In a 1-year multicenter trial with 539 adolescents (Chanoine et al. 2005), BMI had decreased 0.55 kg/m^2 and weight had only increased by 0.51 kg in the drug-treated group compared to an increase of 0.31 kg/m^2 in BMI and 3.14 kg in body weight in the placebo group. In a follow-up, these authors showed that weight loss in the first 12 weeks was predictive of weight loss at the end of 1 year (Chanoine et al. 2006). A meta-analysis of orlistsat treatment of adolescents reported a significantly greater weight loss of –0.29 kg (95% CI –0.46 to –0.12) and a decrease in BMI of 0.7 kg/m^2 (95% CI 0.3 to 1.2 kg/m^2), both favoring orlistat in three studies (McGovern et al. 2008).

TABLE 7.4
Randomized Clinical Trials with Sibutramine Lasting 12 Months or More

Author	Mean Age	Weight (kg)	Number Sibutramine /Placebo	Percent Attrition Sib/Placebo	Weight Loss Sibutramine	Weight Loss Placebo	Study Design and Comments
Trials in Obese Patients							
Hauner 2004	43	100	180 / 182	40% / 48%	8.1 (7.7)	5.1 (6.7)	54-week follow-up; sibutramine 15 mg/day; 2.1–4.2 MJ/day energy deficit diet; exercise; food diary.
Smith 2001	42	87	161 / 161 / 161 15mg / 10mg / placebo	42% / 49% / 51%	6.4 / 4.4 15mg / 10mg (6.6)	1.6 (3.6)	1-year trial; sibutramine 10 mg/day; 15 mg/day; diet counseling
Wirth 2001	43	98	405 / 395 / 201 Cont/Interm	20% / 20% / 27% Cont / Interm / Pla	7.9 / 7.8	3.8	48-week trial with 4-week single blind run-in; sibutramine 15 mg/day; intermittent group ($n = 395$) received drug weeks 1–12, 19–20, and 37–48
Trials in Diabetic Patients							
Kaukua 2004	53	100	114 / 122	8% / 11%	7.1 (10.26)	2.6 (10.26)	1-year trial; type 2 DM; sibutramine 15 mg/day; 700 kcal/day energy deficit
McNulty 2003	49	103	62* / 68 / 64 20mg* / 15mg vs. placebo	28%* / 21% / 28%	8.0* / 5.5 (4.95)	0.2 (4.00)	1-year trial type 2 DM metformin treated; sibutramine 20 mg/day or 15 mg/day; diet counseling
Sanchez-Reyes 2004	47	74	44 / 42	45% / 45%	4.1 (10.45)	1.4 (10.78)	1-year trial type 2 DM treated with diet or sulfonylureas; sibutramine 15 mg/day; diet and exercise counseling

Redmon	54	112			6.5 SE (1.3)	0.8 SE (0.9)	1-year trial; sibutramine 10–15 mg/day; 500–1000 kcal/day with some meal replacements
Rissanen			236				1-year trial sibutramine 15 mg/day; 700 kcal/day deficit
Hypertensive or Dyslipidemic Patients							
McMahon 2000	53	97	170 / 169	22% / 19%	4.40 (5.10)	0.50 (3.80)	1-year trial; sibutramine 20 mg/day; 36% African-American; diet counseling
McMahon 2002	51	98	146 / 74	42% / 51%	4.50 (4.50)	0.40 (3.60)	1-year trial; sibutramine 15 mg/day; diet counseling
Weight Maintenance Trials							
Apfelbaum 1999	38	104	82 / 78	27% / 38%	5.2 (7.5)	+0.5 (5.7)	205 received VLCD; wt loss > 6 kg at 4 weeks randomized to 1-year follow-up; sibutramine 10 mg/day; diet counseling
James 2000	41	103	352 / 115	42% / 50%	8.9 (8.1)	4.9 (5.9)	605 received sibutramine 5 mg/day for 6 months; wt loss > 5% randomized to 18-month trial; sibutramine or placebo 10, 15, or 20 mg/day; 600 kcal/day deficit diet; exercise counseling
Mathus-Vliegen 2005	43	105	94 / 95	35% / 39%	10.7 (7.5)	8.5 (8.1)	VLCD for 8-weeks wt loss > 10% randomized to 18-month trial; sibutramine 10 mg/day; diet and exercise counseling

Orlistat as an over-the-counter preparation. Orlistat at a dose of 60 mg per day is the only over-the-counter preparation currently available for overweight individuals. In pooled data from two published clinical trials of 24 weeks in individuals with a BMI > 28 kg/m^2 and a 16-week trial in individuals with a BMI between 25 and 28 kg/m^2, orlistat at 60 mg three times a day produced significantly more weight loss than placebo (Anderson et al. 2006).

Safety. Safety is a consideration when using any drug. Orlistat is not absorbed from the GI track to any significant degree and its side effects are thus related to the blockade of triglyceride digestion in the intestine (Zhi et al. 1999). Fecal fat loss and related GI symptoms are common initially, but they subside as patients learn to use the drug (Bray and Greenway 1999, 2007). The quality of life in patients treated with orlistat may improve despite concerns about GI symptoms. Orlistat can cause small but significant decreases in fat-soluble vitamins. Levels usually remain within the normal range, but a few patients may need vitamin supplementation. Because it is impossible to tell which patients need vitamins, it is wise to provide a multivitamin routinely with instructions to take it before bedtime. Orlistat does not seem to affect the absorption of other drugs, except cyclosporin.

Sibutramine

Abbott Laboratories removed sibutramine from the market in the United States and Canada on October 8, 2010 at the request of the Food and Drug Administration. It has also been withdrawn in Australia and marketing is suspended in the European Union. The drug is still available in many other countries, including Argentina, Indonesia, Singapore, Azerbaijan, Israel, Brazil, Jamaica, Syria, Cambodia, Kazakhstan, Taiwan, Chile, Korea, Trinidad, Tobago, China, Kuwait, Turkmenistan, Colombia, Kyrgystan, United Arab Emirates, Costa Rica, Lebanon, Venezuela, Dominican Republic, Malaysia, Vietnam, Ecuador, Mexico, Egypt, Nambia, El Savador, New Zealand, Georgia, Nicaragua, Guatemala, Pakistan, Honduras, Panama, Philippines, India and Russia, at the time this book went to press.

Sibutramine is a multiamine neuronal reuptake inhibitor that acts primarily on transporters in the brain for norepinephrine, serotonin, and dopamine. It reduces food intake by increasing "satiety." Part of this effect on feeding may be through modulation of NPY and proopiomelanocortin levels in the hypothalamus and periphery (Levin et al. 2000; Baranowska et al. 2005; Tziomalos et al. 2009). The effects of sibutramine on food intake were assessed in a 2-week double-blind, placebo-controlled trial, where a 30 mg per day dose of sibutramine reduced food intake by 23% on day 7 and 26% on day 14, relative to placebo. The effect of sibutramine on food intake has also been examined in a 10-month trial (Barkeling et al. 2003). The first 2 weeks of this 10-month trial were conducted in a double-blind, randomized, placebo-controlled crossover design. Participants then entered a 10-month open-label trial with repeat food intake at the end. There was a 16% reduction in energy intake at the test lunch in the first part of the study (after 2 weeks). There was still a 27% reduction 10 months later when compared to their pre-weight-loss food intake.

The clinical trials with sibutramine are summarized in Table 7.4. Attrition, or loss to follow-up, was a problem here as it was with orlistat (Fabricatore et al. 2009). For a more detailed discussion of sibutramine, the reader is referred elsewhere (Tzimalos et al. 2009; Bray and Greenway 2007; Ryan 2008).

Sibutramine produces a dose-dependent reduction in body weight (Figure 7.2), and this reduction in weight is primarily body fat (Kamel et al. 2000). In this 6-month study of 1047 patients, the weight loss over 6 months was dose-related. The placebo group lost less than 1 kg. Doses of 5, 10, and 15 mg produced losses of approximately 3.5, 5.5, and 7.0 kg in 6 months. The number of participants losing ≥5% of their body weight was also dose-related, with 19.5% of the placebo patients losing this much, compared to 37.4% in those getting 5 mg per day, 59.6% in those receiving the 10 mg per day dose, and 67.3% in those getting the 15 mg per day dose. A weight loss of ≥10% was also dose-related. None of the placebo-treated patients lost 10%, compared to the 12.1% who received the 5 mg per day dose, 17.2% in those who received the 10 mg per day dose, and 34.7% in those who received the 15 mg per day dose (Bray et al. 1999; Bray and Greenway 1999, 2007).

Treatment with sibutramine for 1 year produced weight losses ranging between 6.4 and 8.1 kg in obese patients, compared with 1.6 to 5.1 kg in the placebo group. Weight loss in the obese diabetic

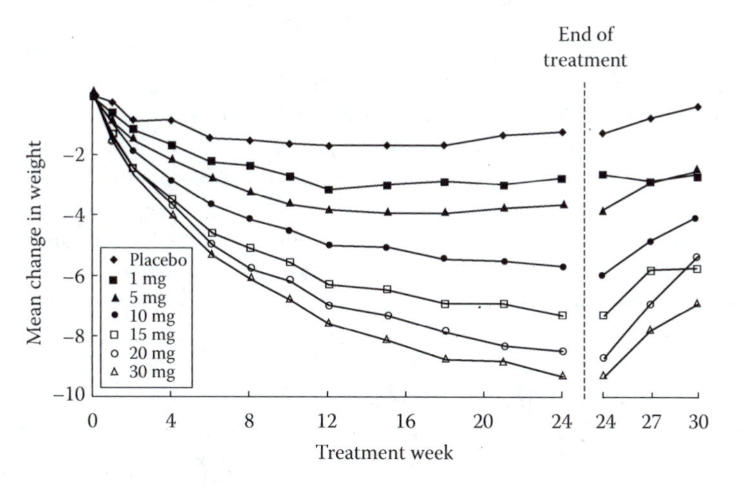

FIGURE 7.2 Six month randomized placebo-controlled dose-ranging trial with placebo and sibutramine at six doses. (Data from Bray et al. *Obes Res* 7(2), 189–198, 1999.)

patients was nearly the same, ranging from 4.1 to 7.1 kg compared to 0.2 to 2.6 kg in the placebo-treated patients. In two trials with obese hypertensive patients receiving different antihypertensive drugs, the weight loss was about 4.5 kg and 0.5 kg in the placebo group.

Another way to look at response to sibutramine is the number of patients who achieve a 5% weight loss or a 10% weight loss compared to placebo. In the meta-analysis of three trials by Padwal et al. (2004), 49% of the patients treated with sibutramine lost more than 5%, compared with 15% in the placebo group. At the 10% weight loss level, 20% of the sibutramine-treated patients achieved this goal, compared to 5% in the placebo group.

Sibutramine can be used intermittently (Wirth and Krause 2001). When a group of patients received continuous treatment with 15 mg per day of sibutramine for 1 year, and the other group had two 6-week periods (weeks 12 to 18 and 30 to 36) when sibutramine was replaced by placebo, there was a small regain in weight following transition to the placebo that was lost when the drug was resumed. At the end of the trial, weight loss was the same in both the intermittent- and continuous-dosed groups and significantly greater than placebo.

The overall effects of sibutramine have been assessed in several meta-analyses, which pool results for placebo and for sibutramine (Haddock and Poston 2002; Rucker et al. 2007; Li Maglioni 2005; Avenell et al. 2004). In the meta-analysis of Li et al. (2005), the overall mean difference after 12 months of therapy in five studies was Fabricatore −4.45 kg (95% CI −5.29 to −3.62 kg) favoring sibutramine. In the meta-analysis of Avenell et al. (2004), the overall effect of sibutramine at 12 months was −4.12 kg (95% CI −4.97 to −3.26 kg). According to the meta-analysis of Rucker et al. (2007), the weighted mean difference in weight was 4.20 kg (95% CI −5.21 to −2.99 kg) favoring sibutramine.

Three studies have evaluated the effectiveness of sibutramine in preventing weight regain. The weight maintenance at 15 months was 3.70 kg (95% CI −5.71 to −1.69 kg) below baseline (Apfelbaum et al. 1999) and at 18 months it was 3.40 kg (95% CI −4.45 to −2.35 kg) below baseline (James et al. 2000). In the three studies using sibutramine for weight maintenance, the mean weighted weight loss was −2.20 kg (95% CI −4.43 to −0.03 kg). Three studies used weight maintenance as the primary endpoint. About 10%–30% more patients treated with sibutramine achieved successful weight loss defined as maintaining 80%–100% of the initial weight loss, compared with placebo ($p < 0.05$ in all three studies) (Rucker et al. 2007).

Diabetic patients respond to sibutramine. A meta-analysis of eight studies in diabetic patients receiving sibutramine (Vettor et al. 2005) found that sibutramine treatment favored changes in body weight, waist circumference, glucose, hemoglobin A1c, triglycerides, and HDL-cholesterol favored sibutramine over placebo. The mean weight loss was –5.53 ± 2.2 for those treated with sibutramine and –0.90 ± 0.17 for the placebo-treated patients. There was no significant change in systolic blood pressure, but diastolic blood pressure was significantly higher in the sibutramine-treated patients (Vettor et al. 2005). In the meta-analysis by Norris et al. (2004), the net weight loss over 12–26 weeks in four trials including 391 diabetics was –4.5 kg (95% CI –7.2 to –1.8 kg), favoring sibutramine. In another meta-analysis, sibutramine reduced both body weight and hemoblogin A1c in diabetic patients (Lloret-Linares et al. 2008).

Sibutramine was also effective when used in patients with dyslipidemia, in patients with the polycystic ovary syndrome (Lindholm et al. 2008), in individuals with binge-eating disorder (Wilfley et al. 2008), those with hypothalamic obesity, and in patients treated with antipsychotic drugs like olanzapine and clozapine (Henderson et al. 2005).

Treatment with sibutramine improves some, but not all, cardiometabolic parameters. Table 7.5 shows these responses and is adapted from Li et al. (2005). Cholesterol, LDL-cholesterol, and triglycerides declined, but HDL-cholesterol and both systolic and diastolic blood pressure along with heart rate were increased (Rucker et al. 2007; Kim et al. 2003; Avenell et al. 2004). Insulin resistance may improve with sibutramine, but this is probably due to the weight loss, since no effect independent of weight loss has been demonstrated. Sibutramine improved a number of other cardiometabolic variables, including fatty liver, inflammatory markers, endothelial function, and left ventricular function (see Tziotmalos et al. 2009).

The likelihood of responding to sibutramine can be predicted from initial weight loss. The likelihood that a patient will achieve a weight loss of >5% when treated with sibutramine is low in patients who do not lose 2 kg (4.4 lb) or more in the first month on 10 mg of sibutramine and these patients should be reevaluated. Pooling data from seven multicenter trials, Finer et al. (2006) found weight loss of 4 kg at 3 months was a better criterion for identifying those who would achieve at least 5% weight loss at 12 months. A younger age, lower depression scores, lower restraint scores, and lower energy intake also appear to predict weight loss with sibutramine (Hainer et al. 2005; Elfhag et al. 2008). Several genotypes have been identified that are associated with better response to sibutramine, but the smaller size of these studies warrants caution (see Tziomalos et al. 2009).

Wadden et al. (2005) have shown that adding a lifestyle program to treatment with sibutramine augments weight loss. With sibutramine alone and minimal behavioral intervention, the weight loss over 12 months was 5.0 ± 7.4 kg (5%). Adding a brief behavioral therapy session to a group that also received sibutramine produced a slightly larger weight loss of 7.5 ± 8.0 kg. When the intensive lifestyle intervention was combined with sibutramine, the weight loss increased to 12.1 ± 9.8 kg.

Sibutramine has been used in adolescents (Berkowitz et al. 2003; Godoy-Matos et al. 2005; Berkowitz et al. 2006). In a 12-month multicenter, randomized, placebo-controlled trial, 498

TABLE 7.5
Effects of Sibutramine on Waist Circumference, Blood Pressure, Heart Rate, and Lipids

Outcome	Number of Studies	Number in Population	Weighted Mean Difference	95% Confidence Interval
BMI (kg/m^2)	5	956	–1.54	–1.79 to –1.30
Waist circumference (cm)	8	1837	–3.99	–4.70 to –3.28
Systolic BP (mmHg)	7	1906	1.69	0.11 to 3.28
Diastolic BP (mmHg)	7	1906	2.42	1.51 to 3.32
Heart rate (beats/minute)	7	1658	4.53	3.49 to 5.57
HDL-cholesterol (mmol/l)	5	977	0.04	0.01 to 0.08
Triglycerides (mmol/l)	4	785	–0.18	–0.30 to –0.07

adolescents aged 12–16 were treated with sibutramine or placebo (Berkowitz et al. 2006). The dose of sibutramine was 10 mg per day for 6 months, and then increased to 15 mg per day in those who had not lost >10% of their baseline BMI. After 12 months, the mean absolute change in BMI was −2.9 kg/m^2 (8.2%) in the sibutramine group, compared with −0.3 kg/m^2 (−0.8%) in the placebo group ($p < 0.001$). Triglycerides, HDL-cholesterol, and insulin sensitivity improved, but there was no significant difference in the changes in either systolic or diastolic blood pressure. A meta-analysis of sibutramine in adolescents reported significantly greater weight loss favoring sibutramine of −1.01 kg (95% CI −1.28 to −0.73) in three studies, which was consistent with a decrease in BMI of 2.4 kg/m^2 (95% CI 1.8 to 3.1 kg/m^2) (McGovern et al. 2008).

Safety. Safety is a primary consideration with any drug. The rise in blood pressure reported with sibutramine is the major concern. A meta-analysis of 21 studies by Kim et al. (2003) found that sibutramine produced a significant weight loss and a significant increase in both systolic and diastolic blood pressure. In a subgroup analysis, they found the effect on systolic blood pressure to be greater with higher doses of sibutramine, in individuals weighing 92 kg or more and in younger individuals (<44 years of age). In another analysis of two studies using sibutramine for 48 weeks, Jordan et al. (2005) reported that sibutramine significantly reduced body weight but did not lead to a difference in systolic blood pressure after 48 weeks (−0.1 ± 15.5 mmHg for placebo and −0.2 ± 1.52 mmHg for the sibutramine group). However, diastolic blood pressure was significantly increased by 0.3 ± 9.5 mmHg in the sibutramine group, but decreased by 0.8 ± 9.2 mmHg in the placebo group (p = 0.049) (Birkenfeld et al. 2002, 2005). Treatment with sibutramine raises bilirubin slightly and low bilirubin levels are predictors of cardiovascular disease (Andersson et al. 2009; Maggioni et al. 2008).

Uncertainties about the cardiovascular safety of sibutramine led to the SCOUT (Sibutramine Cardiovascular OUTcomes Trial) trial that is investigating sibutramine plus weight management in high risk, overweight/obese patients. A 6-week lead-in period during which all patients received sibutramine permitted an initial assessment of tolerability. A total of 10,742 patients received sibutramine and 3.1% of these discontinued due to an adverse event; issues affecting more than 10 patients were drug intolerance, headache, insomnia, nausea, dry mouth, and constipation-, tachycardia-, and hypertension-related events. Serious adverse events, most commonly associated with the system organ class, cardiac disorders, were reported by 2.7% of patients; however, the majority was not considered sibutramine-related. Adverse events relating to high blood pressure and/or pulse rate, whether reported as adverse events leading to discontinuation, or serious adverse events were reported by less than 0.2% of patients. No serious or individual events leading to discontinuation occurred in more than 25 patients. There were 15 (0.1%) deaths; 10 were attributed to a cardiovascular cause. Discontinuations for adverse events were lower than anticipated. In a bulletin from the FDA, they notified health professionals that they were evaluating a report that the sibutramine-treated group in the SCOUT trial had more deaths than the control group. Based on these data, the FDA has put a warning on the drug label for sibutramine.

Increased heart rate is a consistent finding with sibutramine treatment and is part of the reason for avoiding its use in people with active heart disease, previous stroke, heart failure, or cardiac arrhythmias (Torp-Pedersen et al. 2007).

Sibutramine was approved by the FDA in 1997, and is available in 5-, 10-, and 15-mg doses; 10 mg per day as a single dose is the recommended starting level, with titration up or down depending on response. Along with other sympathomimetic drugs, it produced dry mouth, constipation, nausea, and constipation. Doses higher than 15 mg per day are not recommended. Head-to-head comparison of orlistat and sibutramine, as well as the effect of adding the two together, have also been reported. In three studies using sibutramine 10 to 20 mg per day for 3 to 12 months, the reduction in BMI was more with sibutramine than orlistat (Kaya et al. 2004; Sari et al. 2004; Gokcel et al. 2002), but in two other studies, body weight loss or decrease in BMI were similar (Erondu et al. 2007; Kiortsis 2008). A meta-analysis of seven head-to-head trials reported a 2.2-kg greater weight loss with sibutramine (Neovius et al. 2008). As might be anticipated, orlistat was associated with a fall in blood pressure, whereas it increased with sibutramine. Changes in lipid profiles were similar, but the sibutramine group had fewer side effects.

Combination of Sibutramine and Orlistat

In an open-label, randomized 12-week study, 86 overweight patients were assigned to treatment with orlistat 120 mg three times a day, to treatment with sibutramine 10 mg per day, the combination of orlistat and sibutramine, or to a diet group. During the 12 weeks, sibutramine produced more weight loss than orlistat alone. Adding orlistat to sibutramine did not significantly enhance weight loss, confirming the observations of Wadden et al. (2000; Kaya, Aydin et al. 2004).

Sympathomimetic Drugs

The history of sympathomimetic drugs began with the discovery of amphetamine in 1885 and its eventual clinical trials in the 1930s. Amphetamine is a name derived from the chemical structure alpha-methylphenethylamine, and the underlined letters spell its name. α-phenethylamine is the chemical backbone of most of the compounds in this group, except mazindol, which is a tricyclic. In animals and human beings, amphetamine has many properties of the naturally occurring amines norepinephrine and epinephrine, which are released from nerve endings and activate sympathetic tissues. As the use of amphetamine for treating overweight patients increased, it became clear that amphetamine and closely related metamphetamine were addictive. Because of the risk for addiction, organic chemists synthesized a large number of other sympathomimetic molecules that reduced food intake but were less subject to abuse.

Four sympathomimetic amines are approved by the FDA for short-term treatment of obesity. Two of them, phentermine and diethylpropion, are listed as schedule IV by the U.S. Drug Enforcement Agency and the other two, benzphetamine and phendimetrazine, are listed as schedule III. This regulatory classification indicates the U.S. government's belief that they have the potential for abuse, although this potential appears to be very low. These drugs are approved for only a "few weeks," which is usually interpreted as up to 12 weeks. Weight loss with phentermine and diethylpropion persists for the duration of treatment, suggesting that tolerance does not develop to these drugs. If tolerance were to develop, the drugs would be expected to lose their effectiveness, and patients would require increased amounts of the drug to maintain weight loss. This does not appear to occur. These drugs may "release" norepinephrines from their storage vesicles in nerve endings, and they may also act to inhibit reuptake of norepinephrine and dopamine at nerve endings.

Most of the data on the sympathomimetic amines come from short-term trials conducted in the 1960s and 1970s (Bray and Greenway 1999; Padwell et al. 2004). One of the longest clinical trials lasted 36 weeks and compared placebo treatment with phentermine, given either continuously or intermittently (Munro et al. 1968). Both continuous and intermittent phentermine produced similar weight loss, which was significantly greater than placebo. When placebo replaced phentermine every other month, patients' weight loss slowed or they regained a small amount of weight, only to lose weight more rapidly when the drug was reinstituted. In six studies, phentermine produced a mean weight loss of 6.3 kg (range –3.6 to –8.8 kg) compared to a placebo-induced weight loss of 2.8 kg (range –1.5 to –5.2kg) (Haddock et al. 2002). For diethylpropion, the mean weight loss in nine studies was 6.5 kg (range 1.9 to 13.1 kg) and for the placebo group it was 3.5 kg (range 0.4 to 10.5 kg). Data for benzphetamine found a weight loss of 4.03 kg (range 1.6 to 7.3 kg) and for placebo 0.73 kg (range 1.3 to 2.0 kg).

Summary and Pragmatic Trial

The drugs already described and three drugs described in the next section are included in the *Guidelines of the American College of Physicians for Treatment of Obesity.* The table from the *Guidelines* has been summarized below (Table 7.6). The indications and use of the drugs approved by the FDA are discussed above. The others are described below and although not specifically approved for obesity, may be useful in obese patients who have diabetes (metformin and exenatide),

TABLE 7.6
Summary of Drugs in the American College of Physicians Guidelines

Medication	Type of Data Used in the Analysis	Study Population	Weeks of Treatment	Weight Change in kg and 95% Confidence Interval
Drugs Approved by the FDA for Short and Long-Term Treatment of Obesity				
Orlistat (approved for long-term use)	Meta-analysis of 29 RCT	Age 48 years; 73% female; BMI 36.7 kg/m^2	52	−2.75kg 95% CI (−3.31 to −2.20)
Sibutramine (approved for long-term use)	Meta-analysis of 22 RCT	Age 34–54 years; 53% to 100% female	52	−4.45 kg 95% CI (−5.29 to −3.62)
Phentermine (approved for short-term use)	Meta-analysis of 9 studies	Age N/A; 78% female; BMI N/A	2 to 24	−3.6 kg 95% CI (−6.0 to −0.06)
Diethylpropion (approved for short-term use)	Meta-analysis of 13 studies	Age N/A; 80% female; BMI N/A	6 to 52	−3.0 kg 95% CI (−11.5 to 1.6)
Drugs Approved by the FDA but Not for Treatment of Obesity				
Bupropion	Meta-analysis of 3 RCT	Age 43 years; 81% female; wt 94.3 kg	24 to 52	−2.77 kg 95% CI (−4.5 to −1.0)
Fluoxetine	Narrative Synthesis of 9 RCT	Age 48 years; 69% female; BMI 35.5 kg/m^2	52	Range of wt change −1.45 kg lost to 0.5 kg gained
Topiramate	Meta-analysis of 6 RCT	Age 47 years; 68% female; wt 102 kg	24	6.5% 95% CI (4.8% to 8.3%)

Source: Adapted from Li Z, et al., *Ann. Int. Med.*,142, 532–546, 2005.
Note: Sibutramine is not available in the United States, Canada, Australia or Europe.

depression (bupropion or fluoxetine), or migraine headache (topiramate) since each of these drugs is approved by the FDA for that indication, and the obesity is thus a side effect.

To examine the effectiveness of the FDA-approved agents, along with the strategies outlined in Chapter 6, Ryan et al. (2010) conducted a clinical trial using strategies available to every physician. Eight primary care clinics around the State of Louisiana were selected for this study. The physician and staff personnel from each clinic had two sessions designed to acquaint them with *Guideline*-based approaches to obesity, including the use of low calorie diets, behavior therapy, and drugs. During these training sessions there were "practice sessions" to learn how to deliver behavioral strategies and other therapeutic skills.

The trial was divided into three phases. Phase 1 lasted for the first 3 months. During this time, participants received a low calorie diet supplemented with 10 g of fat based on the HealthOne formula, which provided 890 kcal, 75 g protein, 15 g fat, and 110 g carbohydrates. An electrocardiogram was performed and electrolytes were measured every week or so. Phase 2 began at the end of Phase I and lasted to the eighth month. It included a highly structured diet consisting of two meal replacements per day using the HealthOne, Slim Fast, Glucerna, or Boost formulas and other foods to bring the total calories to 1200 for women and 1600 kcal for men. Weekly group sessions with about 15 individuals in each group met for four weekly sessions and then biweekly for 3 months. Medications were introduced in this phase. They included the FDA-approved agents

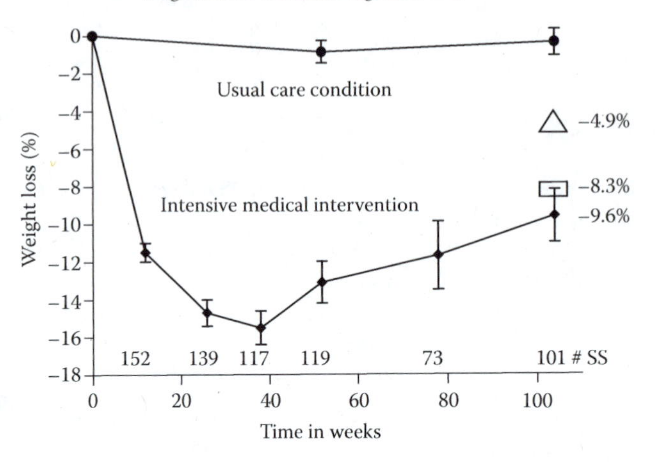

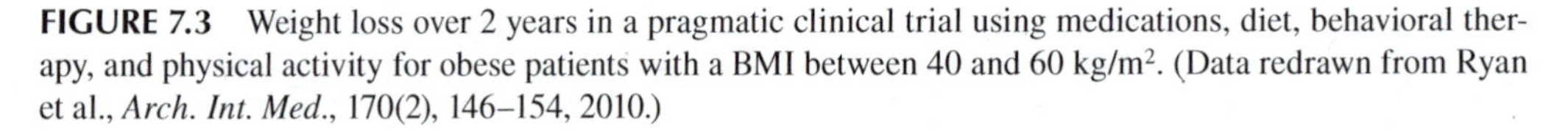

FIGURE 7.3 Weight loss over 2 years in a pragmatic clinical trial using medications, diet, behavioral therapy, and physical activity for obese patients with a BMI between 40 and 60 kg/m^2. (Data redrawn from Ryan et al., *Arch. Int. Med.*, 170(2), 146–154, 2010.)

such as sibutramine, orlistat, or diethylpropion, which were used intermittently in some patients. For depression, the physicians were encouraged to use weight-neutral drugs such as bupropion or venlafaxine. Phase 3 began at the ninth month and continued to the twenty-fourth month. Weight loss medications were used during this phase, and one meal replacement per day was recommended. The behavioral groups met monthly for their sessions. Repeat cycles with low calorie liquid diets lasting from 4 to 12 weeks were reinstituted. Other diets, including high protein diets, the DASH diet, and a low glycemic index diet were also available. Physical activity was encouraged as a help in maintaining their weight loss.

A total of 390 subjects with BMIs between 40 and 60 kg/m^2 were randomized, 200 received "intensive medical intervention" and 190 were assigned to "usual care conditions." At 2 years, those who completed the trial lost 9.7% vs. 0.4% in "usual care conditions." Of this group, 31% lost >5% and 9% lost >20%. Cardiometabolic risks improved with weight loss (Ryan 2010). A comparison of the "intensive medical intervention" and "usual care" arms of the trial is shown in Figure 7.3.

DRUGS APPROVED FOR OTHER USES THAT HAVE EFFECTS ON BODY WEIGHT

Metformin

Metformin is a biguanide that is approved by the FDA for the treatment of diabetes mellitus. This drug reduces hepatic glucose production, decreases intestinal glucose absorption from the gastrointestinal tract, and enhances insulin sensitivity. One mechanism for the reduction in hepatic glucose production by metformin may depend on the phosphorylation of a nuclear binding protein [cAMP response element binding (CREB) binding protein (CBP) at Ser436) AMPK]. This disrupts a number of other signals, including a master transcription factor, peroxisome proliferator activated receptor–γ coactivator 1A (PPARGC1A), which in turn leads to the suppression of hepatic glucose output (He et al. 2009).

Most of the clinical literature on metformin deals with its use in treatment and prevention of diabetes (Setter et al. 2003; Crandall 2008; Gillies et al. 2007). Only a relatively few studies have focused on weight loss with metformin (Bray and Greenway 2007; Park et al. 2009). In one French trial called BIGPRO, metformin was compared to placebo in a 1-year multicenter study involving 324 middle-aged subjects with upper body adiposity and the insulin resistance syndrome (metabolic

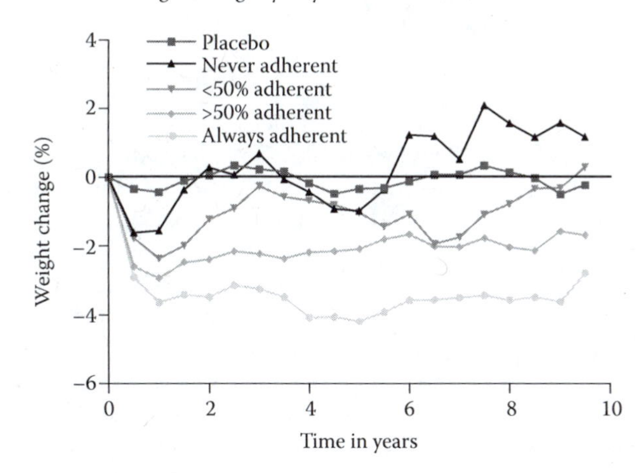

FIGURE 7.4 Ten-year weight change curves for metformin treatment in the Diabetes Prevention Program divided by adherence to medication. (Data from Bray et al., unpublished.)

syndrome). The subjects treated with metformin lost significantly more weight (1–2 kg) than the placebo group, and the study concluded that metformin may have a role in the primary prevention of Type 2 diabetes (Fontbonne et al. 1996). In a meta-analysis of weight loss in three studies with metformin, Avenell et al. (2004) reported a nonsignificant weight loss at 12 months of −1.09 kg (95% CI −2.29 to 0.11 kg). A meta-analysis of three studies with metformin in children and adolescents also found a nonsignificant loss of body weight of −0.17 kg (95% CI −0.62 to 0.28) (Park and Kinra 2009).

The longest and best study of metformin on body weight comes from the Diabetes Prevention Program (2009). During the first 2.8 years of the double-blind, placebo-controlled trial, the metformin-treated group lost 2.9 kg (2.5 %) of their body weight vs. 0.42 kg in the placebo group ($p < 0.001$). The degree of weight loss was related to the adherence to metformin. Those who were the most adherent lost 3.5 kg at 2 years, compared with a small weight gain of 0.5 kg in those who were assigned to, but never took, metformin. This differential weight loss persisted throughout the 8 years of follow-up with highly adherent patients remaining 3–4 kg below baseline and those who were not adherent being no different from placebo (Knowler et al. 2002). This is shown in Figure 7.4.

Glucagon-Like Peptide-1 Agonists

Glucagon-like peptide-1 (GLP-1) is derived from the processing of the proglucagon peptide secreted by intestinal L-cells that increase in density in the lower intestine (Neff and Kushner 2010). It is one of two incretins, the other is GIP (glucose-dependent insulin-stimulatory peptide). These two peptides by themselves have little effect on insulin secretion from the pancreas, but in the presence of glucose, each produces a synergist increase in insulin—thus the name "incretin." GLP-1 also inhibits glucagon secretion and stimulates hepatic gluconeogenesis and delays gastric emptying (Patriti et al. 2004). It may contribute to the superior weight loss and superior improvement in diabetes seen after gastric bypass surgery (Greenway et al. 2002; Small and Bloom 2004). GLP-1 is rapidly degraded by dipeptidyl peptidase-4 (DPP-4), an enzyme that is elevated in the obese. Treatment with DPP-4 inhibitors does not modify body weight, in contrast to GLP-1 agonists, probably because the changes in GLP-1 concentrations are closer to the physiological range. Gastric bypass operations for obesity increase GLP-1, but do not change the levels of DPP-4 (Lugari et al.

2004; Riddle and Drucker 2006). There are two commercially available GLP-1 agonists that act like high doses of native GLP-1 to reduce body weight.

Exenatide

Exenatide (Exendin-4) is a 39-amino-acid peptide that is produced in the salivary gland of the Gila monster lizard. It has 53% homology with GLP-1, but it has a much longer half-life. Exenatide decreases food intake and body weight gain in genetically obese rats while lowering HgbA1c (Szayna et al. 2000). It also increases beta-cell mass to a greater extent than would be expected for the degree of insulin resistance (Gedulin et al. 2005). Exendin-4 crosses the blood–brain barrier and may act in the central nervous system (Rodriquez de Fonseca et al. 2000; Kastin and Akerstrom 2003). Exenatide has been approved by the FDA for treatment of type 2 diabetics who are inadequately controlled while being treated with either metformin or sulfonylureas.

In humans, exenatide reduces fasting and postprandial glucose levels, slows gastric emptying, and decreases food intake by 19% (Edwards et al. 2001). The side effects of exenatide in humans are headache, nausea, and vomiting and are lessened by gradual dose escalation (Fineman et al. 2004). Several clinical trials of 30 weeks or more have been reported (DeFronzor et al. 2005; Kendall et al. 2005; Buse et al. 2004). In one trial with 377 type 2 diabetic subjects who were failing maximal sulfonylurea therapy, exenatide produced a fall in HgbA1c of 0.74% more than observed with placebo. Fasting glucose decreased and there was a progressive weight loss of 1.6 kg (Buse et al. 2004). The interesting feature of this weight loss is that it occurred without prescribing lifestyle, diet, or exercise. A 26-week randomized control trial of exenatide produced a 2.3 kg weight loss compared to a gain of 1.8 kg in the group receiving the glargine form of insulin (Heine et al. 2005).

A systematic review of incretin therapy in type 2 diabetes (Amori et al. 2007) showed a weight loss of 2.37 kg for all GLP-1 analogues vs. control, 1.44 kg for exenatide vs. placebo injection, and 4.76 kg for exenatide vs. insulin (which often leads to weight gain). A 24-week multicenter, randomized, placebo-controlled clinical trial of exenatide enrolled diabetics poorly controlled with either metformin or sulfonylurea with a HgbA1c between 6.6% and 10.0% and a BMI between 25.0 and 39.9 kg/m². The decrease in caloric intake by exenatide (–378 ± 58 kcal per day) was not significantly different from placebo (–295 ± 58 kcal per day, $p = 0.27$). Weight loss was significantly greater and HgbA1c and blood pressure were reduced more in the exenatide-treated patients (Apovian et al. 2009).

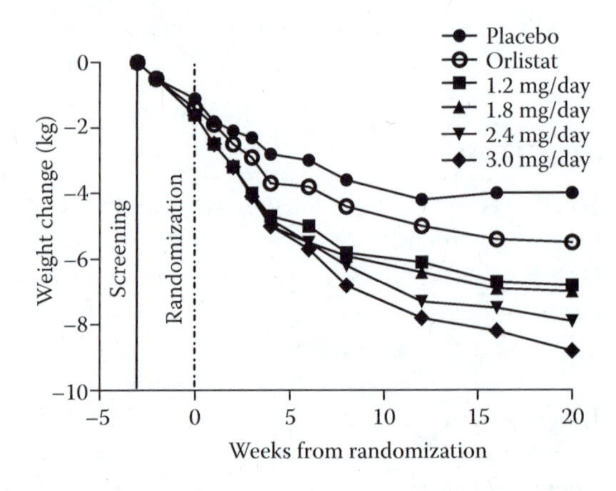

FIGURE 7.5 Effect of liraglutide and orlistat on body weight. (Data from Astrup, A., et al., *Lancet* 374, 1606–1616, 2009.)

Liraglutide

Liraglutide is another GLP-1 agonist that has a 97% homology to GLP-1. This molecular change extends the circulating half-life from 1–2 minutes to 13 hours. Liraglutide reduces body weight. In a 20-week, multicenter European clinical trial, Astrup et al. (2009) reported that daily injections of liraglutide at 1.2, 1.8, 2.4, or 3.0 mg produced weight losses of 4.8, 5.5, 6.3, and 7.2 kg, respectively, compared to 2.8 kg in the placebo-treated group and 4.1 kg in the orlistat-treated comparator group. In the group treated with 3.0 mg per day, 76% achieved a >5% weight loss compared to 30% in the placebo group. Blood pressure was significantly reduced, but there was no change in lipids. The prevalence of prediabetes was reduced 84% to 96% across groups. In a head to head comparison, liraglutide and exenatide produced similar amounts of weight loss (3.24 kg with liraglutide vs. 2.87 kg with exenatide). In poorly controlled type 2 diabetics on maximally tolerated doses of metformin and/or sulfonylurea, iraglutide reduced mean HbA(1c) significantly more than did exenatide (–1.12% vs. –0.79%) (Figure 7.5) (Buse et al. 2009).

Liraglutide has been approved by both the European Medicines Agency and the FDA for treatment of diabetes. The principal concern about liraglutide is the report of C-cell thyroid tumors in animals and the appearance of more thyroid tumors in treated placebo patients. These concerns are currently being evaluated.

Other GLP-1 Agonists

Several other GLP-1 agonists are in development (e.g., albiglutide and taspoglutide). In an 8-week trial, taspoglutide at 20 mg weekly produced a weight loss of 2.8 ± 0.3 kg compared to 0.8 ± 0.3 kg for those treated with placebo (Nauck et al. 2009).

Bupropion

Bupropion is a norepinephrine and dopamine reuptake inhibitor that is approved by the FDA for the treatment of depression and smoking cessation. Two multicenter clinical trials have examined the effect of bupropion in obese subjects with depressive symptoms and in uncomplicated overweight patients. In one study, 421 overweight patients with depressive symptoms and scores of 10 to 30 (normal to abnormal values) on a Beck Depression Inventory were randomized with 213 receiving the 400 mg per day dose of bupropion and 209 receiving the placebo for 24 weeks. The 121 subjects in the bupropion group who completed the trial lost 6.0% ± 0.5% of initial body weight compared to 2.8% ± 0.5% in the 108 subjects in the placebo group ($p < 0.0001$) (Jain et al. 2002). A study in uncomplicated overweight subjects randomized 327 subjects in equal proportions to bupropion 300 mg per day, bupropion 400 mg per day, or placebo. At 24 weeks, the 69% who remained in the study lost 5% ± 1%, 7.2 ± 1%, and 10.1 ± 1% in the placebo, bupropion 300-mg, and bupropion 400-mg groups, respectively ($p < 0.0001$). At 24 weeks, the placebo group was further randomized to either the 300-mg or 400-mg group and the trial was extended to week 48. By the end of the trial, the attrition rate was 41%, and the weight loss in the bupropion 300-mg and bupropion 400-mg groups were not significantly different (6.2% ± 1.25% in the 300-mg-per-day group and 7.2% ± 1.5% of initial body weight in the 400-mg-per-day group) (Anderson et al. 2002). In this trial the nondepressed subjects responded better to bupropion than those with depressive symptoms.

Fluoxetine

Fluoxetine is a selective serotonin reuptake inhibitor approved by the FDA to treat depression. Fluoxetine at a dose of 60 mg per day (three times the usual dose for treatment of depression) produced dose-related weight loss in overweight patients. A meta-analysis of six studies showed a wide range of weight losses. In one study, there was a loss of –14.5 kg and in another a weight gain of +0.40 kg (Li et al. 2005). Another meta-analysis also showed no significant difference between fluoxetine and placebo (Avenell et al. 2004). The mean difference in weight loss at 12 months of −0.33 kg (95% CI −1.49 to 0.82 kg) favoring fluoxetine. The problem with this drug is that after 16 to 24 weeks of treatment, patients began to regain weight, even while continuing the drug (Goldstein et al. 1995). In a review of six studies with 719 patients randomized to fluoxetine and 722 randomized to placebo, weight loss at 6 months in the placebo group was 2.2 kg vs. 4.8 kg in the fluoxetine-treated group. At 1 year, however, the weight losses were almost identical at 1.8 kg in the placebo group and 2.4 kg in the fluoxetine-treated group. Regaining 50% of the lost weight during the second 6 months of treatment on fluoxetine terminated clinical trials for weight loss with fluoxetine. However, fluoxetine may still be a useful short-term treatment in the depressed obese patient.

Topiramate

Topiramate is an antiepileptic drug that was discovered to give weight loss in the clinical trials for epilepsy (Astrup and Toubro 2004). It is a carbonic anhydrase inhibitor, blocks $GABA_A$ receptors, and is a modulator of ion channels. Weight losses of 3.9% were seen after 3 months of treatment and losses of 7.3% after 1 year (Ben-Menachemn et al. 2003). Bray et al. (2003) reported a 6-month, placebo-controlled, dose-ranging study in 385 obese subjects who were randomized to placebo or topiramate at 64 mg per day, 96 mg per day, 192 mg per day, or 384 mg per day. At 24 weeks, weight loss was 2.6%, 5%, 4.8%, 6.3%, and 6.3% in the placebo, respectively. The most frequent adverse events were paresthesias, somnolence, and difficulty with concentration, memory, and attention (Bray et al. 2003). Two multicenter trials followed that showed that subjects who completed 1 year lost 1.7%, 7%, 9.1%, and 9.7% of their initial body weight in the placebo, 89 mg per day, 192 mg per day, and 256 mg per day groups, respectively (Wilding et al. 2004). Results of the second trial were similar.

Three trials have evaluated topiramate treatment of diabetics (Rosenstock et al. 2007; Stenlof et al. 2007; Toplak et al. 2007). In a multicenter, randomized clinical trial in obese type 2 diabetic patients treated with metformin (Toplak et al. 2007), the highest dose of topiramate (192 mg per day) produced 6.5% weight loss after 24 weeks, the 96 mg per day dose produced 4.5% weight loss as compared to 1.7% in the placebo-treated group. Hemoglobin A1c also showed a dose-related decrease. Side effects included paresthesias and events related to the central nervous system.

Topiramate has also been used to treat patients with the Prader–Willi syndrome. Three subjects with Prader–Willi syndrome were treated with topiramate and had a reduction in the self-injurious behavior that is associated with this uncommon genetic disease (Chapter 5) (Shapira et al. 2002). A second study in seven additional subjects confirmed these findings (Smathers et al. 2003). A third study evaluated appetite, food intake, and weight. Although the self-injurious behavior improved, there was no effect on these other parameters (Shapira et al. 2004). Topiramate was also used to treat two subjects with nocturnal-eating syndrome and two subjects with sleep-related eating disorder. There was an improvement in all subjects and there was an 11-kg weight loss over 8.5 months with an average topiramate dose of 218 mg per day (Winkelman 2003).

COMBINATIONS OF DRUGS USED FOR WEIGHT LOSS

Development of Combination Drugs for Obesity

The concept of combining drugs that act on different biological mechanisms is well-established for many diseases. For obesity, this concept was first tried in a landmark study by Weintraub and his colleagues (Weintraub et al. 1992). When this study was conceived, drug treatment for obesity used one or another of the sympathomimetic drugs, like phentermine, or the single serotonergic drug, fenfluramine, that were approved by the FDA as treatment for obesity (Guy-Grand et al. 1988). Since both serotonergic and noradrenergic receptors modulate food intake, Weintraub reasoned that combining phentermine and fenfluramine might produce greater weight loss or reduce the side-effect profile. This new pharmacologic approach to treating obesity came to an abrupt end in 1997 when heart-valve lesions were reported in patients treated with phentermine and fenfluramine, popularly known as Fen/Phen (Connelly 2009). Within 2 months after this report, fenfluramine and dexfenfluramine were withdrawn from the market. The Fen/Phen combination was more effective than either agent alone and produced weight losses of 15% or more. The use of Fen/Phen as a treatment for obesity increased rapidly to reach a peak never seen before or since with antiobesity drugs. When fenfluramine and dexfenfluramine were withdrawn, drug prescriptions for obesity dropped precipitously (Stafford et al. 2003).

The second combination drug to be developed sprang from the observation in Denmark that a preparation used by asthmatics containing both theophylline and caffeine that was used to treat asthma also produced weight loss. In a randomized clinical trial with ephedrine and caffeine, those receiving the combination lost up to 18% of their body weight (Astrup et al. 1992). The combination was, again, significantly greater than placebo or either agent alone. Since ephedrine-like drugs and caffeine can be readily obtained from botanical sources, herbal sources of ephedra and caffeine were soon widely marketed with one company selling more than a billion dollars in 1 year until ephedra was removed from the market by the FDA because of alleged deaths from heart problems. They are no longer marketed.

Bupropion and Naltrexone

Bupropion reduces food intake by acting on adrenergic and dopaminergic receptors in the hypothalamus. Naltrexone is an opioid receptor antagonist with minimal effect on weight loss on its own. The rationale for combining bupropion with naltrexone is the idea that bupropion, acting on adrenergic receptors in the hypothalamus stimulates the production of a prohormone, proopiomelanocortin (POMC) that contains several other peptides in its amino acid sequence, including α–melanocyte-stimulating hormone (α-MSH), which reduces food intake, and β-endorphin, which stimulates food intake by acting on opioid receptors in the brain. Naltrexone blocks this inhibitory feedback by β-endorphin and increases the release of α-MSH, which can continue to inhibit feeding rather than being shut off (Greenway et al. 2009). In experimental animals, naltrexone was shown to modify the activity of the neurons in the brain that affect feeding and to enhance the amount of weight loss produced by bupropion.

With this rationale, the combination of bupropion and naltrexone were tested to validate the concept and then to show long-term effects. Bupropion has been used at a dose of 360 mg per day, halfway between the doses described earlier. Naltexone has been tested at 16, 32, and 48 mg per day in a dose-ranging study, but in later trials was used in doses of 32 and 48 mg per day. In a 24-week dose-ranging study, 419 obese subjects were randomized, but only 244 (64%) completed the 24-week trial. Among the completers, weight loss was 1.2 kg in the placebo group, 3.1 kg in the bupropion-treated group, and 1.6 kg with the 48 mg per day dose of naltrexone. When combined with bupropion, weight loss was greater and similar at all three doses of naltrexone (7.1 kg at 16 mg per day naltrexone and bupropion, 6.6 kg at 32 mg per day naltrexone and bupropion, and 6.9 kg at 48 mg per day naltrexone and bupropion). Nausea was the predominant side effect (Greenway et al. 2009b).

The clinical program designed to establish the use of this combination consists of four main trials, called Contrave Obesity Research Trials or COR trials. COR-I used both 16 and 32 mg of naltrexone with 360 mg per day of bupropropion; COR II used a single 32-mg dose of naltrexone with 360 mg of bupropion, with rerandomization at 28 weeks to 32 mg per day or 48 mg per day of naltrexone and bupropion for nonresponders. The other two trials are COR-diabetes and COR-BMod, which examine the effect of the drug combination in diabetics and for maintenance of weight loss. Some data on COR-I and COR-II are summarized in Table 7.7. In a 52-week multicenter randomized, placebo-controlled trial, the participants were predominantly younger women whose body weight was nearly 100 kg. The combination of bupropion (360 mg) and naltrexone at 16 or 32 mg

TABLE 7.7
Randomized Clinical Trials with the Combination of Bupropion and Naltrexone

Variable	Placebo	Obesity Trial	Obesity with Comorbidities
Age	44 (85% F)	44 (85% F)	
Weight	99	99	
BMI	36	35	
Completers	50%–54%	49%–54%	
Wt Loss (ITT)	1.3	5.0	6.1
Completers	1.9	6.8	8.2
Categorical > 5%	16	48	56
Waist Decrease	2.7	6.9	7.1

Source: Adapted from data presented at the 27th Annual Scientific Meeting of the Obesity Society, Washington, D.C., October 24–28, 2009.

produced greater weight loss and decrease in waist circumference than placebo. The decrease in blood triglycerides, HDL-cholesterol, glucose, and insulin improved with the degree of weight loss. Only with weight losses of >10% did blood pressure and pulse show a significant decrease. Nausea, constipation, and headache were among the more prominent side effects. There was no evidence of increased suicidal thoughts. A second trial combining naltrexone 32 mg with bupropion 360 mg and behavior modification or placebo and behavior modification reported a 9.3% ± 0.4% weight loss at 56 weeks in the drug-treated patients, compared to 5.1% ± 0.6% in the placebo group. Among completers, the weight loss was 11.5% ± 0.6% in those treated with the drug combination against 7.3% ± 0.9% in the placebo group. The fall in blood pressure was less in the drug-treated patients than in those treated with placebo. At week 56, SBP/DBP fell by 3.9 ± 0.7 / 2.8 ± 0.5 mmHg in the drug group vs. 1.3 ± 0.5 / 1.4 ± 0.3 mmHg in the placebo group. This blunting of the fall in blood pressure may offset the beneficial effects noted on the fall in triglycerides and rise in HDL-cholesterol (Wadden et al. 2010).

Topiramate and Phentermine

Topiramate is an anticonvulsant drug that was shown to reduce food intake, but was not developed clinically because of the side effects at the doses selected. Phentermine is a long-established sympathomimetic drug approved for the short-term treatment of obesity in 1959. It is a "scheduled" drug meaning that the U.S. Drug Enforcement Agency has concluded that this drug carries a low risk for potential abuse. Topiramate and phentermine have been combined in one of three combinations: 3.75, 7.5, or 15 mg of phentermine combined, respectively, with 23, 46, or 92 mg of controlled-release topiramate.

Two clinical trials have been conduced to evaluate long-term efficacy and safety of these combinations compared to placebo. One is in obese individuals with a BMI ≥ 35 kg/m^2 and a normal cardiometabolic profile (BP < 140/90, FPG < 110 mg/dL, triglycerides < 200 mg/dL) (Obesity Trial). The other is in people with less obesity but with comorbidities (BMI 27–45 kg/m^2, and two or more of the components for the metabolic syndrome, including treatment for hypertension, treatment for diabetes, or treatment for dyslipidemia) (Obesity with Comorbidities Trial). *The LEARN Manual* by Kelly Brownell provided the behavioral program for both trials. In the "Obesity" trial, the low and full dose of topiramate/phentermine were used. In the trial of "Obesity with Comorbidities," topiramate and phentermine were used at the mid and full dose. The medication was titrated over 4 weeks due to the topiramate label. A total of more than 3750 patients were included in these clinical trials (1250 in the "Obesity" trial and 2500 in the "Obesity with Comorbidities" trial). The

TABLE 7.8
Comparison of Treatment with a Combination of Topiramate and Phentermine or Placebo in Two Different Populations of Obese Patients

Variable		Obesity*			Obesity with Comorbidities+	
Age		43			51	
BMI		42.1			36.6	
Weight		256			227	
% Female		83%			70%	
Hypertension		25%			69%	
Dyslipidemia		19%			57%	
Diabetes		0%			16%	
Treatment	**Placebo**	**Low**	**Full**	**Placebo**	**Middle**	**Full**
Wt loss % ITT	1.6	5.1	11.0	1.8	8.4	10.4
Wt loss comp	2.5	7.0	14.7	2.4	10.5	13.2
Categorical >5%	17	45	67	21	62	70
>10%	12	27	60	10	49	64
>15%	5	11	43	4	26	39

Source: Adapted from data presented at the 27th Annual Scientific Meeting of the Obesity Society, Washington, D.C., October 24–28, 2009.

Note: + Obesity + Comorbidities = obese patients with comorbidities; the inclusion criteria were a BMI between 27 and 45 kg/m^2, and two or more comorbidities.

* Obesity = BMI ≥ 35 kg/m2, a BP < 140/90, FBS < 110 mg/dL, TG > 200 mg/dL.

data are summarized in Table 7.8. By design, the Obesity-Comorbidities trial had a population with many more comorbidities that were also older and had a lower BMI than the other trial. Weight loss among those who completed the trial was similar for the full dose in both trials. The categorical response for those losing >5%, greater than 10%, or greater than 15% was also similar between the two trials for the full dose. At the end of 1 year, there was an improvement in all risk factors in the high dose group, and all but diastolic blood pressure and LDL-cholesterol in the middle dose group. Side effects in both trials included dry mouth, constipation, and tingling or paresthesias. The prevalence of mental and behavioral side effects noted with topiramate alone were not prominent in these trials.

Zonisamide Alone and Combined with Naltrexone

Zonisamide is an antiepileptic drug that has serotonergic and dopaminergic activity, is a carbonic anhydrase inhibitor, and inhibits sodium and calcium channels. Weight loss was noted in the clinical trials for the treatment of epilepsy and in a 16-week randomized control trial in 60 obese subjects (Gadde 1999). Subjects eating a calorie-restricted diet were randomized to zonisamide started at 100 mg per day and increased to 400 mg per day or placebo. The zonisamide group lost 6.6% of initial body weight at 16 weeks compared to 1% in the placebo group (Gadde et al. 2003). Zonisamide in doses of 120, 240, or 360 mg per day is combined with bupropion at doses of 240 or 360 mg per day for evaluation in a 24-week trial (www.clintrials.gov NCT00339014). No published data are available for this combination.

Pramlintide and Leptin

Amylin is a peptide found in the beta-cell of the pancreas that is secreted along with insulin and circulates in the blood. Amylin is deficient in type 1 diabetes, where beta cells are immunologically destroyed. Pramlintide is a synthetic amylin analog that has a prolonged biological half-life and was approved in 2005 by the FDA for the treatment of diabetes (Riddle and Drucker 2006; Huda et al. 2006).

Pramlintide is associated with weight loss, unlike some of the other antidiabetic medications that produce weight gain. In a clinical trial with type 1 diabetics, 651 patients were randomized to placebo or subcutaneous pramlintide 60 mcg three or four times a day, along with an insulin injection. Body weight decreased 1.2 kg relative to placebo and the hemoglobin A1c decreased 0.29%–0.34% (Ratner et al. 2004). An analysis of two 1-year-long studies in insulin-treated type 2 diabetics showed a weight loss of 2.6 kg and a decrease in hemoglobin A1c of 0.5% in subjects with pramlintide doses of 120 mcg twice a day or 150 mcg three times a day (Maggs et al. 2003). Interestingly, African-Americans lost more weight (4 kg), than either Caucasians or Hispanics (2.4 kg and 2.3 kg, respectively). The improvement in diabetes correlated with the weight loss, suggesting that pramlintide is effective in ethnic groups with the greatest burden from overweight. The most common adverse event was nausea, which was usually mild and confined to the first 4 weeks of therapy (Chapman et al. 2005, 2007; Aronne et al. 2007).

Leptin is a hormone produced and secreted by the fat cell. When deficient, it causes massive overweight in animals and man. Treatment with leptin reverses the obesity in leptin-deficient people. The discovery of leptin generated hope that leptin would be an effective treatment for obesity, but except for the rare leptin-deficient individual, treatment with leptin has been a disappointment. Leptin injections at doses of 0.01 mg/kg, 0.05 mg/kg, 0.1 mg/kg, and 0.3 mg/kg daily were relatively ineffective in the treatment of obesity in human subjects (Hukshorn et al. 2000, 2003; Heymsfield et al. 1999).

However, leptin therapy does ameliorate many of the symptoms of lipodystrophy (Oral et al. 2002; Chong 2010). During the 4 months of therapy in lipodystrophic patients, triglyceride levels decreased by 60%, liver volume was reduced by an average of 28%, and resting metabolic rate decreased significantly with therapy (Rosenbaum et al. 2002). Leptin also ameliorates many of the effects associated with calorie restriction, including attenuating the decreased 24-hour energy expenditure and thyroid hormone levels. Leptin also reversed many of the changes in the brain as assessed by functional magnetic resonance (fMRI) associated with hunger in subjects stabilized at 10% below their usual weight (Rosenbaum et al. 2008).

The idea of combining leptin and pramlintide was tested in animals and produced additive weight loss (Roth et al. 2009). In a clinical trial to test this concept, 177 patients with a BMI between 27 and 35 kg/m^2 were enrolled in a study with a 4-week run-in, during which amylin (pramlintide) was begun at a dose of 180 mcg twice a day for 2 weeks, then 360 mcg twice a day for 2 weeks, followed by a 24-week randomized double-blind trial with combined pramlintide and metreleptin (metreleptin = recombinant human leptin) (Ravussin et al. 2009). The 139 patients who lost 2%–8% of body weight during the first 4-week run-in were randomized 2:2:1 to treatment with pramlintide 360 mcg/leptin 5 mg, pramlintide 360 mcg/placebo, or metreleptin 5 mg/placebo for the remaining 20 weeks. The pramlintide/placebo group lost 8.4% of their body weight; the pramlintide/metreleptin group lost 12.7%. The additive effect of the two peptides is evident in this trial (Figure 7.6).

Pramlintide and Phentermine or Sibutramine

Since pramlintide and sympathomimetics operate by different mechanisms, combining pramlintide with either sibutramine or phentermine was an obvious step. In a multicenter trial using that strategy, Aronne et al. (2010) showed that over 24 weeks, the weight loss that was 2% with pramlintide alone rose to just over 10% when combined with either phentermine or sibutramine (Figure 7.7). All patients also received lifestyle intervention. Following a 1-week placebo lead-in, 244 obese or overweight, nondiabetic subjects (88% female; 41 ± 11 y; BMI 37.7 ± 5.4 kg/m^2; weight 103 ± 19 kg; mean ± SD) were treated with subcutaneous placebo injections (sc) three times a day, pramlintide subcutaneously (120 μg three times a day), pramlintide subcutaneously (120 μg three times a day)

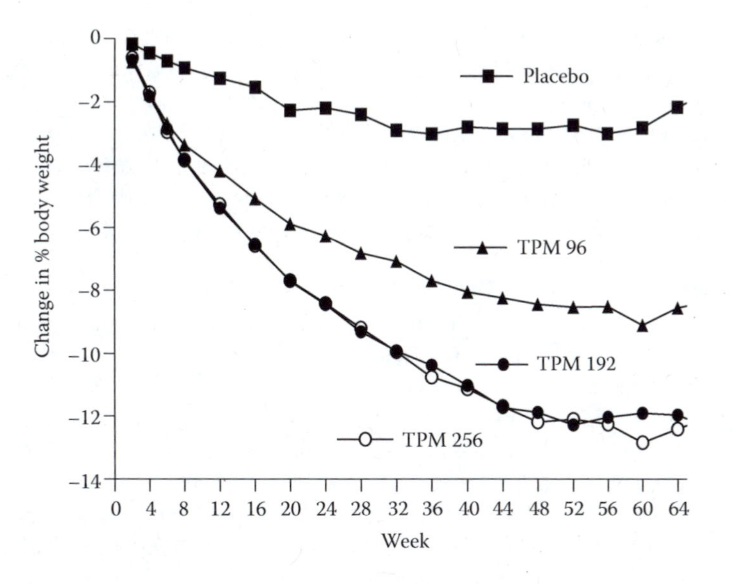

FIGURE 7.6 Weight loss with topiramate in a 6-month trial. (Redrawn from Bray, G., et al., *Obes Res* 11(6), 722–733, 2003.)

+ oral sibutramine (10 mg every morning), or pramlintide subcutaneously (120 μg three times a day) + oral phentermine (37.5 mg every morning) for 24 weeks. Treatment was single-blind for subjects receiving subcutaneous medication only and open-label for subjects in the combination arms. Weight loss achieved at week 24 with either combination treatment was greater than with pramlintide alone or placebo ($p < 0.001$; 11.1% ± 1.1% with pramlintide + sibutramine, 11.3% ± 0.9% with

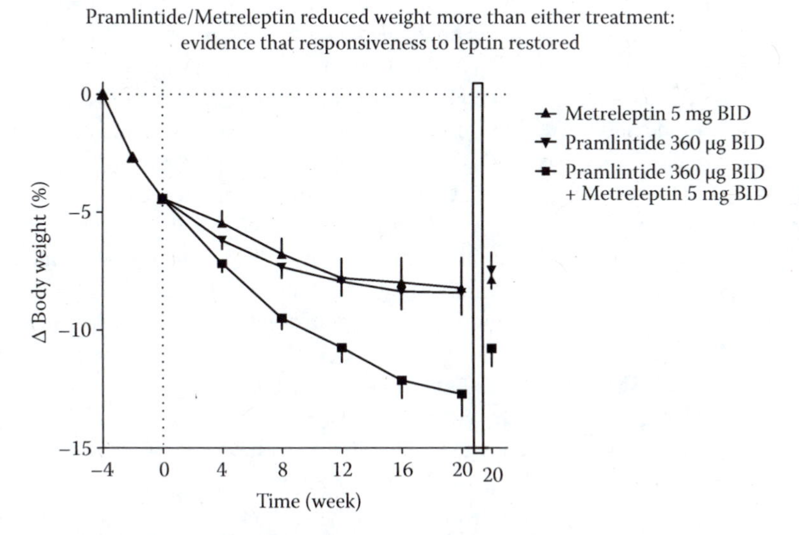

FIGURE 7.7 Weight loss with the combination of pramlintide and sibutamine. (Redrawn from Aronne, L.J., et al., *Obesity (Silver Spring)*, 18(9), 1739–1746, 2010.)

pramlintide + phentermine, 3.7% ± 0.7% with pramlintide alone; and 2.2% ± 0.7% with placebo; mean ± SE). Elevations from baseline in heart rate and diastolic blood pressure were demonstrated with both pramlintide + sibutramine (3.1 ± 1.2 beats per minute [BPM], $p < 0.05$; 2.7 ± 0.9 mmHg, $p < 0.01$) and pramlintide + phentermine (4.5 ± 1.3 BPM, $p < 0.01$; 3.5 ± 1.2 mmHg $p < 0.001$) using 24-hour ambulatory monitoring. However, in the majority of subjects receiving these treatments, blood pressure remained within normal ranges. These results support the potential of combining pramlintide with either sibutramine or phentermine to treat obesity.

Drugs Approved for Attention Deficit Hyperactive Disorder

Ritalin. Ritalin is used in the treatment of attention deficit disorder and also produces weight loss. In a placebo-controlled clinical trial of ritalin and cafilon, a combination of two sympathomimetic drugs, FitzGerald and McElearney (1957) enrolled 31 patients, of whom 25 completed the study. Placebo or drug was assigned by the pharmacist and not known to the patient, although whether they were in the ritalin-placebo or calfilon-placebo group was known. A diet with 1200 kcal per day was prescribed and treatment lasted about two weeks. The difference between ritalin and placebo was a 1.04 ± 0.31 lb (0.47 ± 0.17 kg $p < 0.0001$) weight loss and the difference between cafilon and placebo was a 2.4 ± 0.48 lb (1.1 ± 0.22 kg $p < 0.0001$) weight loss in this short trial.

Atomoxetine. Atomoxetine is a potent inhibitor of norepinephrine reuptake within the central nervous system that is used to treat Attention Deficit-Hyperactive Disorder (ADHD). In a small, 12-week, randomized clinical trial in patients with an average BMI of 36.1 ± 0.6 (m ± SEM), the 12 patients treated with atomoxetine lost 3.6 ± 1.0 kg (–3.7%) vs. a gain of 0.1 ± 0.4 kg (0.2% gain) among the 14 in the placebo group. Side effects were reported as minimal (Gadde et al. 2006).

DRUGS IN LATE STAGES OF CLINICAL EVALUATION

LORCASERIN

The neurotransmitter serotonin is involved in the regulation of food intake and food preference. Mice lacking the serotonin $5HT_{2C}$ receptor have increased food intake because they take longer to become satiated. These mice are also resistant to fenfluramine, a serotonin agonist that causes weight loss. A human mutation of the 5HT-2c receptor has been identified that is associated with early-onset human obesity (Gibson et al. 2004; Nilsson 2005). The precursor of serotonin, 5-hydroxytryptophan, reduces food intake and body weight in clinical studies (Cangiano et al. 1992; Cangiano et al. 1998). Fenfluramine and dexfenfluramine are serotonergic agents and reuptake inhibitors that reduce food intake in human studies (Meguid et al. 2000; Foltin et al. 1996; Guy-Grand et al. 1988; Drent et al. 1995), but were withdrawn from the market in 1997 due to cardiovascular side effects. Meta-chlorophenylpiperazine, a direct serotonin agonist, reduces food intake by 28% in women and 20% in men (Cowen et al. 1995). Another serotoninergic drug, sumatriptan, which acts on the 5-HT1B/1D receptor, also reduced food intake in human subjects (Boeles et al. 1997).

Lorcaserin is a potent, selective serotonin $5\text{-}HT_{2C}$ agonist with ~15-fold and 100-fold selectivity vs. $5\text{-}HT_{2A}$ and $5\text{-}HT_{2B}$ receptors, respectively. In a 12-week, dose-ranging study, a total of 459 male and female subjects with BMIs between 29 and 46 kg/m^2, with an average weight of 100 kg, were enrolled in a randomized, double-blind controlled trial comparing placebo against 10- and 15-mg doses given once daily, and 10 mg given twice daily (20 mg per day). The placebo group lost 0.32 kg (N = 88 completers) compared to 1.8 kg in the 10 mg per day dose given twice daily (N = 86), 2.6 kg in the 15 mg per day dose (N = 82 completers), and 3.6 kg in the 10 mg twice daily (20 mg total) (N = 77 completers). The proportions of completers achieving ≥5% of initial body weight were 12.8%, 19.5%, 31.2%, and 2.3% in the 10 mg once daily, 15 mg once daily, 10 mg twice daily, and placebo groups, respectively. The most frequent adverse events were transient headache, nausea, and dizziness. Echocardiograms showed no apparent drug-related effects on heart valves or pulmonary artery pressure (Smith et al. 2009).

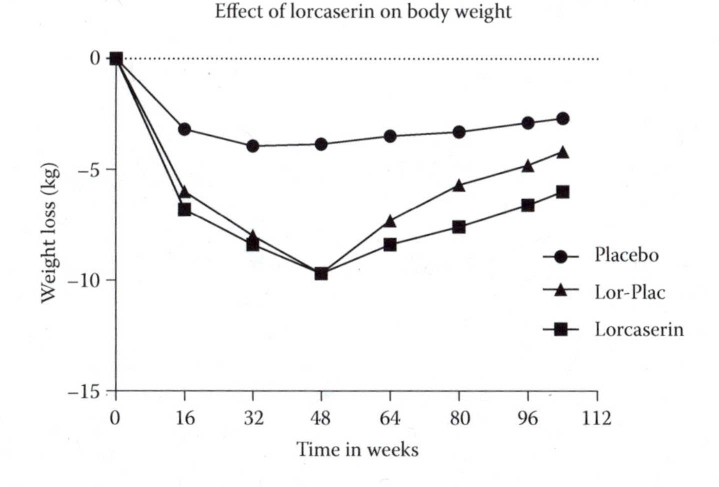

FIGURE 7.8 Weight loss in a 2-year randomized, double-blind, placebo-controlled trial with lorcaserin. (Data plotted from Smith S.R. et al., *N. Engl. J. Med.*, 363, 245–256, 2010.)

In a 2-year, double-blind, multicenter study, 1595 obese men and women were randomized to lorcaserin 10 mg twice daily and 1587 to placebo (Figure 7.8). Participants received a 600 kcal per day deficit diet and a healthy lifestyle program with occasional meetings with a dietitian and a recommendation to walk 30 min per day. Echocardiograms were performed at baseline, weeks 24, 52, 74, and 102. Primary endpoints were weight loss and maintenance of weight loss. Age was 18–65, BMI 27 and up with comorbidities, 30 and up without them. Taking selective serotonin reuptake inhibitors was an exclusion. Of the 883 patients in the Lorcaserin group, 716 entered the second year. Body weight reached a minimum of 9.7 kg below baseline by 48 weeks but had risen to 6.0 below baseline kg at 102 weeks in those who remained on lorcaserin throughout. In those switched to placebo, the weight increase was greater, rising to −4.2kg at 48 weeks, compared to −3.85 at 48 weeks and −2.7 kg at 102 weeks in the placebo group. The weight change and some of the metabolic responses are summarized in Table 7.9. Blood pressure, heart rate, triglycerides,

TABLE 7.9
Effect of Lorcaserin in a 1-Year Clinical Trial

Variable	Placebo	Lorcaserin
N	1587	1595
Age (years)	44	43.8
Weight (kg)	~100	~100
Weight loss ITT	−2.2	−5.8
Per protocol	−3.4	−8.2
Percent losing > 5%	33%	67%
>10%	15%	33%
Waist circum decrease	−3.9 cm	−6.8 cm
hs-CRP	−0.075	−1.378
Fibrinogen	−7.7	−22.3
Quality of life improvement	10.7	12.4

Source: Adapted from data presented at the 27th Annual Scientific Meeting of the Obesity Society, Washington, D.C., October 24–28, 2009.

glucose, HOMA-IR, and C-reactive protein improved, but there was no change in HDL-cholesterol (Smith et al. 2010).

Tesofensine

Tesofensine is a triple monoamine reuptake inhibitor. It blocks the reuptake of serotonin, norepinephrine, and dopamine. Other drugs with this mechanism include sibutramine, a weight loss drug, and venlafaxine, an antidepressant. The initial clinical data on the potential effectiveness of this drug came from "pseudoserendipitous" studies of its effect in neurological diseases. Weight loss was noted in patients with Parkinson's or Alzheimer's disease who were treated with tesofensine (Astrup et al. 2008). This was followed by a randomized double-blind clinical trial in 203 patients who were randomly assigned to placebo or doses of 0.25, 0.5, or 1 mg per day of tesofensine. In 24 weeks, the placebo-treated group lost 2.0% compared to 6.5% in the 0.25-mg-per-day dose, 11.2% in the 0.5-mg-per-day dose, and 12.6% in the 1.0 mg-per-day dose. In the two highest dose groups, tesofensine decreased BMI by 4 units. There were small increases in heart rate and blood pressure, but the clinical profile was relatively free of untoward side effects. The findings about potential cardiovascular risk from the SCOUT trial dealing with sibutramine noted previously may apply to tesofensine and is a potential hurdle for approval of the drug (Figure 7.9).

Cetilistat: A Lipase Inhibitor

Cetilistat (ATL-962), like orlistat, is a gastrointestinal lipase inhibitor. A 5-day trial of cetilistat in 90 normal volunteers showed a three- to seven-fold increase in fecal fat that was dose-dependent, but only 11% of subjects had more than one oily stool. It was suggested that this lipase inhibitor may have fewer gastrointestinal adverse events compared to orlistat (Dunk et al. 2002).

A 12-week study with 372 patients compared placebo with doses of 60, 120, or 240 mg of cetilistat three times a day, and a weight loss between 3.5 and 4 kg compared with a 2-kg loss in the placebo-treated group. In a second phase II study, doses of 40, 80, and 120 mg three times a day were given to type 2 diabetics who showed a dose-related reduction in body weight and in hemoglobin A1c (Bryson et al. 2009; Kopelman et al. 2007; Kopelman et al. 2010).

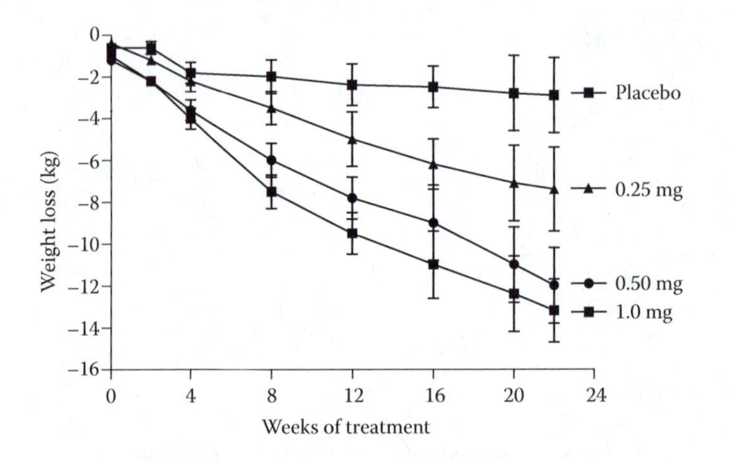

FIGURE 7.9 Weight loss with tesofensine. (Data redrawn from Astrup, A. et al., *Lancet*, 374(9701), 1606–16, 2009.)

CONCEPTS FOR ANTIOBESITY DRUGS IN EARLIER STAGES OF DEVELOPMENT

Gastrointestinal Peptides

PYY 3-36

Polypeptide YY 3-36 (PYY3-36) is a hormone produced by the L-cells in the gastrointestinal tract and is secreted in proportion to the caloric content of a meal. PYY 3-36 levels are lower in obese subjects, both fasting and after a meal than in lean subjects. Caloric intake at a lunch buffet was reduced by 30% in 12 obese subjects and by 29% in 12 lean subjects after a 2-hour intravenous infusion of PYY 3-36 infused intravenously (Batterham et al. 2003). Thrice daily nasal administration over 6 days was well-tolerated and reduced caloric intake by about 30% while giving 0.6 kg weight loss (Brandt et al. 2004). Development of a nasal spray formulation for PYY3-36 has undergone a Phase I clinical trial, but no published data are available.

Oxyntomodulin

Oxyntomodulin is another gastrointestinal peptide that is produced in the L-cells of the intestine from the same peptide precursor that also produces PYY3-36. Oxyntomodulin is released in response to food. Animals injected with oxyntomodulin have a reduction in body fat and food intake. In a short-term clinical study, food intake was reduced by 19.3% after oxyntomodulin compared to a placebo infusion. In a 4-week randomized, double-blind, placebo-controlled trial, overweight volunteers injected oxyntomodulin subcutaneously 3 times a day 30 minutes before meals. Body weight was reduced 2.3 ± 0.4 kg in the group receiving oxyntomodulin compared to 0.5 ± 0.5 kg in the placebo group. Energy intake in the treated group decreased by 170 ± 37 kcal (25% ± 5%) at the beginning study meal and by 250 ± 63 kcal (35% ± 9%) at the final meal (Wynne et al. 2005). Further studies on this intriguing peptide are awaited.

11{beta}-Hydroxysteroid Dehydrogenase Type I Inhibitor

Cortisol, the glucocorticoid secreted by the adrenal gland, can be inactivated through conversion to cortisone in peripheral tissues. Cortisone can be reactivated by the enzyme 11{beta}-hydroxysteroid dehydrogenase type 1. Mice where this enzyme is overexpressed have increased amounts of abdominal fat, suggesting that modulation of this enzyme could be a target to selectively modulate visceral or central adiposity (Hughes et al. 2008; Morton and Seckl 2008).

Ghrelin Antagonists

Ghrelin is a small peptide synthesized in the stomach. Its active form contains an octanoate on the second amino acid. The level rises with fasting and declines after eating, suggesting it may be a signal for eating. Chronic administration produces hyperphagia and weight gain in animals. Moreover, overweight subjects have lower levels than normal weight individuals.

Ghrelin acts at the growth hormone secretogogue receptor (GHSR) to produce its effects. A group of growth hormone stimulating peptides also act on this GHSR to increase food intake in human subjects (Laferrere, Abraham et al. 2005). Antagonists to this receptor might thus be useful drugs for treating overweight patients, and this is supported by suppression of food intake and attenuated weight regain in diet-induced obese (DIO) mice treated with such drugs.

In a 2-year study with a ghrelin-mimetic (Merck's compounds MK-677) 65 men and women aged 60 to 81 were randomized to receive MK-677 25 mg per day or placebo in a double-blind, modified, single-university crossover study. Over 12 months, the ghrelin mimetic enhanced growth hormone pulsatility, increased insulin-like growth factor 1, increased lean body mass by 1.1 kg (95% CI 0.7 to 1.5 kg) vs. a decrease of 0.5 (95% CI −1.1 to 0.2 kg) in the placebo group. No significant changes were observed in visceral fat or total fat mass, but fat mass in the limb was increased.

Body weight increased 0.8 kg in the placebo group vs. 2.7 kg in the MK-677 treated group. Insulin resistance increased (glucose increased 5 mg/dL (0.3mmol/L) and Quicki index was reduced $p < 0.001$). Hemoglobin A1c increased 0.2% in the MK-677 group vs. a fall of −0.1% in the placebo group ($p < 0.002$). Cortisol increased 47 nmol/L in the MK-677 recipients. The increased fat-free mass did not translate into change of strength or function (Nass et al. 2008).

Modulation of Energy Sensing in the Brain

Cells in the body can respond to changes in energy use through monitoring the ratio of adenosine 5′-monophosphate (AMP) to adenosine triphosphate (ATP), which reflect the status of energy storage in high energy phosphate bonds of ATP. In selected regions of the brain changes in the ratio of AMP to ATP may be particularly important in modulating food intake and energy balance. The discovery that blockade of the fatty acid synthase with cerulenin, a naturally occurring product or a synthetic molecule (C-75) opened the door to these insights (Makimura et al. 2001) Fatty acid synthesis and oxidation are coordinately regulated. Adenosine 5′-monophosphate activated kinase (AMPK) phosphorylates acetyl-Co-carboxylase to inhibit the enzyme that converts acetyl-CoA to malonyl CoA in the first step toward long-chain fatty acid synthesis. AMP kinase dephosphorylates malonyl Co-A decarboxylase, which activates this enzyme that lowers malonyl-CoA concentration. The net effect of these phosphorylations by AMP-kinase is to convert substrate to oxidation rather than fatty acid synthesis. Cerulenin or C-75 block fatty acid synthase, which also blocks fat synthesis and activates fatty acid oxidation by activating carnitine palitoyl Co-A transferase-I. Injection of these fatty acid synthase inhibitors into animals produces a reduction in food intake and weight loss, suggesting the potential for future clinical drugs (Xue et al. 2006).

Adiponectin

Adiponectin, also called adipocyte complement-related protein (ACRP), is produced exclusively in fat cells, and is their most abundant protein. It has a long half-life in the blood and is of interest because its production and secretion by the fat cell is decreased as the fat cell increases in size. Higher levels of adiponectin are associated with insulin sensitivity and lower levels of adiponectin, as seen in obesity, are associated with insulin resistance. In experimental studies, adiponectin has been shown to reduce food intake when administered into the brain (Kubota et al. 2007). Although a large molecule, drugs that modulate its production, release, or action may be potential candidates for treating obesity.

Histamine and Histamine H-3 Receptor Antagonists

Histamine and its receptors can affect food intake. Among the antipsychotic drugs that produce weight gain, binding to the H-1 receptor is higher than with any other monoamine receptor and histamine reduces food intake by acting on this receptor (Chiba and Sakata 2009). The search for drugs that can modulate food intake through the histamine system has focused on the histamine H3 receptor, which is an autoreceptor, that is, activation of this receptor inhibits histamine release, whereas blockade of the receptor increases histamine release. Both imidazole and nonimidazole antagonists of the H3 receptor have been published and shown to reduce food intake and body weight gain in experimental animals (Goudie et al. 2003; Kim et al. 2007).

Histamine injected into cat brains reduced food intake (Barak et al. 2008). L-histidine that is converted to histamine also reduced food intake and metoprine that blocks histamine breakdown also suppresses food intake in rats. Conversely, alpha-fluormethylhistidine, which irreversibly inhibits histidine decarboxylase, increases food intake. A clinical trial with betahistine, an orally active histamine agonist enters the central nervous system and is used to treat vestibular disorders. In a randomized, placebo-controlled 12-week clinical trial, 281 obese people were treated with 8, 16, or

24 mg per day of betahistine or placebo twice daily. The overall weight loss was not significantly different between treatment groups, but the subgroup of white women under age 50 lost −4.24 ± 3.87 kg treated with 48 mg ($N = 23$) compared to −1.65 ± 2.96 kg (p −0.005).

COMPLEMENTARY AND HERBAL MEDICINE

The Dietary Supplement Health Education Act of 1994 provided the framework for an expansion in the use of dietary supplements by Americans. Information about the frequency of use was obtained by a random digit-dialed telephone survey of 3500 U.S. adults aged 18 and older with a 28% response rate (Pillitteria et al. 2006). In this survey, females, young, less well-educated, and lower income individuals were more likely to use these products. Many respondents believed that dietary supplements are safer than prescription or over-the-counter medications, and many over-estimated the degree of regulatory screening of these products. Using a cross-sectional population-based telephone survey by health behaviors from Sept 2002 through Dec 2002, Blanck et al. (2007) estimated that 15.2% of adults (women 20.6% and men 9.7%) had ever used a weight-loss supplement, and 8.7% had used one in the past year (11.3% women and 6.0% men). Almost 10% (10.2%) had used them for 12 months or more and almost one-third (30.2%) had used them in the past year with nearly three-quarters of this group (73.8%) using products containing ephedra, caffeine, and/or bitter orange. In this time period, ephedra/ephedrine products topped the list (55%) followed by chromium, hydroxycitrate, and bitter orange. However, since this data was collected in 2002 before the FDA removed the ephedra products, the order of preference is different. Data in this discussion have come largely from two recent reviews, and commentaries have examined randomized clinical trials for complementary therapies for reducing body weight (Dwyer et al. 2005; Pittler and Ernst 2005).

Interventions Requiring Special Training

Acupuncture/Acupressure

Acupuncture consists of placing needles at key points controlling neural connections for relief of pain and other clinical purposes. Pittler and Ernst (2005) identified four randomized, controlled trials in which sham treatments were used. Two of the randomized trials of acupuncture reported a reduction in hunger, whereas two others showed no differences in body weight. Overall the evidence does not support a specific acupuncture procedure that works. A systematic review (Cho et al. 2009) suggests that acupuncture is an effective treatment for obesity, but about two-thirds of the studies were of low quality. Compared to lifestyle, acupuncture produced weight loss of 1.79 kg. When compared with placebo or sham therapy, acupuncture produced a 1.90 kg weight loss. However, the poor quality of many of the studies leaves us with concern.

Homeopathy

Two different preparations have been used in homeopathic doses to treat overweight and they were reflected in two randomized, controlled trials. Helianthus tuberoses D1 was investigated for 3 months in one trial, where those receiving the active ingredient lost 7.1 kg, which was significantly more than in the placebo group. In a second trial, a single dose of Thyroidinum 30cH was given to fasting patients, but it was no more effective than placebo.

Hypnotherapy

Hypnotherapy has been examined in six randomized, controlled trials that compared hypnotherapy plus cognitive behavior therapy to cognitive behavior therapy alone. The addition of hypnotherapy to cognitive behavior therapy adds a small, but significant weight loss to the cognitive behavior therapy (Pittler and Ernst 2005).

Minerals and Metabolites

Chromium Picolinate

Chromium is a trace mineral and a cofactor to insulin. It has been claimed that chromium can cause weight loss and fat loss while increasing lean body mass. A recent meta-analysis of 10 double-blind, randomized controlled trials in participants with a BMI between 28 and 33 kg/m^2 showed a statistically significant weight loss of 1.1 to 1.2 kg over a 6- to 14-week treatment period. There were no adverse events, but the authors pointed out that this weight loss, although statistically significant, was not clinically significant (Pittler and Ernst 2004). This data has to be interpreted cautiously, since it relies heavily on one robust study. Cefalu et al., in a review of the field, have shown that chromium picolinate may have a significant effect in preventing weight regain (Cefalu et al. 2002). Dwyer et al. (2005) conclude that there is little evidence of benefit and few or no adverse events.

Hydroxymethyl Butyrate

β-hydorxy-β-methylbutyrate is a metabolite of leucine. It acts in vivo to inhibit the breakdown of protein. The literature review by Pittler and Ernst (2005) found two randomized, controlled trials that reported significant differences in fat mass reduction and at least a trend toward an increase in lean body mass. Further studies are clearly needed.

Pyruvate

Pyruvate is an intermediary in the metabolism of glucose and also serves as a hydrogen shuttle between liver and muscle. It has been suggested to improve exercise performance and body composition. Pittler and Ernst (2005) identified two randomized, controlled trials that included subjects with a BMI of 25 kg/m^2 or above. There were no significant effects on body weight reduction compared to placebo. They conclude that the case for pyruvate is weak.

Conjugated Linoleic Acid

The word "conjugated" in linoleic acid refers to the position of the double-bond between carbons 9–11 or 10–12. There are differences in effects of each of the isomeric combinations. In an analysis of 13 randomized, controlled trials lasting 6 months or less, Larsen et al. (2003) reported that there was little evidence that conjugated linoleic acid produced weight loss in human beings, although one report suggests it lowers body fat without an effect on body weight (Riserus et al. 2004). There is also concern about liver toxicity from the trans-10, cis-12 isomer. Dwyer et al. (2005) conclude that there is little evidence of benefit.

Calcium

Nearly 20 years ago McCarron et al. (1984) reported that there was a negative relationship between body mass index and dietary calcium intake in the data collected by the National Center for Health Statistics. More recently, Zemel et al. (2000) found that there was a strong inverse relationship between calcium intake and the risk of being in the highest quartile of the BMI. These studies have prompted a reevaluation of studies measuring calcium intake or giving calcium orally. In the prospective trials, subjects receiving calcium had a greater weight loss than those receiving placebos. Increasing calcium from 0 to nearly 2000 g per day was associated with a reduction in BMI of about 5 units (Davies et al. 2000). These data might suggest that low calcium intake played a role in the current epidemic of overweight. However, three controlled clinical trials have failed to show an effect of calcium on weight loss, leaving the issue in limbo (Shapses et al. 2004; Shapses et al. 2001; Barr 2003).

The relationship of calcium and body weight is the most confusing, because there is a patent issued for the effects of dairy products for producing weight loss issued to one of the proponents of this approach. Such a relationship where monetary gain is associated with publication of positive studies raises concerns when reading the published studies. Moreover, there is inconsistency in both the animal and human studies. In one small clinical trial increasing dietary intake of calcium by adding 800 mg per day of supplemental calcium to a diet containing 400–500 mg per day was claimed to augment weight loss and fat loss on reducing diets (Zemel et al. 2004). In two small studies in African-American adults, Zemel et al. (2005) claimed that substitution of calcium-rich foods in isocaloric diets reduced adiposity and improved metabolic profiles during a 24-week trial. In another small study, Zemel et al. (2005) randomized 34 subjects to receive a control calcium diet with 400–500 mg per day ($N = 16$) or a yogurt supplemented diet ($N = 18$) for 12 weeks. In this small, short duration study, fat loss was greater on the yogurt diet (–4.43 kg) than the control diet (–2.75 kg). Based on this data, they claim that yogurt enhances central fat loss (Zemel et al. 2005). In a large multicenter trial that enrolled nearly 100 subjects, the same authors claim that a hypocaloric diet with calcium supplemented to the level of 1400 mg per day did not significantly improve weight loss or body composition when compared to a diet with lower calcium intake (600 mg per day), whereas a diet with three servings per day of dairy products augmented weight and fat loss (Zemel et al. 2005).

Two other studies, however, failed to find any effect of calcium supplementation on body weight or body fat (Shapses et al. 2004; Barr 2003). A large randomized clinical trial examined the effect of 1500 mg per day of calcium (as calcium carbonate) vs. placebo in a double-blind 2-year trial in 340 overweight (39%) or obese (61%) men ($N = 95$) and women ($N = 245$). Of these 75% completed the trial. Calcium supplementation had no effect on body weight, body fat, or BMI, but did reduce circulating parathyroid hormone, as expected (Yanovski et al. 2009). Dwyer et al. (2005) conclude that the evidence of benefit is equivocal and limited to small trials, but there are no major concerns regarding adverse events.

Herbal Dietary Supplements

Green Tea Extract

Green tea contains epigallo-catechin gallates that have been shown to increase energy expenditure by about 4% to 10% in a metabolic ward setting (Dulloo et al.) and in an outpatient setting, but not consistently. In a comparison of green tea extract, tyrosine, and caffeine against a placebo, Belza et al. (2006) found that only caffeine increased energy expenditure over 4 hours. Green tea extract (epigallocatechin gallate or EGCG) and caffeine or placebo were used in a weight maintenance randomized controlled trial in 76 subjects who lost 5.9 kg with a 4-week VLED, followed by 3 months of weight maintenance. High caffeine users lost more weight, fat mass, and waist circumference than low caffeine consumers. In the high caffeine consumers, no effects were seen with the EGCG + caffeine mixture during weight maintenance, but there was further weight loss in the low caffeine consumers (Westerterp-Plantega et al. 2005).

Ephedra sinica

Ephedra sinica is an evergreen that grows in central Asia and its principal ingredient is ephedrine. Ephedrine with caffeine has been shown to produce weight loss in randomized, placebo-controlled clinical trials (Astrup et al. 1992). The ephedra alkaloids from Ma huang contain ephedrine and two randomized, placebo-controlled clinical trials, one of 3 months and one of 6 months showed significantly greater weight loss than with placebo (Boozer et al. 2001). The ephedra-containing herbal preparations were pulled from the market by the FDA in April of 2004 because of alleged harmful cardiovascular side effects (Shekelle et al. 2003), but this, as stated above, has recently been reversed.

Garcinia cambogia

Garcinia cambogia contains hydroxycitric acid, an inhibitor of a citrate cleavage enzyme (ATP; citrate lyase) that inhibits fatty acid synthesis from carbohydrate. Hydroxycitrate was studied by

Roche in the 1970s and was shown to reduce food intake and cause weight loss in rodents (Sullivan and Triscari 1977). Although there have been reports of successful weight loss with small studies in humans, some of which were combined other herbs, the largest and best designed placebo-controlled study demonstrated no difference in weight loss compared to a placebo (Heymsfield et al. 1998; Pittler and Ernst 2004). Thus, there is no evidence for efficacy.

Yohimbine from *Pausinystalia yohimbe*

Yohimbine is an α_2-adrenergic receptor antagonist that is isolated from *Pausinystalia yohimbe*. The three randomized clinical trials that Pittler and Ernst identified (Pittler and Ernst 2005) give conflicting results as to whether there is significant weight loss with this plant extract compared to placebo.

Hoodia

Hoodia gordonii is a cactus that grows in Africa. It has been eaten by Bushmen to decrease appetite and thirst on long treks across the desert. The active ingredient is a steroidal glycoside called P57AS3 or just P57. P57 injected into the third ventricle of animals increases the ATP content of hypothalamic tissue by 50%–150% and decreases food intake by 40%–60% over 24 hours (Phytopharm). Phytopharm is developing P57 in partnership with Unilever. Information on the Phytopharm Web site describes a double-blind, 15-day trial in which 19 overweight males were randomized to P57 or placebo. Nine subjects in each group completed that study. There was a statistically significant decrease in calorie intake and body fat with good safety. Since Hoodia is a rare cactus in the wild and cultivation is difficult, it is not clear what the dietary herbal supplements claiming to contain Hoodia actually contain or if they are effective in causing weight loss.

Citrus aurantium (Bitter Orange)

Since the withdrawal of ephedra from the dietary herbal supplement market, manufacturers of dietary herbal supplements for weight loss have turned to citrus aurantium, which contains phenylephrine. A recent systematic review found only one randomized, placebo-controlled trial involving 20 subjects treated with Citrus aurantium for 6 weeks. This trial demonstrated no statistically significant benefit for weight loss (Bent et al. 2004). There have been reports of cardiovascular events associated with the use of citrus aurantium, including a prolonged QT interval with syncope and an acute myocardial infarction (Nasir et al. 2004; Nykamp et al. 2004). Thus, there is no evidence for efficacy of citrus aurantium in the treatment of overweight, but concern does exist regarding its safety. Dwyer et al. (2005) conclude that there is no adequate evidence for efficacy and that there are safety concerns. Thermogenic compounds from *Citrus aurantium* were administered to 30 healthy normal and overweight men and women. The thermic effect of food was 20% lower in women than in men. The thermogenic response to a single dose of C. aurantium extract was higher in men, but when added to a meal, *C. aurantium* only increased the thermic response in women (Gougeon et al. 2005).

Ayurvedic Preparations

Ayurvedic medicine is the traditional medicine of India. Ayurvedic herbal preparations containing *Triphala guggul* have been assessed in one randomized clinical trial (Pittler and Ernst 2005). Patients in the treated group lost between 7.9 and 8.2 kg, which was significantly greater than placebo (Paranjpe et al. 1990).

In another study examining a combination of tyrosine, capsaicin, catechines, and caffeine, Belza et al. (2007) reported a 24-kcal increase in the drug-treated group.

Fiber

The possibility that fiber might be useful in maintaining lower weight comes from epidemiological studies. A recent reexamination of data from the Seven Countries Studies has shown that the fiber intake within each of the participating countries was inversely related to the body weight. Men eating more fiber had lower body weight. Epidemiological data suggests that countries that have higher fiber consumption have a lower prevalence of obesity (Kromhout et al. 2001). Fiber intake may also be inversely related to the development of heart disease (Wolk et al. 1999) and diabetes (Salmeron et al. 1997).

Chitosan

Chitosan is a partially deacetylated polymer of *N*-acetylglucosamine derived from the polysaccharide chitin. It is a dietary fiber derived from crustaceans that has been advocated as a weight loss agent. A recent systematic review of the randomized clinical trials of chitosan concluded, based on 14 trials longer than 4 weeks involving 1071 subjects, that chitosan gives 1.7 kg weight loss that is statistically significant (Mhurchu et al. 2005). This degree of weight loss falls far short of the 5 kg felt to be clinically significant, however. Dwyer et al. (2005) conclude that there is little evidence of benefit and some adverse gastrointestinal symptoms. In an analysis of 15 trials of chitosan including 1219 people, there was a small but significant weight loss (weighted mean difference from placebo −1.7kg (95% CI −0.3 to −0.1) and a decrease in total cholesterol and blood pressure (Jull et al. 2008).

Glucomannan

Glucomannan is a soluble fiber derived from the root of the *Amorphophallus konjac* plant. Its chemical structure is similar to that of galactomannan found in guar gum. They are both polysaccharide chains of glucose and mannose and serve as water-soluble fibers. In one randomized controlled trial identified by Pittler and Ernst (2005), the subjects were 20% or more overweight and those on the glucomannan lost more weight than the placebo group. In an analysis of 14 studies including 531 subjects, glucomannan slightly but significantly reduced body weight (−0.79 kg (95% CI −1.53 to −0.05)), lowered total cholesterol, LDL cholesterol, triglycerides, and fasting blood glucose (Sood et al. 2008).

Guar Gum

Guar gum is an extract from *Cyamopsis tetragonolobus*. It is the most widely studied of the compounds in this group with 20 randomized placebo-controlled trials. In a meta-analysis of 11 of these trials, the data do not show that guar gum is more effective than placebo (Pittler and Ernst 2005).

Plantago psyllium

The psyllium extracted from the seeds of this plant is a water-soluble fiber. In one randomized placebo-controlled trial identified by Pittler and Ernst (2005), there was no significant change in body weight in either the treatment or placebo group.

Sweetener

Stevia

Stevia rebaudiana is a South American plant that contains stevosides that act as noncaloric sweeteners. Stevia has been used as a sweetener in Brazil and Japan for more than 20 years and has been approved by the FDA as a food additive. There are three clinical trials testing stevia. The first trial was a randomized multicenter, placebo-controlled trial that enrolled 106 hypertensive subjects for 1 year of treatment. Subjects took stevoside 250 mg three times a day or a placebo. After 3 months, the systolic blood pressure dropped from 166 to 153 mmHg and the diastolic blood pressure fell from 105 to 90 mmHg, and maintained this statistically significant reduction for the rest of the year-long trial (Chan et al. 2000). The second trial enrolled 12 diabetic subjects in a crossover design. Glucose and insulin were measured around a standard meal, with stevioside 1 gram or corn starch

1 gram given just prior to the meal. There was a statistically significant 18% reduction in the glucose area under the curve and an increase in insulin sensitivity (Gregersen et al. 2004). The third trial randomized 174 hypertensive subjects took stevioside 500 mg three times a day or placebo for 2 years. The systolic blood pressure fell from 150 to 140 mmHg and the diastolic pressure fell from 95 to 89 mmHg by the end of the first week and this statistically significant difference persisted for the rest of the 2-year study. The stevoside group was protected from left ventricular hypertrophy and, like the other two trials, there were no adverse events or laboratory abnormalities (Hsieh et al. 2003). There was no weight loss in this 2-year trial. Thus, stevia does not appear to give weight loss, but may be useful in the treatment of the metabolic syndrome.

WHY HAS DEVELOPMENT OF EFFECTIVE ANTIOBESITY DRUGS BEEN SO DIFFICULT?

Only two drugs are approved for long-term treatment of obesity and six others can be used for "a few weeks." Contrast this with the large number of antibiotics, antihypertensive drugs, antidiabetic drugs, and drugs to treat hypercholesterolemia. There are a number of potential answers to the question of why we don't have more drugs. First, many drugs have turned out to have unanticipated consequences that have led to their withdrawal. A number of these are listed in Table 5.8 in Chapter 5.

Additional Effects of Drugs That Act on the Receptors

Undesirable side effects from drugs that target the appropriate receptor as well as other receptors sounded the death knell for three different sympathomimetic drugs. The first is the α-1 adrenergic agonist, phenylpropanolamine (PPA). PPA reduces food intake in experimental animals and the effect is blocked by an α-1 adrenergic antagonist. In clinical trials, PPA produced modest weight loss, but it is also a vasoconstrictor and can raise blood pressure. Sporadic reports of stroke allegedly associated with its use led to a case-control study of stroke among people using sympathomimetic drugs. PPA was taken off the market due to its association with hemorrhagic stroke in women (Kernan et al. 2000).

Addiction is a problem associated with some sympathomimetic drugs. Shortly after amphetamine was shown to reduce body weight, it was also shown to produce addiction. This probably reflects its action on both the noradrenergic and dopaminergic receptor systems. It hits two targets, one which is beneficial, and one harmful.

There are 14 serotonin receptors. Activation of one or more of these serotonin receptors reduces food intake, but other receptors modulate a variety of other effects. Fenfluramine has a beta-phenethylamine backbone and is a selective serotonergic drug that was approved for use by the FDA in 1975. In 1997, patients treated with fenfluramine and phentermine were reported to develop aortic regurgitation in up to 25% of the cases (Connelly et al. 1997; Jollis et al. 2000; Gardin et al. 2000; Davidoff et al. 2001). Based on these findings, fenfluramine and its dextro-isometer D-fenfluramine were removed from the market in September of 1997.

Side Effects of Actions on the Target Receptor That Influence Other Systems

Antagonists to the cannabinoid receptor are one example of this problem. Tetrahydrocannabinol is the active ingredient of Cannabis and is known to stimulate food intake. Identification of the cannabinoid receptors and of two endogenous ligands for these receptors stimulated a search for drugs that could block this system. Rimonabant was the first one developed. After extensive trials, it was approved in Europe but was not approved by the FDA because of concerns about suicidality. As this concern grew, marketing of Rimonabant was suspended in Europe on October 23, 2008—just over 2 years after its approval—because of these psychiatric problems.

Inhibition of the dopamine receptors is another example. Dopamine receptors are involved in the hedonic experiences related to eating and other activities. Activation of these receptors may be involved in the addiction associated with amphetamine noted above. A second problem arose from the use of a drug, Ecopipam, which is a selective dopamine D1/D5 antagonist. It produced increased suicidal ideation. This drug was evaluated in four randomized, double-blind, multicenter trials comparing ecopipam (N = 1667) and placebo (N = 1118) in obese subjects including type 2 diabetic subjects. Ecopipam produced a 3.1% to 4.3% greater weight loss than placebo at 52 weeks. Clinical trials were discontinued, however, because of unexpected psychiatric adverse events (ecopipam 31% vs. placebo 15%), including depression, anxiety, and suicidal ideation. Although ecopipam was effective for achieving and maintaining weight loss in obese subjects, the adverse effects on mood precluded its use in management of weight loss (Astrup et al. 2007).

Ecopipam is a selective dopamine D1/D5 antagonist that was evaluated in four randomized, double-blind, multicenter trials that compared ecopipam (N = 1667) and placebo (N = 1118) in obese subjects including type 2 diabetic subjects. In the dose-ranging studies, subjects received 10, 30, or 100 mg daily for 12 weeks and in the 52-week study, 50 or 100 mg daily, combined with a weight loss program. Primary efficacy variables were the proportion of subjects with ≥5% weight loss from baseline at 12 weeks (phase 2) or the distribution of percentage weight loss from baseline at 52 weeks (phase 3). In the phase 2 study, 26% of subjects administered ecopipam 100 mg vs. 6% placebo, subjects lost more than 5% of their body weight after 12 weeks ($p < 0.01$). In the phase 3 studies, ecopipam 100 mg produced a 3.1% to 4.3% greater weight loss than placebo at 52 weeks. More subjects administered ecopipam vs. placebo and achieved a 5% to 10% or >10% weight loss in two nondiabetic phase 3 trials. Clinical trials were discontinued because of unexpected psychiatric adverse events (ecopipam 31% vs. placebo 15%), including depression, anxiety, and suicidal ideation. Although ecopipam was effective for achieving and maintaining weight loss in obese subjects, the adverse effects on mood excluded its projected use in management of weight loss (Astrup et al. 2007).

Effect on Food Intake or Body Weight Is Statistically, but Not Clinically, Significant

Neuropeptide Y is widely distributed and has five receptors, Y-1, Y-2, Y-4, Y-5, and Y-6. Activation of NPY receptors Y-1 or Y-5 dramatically increases food intake in animals, and continued stimulation of the NPY receptor produces obesity, making an antagonist to this receptor an attractive target for an antiobesity drug. MK-0557 is one such drug. It is a highly selective NPY-5 receptor antagonist with 98% receptor occupancy at a 1.25 mg dose vs. 3% for placebo using positron emission tomography (Erondu et al. 2007). In a 12-week dose-ranging study, weight losses were 0.7, 1.6, 2.2, 2.0, and 2.3 kg for P, 0.2, 1, 5, and 25 mg dose, respectively ($p = 0.041$). In a 52-week study, the placebo group had 1.1 kg (−1.5, −0.6 kg) weight loss compared with −2.2 kg (−2.5, 1.8 kg) in the group treated with 1 mg per day. This small, but statistically significant difference was not substantial enough for further drug development. However, it did demonstrate that the NPY-5 receptor was involved in modulating food intake and body weight in human beings.

The limited response to an agonist to the melanocortin-4 receptor is a second example (Krishna et al. 2009). Based on animal and genetic studies, the melanocortin-4 receptor has an important role in the control of food intake. MK-0493 is a selective and novel melanocortin-4 receptor agonist that has been evaluated clinically. Single doses of 200 mg and 500 mg produced only a marginally significant effect on 24-hour food intake vs. placebo. In two subsequent weight loss trials (one following stepped titration), MK-0493 produced a small, but not statistically significant weight loss relative to baseline. These clinical studies suggest that an MC4R agonist alone may not be an easy clinical target. One possible explanation is the redundancy that exists in the control of food intake (Krishna et al. 2009).

The limited response to the beta-3 receptor agonists is another example of where an "on target" effect doesn't produce the anticipated weight loss. The discovery of the beta-3 receptor and the demonstration that activation of this receptor could increase thermogenesis in brown adipose tissue led to the search for drugs to increase energy expenditure in human beings. The initial compounds were made against rodent receptors and were ineffective. When the human receptor was cloned, it served as the basis for developing a new generation of β-3 agonists that were tested in human beings. TAK-677 is a novel beta-3 agonist that was tested over 4 weeks in 65 healthy obese younger men and women with a BMI of 33.9 ± 2.1. Subjects were randomized to three groups and after 28 days of treatment with placebo, given 0.2 mg or 1 mg in two divided doses daily, the 24-hour energy expenditure in a whole room calorimeter fell by 39 kcal per day in the placebo group and rose by 13 kcal per day with the higher dose of TAK-677. Heart rate increased significantly by eight beats per minute in the higher dose group. This drug was not developed further (Redman et al. 2007). The recent identification of brown adipose tissue by positron emission tomography in human beings may have reawakened interest in the idea of enhancing thermogenesis.

Capsinoids are nonpungent compounds with molecular structures similar to capsaicin from red peppers, which is thought to have thermogenic properties. Thirteen healthy subjects received four doses of the capsinoids (1, 3, 6, and 12 mg) and placebo using a crossover, randomized, double-blind trial. RMR was measured by indirect calorimetry for 45 minutes before and 120 minutes after ingesting capsinoids or placebo. Capsinoids had no significant effect on energy expenditure, blood pressure, or axillary temperature (Galgani et al. 2009).

Loss of Effectiveness over Time—Lack of Durability

Fluoxetine produces dose-related weight loss in overweight patients but, even as therapy is continued, the effect wanes, suggesting that its use in obesity can only be short-term. A total of 1441 subjects were randomized to fluoxetine (719) or placebo (722). Of these, 522 subjects on fluoxetine and 504 subjects on placebo completed 6 months of treatment. Weight loss in the placebo and fluoxetine groups at 6 months and 1 year were 2.2, 4.8, 1.8, and 2.4 kg, respectively. The regain of 50% of the lost weight during the second 6 months of treatment on fluoxetine makes it inappropriate for the long-term treatment of obesity, which requires chronic treatment.

Development of Antibodies That Inhibit Drug Action

Peptides are "antigenic" substances and foreign ones are expected to produce antibodies that may vary in their effect on action of the administered peptide. Ciliary neurotrophic factor is a peptide that produces weight loss in animals by acting on hypothalamic receptors. When tested in human beings it also produced modest weight loss, but antibodies developed in up to 70% of those treated and prevented its effects. Drug development was terminated.

Conclusions

Although the drugs presently available for the treatment of overweight are few in number and limited in efficacy, the pipeline for overweight drug development is very rich. Since drug development is more sophisticated today than in the past, we anticipate that the development of safe and effective drugs for the treatment of overweight will proceed at a more rapid pace than was the case for other chronic diseases that presently have safe and effective medications, like hypertension and diabetes.

8 Surgery for Obesity

KEY POINTS

- The number of surgical procedures performed for extreme degrees of obesity now exceeds 200,000 per year. Laparoscopic techniques have largely replaced open surgical procedures.
- Several surgical procedures are currently done—two of which restrict the flow of intestinal contents (gastroplasty and lap-banding) and two that are restrictive and malabsorptive (gastric bypass and biliopancreatic diversion).
- Gastric bypass is the most commonly performed procedure in the United States and produces more weight loss than gastroplasty or gastric lap-banding.
- These operations are associated with reduced food intake and altered gastrointestinal hormones.
- As with all surgical procedures there are short-term and longer-term risks, including death, reoperation, infection, and metabolic derangements.
- Quality of life improves and use of health services decreases following the initial high costs.
- Laparoscopic bariatric surgery has fewer postoperative problems and more rapid postoperative recovery.
- Laparoscopic bariatric surgery involves less pain, fewer infections, and fewer hernias and other complications, and it allows faster postoperative recovery.

INTRODUCTION

Surgical treatment for obesity is growing rapidly. This can be seen in Figure 8.1, which shows the number of surgeries performed to treat obesity over the past 15 years. After about 2000, there was a rapid increase in the number of surgeries, probably reflecting the improvements in surgical procedures. The popularity of the procedure is due to the significant weight reduction that follows the operation and in the long duration of this response for most patients. Once the surgical procedure is done, the patient can't undo it. It is permanent until the surgeon reverses it. Because of this irreversibility, I call it a "noncognitive" treatment. It is similar to the effect on dental cavities of adding fluoride to the drinking water. Fluoride reduces dental cavities over and above what can be done by brushing and flossing your teeth. After surgical treatment for obesity, patients modify their food intake, but with the reduction in size of the stomach or the rerouting of the intestinal contents, only occasionally do patients manage to eat enough to compensate for the surgery. Thus, surgery provides a form of long-term treatment for obesity that lifestyle, diet, exercise, and medications can't yet match. The reduction in body weight reverses diabetes in nearly 80% of the patients who have diabetes, making it a very effective treatment for diabetes, and one that is cost-effective.

Historical Development of Surgical Treatments for Obesity

Surgical intervention for obesity can be dated more than 1000 years ago at a time long before there was anesthesia available to reduce the pain of an operation. According to Preuss (1985), a corpulent rabbi named Eleazar was given a sleeping potion and taken into a marble chamber, where his abdomen was opened and many basketfuls of fat were removed. Plinius also describes a very similar

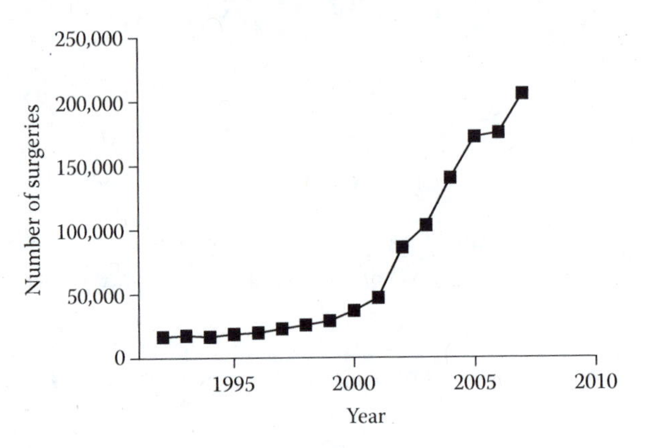

FIGURE 8.1 Growth in number of bariatric operations.

"heroic cure for obesity": "the son of the Consul L. Apronius had fat removed and thus his body was relieved of a disgraceful burden." More recently, in AD 1190, a surgeon cut open the abdomen of Count Dedo II of Groig in order to remove the excessive fat from him (Preuss 1985). Following the advent of anesthesia in 1846 (Bigelow 1846), this procedure has been revived, and many new surgical procedures have been introduced. The events leading up to this important discovery are presented in the context of the times by Fulop-Muller (1938).

Gastrointestinal surgery underwent rapid development in the nineteenth century after the discovery of ether anesthesia in 1846. One of the inventive giants in surgery for the stomach was Billroth (1829–1894), who pioneered the removal of part of the stomach and various techniques to reduce gastric acid secretion that were believed to underlie the peptic ulcer syndrome. The Billroth procedure (Billroth 1881) involved removal of the pylorus. The Billroth II operation involved draining the stomach into the intestine by connecting them together (Hauer 1884). These were clearly the forerunners of the various types of gastrointestinal procedures that were developed after World War II.

Theodor Albert Billroth (1829–1894) is considered to be the father of visceral surgery and is the man who pioneered two operations that involve reconfiguring the flow of stomach contents into the intestine. Billroth was born in Rugen, Germany into a clerical family. In spite of his mother's wishes, he enrolled in the medical faculty at the University of Göttingen. He began his career working with von Graefe, a famous nineteenth-century surgeon, and followed this by a disappointing period of private practice and the final beginnings of his outstanding achievement by being selected for the Langenbeck Clinic and then appointed, at age 31, to the Professorship of Surgery at the University of Zurich. Billroth was a charming man with a genial personality, a strong artistic bent, which is revealed in the few specimens of verse and music that he left, and an outstanding scholar and medical educator. He was a lifelong friend of Johannes Brahms, the great German composer, who performed with colleagues in a quartet at the University of Zurich. His operative successes were captured in the names of the "Billroth I" operation for removal of the pylorus and the "Billroth II" operation in which the contents of the stomach are drained into the jejunum, a procedure that is similar in some respects to the gastric bypass for obesity (Talbot 1970, p. 674; Garrison 1914, pp. 532–533; Porter 1997, pp. 598–599; Bray 2007).

Edward Eaton Mason (b. 1920) is known as the "Father of Bariatric Surgery" because of his seminal contributions to this field of obesity. He was born in Boise, Idaho in October 1920. His education was speeded up by World War II. After finishing high school in 1939, he entered the University of Iowa and received his BA in 1943 and his MD 2 years later in 1945, near the end of the war. He his wife Dordana met while he was in medical school. Mason did his surgical internship and residency at the University of Minnesota where the well-known Orvar Wangensteen, MD, was chair of the Department of Surgery. He returned to the University of Iowa where he spent his academic career. He is a member of many professional societies. He published his first seminal paper on surgical operations for obesity in 1967 (Scott 1991; MacGregor 2002; www.asbms.org).

The operation that introduced bariatric surgery after World War II was a jejuno-ileal bypass reported by Kremen et al. (1954), done on a single patient. Believing that if obese patients lost weight, they would be able to maintain the weight loss, i.e., be cured, Payne and DeWind (1963) performed a series of 11 jejuno-colic anastamoses where the middle of the jejunum was attached to the middle of the transverse colon. This produced major weight loss, but significant diarrhea. When the patients were reanastamosed after losing weight, they all returned to their initial weight, or even more. Realizing that this surgery had not "cured" obesity, they developed the jejuno-ileal bypass that could be maintained for a longer period of time (DeWind and Payne 1976). These jejuno-ileal operations were associated with overwhelming and unacceptable metabolic and infectious complications and this operative procedure for obesity was discontinued in the late 1980s.

While these early operations with their unanticipated side-effects were spreading through the surgical world, Dr. Mason in Iowa was developing an alternative approach that would sweep aside the earlier operations and become the predominant surgical approach to obesity for which the title of "Father of Bariatric Surgery" rightly belongs to Professor Edward E. Mason (b. 1920). In 1967, Mason and Ito (1967) published a seminal paper in which a gastrointestinal bypass was done for treatment of obesity. This procedure proved to be durable and is currently the leading operation that is performed. Over the next few years, Mason developed a number of other procedures for reducing the size and flow of gastrointestinal contents through the stomach, but none has been as successful nor widely copied as the gastric bypass.

Surgical Operations

The operations used to treat obesity are generally referred to as "bariatric" operations, a word derived from the Greek meaning "heavy." All of them involve some manipulation of the plumbing that we call the gastrointestinal track. Figure 8.2 shows some of the operations that are used or have been used to treat obesity. The initial operation by Payne and Dewind separated the intestine at the mid-jejunum and connected the proximal end to the colon so that the content of the upper GI track was emptied into the colon (not shown). Weight loss with this procedure was rapid and subjects returned to nearly normal weight. However, there were serious problems with diarrhea and loss of potassium and other minerals. Believing that their patients had been "cured" of their obesity, the operations were reversed with rapid regain of the lost weight. The next approach was by the same group (DeWind and Payne 1976) who pioneered a less drastic rearrangement of the GI-track by coupling the jejunum to the distal segment of the ileum. These operations were very popular during the 1970s but fell into disuse as the number of complications continued to rise and alternative gastric operations came into use.

Restrictive operations were pioneered and developed by Mason and his associates. These appeared in 1979 and 1980 and involved reducing the volume of the stomach with various stapling procedures, but leaving the flow of food from esophagus to duodenum (Pace et al. 1979; Gomez

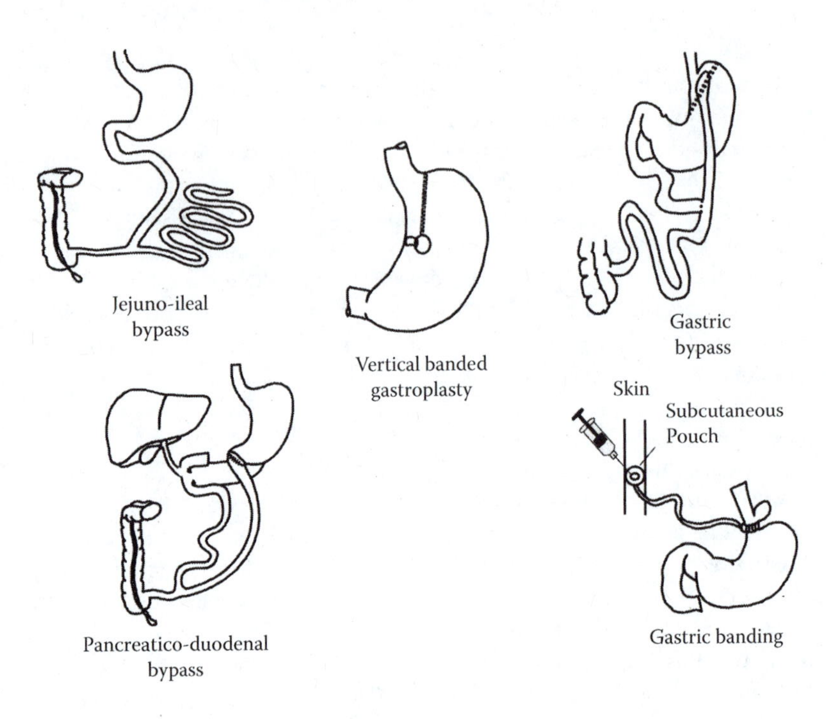

FIGURE 8.2 Illustrations of operative procedures.

1979). They consisted of both transverse staple lines as well as vertical staple lines that in effect prolonged the esophagus in a procedure called the vertical-banded gastroplasty (Mason 1982).

An alternative restrictive procedure consists of placing a plastic band around the stomach and, in some of the systems, providing a way to inflate it from a subcutaneous reservoir. The initial procedure was performed in 1976, but not published until 8 years later (Bo and Modalsli 1983). This procedure is now widely used in Europe and has been approved by the Food and Drug Administration in the United States.

Three procedures have been developed that involve combinations of gastric and intestinal operations. The first of these is the gastric bypass, originally developed by Mason and Ito (Mason and Ito 1967, 1969). In this procedure, a small gastric pouch is anastamosed to the distal limb of the jejunum, while the proximal limb is attached to the side of this loop a short ways below the connection of the jejunum to the stomach. This operation is both a restrictive and modestly malabsorptive procedure. The next procedure is the biliopancreatic diversion, which was developed by Scopinaro and consists of two long intestinal segments, one draining contents from the stomach and the other delivering the duodenal juices. They are connected near the ileo-cecal valve, thus reducing the length of the intestine where food and intestinal juices are brought together, thus reducing absorption. The final procedure in this group is the distal gastric bypass where the jejunum replaces the duodenum in draining the lower stomach—the so-called biliopancreatic diversion with duodenal switch (Marceau et al. 1993).

All of these operations can now be done laparoscopically, which has significantly reduced the operative morbidity and allowed more patients to have these procedures. Laparoscopic procedures were first undertaken by Fried and Peskova (1997) and by Belachew et al. (1995).

RATIONALE FOR SURGICAL INTERVENTION FOR OBESITY

Obesity viewed as a problem of energy balance isn't initially an obvious target for surgery. However, when you consider that the "cornerstones" of treatment of overweight as discussed in Chapters 6 and

7 produce only modest weight loss, which is often regained, some more definitive kind of procedure seems worth considering. The magnitude of the weight loss that can be achieved with behavioral, dietary, exercise, and pharmacological approaches is limited to about 10% of initial body weight. For an individual weighing 150 kg (330 pounds), this is a 15-kg weight loss, which is only modest at best. When treatment is "stopped" because the patient is dissatisfied with the failure to lose enough weight or the cost is more than they want to pay, weight is usually regained over several months to or above the baseline weight. This observation reinforces the notion treatments for obesity only work when used. The Nationwide Inpatient Sample from 1998 to 2002 showed that the number of bariatric operations increased from 13,365 to 72,177, a more than 5-fold increase in 5 years. More than 80% of these were the gastric bypass operation pioneered by Mason. Several other trends were also noted: Operations on women increased from 81% to 84% of the total; privately insured patients increased from 75% to 83% of the patients; and the proportion of patients aged 50 to 64 rose from 15% to 24%. Length of hospitalization decreased from 4.5 to 3.3 days, and operative mortality ranged from 0.1% to 0.2%. Thus, consideration of bariatric surgery as a treatment for obesity is occurring more frequently both for the patient and for the physicians and other health professionals who take care of these patients.

Bariatric surgery has come of age. On February 21, 2006, the Center for Medicare and Medicaid Services agreed to expand financial coverage to include bariatric surgery as a treatment for obesity. We can thus expect even more procedures to be done in the future. There are several sources of information that the reader can consult for additional details (Sjostrom 2004; Buchwald et al. 2004; Shekelle et al. 2004; Inge et al. 2004; Bray 2007; Colquitt et al. 2005; Mechanick et al. 2008).

INDICATIONS

The current criteria for bariatric surgical procedures were originally outlined by a consensus development panel at the National Institutes of Health (NIH) in 1991 and are summarized in Table 8.1. Adult patients are eligible to be considered for these procedures if they have a BMI > 40 kg/m^2 or a BMI > 35 kg/m^2 if they have serious comorbidities such as sleep apnea, diabetes mellitus, or joint disease. For individuals less than 16 years of age, surgical and pediatric consultants should review each case individually (Inge et al. 2004), since operations that reduce caloric intake can slow weight gain when performed before an adolescent has achieved full adult height. Similarly, bariatric surgery for people older than 65 years of age should be considered on an individual basis, since adaptation to the postoperative effects of the procedure may be more troublesome and difficult. Potential patients must have tried and failed nonsurgical procedures for weight loss. The patient and their significant others must understand the procedure and its complications and the patient must have acceptable surgical risks.

TABLE 8.1
Indications and Contraindications for Bariatric Surgery

Indications

1. BMI > 40 kg/m^2 or BMI 35–39.9 kg/m^2 and life-threatening cardiopulmonary disease, severe diabetes, or lifestyle impairment
2. Failure to achieve adequate weight loss with nonsurgical treatment

Contraindications

1. History of noncompliance with medical care
2. Certain psychiatric illnesses: personality disorder, uncontrolled depression, suicidal ideation, or substance abuse
3. Unlikely to survive surgery

CONTRAINDICATIONS

Patients with major depression or psychosis should be carefully reviewed by a behavioral specialist before being accepted. Binge-eating disorders, current drug and alcohol abuse, severe cardiac disease with prohibitive anesthetic risks, severe coagulopathy, or inability to comply with nutritional requirements including lifelong vitamin replacement are other contraindications.

A large number of complications can occur in the postoperative period and it is thus desirable to have bariatric operations performed in a setting that can provide comprehensive medical and nutritional support. Guidance in how to do this has been developed by the American Society of Bariatric Surgeons (ASBS) through their guidelines for establishing Centers of Excellence (COE) for bariatric clinics (ASBS 2003). A number of NIH-funded surgical centers have been established to advance the science and care of patients needing bariatric surgery (Flum et al. 2007) since they note that fewer men, Blacks, and Hispanics are operated on for obesity than White, more affluent individuals.

BARIATRIC SURGERY FOR PEDIATRIC PATIENTS

The rising prevalence of obesity among children and adolescents has seen an increased interest in bariatric surgery for this age group (Inge et al. 2004). The principal concern in this age group is the potential for reducing linear growth if a patient is operated on before their adult height is reached. The criteria for adolescent patients are given in Table 8.2. The largest study in adolescents contained only 33 patients who underwent several different procedures, thus providing little guidance (Sugerman et al. 2003). The review of pediatrics suggests that, at the present time, the gastric bypass may be the most appropriate procedure.

EFFECTIVENESS OF SURGICAL PROCEDURES

Criteria for establishing success with bariatric surgery are often done using the loss of excess body weight. This concept calculates the amount of weight above some appropriate level, such as a BMI of 25 kg/m^2, and determines the fraction lost after surgery. This provides the patient and doctor with an idea of how much of the excess weight has actually been shed. Using the percentage of actual

TABLE 8.2
Criteria for Bariatric Surgery in Adolescents

Adolescents being considered for bariatric surgery should

1. Have failed ≥6 months of organized attempts at weight management, as determined by their primary care provider.
2. Have attained or nearly attained physiologic maturity.
3. Be very severely overweight (BMI ≥ 40 kg/m^2) with serious obesity-related comorbidities or have a BMI of ≥50 with less severe comorbidities.
4. Demonstrate commitment to comprehensive medical and psychological evaluations both before and after surgery.
5. Agree to avoid pregnancy for at least 1 year postoperatively.
6. Be capable of and willing to adhere to nutritional guidelines postoperatively.
7. Provide informed assent to surgical treatment.
8. Demonstrate decisional capacity.
9. Have a supportive family environment.

TABLE 8.3
Comparison of Actual Weight Loss and Percentage Excess Weight Loss with Various Bariatric Procedures

	Weight Loss		Excess Weight Loss	
	Mean	95% CI	Mean	95% CI
Gastric banding	32.4 kg	(−45.4, −13.1 kg)	49.6%	(−70.0, −32.0%)
Gastric bypass	47.1 kg	(−62.7, −21.0 kg)	68.1%	(−77.0, −33.0%)
Gastroplasty	39.4 kg	(−70.0, −9.0 kg)	69.2%	(−93.0, −48.0%)
BPD	46.0 kg	(−54.2, −33.0 kg)	72.1%	(−75.0, −62.0%)

Source: Adapted from Buchwald, H., et al., *JAMA*, 292(14), 1724–1737, 2004.
Note: BPD, biliopancreatic diversion.

weight loss suffers in comparison, since losing more than one-third of actual body weight is often undesirable, but a third or half of excess body weight is usually achieved after bariatric surgery (Bray et al. 2009). A comparison of the percentage of excess weight loss and weight loss is shown in Table 8.3, which provides the actual weight loss (weighted for number of patients in the study) for four different procedures next to the percent of excess weight loss. The percent excess weight loss is about one-third higher since it calculates the loss from actual weight to the upper limit of normal rather than zero.

No-Longer-Used Intestinal Bypass Procedures

The jejuno-ileal bypass was in use for over a decade following its development by DeWind and Payne, but the complications made it an unsatisfactory long-term procedure. In a comparative trial, weight loss with the jejuno-ileal bypass was 33% against 16% for the horizontal gastroplasty, but the side-effects were less severe with the gastroplasty. In a 2-year comparison of jejuno-ileal bypass in 130 patients against 66 patients treated by diet in the Danish Obesity Project (1979), Stokholm et al. (1982) favored the surgical group with a weight loss of 42.9 kg vs. 5.9 kg in the diet group. The surgically operated patients had significant postoperative problems, but also had more improvement in blood pressure and quality of life.

Gastroplasty

Gastroplasty in its many forms was a very popular procedure, and one pioneered by Mason. In a study of 204 patients weighing 112 kg who were assigned to either horizontal gastroplasty or gastric bypass, weight loss at 3 years was 39 kg after gastric bypass compared to 17 kg after horizontal gastroplasty (Hall et al. 1990; Sjostrom et al. 1999). The horizontal gastroplasty has also been compared with a very low calorie diet (VLCD) in a 2-year study with a 5-year follow-up, but a drop-out rate in excess of 50%. After 2 years, the weight loss was 8.2 kg in the VLCD group compared with 30.6 kg in the surgically treated group (Andersen et al. 1984; Andersen et al. 1988). After 5 years, the percentage losing more than 10% of initial weight was 16% in the surgical group, but only 3% in the VLCD group.

Gastric Bypass

Gastric bypass is one of the most widely accepted procedures. In one trial comparing laparoscopic Roux-en-Y (RYGB) gastric bypass vs. a mini gastric bypass, 40 subjects were randomized to each procedure and followed for a mean of 31.3 months (Lee et al. 2005). As expected, the operative time

TABLE 8.4
A Meta-Analysis of Weight Loss with Laparoscopic Gastric Bypass and Laparoscopic Adjustable Gastric Band

	Laparoscopic Gastric Bypass		Laparoscopic Adjustable Gastric Band	
Years after Surgery	# Studies	% EWL	# Studies	% EWL
1	10	61.5	15	42.6
2	5	69.7	12	50.3
3	2	71.2	9	55.2

Source: Adapted from Garb, J., *Obes. Surg.*, 19, 1447–1455, 2009.
Note: % EWL, percent excess weight lost.

was shorter with the mini bypass procedure and the operative morbidity was higher in the RYGB procedure. Weight losses at 1 and 2 years were similar in the two groups. The authors concluded that the mini gastric bypass is simpler and safer than the RYGB procedure. However, a meta-analysis of studies using laparoscopic techniques to perform either the gastric bypass or the adjustable lap-band found that weight loss favored the gastric bypass (Table 8.4). This data is expressed as percent excess weight loss, which is about 50% higher for the gastric bypass studies than for the lap-band studies (Garb et al. 2009).

The Swedish Obese Subjects (SOS) study is a controlled but nonrandomized trial directly comparing surgical and nonsurgical treatment for obesity, and is the largest trial comparing surgical vs. medical treatment of morbid obesity (Sjostrom et al. 2004; Karlsson et al. 1998; Torgerson and Sjostrom 2001; Sjostrom et al. 1992; Sjostrom 2004). A total of 6328 obese subjects with a BMI > 34 kg/m^2 for men and >38 kg/m^2 for women were recruited. Of these, 2010 chose surgical intervention for obesity (gastric banding, gastroplasty, or gastric bypass), while 2037 matched controls received conventional treatment. Operated participants were matched on a number of criteria to a group of 6322 overweight men and women in the SOS registry who were not operated on. The SOS study began slowly in 1987 but has contributed significant new information about overweight individuals and the effects of surgical intervention. Prior to surgery there were an average of 7.6 weight loss attempts for the men and 18.2 for the women. The mean for the largest weight loss prior to surgery was 17.7 kg for the men and 18.2 kg for the women, but they were only able to maintain this for 7 to 10 months. When the banding operation was compared with vertical-banded gastroplasty and gastric bypass in the Swedish Obese Subjects study, Sjostrom et al. (2004) reported similar weight losses out to 10 years in the lap-band and vertical-banded gastroplasty that were significantly less than those seen with the gastric bypass (Figure 8.3).

Biliopancreatic Diversion

No randomized comparisons of the biliopancreatic diversion with other procedures have yet been published. However, there are two nonrandomized comparisons. When 142 patients with the biliopancreatic diversion were compared with 93 patients undergoing a lap-band procedure, excess weight loss was 60% with the diversion operation against 48% for the lap-band (Bajardi et al. 2000). In a comparison of the biliopancreatic diversion with a long-limb gastric bypass, BMI was reduced from 64 to 37 kg/m^2 in the diversion group, compared to a decrease from 67 to 42 kg/m^2 (Murr et al. 1999). The biliopancreatic diversion appears to have more side-effects than the other procedures. Scopinaro, who originated the procedure, reported a low mortality of 0.5% with an excess body weight loss of 75%. Anemia occurring in spite of iron and folate replacement occurred in <5%, stomach ulcers during H_2-blocker therapy in 3.2%, and protein malnutrition in 3% (Scopinaro et al. 1996).

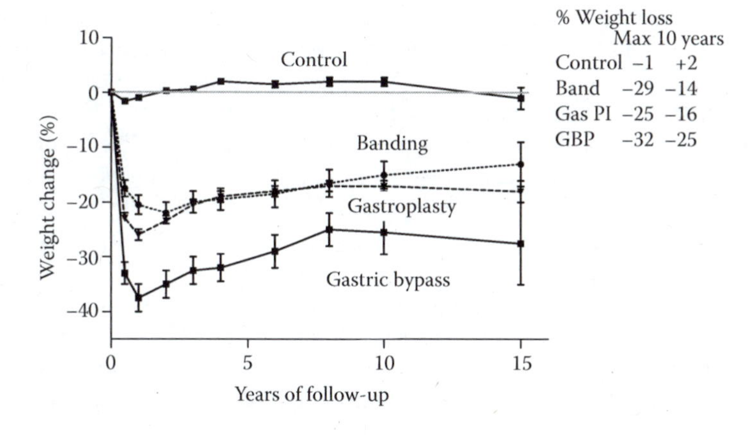

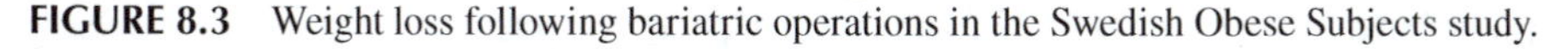

FIGURE 8.3 Weight loss following bariatric operations in the Swedish Obese Subjects study.

Laparoscopic Banding of the Stomach

One randomized clinical trial compared intensive medical management vs. laparoscopic insertion of an adjustable gastric band (LAP-BAND system). Included in the trial were individuals who had a BMI between 30 and 35 kg/m^2, who also had comorbid conditions such as hypertension, dyslipidemia, diabetes obstructive sleep apnea, or gastroesophageal reflux disease, severe physical limitations, or clinically significant psychosocial problems. The intensive medical program consisted of a VLCD and lifestyle changes for 12 weeks, followed by a transition phase over 4 weeks combining some VLCD meals with 120 mg of orlistat, and then orlistat 120 mg before all meals. Surgery was performed by two surgeons. Of the 40 patients in each group, one withdrew before surgery, leaving 39 at the end of 2 years. Seven dropped out of the intensive intervention, leaving 33 patients who completed treatment. Both groups had an identical 13.8% weight loss at 6 months. The surgical group continued to lose weight and were 21.6% below baseline at 2 years. The nonsurgical group regained weight from 6 to 24 months, at which time they were on average only 5.5% below baseline weight. At 2 years, the surgically treated group had significantly greater improvements in diastolic blood pressure, fasting plasma glucose level, insulin sensitivity index, and HDL-cholesterol level. Quality of life improved more in the surgical group. Physical function, vitality, and mental health domains of the SF-36 were improved in the surgical group. Thus, laparoscopic insertion of an adjustable gastric band may be beneficial to some patients with weights below those usually recommended for bariatric surgery (O'Brien et al. 2006).

Gastric banding is also widely used. A systematic review of 14 comparative studies, including one randomized trial, compared banding with gastric bypass in trials that lasted 1 year or more (Tice et al. 2008). All but two trials were of very low quality. At 1 year, excess weight loss was 26% greater with gastric bypass (19%–34%). In the highest quality study, the excess body weight loss with the RYGB gastric bypass was 76% vs. 48% for the gastric banding procedure. In this study, diabetes resolved in 78% of the gastric bypass group compared to 50% in the gastric banding group, but perioperative complications were more common with gastric bypass (9% vs. 5%), but long term reoperation rates were lower with gastric bypass (16% vs. 24%). This study favors the gastric bypass.

MECHANISMS FOR WEIGHT LOSS

There are at least two mechanisms that can account for the weight loss after bariatric surgery. The first of these is malabsorption. This was clearly an important component of the jejuno-ileal bypass (Bray 1976), and is a prominent feature of the biliopancreatic diversion procedures. A second mechanism is a reduction of food intake due to altered hormonal secretion from the gastrointestinal track or the mechanical changes in GI anatomy. Two GI hormones have received the most attention as potential candidates for modulating postsurgical effects on food intake. Glucagon-like peptide-1 (GLP-1 or enteroglucagon) is secreted from the L-cells in the lower intestinal track and has effects on GI function and on food intake. The supply of nutrients to the lower GI track may well enhance its release. More interest has been sparked by ghrelin. Ghrelin is a small peptide released primarily from the stomach that stimulates food intake. Cummings et al. reported that after bariatric surgery, the level of this peptide was significantly reduced (Cummings et al. 2002; Tritos et al. 2003). However, there have been contradictory reports since.

The other mechanism that could decrease food intake is the reduced volume of the stomach or the altered anatomy of the GI track. In one report. Lindroos et al. (1996) found no difference in energy intake between patients with a gastric bypass and those with a gastroplasty, although those with a gastroplasty lost less weight. In the SOS study, food intake in the operated groups was less than in the control group at all time intervals (Figure 8.4).

Another way to look at mechanisms for weight loss is as a "foregut" and a "hindgut" hypothesis. The foregut hypothesis is based on the concept that it is peptides in the enteroinsulin axis that are related to the reduction in food intake. The two principal peptides in this axis are glucagon-like peptide-1 (GLP-1, also called enteroglucagon) and gastric inhibitory peptide or, more appropriately, glucose-dependent insulinotrophic peptide (GIP). GLP-1 is released from the "L" cells in the gut, most of which are located in the ileum, colon, and rectum. It reduces food intake and slows gastric emptying and may be increased after bariatric surgery. GIP is secreted from the "K" cells located in the jejunum. It is a potent stimulator of insulin in the presence of glucose and is released by food intake. It also inhibits gastric acid. In the GK rat, a diabetic animal model, Rubino et al. (2006) showed that excluding the duodenum with a gastric bypass worsened glucose tolerance compared to animals where food could flow through the pylorus, as well as enter the GI track through a gastric-jejunal anatamosis.

The hind-gut hypothesis focuses on the role of GLP-1, which will be increased by the enhanced flow of GI contents to the lower bowel. Patriti et al. (2005) showed that moving a segment of ileum up between the duodenum and jejunum improved glycemia in the diabetic GK rat independent of weight loss or food intake. Intestinal transposition also increased the blood concentration of GLP-1.

The lap-band procedure reduces food intake and feelings of satiety. In one trial, Dixon et al. (2005) gave a test meal to individuals with a lap-band on two occasions, one with optimal restriction and one with reduced restriction. In the overweight control subjects with no bariatric procedure, the baseline levels of glucose, insulin, and leptin were higher, whereas the ghrelin level was lower.

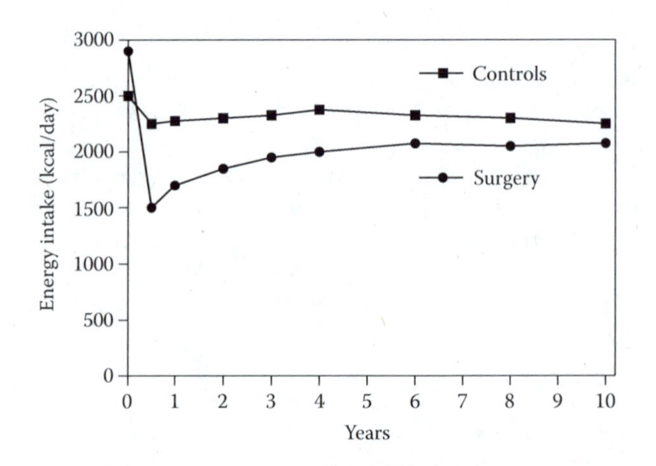

FIGURE 8.4 Food intake following bariatric operations in the Swedish Obese Subjects study.

When they ate the test meal, the control subjects had a larger response of glucose and insulin, whereas the subjects with the lap-band had similar responses to both meals. Satiety, however, was less when the band was at the optimal restriction and there was less reduction in satiety when the band was not optimally inflated.

BENEFITS FROM BARIATRIC SURGERY

Weight Loss

Weight loss is a major motivator for choosing bariatric surgery, and its effectiveness is clear. Weight loss is a major benefit, but there are many other benefits, some tangible and some less so.

Reduced Mortality

Bariatric surgery produces more weight loss than conventional therapy for overweight, and the weight loss is more durable. It also prolongs life. The first clear-cut suggestions that bariatric surgery might reduce mortality came from Flum and Dellinger (2004) and Christou et al. (2005). In a large series of patients from the state of Washington, a 15-year follow-up showed that 16.3% of 66,109 obese, nonoperated patients had died, compared with 11.8% of 3328 operated obese patients. When survival was compared beginning 1 year after the procedure, the adjusted hazard for death in the operated patients was 33% lower than in the nonoperated patients (hazard ratio 0.67; 95% CI 0.54–0.85) (Flum and Dellinger 2004). In a 5-year Canadian study of two cohorts, one with bariatric surgery and one without, the mortality rate in the surgical cohort was 0.68% compared with 6.17% in controls (relative risk 0.11, 95% CI 0.04–0.27). This translates into an 89% risk reduction for death (Christou 2005). Mortality rates are influenced by the experience of the surgeon (Schauer et al. 2003; Wittgrove and Clark 2000; Flum and Dellinger 2004).

Bariatric surgery has also been shown to reduce mortality in two more recent trials (Sjostrom et al. 2008; Adams et al. 2008). One was a retrospective cohort study from the State of Utah and the other was the SOS study, which was based on a matched prospective cohort. In the Utah study, during a mean follow-up of 7.1 years, adjusted long-term mortality from any cause in the surgery group decreased by 40%, as compared with that in the control group (37.6 vs. 57.1 deaths per 10,000 person-years, $p < 0.001$). The specific causes of mortality in the surgery group decreased 56% for coronary artery disease (2.6 vs. 5.9 per 10,000 person-years, $p = 0.006$), 92% for diabetes (0.4 vs. 3.4 per 10,000 person-years, $p = 0.005$), and 60% for cancer (5.5 vs. 13.3 per 10,000 person-years, $p < 0.001$) (Adams et al. 2007).

In the SOS study, the average weight change in the 2037 matched control subjects was less than ±2% in the 15 years during which weights were recorded. Maximum weight losses in the surgical subgroups were observed after 1 to 2 years. They were 32% for the gastric bypass group, 25% for the vertical-banded gastroplasty group, and 20% in the banding group. After 10 years, weight losses from baseline stabilized at 25%, 16%, and 14%, respectively. There were 129 deaths in the control group and 101 deaths in the surgery group. The unadjusted overall hazard ratio for death was 0.76 in the surgery group ($p = 0.04$), as compared with the control group, and 0.71 after adjustment for sex, age, and risk factors ($p = 0.01$). The most common causes of death were myocardial infarction (control group, 25 subjects; surgery group, 13 subjects) and cancer (control group, 47; surgery group, 29) (Sjostrom et al. 2007).

Cost Effectiveness

Several studies show that bariatric surgery is a cost-effective procedure (Cremieux et al. 2008; Sampalis et al. 2004; Salem et al. 2008; Picot 2009). The modeled cost-effectiveness analysis showed that both operative interventions for severe obesity were cost effective. Using a modeling technique,

Salem et al. found that both laparoscopic adjustable gastric banding and RYGB gastric bypass were cost-effective at <$25,000. Laparoscope gastric bypass was more cost-effective than RYGB for all scenarios (Salem et al. 2008). In the study by Christou et al. (2008), bariatric surgery patients had higher total costs for hospitalizations (per 1000 patients) in the first year following cohort inception (surgery cohort = CDN $12,461,938; control cohort = CDN $3,609,680), but after 5 years, average cumulative costs for operated patients were CDN $19,516,667 vs. CDN $25,264,608, for an absolute difference of almost CDN $6,000,000 per 1000 patients. Moreover, the initial costs of surgery can be amortized over 3.5 years (Sampalis et al. 2004). In a third study, the mean bariatric surgery investment ranged from approximately $17,000 to $26,000. After controlling for observable patient characteristics, we estimated all costs to have been recouped within 2 years for laparoscopic surgery patients and within 4 years for open surgery. Downstream savings associated with bariatric surgery are estimated to offset the initial costs in 2 to 4 years (Cremieux et al. 2008). Finally, bariatric surgery appears to be a clinically effective and cost-effective intervention for moderately to severely obese people compared with nonsurgical interventions. Uncertainties remain and further research is required to provide detailed data on patient quality of life, impact of experience of the surgeon on the outcome, late complications leading to reoperation, duration of comorbidity remission, and resource use. Good-quality RCTs will provide evidence on bariatric surgery for young people and for adults with class I or class II obesity. New research must report on the resolution and/or development of comorbidities such as type 2 diabetes and hypertension so that the potential benefits of early intervention can be assessed (Picot et al. 2009).

Prevention and Reversal of Diabetes

The prevention and reversal of diabetes probably plays an important role in the reduced mortality and cost-effectiveness of bariatric surgery. Historically, improvement in diabetes was first shown in 1955, following subtotal gastrectomy (Friedman et al. 1955). However, it was a paper by Pories et al. in 1992 titled, "Is Type II Diabetes Mellitus (NIDDM) a Surgical Disease?" published in the Annals of Surgery that caught people's attention. They were the first to note the marked effect of bariatric surgery on diabetes (Pories et al. 1992a; Pories et al. 1992b). The title of a later paper was equally provocative, "Who Would Have Thought It? An Operation Proves to Be the Most Effective Therapy of Adult-Onset Diabetes Mellitus" (Pories et al. 1995). Although there were design issues with these retrospective studies, they showed an annual incidence of 4.5% in the control group compared with only 1% in the surgically operated group. A beneficial effect on reversal of existing diabetes and prevention of its development has been confirmed in a number of other studies (Long et al. 1994; Torquati et al. 2005; Mari 2006; Schauer et al. 2003; Sugerman et al. 2003; Buchwald 2009). Data from a meta-analysis of weight loss and reversal of diabetes is shown Table 8.5. The percentage of reversal is related to the degree of weight loss, which is consistent with improvements in insulin sensitivity (Mari and Manco 2006).

The SOS, a prospective controlled study, has also reported impressive improvement in diabetes. After 2 years of follow-up, the incidence of diabetes was 8% in the matched control group and 1% in the surgical group. After 10 years, the incidence of diabetes in the control group was 24% compared to only 7% in the operated group. The incidence rate was related to the amount of weight lost. In the subgroup losing more than 12% of their initial body weight, there were no new cases of diabetes, compared to 7% in those losing 2%, and 9% in those gaining 4% (Sjostrom 2004). The rate of recovery from diabetes was 72% in the operated group and 21% in the control group. By 10 years, the recovery rate was still substantial at 36% in the operated group compared to 13% in the control group (Sjostrom et al. 2004). This was reflected in the low odds ratio [OR] for diabetes (OR 0.10) and hyperinsulinemia (OR 0.1). In an unblinded, randomized, controlled trial, Dixon et al. (2008) enrolled 60 diabetic patients with a BMI between 30 and 40 kg/m^2 into either a lap-band operation or a lifestyle program. At 2 years, the lap-band group had lost –20.0% of their body weight compared to –1.4% in the lifestyle group. Remission of diabetes occurred in 73% (22/30) of those in the

TABLE 8.5
Efficacy of Bariatric Surgical Operation of Weight Loss and Resolution of Diabetes Mellitus

Procedure	Percent Excess Weight Loss	Percent Resolution of Type 2 Diabetes
Biliopancreatic diversion/ duodenal switch	63.6%	95.1%
Gastric bypass	59.7%	80.3%
Gastroplasty	55.5%	79.7%
Gastric banding	46.2%	56.7%

Source: Adapted from Buchwald, H., et al., *Am. J. Med.*, 122(3), 248–256, 2009.

surgical group and 13% (4/30) in the diet-treated group. The relative risk of remission from diabetes was 5.5 (95% CI 2.2–14.0) and was related to weight loss.

Based on these findings, the Diabetes Surgery Summit held in Rome on March 29–31, 2007 concluded that the surgical procedures may contribute to improvement in diabetes beyond the weight loss and that the procedure may be appropriate for individuals with a BMI of 30 to 35 kg/m^2 (Burguera et al. 2007).

Improvement in Quality of Life

Quality of life is improved after bariatric surgery in both adults (Ryden and Sullivan 2004; Basis and Lopez-Jimenez 2009; Muller and Wenger 2008; Nguyen et al. 2009; Karlsson et al. 2007) and in adolescents (Loux and Hariacharan 2008). In a prospective randomized trial comparing laparoscopically performed gastric bypass and adjustable gastric banding, Nguyen et al. (2009) found that quality of life, measured by the widely used SF-36 questionnaire of eight health concepts including physical functioning, emotional pain, bodily pain, vitality, social functioning, mental health, and general health, improved in both groups. In a prospectively matched-pair analysis using age, BMI, and gender, 52 consecutive patients who had a laparoscopic gastric bypass were matched with 52 patients who had received a gastric band laparoscopically. After 3 years, BMI fell from 45.7 kg/m^2 to 30.4 kg/m^2 in the gastric bypass group, and from 45.3 kg/m^2 to 33.1 kg/m^2 in the banding group. The SF-36 scores were the same before surgery and follow comparably after surgery to values within the normal range for the population under study (Muller and Wenger 2008). In a small group of adolescents, there was also a prompt fall in SF-36 scores (Loux and Harichrahan 2008).

Reduced Risk of Cancer

Bariatric surgery resulted in a significant reduction in the mean percentage of excess weight loss (67.1%, $p < .001$). The surgery patients had significantly fewer physician and hospital visits for all cancer diagnoses ($n = 21$, 2.0%) compared with the controls ($n = 487$, 8.45%; RR .22, 95% CI .143 to –.347; $p = .001$). The physician/hospital visits for common cancers such as breast cancer were significantly reduced in the surgery group ($p = .001$).

In a retrospective case-control study (McCawley 2009), there were 1482 women who had bariatric surgery, and 53 of these (3.6%) were diagnosed with cancer. The most common cancer site was the breast ($n = 15$, 28.3%) followed by the endometrium ($n = 9$, 17%) and the cervix ($n = 6$, 11.3%). The mean age at cancer diagnosis was 39.4 years. Most cancers ($n = 34$, 64.1%) were diagnosed before the bariatric surgery. Bariatric surgery patients with cancer were older than noncancer patients at time of surgery (mean age 44.7 vs. 41.6 years; $p = 0.019$), but otherwise did not differ significantly with regard to race, body mass index, or comorbid conditions. Compared with a control group of 3495 morbidly obese women who had not undergone bariatric surgery, the surgery patients had fewer cancers (3.6% vs. 5.8%, $p = 0.002$), were younger (41.7 vs. 46.9 years, $p < 0.001$), and were younger at cancer diagnosis (45.0 vs. 56.8 years, $p < 0.001$). The most frequent cancers in the control obese women were endometrial, ovarian, and breast cancer. Both groups of obese women with endometrial, breast, ovarian, and colorectal cancers were younger at diagnosis compared with Virginia Cancer Registry means.

Conclusions. Breast and endometrial cancers remain the most common types in obese women and may occur at young ages; bariatric surgery may decrease cancer development in obese women. The SOS study also showed a reduction in cancer risk in women, but not men. The cancer follow-up rate was 99.9% and the median follow-up time was 10.9 years (range 0–18.1 years). Bariatric surgery resulted in a sustained mean weight reduction of 19.9 kg (SD 15.6 kg) over 10 years, whereas the mean weight change in controls was a gain of 1.3 kg (SD 13.7 kg). The number of first-time cancers after inclusion was lower in the surgery group ($n = 117$) than in the control group ($n = 169$; HR 0.67, 95% CI 0.53–0.85, $p = 0.0009$). The sex-treatment interaction p value was 0.054. In women, the number of first-time cancers after inclusion was lower in the surgery group ($n = 79$) than in the control group ($n = 130$; HR 0.58, 0.44 to 0.77; $p = 0.0001$), whereas there was no effect of surgery in men (38 in the surgery group vs. 39 in the control group; HR 0.97, 0.62 to 1.52; $p = 0.90$). Similar results were obtained after exclusion of all cancer cases during the first 3 years of the intervention. Bariatric surgery was associated with reduced cancer incidence in obese women but not in obese men.

Cardiometabolic and Other Benefits

Other benefits from the weight loss associated with bariatric surgery include reduced prevalence of sleep apnea, and improved cardiovascular function. Sleep apnea is markedly improved by even a modest weight loss (Dixon et al. 2001; Buchwald et al. 2004; Fritscher et al. 2009; Haines and Nelson 2007; Grunstein et al. 2007). In a polysomnographic study comparing before and after data, Haines et al. (2008) found that preoperatively 33% of 289 patients had severe sleep apnea, 18% had moderate sleep apnea, 32% had mild sleep apnea, and only 17% were free of this complication. In a follow-up to 11 months, there was a significant reduction in sleep apnea. The preoperative BMI correlated with the severity of sleep apnea, and surgically induced weight loss produced significant improvement.

The metabolic syndrome and its components are improved by weight loss after bariatric surgery. There was an initial linear reduction in the systolic and diastolic blood pressure with the degree of weight loss (Sjostrom et al. 1997) and the odds ratio for incident hypertension was 0.38. This decline only persisted for the first 2–4 years and was followed by a return to baseline levels (Sjostrom et al. 1999). Triglyceride and insulin levels also showed a linear decrease with weight loss (OR 0.28 for hypertriglyceridemia). The concentration of HDL-cholesterol increased linearly with weight loss (OR 0.28), but cholesterol did not decline significantly until weight loss had exceeded 25 kg (OR 1.24) (Sjostrom et al. 1999).

Surgically treated patients required less medication for cardiovascular disease or diabetes than matched controls (Agren et al. 2002). Among those not already requiring such medications, surgery reduced the proportion who required initiation of treatment, as well as the costs of medications (Narbro et al. 2002).

COMPLICATIONS

All bariatric procedures have complications, but the type and frequency vary with the type of surgery. The early problems have been summarized in Table 8.6, adapted from the Longitudinal Analysis of Bariatric Surgery (Flum et al. 2009). In this pooled data set, death occurred in 2.1% of those with open RYGB gastric bypass, 0.2% of those with a laparoscopic gastric bypass, and in none of the 1198 patients who had an adjustable lap-band ($p < 0.001$). Most other complications were significantly different between groups, the insertion of a percutaneous drain being the one exception.

TABLE 8.6
Adverse Outcomes during the First 30 Days after Bariatric Surgery

	Open	Laparoscopic Procedures		
Outcome	**RYGP**	**RYGP**	**Gastric Band**	**P Value**
Number	437	2975	1198	
Death	2.1%	0.2%	0	<0.001
Deep-vein thrombosis	1.1%	0.4%	0.3%	0.05
Tracheal reintubation	1.4%	0.4%	0.4%	0.004
Endoscopy	1.1%	1.5%	1.1%	<0.001
Tracheostomy	1.1%	0.2%	0	0.001
Percutaneous drain	0.7%	0.4%	0	0.48
Abdominal operation	3.4%	3.2%	0.8%	<0.001
In hospital after 30 days	0.9%	0.4%	0	0.02
Composite endpoint	7.8%	4.8%	1.0%	<0.001

Source: Adapted from LABS Consortium, *N. Engl. J. Med.*, 361, 445–454, 2009.

Most complications were more frequent in the open RYGB, the exceptions being endoscopy and abdominal reoperation within the first 30 days where open and laparoscopic RYGB were the same (Flum et al. 2009).

The mortality appears to relate, at least in part, to the complexity of the bariatric procedure. Using pooled data, the 30-day mortality is about 0.2%–0.3% with banding procedures, about 0.9%–1.0% with gastric bypass, and a little over 1% with the "switch" types of operative procedures (Buchwald et al. 2004; Maggard et al. 2005).

Leaks around staple lines are a major life-threatening complication of the gastric bypass and the biliopancreatic diversion. Leaks from the staple lines are the most serious complication and require immediate surgical intervention. They may be responsible for up to 50% of deaths (Regan et al. 2003). The quoted leak rate following gastric bypass is between 0% and 5.1%, with the average leak rate between 2% and 3% (Wittgrove and Clark 2000; Schauer et al. 2000; Nguyen et al. 2001; Westling and Gustavsson 2001). Early symptoms of a leak in the suture line may be subtle, including a low-grade fever, respiratory distress, or an unexplained tachycardia (Hamilton et al. 2003). Exploratory surgery should be performed without delay.

Hospitalization following RYGB gastric bypass is significantly increased. Between 1995 and 2004, there were 60,077 gastric bypass operations performed in California with 11,659 performed in 2004 alone (Zingmond et al. 2005). The hospitalization rate was 7.9% in the year preceding the RYGB and 19.3% in the year following. Among the 24,678 patients for whom 3-year data are available, 8.4% were admitted to the hospital in the year before surgery, 20.2% in the first year after bariatric surgery, 18.4% in the second year, and 14.9% in the third year. The authors conclude that hospitalization in the years following gastric bypass is related to the surgery.

Another early postoperative risk common to all procedures is pulmonary embolus (Melinek et al. 2002). The incidence of deep vein thrombosis and pulmonary embolism varies between 0% to 3.3% with laparoscopic bypasses (Wittgrove and Clark 2000; Schauer et al. 2000; Nguyen et al. 2001; Westling and Gustavsson 2001) and 0.3% to 1.9% with open bypasses (Griffen 1979; Fobi et al. 1998; Hall et al. 1990). In an autopsy series (Melinek et al. 2002), pulmonary embolism was the cause of death in 30% of patients. In addition, 80% had silent pulmonary emboli despite prophylactic treatment with anticoagulants. Risk factors associated with fatal PE include severe venous stasis disease, BMI > 60, truncal adiposity, and obesity-hypoventilation syndrome (Sapala et al. 2003). Use of heparin prophylactically would appear to be a desirable postoperative procedure in obese patients having this operation.

Ventral hernias occur in up to 24% of patients who have open operations, but with laparoscopic surgery, it is reduced to an incidence of 0% to 1.8% (Pories et al. 1995; Wittgrove and Clark 2000; Nguyen et al. 2001; Nguyen et al. 2000; Higa et al. 2000). The RYGB procedure also carries a risk of internal hernias, since the anatomical changes provide new holes through which bowel can be squeezed (Champion and Williams 2003). These internal hernias have been described in 0% and 5% of patients undergoing laparoscopic bariatric surgery (Nguyen et al. 2001; Higa et al. 2000); surgical intervention is required.

The obese have an increased risk of gallstones, and bariatric surgery increases this risk further (Ko et al. 2004). In a meta-analysis of five randomized clinical trials (Uy et al. 2008), urosdeoxycholic acid reduced the incidence of gallstones from 27.7% to 8.8% [RR 0.43 (95% CI 0.22–0.83)].

The metabolic and nutritional derangements can pose significant problems following malabsorptive procedures. Lifelong use of vitamins and minerals is important. Malabsorption of iron, vitamin B12, and folate are the most likely problems. Malabsorption of fat-soluble vitamins, protein, and thiamine may also occur and can manifest itself clinically.

OTHER PROCEDURES

Duodenal Sleeve

The duodenal sleeve is a strategy for reducing absorption of nutrients from the stomach by placing an impermeable liner from the entrance to the stomach down a variable length of the duodenum. In one trial with this technique (Schouten et al. 2009), the device was placed in 30 out of 41 individuals with the remaining 11 serving as a dietary control. Four implantations were not successful, leaving 26 implantations. Four were removed before the end of the 12-week trial. There were adverse events in 100% of the implanted patients compared to 27.3% ($n = 3$) in the diet group. Nausea, upper abdominal pain (first week), a pseudopolyp formation, and inflammation at the implant site were the most common. More information about this new procedure is awaited.

Intragastric Balloon

The intragastric balloon (Bioenterics Intragastric Balloon, Inamed) is a temporary alternative to produce weight loss in moderately obese individuals. It consists of a soft, saline-filled balloon placed in the stomach endoscopically that promotes a feeling of satiety and restriction. It is currently not available for use in the United States, but is undergoing extensive testing in Europe and Brazil. Mean excess weight loss is reported to be 38% and 48% for 500 and 600 mL balloons, respectively (Roman et al. 2004). However, the results of a Brazilian multicenter study indicate weight loss is transient, with only 26% of patients maintaining over 90% of the excess weight loss over one year (Salletesini et al. 2004). Side-effects include nausea, vomiting, abdominal pain, ulceration, and balloon migration. A review of 30 studies with the Bioenterics Intragastric Balloon included 18 prospective studies, among which five were randomized trials, and 12 retrospective studies. Only 1 of the 3 sham-controlled studies favored the balloon. In the nonrandomized studies, weight loss averaged 17.8 kg (range 4.9 to 28.5kg). Gastric perforation and intestinal obstruction each occurred with a frequency of 0.2%. Early removal was required in 2.5% (Dumonceau 2008).

Gastric Stimulation or Gastric Pacing

Gastric pacing as a technique for weight loss was pioneered in pigs, where repeat stimulation produced significant weight loss (Cigaina et al. 1996). The first clinical trial included 24 overweight human beings with a BMI > 40 kg/m^2. Over 9 months of the trial, the BMI was reduced 4.7 kg/m^2 with no significant side-effects (Cigaina et al. 1996). In a follow-up study of 11 patients with an initial BMI of 46.0 kg/m^2 who lost 3.6 kg in the 2 months after implantation of the pace maker, but before it was turned on, there was a further 6.8 kg weight loss after 6 months of electrical stimulation. Following a test meal, there was a smaller rise in cholecystokinin, and lower levels of somatostatin, GLP-1, and leptin, although it is unclear whether this was secondary to the stimulation or weight loss. In a summary of experience on more than 200 patients who had gastric implantation, Shikora (2004) noted that some patients responded well, whereas others did not. An algorithm was developed based on baseline age, gender, body weight, BMI, and response to preoperative questionnaires. With this algorithm, the selection rate for the procedure was 18% to 33%. When this algorithm is applied, excess weight loss is up to 40% in 12 months, compared to a 4% excess weight gain in the control group. More data is needed.

Liposuction

Liposuction, which is also known as lipoplasty or suction-assisted lipectomy, is the most common esthetic procedure performed in the United States with over 400,000 cases performed annually (Klein et al. 2004). Although not generally considered to be a bariatric procedure, removal of fat by aspiration after injection of physiologic saline has been used to remove and contour subcutaneous fat. As the techniques have improved, it is now possible to remove significant amounts of subcutaneous adipose tissue without affecting the amount of visceral fat. In a study to examine the effects of this procedure, Klein et al. (2004) studied seven overweight diabetic women and eight overweight women with normal glucose tolerance before and after liposuction. One week after assessing insulin sensitivity, the subjects underwent large volume tumescent liposuction, which consists of removing more than 4 liters of aspirate injected into the fat beneath the skin. There was a significant loss of subcutaneous fat, but no change in the visceral fat. Subjects were reassessed 10–12 weeks after the surgery, when the nondiabetic women had lost 6.3 kg of body weight and 9.1 kg of body fat, which reduced body fat by 6.3%. The diabetic women had a similar response with a weight loss of 7.9 kg, a reduction in body fat of 10.5 kg, and a reduction in percent fat of 6.7%. Waist circumference was also significantly reduced. In spite of these significant reductions in body fat, there were no changes in blood pressure, lipids, or cytokines (tumor necrosis factor-a, interleukin-6) or C-reactive protein. There was also no improvement in insulin sensitivity, suggesting that removal of subcutaneous adipose tissue without reducing visceral fat has little influence on the risk factors related to being overweight.

Omentectomy

The omentum is the fat that laps over the intestines and is a component of the total visceral fat, but one that exclusively drains into the portal vein. The quantity is sufficiently small that its removal in dogs could not be detected with imaging techniques or measurement of total body fat. However, omentectomy did alleviate insulin resistance by augmenting the sensitivity to insulin in peripheral tissues. This finding makes this small fat tissue one of the more important metabolic regulators of insulin sensitivity that is known (Lottati and Kolka 2009).

Omentectomy is the direct removal of the intra-abdominal fat by surgical means. One randomized controlled trial in 50 overweight subjects compared the effect of an adjustable lap-band alone or a lap-band plus removal of the omentum (Thorne et al. 2002). Of the original 50 operated patients, 37 were reevaluated at the end of 2 years after surgery. The reduction in body weight was 27 kg in the lap-band group and 36 kg in the lap-band + omentectomy group ($p = 0.07$). Both glucose and insulin improved more in the subjects with omentectomy than in those without it. This study complements the one by Klein described above by showing that removal of extra visceral fat can have a small but significant effect, while decreasing subcutaneous fat alone has little impact. Another clinical trial did not find any effect of randomly removing the omentum in some patients who had a gastric bypass (Csendes et al. 2009). In this study, 35 patients had omentectomy and 35 did not. Two years after the operation, the glucose, insulin, cholesterol, triglycerides, and weight changes were similar in the two groups.

9 Postscript *Obesity in the Twenty-First Century*

LESSONS WE HAVE LEARNED IN THIS BOOK

Obesity Is an Ancient Problem

Statuettes with prominent obesity date from more than 30,000 years ago in the Paleolithic or Old Stone Age (Conrad 2009), and indicate that humans have been aware of excess fat for a very long time. In spite of this long history, understanding this problem required a large base of scientific knowledge that took centuries to develop. To depict this growth of knowledge, I have constructed an inverted triangle (Figure 9.1) designed to indicate that from a small base there is a steady growth of knowledge (Ziman 1976). At the tip of the pyramid, 30,000 years, are the Paleolithic figurines found throughout Eurasia. It took nearly 28,000 of these 30,000 years before a sound clinical base for obesity began to appear in medical cultures around the world, and an additional 1500 years before there was enough knowledge to begin to understand the problem in any detail.

The scientific beginnings of obesity can be dated to the seventeenth century. Even these beginnings that included a scale used by Santorio (1614) to weigh himself and detect what we now call "insensible" weight loss, that is, the loss of water through the air we expire and perspiration. It was almost two centuries before real progress began in the early nineteenth century.

Lessons Learned in the Nineteenth Century

Concept of Energy Balance

One major nineteenth-century conceptual base for the science of obesity was the discovery of oxygen by Lavoisier (1789), formulation of the energy balance concept (Helmholtz 1847), and its application to human beings living in a metabolic chamber by Atwater and Rosa (1896). This century-long journey was punctuated by all of the false starts and major breakthroughs that characterize scientific revolutions (Kuhn 1962).

The Body Mass Index

The body mass index was a second lesson from the nineteenth century. It was introduced by Quetelet (1835) from his studies on the development of the human being. Although it was not widely used during the next century as a way to evaluate obesity, over the last 50 years of the twentieth century, it has become the main way of relating height, weight, and the prevalence of obesity around the world.

The First Diet Reaches World-Wide Popularity

The third noteworthy event in the nineteenth century was the beginning of popular diets for weight loss. It started in 1863, at the time of the American Civil War, when a small pamphlet was published in England by William Banting. It was quickly republished and went through editions for the next 40 years. It was widely translated and the word "banting" became synonymous with dieting. The list of popular diets that followed come like crops of new eggs each year and will continue into the twenty-first century.

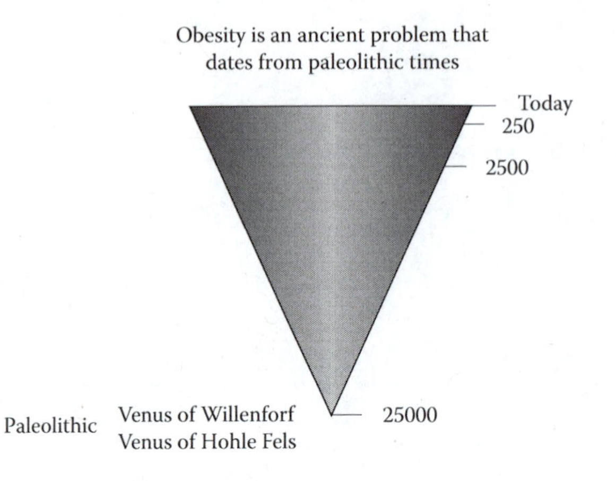

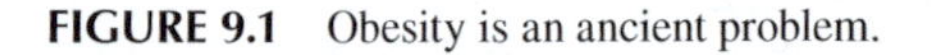
FIGURE 9.1 Obesity is an ancient problem.

Lessons Learned in the Twentieth Century

As we can see from the second triangle in Figure 9.2, most of the action has been in the twentieth century. This triangle begins very near the broad top of the first figure, showing how much scientific background we started with. This triangle is still expanding—can we glimpse what it will show in the twenty-first century?

Obesity Is Hazardous to Health

The most important lesson of the twentieth century was that obesity is hazardous to health and that losing weight intentionally can prolong life. At the beginning of the twentieth century, the Life Insurance Industry (Association of Life Insurance 1913) established that overweight individuals with insurance policies had earlier deaths than people of normal weight. Although major deviations in weight were recognized as hazardous, there was reluctance to accept that modest degrees of overweight were hazardous. It took the Framingham Study (Hubert et al. 1983) to finally establish in the 1980s that obesity was an independent predictor of early death. This was followed by an ever-growing number of studies that buttressed this finding and refined its limits.

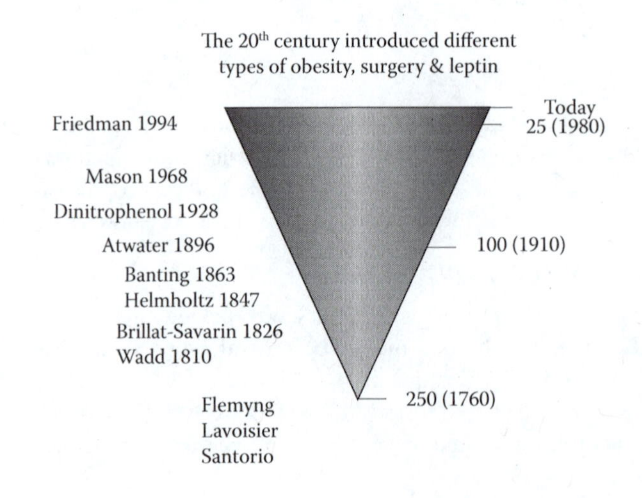

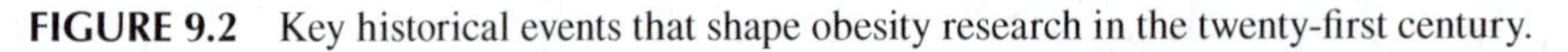
FIGURE 9.2 Key historical events that shape obesity research in the twenty-first century.

Intentional Weight Loss Prolongs Life

If being overweight is hazardous to your health, one might presume that weight loss would be beneficial. However, it has been known from ancient times that weight loss can be a harbinger to underlying disease and this was confirmed in the twentieth century (Pamuk et al. 1992). Separating this "unintentional" weight loss caused by underlying disease and "intentional" weight loss has been one of the successes of the late twentieth century. The detrimental associations with obesity such as diabetes, high blood pressure, sleep apnea, and other illnesses could be mitigated or reversed by weight loss. It was the use of bariatric surgery in a controlled trial beginning in the 1980s that provided the most convincing evidence for improved longevity with weight loss. After an 11-year follow-up, the Swedish Obese Subjects (SOS) study showed a significant reduction in mortality among the group that lost weight compared to the obese individuals who did not lose weight (Sjostrom et al. 2007).

There Are Many Types of Obesity

The twentieth century dawned with the publication of two seminal papers, one by Josef Babinski (1900), a leading neurologist and the other by Alfred Frohlich (1901) a budding young endocrinologist. They each described a single patient whose obesity resulted from injury to the hypothalamus producing short stature, obesity, and impaired sexual development. This syndrome was known for many years as "The Frohlich Syndrome" or the "Adiposo-genital Syndrome" and lead to a century-long series of studies on the mechanisms by which the hypothalamus controlled food intake and body fat stores (King 2006; Bray and York 1979).

A second type of obesity was identified in 1912 Harvey Cushing (1932), the famous neurosurgeon. He described individuals who had obesity due to a disease of the pituitary gland. This resulted, as we now know, because a small tumor in this gland secreted a hormone that stimulated the production of excessive amounts of adrenal steroids. The publication of the syndrome that came to be known as "Cushing's Syndrome" occurred at the time when the first genetically inherited strains of obesity were identified. At about the same time, the first strain of mice with "inherited" obesity was described. As the twentieth century passed, several other types of obesity in mice and rats were described that inherited their obesity. Discovery of these mice set the stage for one of the key discoveries of the twentieth century—the discovery of leptin in 1994 (Zhang et al. 1994).

The identification of different types of obesity continued throughout the twentieth century. In 1956, for example, Prader, Labhart, and Willi (1956) reported a syndrome that bears their name. It is rare, but distinctive. A number of other rare but distinctive types of obesity have now been described. The stage was thus set for the growth of genetic and epigenetic studies into the causes of obesity in the twenty-first century.

Not All Fat Is the Same

The concept of the "cell" as a distinct entity came in the early nineteenth century (Schwann 1839), and it was shortly after that we recognized that it is where fat is stored (Hassall 1849). The fat cell plays a part in the daily orchestra of life. It makes music through the chemicals it produces. Sometimes the notes are beautiful, but they can also be discordant (Flier 2004). With the discovery that leptin is made almost entirely in the fat cell, it has become clear that the fat cell has very significant functions besides storing fat (Zhang et al. 1994). Fat cells are part of the largest glandular (endocrine) tissue in the body. They produce numerous products that are released into the circulation and that act on other cells. Among these are molecules that cause inflammation, molecules that are involved in controlling blood pressure or influencing cell growth, and molecules that regulate fat metabolism and blood clotting. What a powerhouse fat tissue is in the human body!

The commonly called "beer-belly" or "apple shape" is medically termed "central adiposity" (Vague 1947). The twentieth century shows us that central adiposity is a risk to your health. This was first noted nearly 100 years ago and again right after World War II, but it wasn't until 1982 that it became widely appreciated that people with central adiposity were at high risk for diabetes and heart disease (Lapidus et al. 1984; Larsson et al. 1982; Kissebah 1982). Waist circumference is a useful way to measure central adiposity and is one criterion for diagnosing the metabolic syndrome. The other signs and symptoms that are used in diagnosing the metabolic syndrome include high blood pressure, high blood sugar, low levels of HDL-cholesterol, and high levels of triglycerides that are collectively related to the risk of developing heart disease and diabetes.

Food Intake Drives the Obesity Epidemic

The issue of whether rising food intake or reduced physical activity was the cause of obesity has raged since the epidemic began in the late twentieth century. Providing answers to this question was greatly facilitated by the discovery that stable isotopes of oxygen and hydrogen could be used to estimate energy expenditure in free living people (Lipson 1949; Schoeller 1998). With this technique, it became clear that food intake records often underestimated the amount of energy that was needed to provide for daily energy expenditure (Lichtman 1986). It also made possible the measurement of changes in physical activity level (Westerterp and Speakman 2008). What they found was that the physical activity level (PAL) had not changed over about 20 years. Putting this data together, Swinburn et al. (2009) concluded that the increase in food intake could account for all of the weight gain identified in the obesity epidemic of the last 25 years of the twentieth century.

Aniline Dyes and Drug Development

The late nineteenth century was the heyday for the textile industry and the chemical dyes that made these mass-produced fabrics so colorful. As the dye industry grew, organic chemistry expanded and the introduction of new drugs for treatment of many diseases was one important outcome. Amphetamine, a product of this industry, was the first drug used systematically to treat obesity in clinical studies just before World War II.

Obesity Becomes Organized

As the field of obesity began to mature as a field of scholarly work, a number of things happened. First, groups of scientists interested in obesity began to form local organizations to promote interest in the problem. The first of these was in the United Kingdom called The Association for the Study of Obesity. It held its first meeting in 1968 (Howard 1975). This was followed in 1973 by the first NIH Fogarty Center Conference on Obesity held in Washington, DC (Bray 1976). One year later the First International Congress on Obesity was held in London (Howard 1975). Following these congresses, it was clear that a journal devoted to papers dealing specifically with obesity was needed, and the *International Journal of Obesity* was founded. Publication began in 1976 under the editorship of Dr. Alan Howard and Dr. George Bray. Subsequent international congresses were held in 1977 in Washington, DC (Bray 1978), in 1980 in Rome (Bjorntorp et al. 1981), in 1983 in New York City (Hirsch and Van Itallie 1984), in 1986 in Jerusalem (Blondheim et al. 1987), in 1990 in Kobe, Japan (Oomura et al. 1991), in 1994 in Toronto (Angel et al. 1995), in 1998 in Paris (Guy-Grand et al. 1999), in 2002 in Sao Paulo (Medeiros-Neto and Halpern 2003), in 2006 in Sydney, Australia, and in 2010 in Stockholm, Sweden. In 1986, the International Association for the Study of Obesity was formed under the leadership of Dr. Barbara Hansen. As growth continued, a second journal appeared in 1980 under the title *Obesity and Weight Regulation*. This journal, like so many others, succumbed, in part, because it was not part of one of the national associations (Bray 1995). *Obesity Surgery* was the third journal to be founded and was followed in 1993 by *Obesity Research*, published by the North American Association for the Study of Obesity. This rapid growth of scientific journals surrounding a scientific discipline is characteristic of developments that have sprung up throughout the scientific sphere to provide a way of focusing the activities of scientists in a manageable way. It is part of the expanding triangle illustrated in Figure 9.2.

Two events in the 1970s impacted the development of obesity. One was the development of the "isomerase" process for converting corn starch into high-fructose corn syrup (HFCS), which is cheap to make and which has displaced much of the sugar (sucrose) in foods and essentially all of the sugar (sucrose) used to sweeten soft drinks in America. At the same time, and without adequate recognition at the time, agricultural policies in the United States were undergoing changes that made some food products, including corn, cheaper. As food prices fell, they represented a smaller fraction of the household budget, and this allowed more people to eat away from home and to enjoy the tasty, high-energy-density foods provided by the increasing number of fast-food and other restaurants (Bray 2010). Tucked away at the same time was the first edition of my first book about obesity, *The Obese Patient*, published in 1976.

The last decade of the twentieth century also saw the birth of the Pennington Biomedical Research Center in Baton Rouge, LA, made possible by a donation from Claude Bernard Pennington, a philanthropic oilman. The recruitment of George A. Bray, MD as its first director and Claude Bouchard, PhD as its second director focused the research agenda of this institution on obesity. At the celebration of the twentieth anniversary of the PBRC in 2009, a symposium was organized on the 20 most important contributions to the field of obesity in the past 20 years. These included talks on leptin and its receptor, adiponectin and its receptor, the melanocortin receptors, signals arising from the GI tract, the uncoupling proteins in brown adipose tissue, the inflammatory aspects of fat tissue, the role of epigenetic factors in the obesity epidemic, the newer imaging techniques as they apply to obesity, bariatric surgery, regulation of body weight, the global problem of obesity, fructose as a dietary factor, television as a sedentary activity, and the built environment as it influences obesity. Clearly, many of these topics will be fruitful subjects for research programs in the twenty-first century (Bouchard et al. 2009).

Leptin Is Discovered in the Last Decade of the Twentieth Century

The most important advance in obesity in the last half of the twentieth century was the discovery of leptin (Zhang 1994). This peptide hormone is made predominantly in the fat cells. When leptin is absent, massive overweight occurs in human beings and in research animals. Defects in the leptin receptor, the "lock" that the leptin molecule "key" fits into, are responsible for a small number of massively overweight people. In addition to derangements in the leptin genes, defects in other genes can produce obesity in human beings. One of these genes, called the melanocortin-4 receptor gene, is defective in up to 5% of markedly overweight youngsters. This is one of the most frequent genetic causes for a chronic human disease yet reported. Yet, collectively, these individuals are only a tiny fraction of all obese people.

Lifestyle Strategies Introduced into Treatment

Behavior modification could be used to treat overweight subjects (Stuart 1967). As this technique was developed in detail, it became one of the "three pillars," along with diet and exercise, for the treatment of obesity. Because of the response to behavioral strategies, obesity has been labeled a "lifestyle disease." Efforts have been made to adapt these behavioral techniques to prevent development of weight gain in larger groups of people, but they have been disappointing.

Clinical Trials Come of Age

Diets can reduce your risk of disease and prove a way to treat some of them effectively. This was shown elegantly in a study comparing the effects on blood pressure with one of three different dietary patterns (Appel et al. 1997; Sacks et al. 2001). The first diet, the reference diet, was a standard American diet or Western-type diet, with plenty of fat, meat, and normal amounts of fruits and vegetables. The second diet, one of the two experimental diets, was called the "fruits and vegetables diet" because it was enriched with fruits and vegetables. The aim was to increase dietary intake of magnesium and potassium from fruits and vegetables to the seventy-fifth percentile of normal, that is, a level above what three out of four people would normally get in their diet. The third diet—the Combination or DASH Diet—was enriched to the same degree as the second diet with fruits and vegetables. In addition, it had more low fat dairy products to increase calcium intake and also had lowered total fat intake (27% vs. 33% in the control diet), more fiber, higher protein (18%) with the extra 3% from vegetable sources, and reduced intake of calorically sweetened beverages and other sweets. Blood pressure was significantly reduced in people eating the fruits-and-vegetables diet and reduced even more in the people eating the Combination (fruits-vegetables-low-fat dairy products) or DASH diet (Chapter 6).

Another large clinical trial, called the Diabetes Prevention Program, showed that weight loss with a reduction of fat and more activity could significantly reduce the risk of diabetes mellitus in people at high risk for this disease (Diabetes Prevention Program 2002).

Surgery for Obesity Expands

Surgical treatment for obesity began in the 1960s (Mason and Ito 1967). The current popularity of these procedures is the result of the lowered risk from surgery with the use of newer, so-called laparoscopic surgeries. Using laparoscopic techniques reduces the risk and has increased the number of treated patients. It is estimated that more than 200,000 people have this surgery each year. The mortality has been reduced and many of the complications associated with surgery have been reduced.

WHERE DO WE GO IN THE TWENTY-FIRST CENTURY?

This book began with an historical review of the field, and it is appropriate as I draw it to a close to bring the past to the future. In his beautifully written book from 1826 titled *The Physiology of Taste* (*Le Physiology du Gout*), Brillat-Savarin made the following prescient comments that may point the way forward when he said:

> "Any cure of obesity must begin with the three following and absolute precepts: discretion in eating, moderation in sleeping, and exercise on food or on horseback."
> But, ". . . it needs great strength of character for a man to get up from the table while he is still hungry . . ." "it is a painful insult to fat people to tell them to get up early in the morning. . ." "Exercise on foot . . . is horribly tiring, and the perspiration it rings out places one in grave danger of false pleurisy . . ."
> "Therefore, while it is admitted that anyone who wishes to reduce his weight should eat moderately, sleep but little, and exercise as much as possible, another method must be sought to attain the same end." (Brillat-Savarin 1826)

This was a call to creative thinking about the problem of obesity—a problem that still needs this kind of thinking.

Future Trends

Genetics and Epigenetics

As we have seen, understanding the genetic basis of obesity has made much progress in the last decade of the twentieth century and the first decade of the twenty-first century. However, much remains to be done to get a clear picture of all of the genes that have small effects on body weight, which collectively make it easier to become obese. We also have begun to scratch the surface of understanding how genes are regulated and this may be even more important for the ordinary types of obesity. From animal studies, we know that changing the composition of the diet to provide more "methyl" groups can change both the coat color and body fat content of specific strains of animals. The so-called "epigenetic programming" has been discussed in relation to the effects of smoking in pregnant women on the future risk for obesity in their children. There are almost certainly many more environmental factors—some call them endocrine disruptors—that can modify the risk of obesity during pregnancy and later in life.

Energy Balance—Long-Term Signals

The recent analysis of the obesity epidemic to try to decide whether food intake has risen, exercise fallen, or both, has been quite definitive in my judgment. It is the rise in food intake. Yet even in this surfeit of food, not everyone gets fat. This means that there are internal and/or external signals that help regulate body weight. Although we have mapped out the signals that affect meal to meal food intake, we still have only rudimentary understanding of what regulates food intake and body fat stores over longer periods of time (Bray et al. 2008). This is clearly an important research item for the agenda of the twenty-first century.

Hedonic Influences—Is Food Addictive?

Eating is a pleasurable experience most of the time. Food companies know that foods need to "taste" good for them to sell well. The fast food companies are masters at providing "tasty" palatable foods that people like and at an affordable price. For some people, these "pleasurable" responses to overeating stimulate eating of more than is needed. The relationship of pleasurable eating and pleasure from other senses was demonstrated by the failure of two drugs that acted to attenuate food intake through receptor systems that are involved with pleasure. In both cases there was increased suicidal ideation leading to termination of these products.

Behavior Change—Influence of Neighbors

One of the surprising findings at the transition from the twentieth to the twenty-first century is that neighbors influence one another's weight status. Neighbors in this context are not just the people living next door, but people even at a distance with whom an individual has a relationship (Christakis and Fowler 2007). The data showing this came from the long-standing Framingham Study started in Framingham, MA in 1948, which has contributed so much to our understanding of heart disease and obesity. The message is that we may be able to influence the "obesity epidemic" on a population basis.

Neural Plasticity—Changing Networks

One of the interesting facts about leptin, the hormone from adipose tissue that attenuates food intake, is that it also influences neural development in the brain. In mice that are deficient in leptin, the neural network in the base of the brain remains immature. When these animals are treated with leptin, the neural networking increases (Pinto 2004). Unraveling the meaning of this type of neural plasticity, and how the neural networks talk to one another in response to the environment, is another key way for affecting the epidemic of obesity.

Price and Palatability

We are all price sensitive; that is, we look for bargains. One way to get a bargain in food is through the amount of energy you get for your dollar. I described in Chapter 3 that the cheapest foods were ones with federal subsidies that are mass produced and can provide sugar and fat cheaply. You can get a day's worth of calories (2000–3000) for a small amount of money. Fruits and vegetables, for which we aren't using taxpayer dollars to support farm prices, are more expensive. However, the cheapest food, in my judgment, is not the best food. Getting chicken and fish, fruits and vegetables, and unrefined whole grains is worth the extra money—it will reduce the intake of the high fat, high sugar (fructose), highly refined foods that most experts think are related to the current epidemic.

Cognitive Theories and Success

The Fluoride Hypothesis

Behavioral strategies are cognitive strategies, that is, they require you to do something active, such as dieting, exercising, or modifying the way you live. We are slowly learning that these cognitive strategies do not translate into the prevention of obesity, and that the weight that people initially lose using them is often regained. The alternative to "cognitive" approaches is the use of "noncognitive" approaches, that is, ways of dealing with overweight that do not require much active individual involvement. This is one answer to Brillat-Savarin's challenge. In the prevention of dental caries ("cavities"), the addition of fluoride to the drinking water supply will reduce cavities and is a good example of a noncognitive strategy. When our water is fluoridated, dental caries are dramatically reduced, without our intentional activity.

There are several things that may help prevent overweight and that don't require much effort. Taking more calcium may be one of them. People with higher intakes of calcium have lower body weight in some, but not all, studies. Low fat dairy products are good sources of calcium and can help lower blood pressure. I recommend the use of fruits and vegetables as sources of "good fructose," and low-fat dairy products unless you are susceptible to kidney stones. Calcium can help your bones and may have some benefit for your body weight.

Less sleep is associated with higher body weights. Children who sleep less gain more weight in their preschool years (Al Mamun et al. 2007). This also applies to adults, and there is now a potential explanation for this effect in the changes of sleep-influencing hormones—changes that occur with too little sleep. Try to get your 8 hours of sleep each night, and even more sleep for the children.

Another low-effort strategy for weight loss would be to buy foods for "health," not for "price." Turning off that natural desire to get more for your money when buying food may be hard. But what you get for your money when you buy cheap food may be "bad fructose" and fat, which may simply become "waste on your waist." My conclusion is that it is better to eat well than to eat cheaply.

The Oil Price and Oil Equivalents for Calories

Oil comes in two forms—the oil from the ground that is used to make gasoline and other petroleum products, and the oil(s) in food that are largely composed of triacylglycerols that can be digested in the intestinal tract. For most of the twentieth century, the price of oil, and thus the products produced from it, was low allowing it to be used for many things. We have done this by purchasing oil from the "oil-producing" countries as our own supply of oil from oil wells on American soil has decreased. The economic benefits of this are evident when visiting any of their "oil-rich" countries and contrasting them with their "oil-poor" neighbors. The impact on our food supply is also evident. Oil-based products provide the fertilizer that allows farmers to grow bumper crops. It provides the chemicals to make the packaging for this food. It allows shipment of fresh food to all parts of the world. In the latter half of the twentieth century, the supply of fresh fruits and vegetables during winters months increased in all wealthy countries in the northern hemisphere as a result of air-shipment, which uses oil-based products. In a discussion of the food supply, Pollan (2008) pointed out that from 1940 to 2005 the amount of oil used for each calorie of food we grow has increased over 20-fold! The food industry is now strongly oil-based.

As the world demand for oil and other energy sources rises in the twenty-first century, oil prices are likely to rise substantially. Early in the twenty-first century we saw oil prices rise to over $160/barrel and then fall with the recession of 2008–10. As world demand rises again, the supply of oil will remain stable or decline, driving the price of oil upward. This will produce profound changes in the food supply just as the cheap oil did in the late twentieth century: more local foods, fewer exotic raspberries in the winter, and higher prices for food. These changes in the price of oil and the ensuing changes in the food supply and its cost, may provide the kind of "fluoride" for obesity that I discussed earlier.

We will all have to wait and see.

Appendix
Dissertations Relating to Obesity from the Sixteenth, Seventeenth, and Eighteenth Centuries

SIXTEENTH CENTURY

Forrest, Pierre 1570 (See Regneller Book)

Erastus, Thomas de. Pinguedinis in animalibut generatione et concretione. In MM Schenkio, Philosophi et medici celeberrimi disputationum et episolarum medicnalium, volumen doctissimum. Tiguri: Johan Wolphium, 1595.

SEVENTEENTH CENTURY

Ettmueller, M. Pratique de medicine speciale . . . sur les maladies propres des hommes, des femmes & des petits enfans, avec des Dissertations . . . sur l'epilepsie, l'yvresse, le mal hypochondriaque, la douleur hypochondriaque, la corpulence, & la morsure de la vipere (trad. nouv). Lyon: Thomas Amaulry, 1691.

Gosky, A.U. Disputatio solennis de marasmo, sive marcore: macilentia item & gracilitate sanorum; macilentia & gracilitate aegrotatium; crassitie & corpulentia sanorum naturali; crassitie & magnitudine corporis morbosa aegrorum. Argentinae: Typis Eberhardii Welperi, 1658.

Held, J.F. Disputationem medica de corpulentia nimia. Publicae . . . censurae . . . submittit. Jenae: Nisianis, 1670.

Leisner, K.C. Dissertatio medica de obesitate exsuperante. Jenae: Typ Gollnerianis, 1683.

Widemann, G.M. Disputatio medica de corpulaentia nimia. Lipsiae: typ Krugerianus, 1681.

EIGHTEENTH CENTURY

Bass, G. Dissertationem inauguralem medicam de obesitate nimia. Erfordiae: Preolo Heringii, 1740.

Bertram, J.W. Dissertatio inauguralis medica de pinguedine. Halae Magdeb: J.C. Hilligeri, 1739.

Bon, J. Dissertatio medica inauguralis. De mutatione pinguedinis. Harderovici: Apud Johannem Moojen, 1742.

Bougourd, O. An obesis somnus brevis salubrior? Paris: 1733.

Dissertatio inauguralis medica de obesitate: Viennae: Typis Joan Thomae Nobil. de Trattnern, 1776.

Ebart, F.C.W. Dissertatio inauguralis medica de obesitate nimia et morbis inde orindus. small quarto ed. Gottingen: Lit J.H. Schulzii, 1780.

Fecht, E.H. Disputatio medica inauguralis de obesitate nimia. Rostochi: J. Wepplingii, 1701.

Hoelder, F.B. Obesitatis corporis humani nosologia. Tubingae: Lit Schrammianis, 1775.

Homeroch, C.F. De pinguidine ejusque sede tam secundum quam preaeter naturam constitutis. Lipsiae: Ex Offician Langenhemiana, 1996.

Hulsebusch, J.F. Dissertatio inauguralis medica sistens pinguedinis corporis humani, sive panniculi adiposi veterum, hodie membranae cullulosae dictae fabricam, ejusque, & contenti olei historiam, usum, morbos. Lugduni Batavorum: Joh Arnold Langerak, 1728.

Jansen, W.X. Pinguedinis animalis consideratio physiologica et pathologica. Lugduni Batavorum: J. Hazebroek, A. van Houte et Andream Koster, 1784.

Kroedler, J.S. Theses inauguralis medicae de eo quod citius moriantur obesi, quam graciles secundum Hippocratis aphorismum XLIV. Sect II. Erfordiae: Typis Groschianis, 1724.

La Sone, J.M.F. An in macilentis liberior quam in obesis circulatio. Paris: Quillau, 1740.
Locke, S.C.J. De celeri corporum incremento causa debilitatis in morbis. Lipsiae: ex officina Langenhemia, 1760.
Lohe, A.W. Exhibens de morbis adipis humani principia generalia. Duisburg, 1772.
Muller, P.A. Dissertatio physiologica de pinguedine corporis. Hafniae: Typis Andreae Hartvigi Godiche, 1766.
Oswald, J.H. Obesitatis corporis humani therapia. Tubingae: Litteris Schrammianis, 1775.
Person, C. An parcior obesis, quam macilentis sanguinis missio. Paris: Quillau, 1748.
Pohl, J.C. Dissertationem inauguralem de obesis et voracibus eorumque vitae incommodis ac morbis. Lipsiae: J.C. Langenhemii, 1734.
Polonus, S.I. Dissertatio medica inauguralis de pinguedine. Harderovici: Typis Everardi Tyhoff, 1797.
Quabeck, K.J. Dissertatio inauguralis medica de insolito corporis augmento frequenti morborum futurorum signo. Halae Magdeb: J.C. Hendelii, 1752.
Redhead, J. Dissertatio physiologica-medica, inauguralis, de adipe, quam annuente summo numine. Edinburgh: Balfour et Smellie, 1789.
Riegels, N.D. De usu glandularum superrenalium in animalibus nec non de origine adipis. Hafniae, 1790.
Reussing, H.C.T. Dissertatio inauguralis medica de pinguedine sana et morbosa. Jenae: ex officina Fiedleriana, 1791.
Riemer, J.A. De obesitatis causis praecipuis. Halae and Salem: Stanno Hendeliano, 1778.
Schroeder, P.G. Dissertatio inauguralis medica de obesitate vitanda. Rintelii. J.G. Enax, 1756.
Schulz, C. Disputatio medica inauguralis de obesitate quam, annuente summo numine. Lugduni Batavorum: Conradum Wishoff, 1752.
Seifert, P.D.B. Dissertatio phyiologico-pathologico de pinguedine. Gryphiswaldiae: I.H. Eckhardt, 1794.
Steube, J.S. Dissertatio medica de corpulentia nimia. Jenae: Litteris Mullerianus, 1716.
Tralles, B.L. Dissertatio de obesorum ad morbos mortemque declivitte. Halae Magdeb: Litteris Hilligerianis, 1730.
Triller, D.W. De pinguedine seu succo nutritio superfluo. Halae: Type C. Henklii, 1718.
Trouillart, G. Dissertatiio physiologico-practica inauguralis de pinguedine, et morbis ex nimia ejus quantitate. Harderovici: Apud Joannem Moojen, 1767.
Vaulpre, J.M. De obesitate, comodis et noxis. Montepellier: Joannem-Franciscum Picot, 1782.
Verdries, J.M. Dissertatio medica inauguralis de pinguedinis usibus et nocumentis in corpore humano. 8th ed. Giessae Hassorum: J.R. Vulpius, 1702.

Bibliography

Ackerknecht, E.H. *Medicine at the Paris Hospital.* Baltimore: The Johns Hopkins University Press, 1967.

Beller, A.S. *Fat and Thin: A Natural History of Obesity.* New York: Farrar Giroux and Straus, 1978.

Bray, G.A. *The Obese Patient.* Philadelphia: W.B. Saunders, 1976.

Bray, G.A. *An Atlas of Obesity and Weight Control* (The Encyclopedia of Visual Medicine series). New York: The Parthenon Publishing Group, 2003.

Bray, G.A. *The Battle of the Bulge.* Pittsburgh, PA: Dorrance Publishing, 2007.

Bray, G.A. *The Metabolic Syndrome and Obesity.* Totowa, NJ: The Humana Press, 2007.

Bray, G.A., Bouchard, C. (eds). *The Handbook of Obesity: Clinical Applications,* 3rd ed. New York: Informa HealthCare, 2008.

Bray, G.A. (ed.) *Obesity in Perspective.* A conference sponsored by the John E. Fogarty International Center for Advanced Study in the Health Sciences. National Institutes of Health, Bethesda, MD, October 1–3, 1973. Washington, DC: U.S. Government Printing Office, DHEW Publ No (NIH) 75-708, Parts I and II.

Bray, G.A. *The Low-Fructose Approach to Weight Control.* Pittsburgh, PA: Dorrance Publishing, 2009.

Brillat-Savarin, J.A. *Physiologie du gout, ou meditations de gastronomie transcendante; ouvrage theorique, historique et a l'ordre du jour, dedie aux gastronomes parisiens.* Paris: Sautelet et Cie, 1826.

Brillat-Savarin, J.A. *The Physiology of Taste or, Meditations on Transcendental Gastronomy* (A new translation by M.F.K. Fisher with illustrations by Sylvain Sauvage). New York: The Limited Editions Club, 1949.

Bruch, H. *The Importance of Overweight.* New York: W.W. Norton & Company, Inc., 1957.

Cannon, W.B. *The Wisdom of the Body.* New York: W.W. Norton & Company, 1932.

Carel, R. *Obesite. Ante-hypophyse et Metabolisme des Lipides.* Paris: Vigot Freres, editeurs. 1936.

Chambers, T.K. The Gulstonian lectures on corpulence. *Lancet* 1850;2:11–19, 342–350, 438–445.

Duffin, J. *History of Medicine. A Scandalously Short Introduction.* Toronto: The University of Toronto Press, 1999.

Garrison, F. *An Introduction to the History of Medicine.* Philadelphia: W.B. Saunders and Co., 1914.

Garrow, J.S. *Energy Balance and Obesity in Man.* Amsterdam: Elsevier/North Holland Press, 1978.

Garrow, J.S. *Treat Obesity Seriously. A Clinical Manual.* Edinburgh and London: Churchill Livingstone, 1981.

Guerini, A. *Obesity and Depression in the Enlightenment. The Life and Times of George Cheyne.* Norman, OK: University of Oklahoma, 2000.

Haslam, D., Haslam, F. *Fat, Gluttony and Sloth: Obesity in Literature, Art and Medicine.* Liverpool: University of Liverpool, 2008.

Hautin, R-J-R. *Obesite. Conceptions Actuelle.* These pour le Doctorat en Medecin. Bordeaux: Imprimerie Biere, 1939.

Kleiber, M. *The Fire of Life. An Introduction to Animal Energetics.* New York: John Wiley & Sons, Inc., 1961.

Lusk, G. *The Elements of the Science of Nutrition.* Philadelphia: W.B. Saunders Company, 1928.

Medvei, V.C. *A History of Endocrinology.* Lancaster: MTP Press, 1982.

Mintz, S.W. *Sweetness and Power. The Place of Sugar in Modern History.* New York: Penguin Books, 1986.

Oliver, J.E. Fat Politics. *The Real Story behind America's Obesity Epidemic.* New York: Oxford University Press, 2006.

Ostman, J., Birtton, M., Jonsson, E. *Treating and Preventing Obesity. An Evidence Based Review.* Weinheim: Wiley-VCH Verlage GmbH & Co. KGaA, 2004.

Pollen, M. *The Omnivore's Dilemma. A Natural History of Four Meals.* New York: The Penguin Press, 2006.

Porter R. *For the Greater Good.* New York: W.W. Norton and Company, 2007.

Power, M.L., and Schulkin, J. *The Evolution of Obesity.* Baltimore: Johns Hopkins University Press, 2009.

Rony, H.R. *Obesity and Leanness.* Philadelphia: Lea and Febiger, 1940.

Schwartz, H. *Never Satisfied. A Cultural History of Diets, Fantasies and Fat.* New York: The Free Press, 1986.

Stearns, P.N. *Fat History. Bodies and Beauty in the Modern West.* New York: New York University Press, 1997.

Talbot, J.H. *A Biographical History of Medicine. Excerpts and Essays on the Men and Their Work.* New York: Grune and Stratton, 1970.

Taubes, G. *Good Calories Bad Calories. Challenging the Conventional Wisdom on Diet, Weight Control, and Disease*. New York: Alfred A. Knopf, 2007.

Wadd, W. *Cursory Remarks on Corpulence; or Obesity Considered as a Disease: with a Critical Examination of Ancient and Modern Opinion, Relative to its Causes and Cure*, 3rd ed. London: J. Callow, 1816.

Wadd, W. *Comments on Corpulency Lineaments of Leanness Mems on Diet and Dietetics*. London: John Ebers & Co., 1829.

World Health Organization. Obesity: Preventing and Managing the Global Epidemic. Report of a WHO Consultation. Geneva: World Health Organization Technical Report Series # 892, 2000.

Worthington, L.S. *De l'obesite. Etiologie, Therapeutiques et Hygiene.* These presentee et soutenir le 12 Aout, 1875. Paris: I. Martinet, 1875, Pp. 1–188.

References

PREFACE

Adams T.D. Gress R.E., et al. 2007. Long–term mortality after gastric bypass surgery. *N Engl J Med* 357: 753–761.

Appel L.J. Moore T.J., et al. 1997. A clinical trial of the effects of dietary patterns on blood pressure. *N Engl J Med* 338:1117–1124.

Association of Life Insurance Medical Directors and Actuarial Society of America. 1913. *MedicoActuarial Mortality Investigation*. New York: The Association of Life Insurance Medical Directors and The Actuarial Society of America.

Atwater W.O., Rosa E.B. 1899. *Description of a New Respiration Calorimeter and Experiments on the Conservation of Energy in the Human Body*. USDA Bull. 63, Washington, D.C.: USDA Office of Experimental Station.

Babinski M.J. 1900. Tumeur du corps pituitaire sans acromégalie et avec de développement des organes génitaux. *Revue Neurologique* 8:531–533.

Banting W. 1864. *Letter on Corpulence Addressed to the Public*, 3rd ed. London: Harrison.

Boyle R. 1764. *The Works of the Honourable Robert Boyle*. London: A. Millar.

Bray G.A. 1976a. *The Obese Patient*. Major Problems in Internal Medicine, Vol 9, Philadelphia: WB Saunders Company, pp. 1–450.

Bray G.A. (Ed). 1976b. *Obesity in Perspective*. Fogarty International Center Series on Preventive Med. Vol 2, parts 1 and 2, Washington, DC: U.S. Government Printing Office, DHEW Publication #75-708.

Bray G.A. ©1982. *The Physicians Diet Plan*. Unpublished manuscript, pp. 1–249.

Bray G.A. 1998. *Contemporary Diagnosis and Management of Obesity*. Newton, PA: Handbooks in Health Care.

Bray G.A. 2009. Soft drink consumption and obesity: It's all about fructose. *Curr Opin Lipidology* 21(1): 51–57.

Bray G.A, Nielsen S.J., Popkin B.M. 2004. High fructose corn syrup and the epidemic of obesity. *Am J Clin Nutr* 79:537–544.

Bray G.A. 2007a. *The Battle of the Bulge*. Pittsburgh: Dorrance Publishing Co.

Bray G.A. 2007b. *The Metabolic Syndrome and Obesity*. Totowa NJ: Humana Press.

Cushing H.W. 1912. *The Pituitary Body and its Disorders. Clinical States Produced by the Disorders of the Hypophysis Cerebri*. Philadelphia: Lippincott.

DPP Research Group. 2002. Reduction in the incidence of type 2 diabetes with lifestyle intervention or metformin. *N Engl J Med* 346:393–403.

Farooqi I.S., O'Rahilly S. 2007. Genetic factors in human obesity. *Obes Rev* 8(Suppl 1):37–40.

Flemyng M. 1760. *A Discourse on the Nature, Causes, and Cure of Corpulency. Illustrated by a Remarkable Case*. Read before the Royal Society November 1757. London: L. Davis and C. Reymers.

Flier J. 2004. Obesity wars: Molecular progress confronts and expanding epidemic. *Cell* 116:337–350.

Franco M., Ordunez P., et al. 2007. Impact of energy intake, physical activity, and population-wide weight loss on cardiovascular disease and diabetes mortality in Cuba, 1980–2005. *Am J Epidemiol* 166:1374–1380.

Frohlich A. 1901. Ein Fall von Tumor der hypophysis ceribri ohne Akromegalie. *Wien Klin Rdsch* 15: 883–886.

Harvey W. 1872. *On Corpulence in Relation to Disease: With Some Remarks on Diet*. London: Henry Renshaw.

Haslam D., Haslam F. 2008. *Fat, Gluttony and Sloth: Obesity in Literature, Art and Medicine*. Liverpool: University of Liverpool.

Howard A.N. (ed). 1975. *Recent Advances in Obesity Research: I. Proceedings of the 1st International Congress on Obesity* October 8–11, 1974 held at the Royal College of Physicians, London. London: Newman Publishing Ltd.

Larsson B., Svardsudd K., et al. 1984. Abdominal adipose tissue distribution, obesity and risk of cardiovascular disease and death: 13 year follow up of participants in the study of 792 men born in 1913. *Br Med J* 288:1401–1404.

Lavoisier A.L. 1789. *Traité Elémentaire de Chimie, Présenté dans un Ordre Nouveau et d'après les Découvertes Modernes. . . ; avec figures*. Paris: Chez Cuchet.

Malik V.S., Popkin B.M., Bray G.A., Despres J.-P., Hu F.B. 2009. Sugar-sweetened beverages, obesity and cardiometabolic risk: A systematic review and meta-analysis. *Diabetes Care* 33:2477–2483.

NHLBI Obesity Education Initiative Expert Panel on the Identification, Evaluation, and Treatment of Overweight and Obesity in Adults. Clinical guidelines on the identification, evaluation, and treatment of overweight and obesity in adults—The evidence report. 1998. *Obes Res* 6:51S–63S.

Ogden C.L., Yanovski S.Z., et al. 2007. The epidemiology of obesity. *Gastroenterology* 132:2087–2102.

Olsen N.J., Heitmann B.L. 2009. Intake of calorically sweetened beverages and obesity. *Obes Rev* 10(1):68–75.

Ravelli A.C., van Der Meulen J.H., et al. 1999. Obesity at the age of 50 y in men and women exposed to famine prenatally. *Am J Clin Nutr* 70:811–816.

Rony H.R. 1940. *Obesity and Leanness*. Philadelphia: Lea and Febiger.

Sacks F.M., Svetkey L.P., et al. 2001. For the DASH–Sodium collaborative research group. A clinical feeding trial of the effects on blood pressure of reduced dietary sodium and the DASH dietary pattern (The DASH–Sodium Trial). *N Engl J Med* 344:3–10.

Short T. 1727. *A Discourse Concerning the Causes and Effects of Corpulency Together with the Method for Its Prevention and Cure*. London: J. Roberts.

Sjostrom L., Narbro K., et al. 2007. Swedish Obese Subjects Study. Effect of bariatric surgery on mortality in Swedish obese subjects. *N Engl J Med* 357:741–772.

Stuart R.B., Davis B. 1972. *Slim Chance in a Fat World: Behavioral Control of Obesity*. Champaign, IL: Research Press Company.

Swinburn B., Sacks G., Ravussin E. 2009. Increased food energy supply is more than sufficient to explain the US epidemic of obesity. *Am J Clin Nutr* 90(6):1453–1456.

Vartanian L.R., Schwartz M.B., Brownell K.D. 2007. Effects of soft drink consumption on nutrition and health: A systematic review and meta-analysis. *Am J Public Health* 97:667–675.

von Helmholtz H. 1847. *Über die Erhaltung der Kraft, eine physikalische Abhandlung: vorgetragen in der Sitzung der physikalischen Gesellschaft zu Berlin am 23sten Juli*. Berlin: G. Reimer, 1847.

von Mayer J.R. 1842. Bemerkungen uber die Krafte der unbelebten Natur. *Ann Chem Pharm (Lemgo)* 42: 233–240.

Whitlock G., Lewington S., Sherliker P., Clarke R., Emberson J., Halsey J., Qizilbash N., Collins R., Peto R. 2009. Body–mass index and cause–specific mortality in 900,000 adults: collaborative analyses of 57 prospective studies. Prospective Studies Collaboration. *Lancet* 373(9669):1083–1096.

WHO. 2000. Obesity: preventing and managing the global epidemic. Report of a WHO consultation. *World Health Organ Tech Rep Ser* 894:i–xii, 1–253.

Winett R.A., Tate D.F., et al. 2005. Long-term weight gain prevention: A theoretically based Internet approach. *Prev Med* 41:629–641.

Worthington L.S. 1875. *De l'Obésité. Étiologie, Thérapeutique et Hygiene*. Paris: E. Martinet.

Zhang Y., Proenca R., et al. 1994. Positional cloning of the mouse obese gene and its human homologue. *Nature* 372:425–432.

INTRODUCTION

Alphen J.V., Aris A. 1996. *Oriental Medicine: An Illustrated Guide to the Asian Arts of Healing*. Boston: Shambhala.

Angell W. 1989. *Die Venus von Willendorf*. Wien: Editions Wien.

Archeological Catalogue of China.

Beller A.S. 1977. *Fat & Thin: A Natural History of Obesity*. New York: Farrar, Straus and Giroux.

Bernal I. 1999. *The Mexican National Museum of Anthropology*. Transl. C.B. Czitrom. Panorama Editorial S.A.

Bienkowski P. (ed) 1991. *Treasures from an Ancient Land. The Art of Jordan*. Gloucestershire: Alan Sutton Publishing.

Bray G.A. 2004. Obesity in historical perspective. In *Handbook of Obesity*. G.A. Bray, C. Bouchard, eds. New York: Elsevier.

Bray G.A. 1990. Obesity: Historical development of scientific and cultural ideas. *Int J Obes* 14:909–926.

Bray G.A. 2007. *The Battle of the Bulge*. Pittsburgh PA: Dorrance Publishing.
Campbell D. 1926. *Arabian Medicine and Its Influence on the Middle Ages*. London: Kegan Paul, Trench, Trubner & Co. Ltd.
Castiglioni A. 1941. *A History of Medicine*. Transl. EB Krumbhaar. New York: Alfred A. Knopf.
Clark G. 1967. *The Stone Age Hunters*. London: Thames and Hudson Ltd.
Coe M.D., Diehl R.A., Furst P.T., Reilly III F.K., Schele L., Tate C.E., Taube K.A. 1995. *The Olmec World. Ritual and Rulership*. Princeton: The Art Museum.
Conrad N.J. 2009. A female figurine from the basal Aurignacian of Hohle Fels Cave in southwestern Germany. *Nature* 459:248–252.
Contenau G. 1938. *La médecine en Assyrie et en Babylonie*. Paris: Librairie Maloine.
Darby W.J., Ghalioungui P., Grevetti L. 1977. *Food: The Gift of Osiris*. London: Academic Press.
Duffin J. 1999. *History of Medicine—A Scandalously Short Introduction*. Toronto, University of Toronto Press.
Filer J. 1995. *Egyptian Bookshelf Disease*. London: British Museum Press.
Gaarder J. 1995. *Sophie's World. A Novel about the History of Philosophy*. Transl. P Moller. London: Phoenix House.
Gamble C. 1986. *The Paleolithic Settlement of Europe*. Cambridge: Cambridge University Press.
Garrison F. 1929. *An Introduction to the History of Medicine*. Philadelphia: W.B. Saunders and Co.
Garrison F.H. 1914. *An Introduction to the History of Medicine with Medical Chronology Bibliographic Data and Test Questions*. Philadelphia: W.B. Saunders Co.
Gimbutas M. 1989. *The Language of the Goddess*. London: Thames & Hudson.
Gimbutas M. 1999. *The Living Goddesses*. MR Dexter, ed. Berkeley: University of California Press.
Goodison L., Morris C. 1998. Beyond the Great Mother: The sacred world of the Minoans. In *Ancient Goddesses: The Myths and the Evidence*. London: British Museum.
Green R.M. 1951. *A Translation of Galen's Hygiene (De Sanitate Tuenda)*. Springfield, IL: Charles C. Thomas.
Gruner O.C. 1930. *A Treatise on the Canon of Medicine of Avicenna Incorporating a Translation of the First Book*. London: Luzac.
Hautin R.J.R. 1939. *Obésité. Conceptions actuelle. Thèse pour le Doctorat en Médecine*. Bordeaux: Imprimerie Bier.
Hippocrates. 1839. *Oeuvres complètes d'Hippocrate: traduction nouvelle avec le texte grec en regard, collationné sur les manuscrits et toutes les éditions; accompagnée d'une introduction, . . . suivie d'une table générale des matières / par É. Littré*. Paris: J.B. Balliere.
Huang Ti. 1966. *Nei ching su wen: The Yellow Emperor's Classic of Internal Medicine*, E. Veith, trans. Berkeley: Univ. of California Press.
Husain S. 1997. *The Goddess. An Illustrated Guide to the Divine Feminine*. London: Duncan Baird Publishers.
Iason A.H. 1946. *The Thyroid Gland in Medical History*. New York: Frobin Press.
Kryger M.H. 1983. Sleep apnea: From the needles of Dionysius to continuous positive airway pressure. *Arch Intern Med* 143:2301–2303.
Kryger M.H. 1985. Fat, sleep and Charles Dickens: literary and medical contributions to the understanding of sleep apnea. *Clin Chest Med* 6:555–562.
Kulacoglu B. 1992. *Museum of Anatolian Civilizations. Gods and Goddesses*. Transl. J. Ozturk. Anhara: Museum of Anatolian Civilizations.
Leppmann W. 1968. *Pompeii in Fact and Fiction*. Transl. Melmoth–Hutchinson. London: Elek.
Lloyd G.E.R. 1978. *Hippocratic Writings*. New York: Penguin Books, pp 212.
Major R.H. 1954. *A History of Medicine*. Springfield, IL: Charles C. Thomas.
Malone C. 1998. God or goddess. The temple art of ancient Malta. In *Ancient Goddesses: The Myths and the Evidence*. C. Goodison, L. Morris, eds. London: British Museum.
Martinie J. 1934. *Notes sur l'histoire de l'obésité. Thèse de Paris 1934*. Paris: Les Presses Universitaires de France.
Melaart J. 1965. *Earliest Civilizations of the Middle East*. London: Thames and Hudson, Ltd.
Meskell L. 1998. Twin peaks. The archeologies of Çatalhöyük. In *Ancient Goddesses: The Myths and the Evidence*. C. Goodison, L. Morris, eds. London: British Museum.
Mettler C.C., Mettler F.A. 1947. *Philadelphia History of Medicine. A Correlative Text, Arranged According to Subjects*. Philadelphia: The Blakiston Co.
Moll R.G., Cuesta M.S. 1998. *Tlatilco de muheres bonitas, hombres y dioses*. Mexico: Circolo de Arte.
Neumann E. 1972. *The Great Mother. An Analysis of the Archetype*. 2nd edition. Transl. R. Manheim. Princeton: Princeton Bollingen.

Nunn J.F. 1996. *Ancient Egyptian Medicine*. London: British Museum Press.
Ohrbach S. 1978. *Fat Is a Feminist Issue: The Anti-Diet Guide to Permanent Weight Loss*. New York: Paddington Press Ltd.
Osler W. 1921. *The Evolution of Modern Medicine*. New Haven: Yale University Press.
Precope J. 1952. *Hippocrates on Diet and Hygiene*. London: Zeno.
Reeves C. 1992. *Egyptian Medicine*. London: Shire Publications Ltd.
Selwyn-Brown A. 1928. *The Physician throughout the Ages*. New York: Capehard-Brown Co., Inc.
Seton L. 1967. *Early Highland Peoples of Anatolia*. London: Thames and Hudson Ltd.
Sigerist H.E. 1961. *A History of Medicine*. New York: Oxford University Press.
Smith E. 1930. *The Edwin Smith Surgical Papyrus. Published in Facsimile and Hieroglyphic Transliteration with Translation and Commentary in Two Volumes by James Henry Breasted. Classics of Medicine*, Special Edition, 1984. Chicago: University of Chicago Press.
Spycket A. 1995. Kassite and Middle Elamite sculpture. In *Later Mesopotamia and Iran. Tribes and Empires 1600–538 BC*. London: British Museum Press.
Stephen–Chauvet. 1936. *La médecine chez les peuples primitifs*. Paris: Librairie Maloine.
Tibetan medical paintings. 1992. *Illustrations to the Blue Beryl Treatise of Sangye Gyamtso. (1635–1705)*. New York: Henry N. Abrams Inc.
Ullmann M. 1978. *Islamic Medicine*. Edinburgh: University Press.
Wheeler M. 1966. *Civilizations of the Indus Valley and Beyond*. London: Thames and Hudson Ltd.
Witcombe C.L.C.E. 2000. Women in prehistory: The Venus of Willendorf. http://witcombe.sbc.edu/willendorf/willendorfdiscovery.html.
Yang X. 1999. *The Golden Age of Chinese Archeology. Celebrated Discoveries from the People's Republic of China*. Washington, DC: National Gallery of Art.

CHAPTER 1

Ackerknecht E.H. 1967. *Medicine at the Paris Hospital*. Baltimore: Johns Hopkins University Press.
Addison T. 1855. *On the Constitutional and Local Effects of Disease of the Suprarenal Capsules*. London: Samuel Highley.
Albala, K. 2005. Personal communication presented at Experimental Biology in 2005 in Symposium on the History of Obesity.
Anonymous. 1818. *The Life of that Wonderful and Extraordinarily Heavy Man, Daniel Lambert, from His Birth to the Moment of His Dissolution; with an Account of Men Noted for Their Corpulency, and Other Interesting Matter*. New York: Samuel Wood & Sons.
Atwater W.O., Benedict F.G. 1903. Experiments on the metabolism of matter and energy in the human body. 1900–1902. Washington, DC: U.S. Government Printing Office. Office of the Experiment Station–Bulletin no.136.
Atwater W.O., Rosa E.B. 1899. Description of a new respiration calorimeter and experiments on the conservation of energy in the human body. USDA Bull. 63, Washington, D.C.: USDA Office of Experimental Station.
Auenbrugger L. 1761. *Inventum novum ex percussione thoracis humani et signo abstnisos*. Vindobonae: Trattner JT.
Babinski M.J. 1900. Tumeur du corps pituitaire sans acromégalie et avec de développement des organes génitaux. *Rev Neurol.* 8:531–533.
Barkhausen. 1843. Merkwurdige allgemeine Fettablagerung bei einem Knaben von 5 1/4 Jahren. *Hannov Ann f ges Heilk*. 8:200–203.
Beaujouan G. 1963. Motives and opportunities for science in the medieval universities. In *Scientific Change. Historical Studies in the Intellectual, Social and Technical Conditions for Scientific Discovery and Technical Invention, from Antiquity to the Present*. AC Crombie, ed. New York: Basic Books.
Beddoes T. 1802. *Hygeia: or Essays Moral and Medical, on the Causes Affecting the Personal State of Our Middling and Affluent Classes*. Bristol: J. Mills.
Benedict F.G., Miles W.R., Roth P., Smith H.M. 1919. *Human Vitality and Efficiency under Prolonged Restricted Diet*. Washington, DC: Carnegie Institution of Washington.
Benedict F.G. 1915. *A Study of Prolonged Fasting*. Washington, DC: Carnegie Institution of Washington. Report Num. 203.
Benivieni A. 1507. *De abditis nonnullis ac miran dis morbor vm et sa nationaum cavsis*. Florence: Klas Octobris.

Benivieni A. 1954. *De abditis nonnullis ac morandis morboum et sanationum causes.* Transl. Charles Singer. With a biographical appreciation by Esmond R. Long. Springfield, IL: Charles C. Thomas.

Bernard C. 1865. *Introduction a l'etude de la medicine experimentale.* Paris: J.B. Bailliere et fils.

Bernard C. 1848. De l'origine du sucre dans l'économie animale. *Arch Gen Med* 18(4th ser):303–319.

Bernard C. 1855. Sur le mécanisme de la formation du sucre dans le foie. *C R Acad Sci* 41:461–469.

Bichat X. 1801. *Anatomie générale, appliquée à la physiologie et à la médecine.* Paris: Chez Brosson, Gabon et Cie.

Bigelow H.J. 1846. Insensibility during surgical operations produced by inhalation. *Boston Med Surg J* 35:309–317.

Boerhaave H. 1757. *Opera omnia medica, quorum sries post praefationem.* Venetiis: Laurentium Basilium.

Bonetus T. 1700. *Sepulchretum, sive anatomia practica, ex cadaveribus morbo denatis, proponens historias omnium humani corporis affectum.* Genevae: Sumptibus Cramer & Perachon.

Bowditch N.L. 1848. *The Ether Controversy. Vindication of the Hospital Report of 1848.* Boston: John Wilson.

Boyle R. 1764. *The Works of the Honourable Robert Boyle.* London: A. Millar.

Bray G.A. 1990. Obesity: Historical development of scientific and cultural ideas. *Int J Obes* 14:909–926.

Bray G.A. 2004. Obesity is a chronic, relapsing neurochemical disease. *Intern J Obes* 28:34–38.

Bray G.A. 2007 *The Battle of the Bulge.* Pittsburgh: Dorrance Publishing Co.

Bray G.A. 2009. History of obesity. In *Obesity Science to Practice.* G. Williams and G. Fruhbeck, eds. Chichester: Wiley-Blackwell, pp 2–18.

Bright R. 1827. *Reports of Medical Cases, Selected with a View of Illustrating the Symptoms and Cure of Diseases by Reference to Morbid Anatomy.* London: Longman, Rees, Orme, Brown and Green.

Brillat-Savarin J.A. 1826. *Physiologie du gout, ou meditations de gastronomie transcendante; ouvrage theorique, historique et a l'ordre du jour, dedie aux gastronomes parisiens.* Paris: Sautelet et Cie.

Brillat-Savarin J.A. 1970. *The Physiology of Taste.* London: Penguin Books.

Brillat-Savarin J.A. 1994. *The Physiology of Taste or, Meditations on Transcendental Gastronomy.* Transl. MFK Fisher. Drawings and color lithographs by Wayne Thiebaud. San Francisco: Arion Press.

Burwell C.S., Robin E.D., Whaley R.D., Bickelman A.G. 1956. Extreme obesity associated with alveolar hypoventilation: A Pickwickian syndrome. *Am J Med.* 21:811–818.

Burton W. 1743. *An Account of the Life and Writings of Herman Boerhaave, Doctor of Philosophy and Medicine; Professor of the Theory, and Practice of Physic; and also of Botany, and Chemistry in the University of Leyden.* London: Henry Lintot.

Bynum W.F., and Wilson J.C. 1992. Periodical knowledge: Medical journals and their editors in nineteenth-century Britain. In W.F. Bynum, S. Lock, R. Porter, eds. *Medical Journals and Medical Knowledge: Historical Essays.* New York: Routledge, pp 29–48.

Canguilhem G. 1988. *Ideology and Rationality in the History of the Life Sciences.* Transl. A Goldhammer. Cambridge: MIT Press.

Castiglione A. 1931. *Life and Work of Sanctorius.* Transl. by E. Techt New York: Medical Life.

Celsus A.A.C. 1935. *De Medicina with an English Translation by W.G. Spencer.* London: Heinemann.

Chambers T.K. 1850. The Gulstonian lectures on corpulence. *Lancet* 2:11–19, 342–350, 437–445.

Cheyne G. 1733. *The English Malady: or, a Treatise of Nervous Diseases of All Kinds, as Spleen, Vapours, Lowness of Spirits, Hypochondriacal, and Hysterical Distempers & C.* London: For Strahan and Leake.

Cheyne G. 1724. *An Essay of Health and Long Life.* London: George Strahan and J. Leake.

Coe T. 1751–1752. A letter from Dr. T. Coe, Physician at Chelmsford in Essex, to Dr. Cromwell Mortimer, Secretary R.S. concerning Mr. Bright, the Fat man at Malden in Essex. *Phil Trans* 47:188–193.

Copernicus N. 1543. *De Revolutionibus Orbium Colestium.* Libri VI. (2)

Cornaro L. 1558. *Trattato de la vita sobria.* Padoua: Gratioso Perchiacino

Cornaro L. 1737. *Sure and Certain Methods of Attaining a Long and Healthful Life: With Means of Correcting a Bad Constitution.* London: D. Midwinter (English Translation).

Cornaro L. 1916. *Introduction to the Discourses on the Sober Life.* New York: Thomas Y. Crowell Company, Publishers.

Corvisart J.-N. 1984. *An Essay on the Organic Diseases and Lesions of the Heart and Great Vessels.* Bound with L. Auenbrugger. *On Percussion of the Chest.* Birmingham: Classics of Medicine Library.

Cullen W. 1793. *Synopsis and Nosology, Being an Arrangement and Definition of Diseases* (The second edition translated from Latin to English). Springfield, CT: Edward Gray.

Cullen W. 1810. *First Lines of the Practice of Physic, by William Cullen, M.D. Late Professor of the Practice of Physic in the University of Edinburgh, and Including the Definitions of the Nosology; with Supplementary Notes Chiefly Selected from Recent Authors, Who Have Contributed to the Improvement of Medicine by Peter Reid, M.D.* Edinburgh: Abernethy and Walker.

Davy H. 1800. *Researches, Chemical and Philosophical: Chiefly concerning Nitrous Oxide or Dephlogisticated Nitrous Air, and its Respiration*. London: Printed for J. Johnson.

Don W.G. 1859. Remarkable case of obesity in a Hindoo boy aged twelve years. *Lancet*. I:363.

Dubourg L. 1864. *Recherches sur les causes de la polysarcie*. Paris: A. Parent.

Duffin J. 1999. *History of Medicine. A Scandalously Short Introduction*. Toronto: University of Toronto Press.

Dupytren. 1806. Observation sur un cas d'obésité, suivie de maladie du coeur et de la mort. *J Med Chir Pharm* 12:262–273.

Ehrlich P., Hata S. 1910. *Die experimentelle Chemotherapie der Spirillosen*. Berlin: Julius Springer.

Eknoyan, G. 1999. Santorio Sanctorius (1561–1636). Founding father of metabolic balance studies. *Am J Nephrol* 19:226–233.

Eschenmeyer. 1815. Beschreibung eines monstrosen fett Mädchen, das in einem Alter von 10 jahren starb, nach dem es eine hohe van 5 fuss 3 zoll und ein Gewicht von 219 pfund erreicht hatte. *Tubing Bl f Naturw u Arznk* 1:261–285.

Flemyng M. 1760. *A Discourse on the Nature, Causes, and Cure of Corpulency. Illustrated by a Remarkable Case. Read before the Royal Society November 1757*. London: L. Davis and C. Reymers.

Foster M.L. 1926. *Life of Lavoisier*. Northampton, MA: Smith College.

Frank, R.G, Jr. 1980. *Harvey and the Oxford Physiologists. A Study of Scientific Ideas*. Berkeley: University of California Press.

Frohlich A. 1901. Ein fall von tumor der hypophysis cerebri ohne akromegalie. *Wiener Klin Rdsch*. 15:883–886.

Galen C. 1531. *Pergameni opera, iam recens ver sa; quorum catalogum proxima indicabit pagina*. Basileae ex aedivus.

Garrison F.H. 1914. *An Introduction to the History of Medicine with Medical Chronology Bibliographhic Data and Test Questions*. Philadelphia: W.B. Saunders Co.

Glais J. 1875. *De la grossesse adipeuse*. Paris: A. Parent.

Gordon S. 1862. Art. XV.–Reports of rare cases. IV. Case of extensive fatty degeneration in a boy 14 years of age. Death from obstructed arterial circulation. *Dublin Q J Med Sci* 33:340–349.

Gould G.M., Pyle WL. 1956. *Anomalies and Curiosities of Medicine*. 1896. New York: Julian Press.

Gruner O.C. 1984. *Avicenna. The Canon of Medicine of Avicenna*. London: Luzac & Co., 1930; Birmingham, AL: The Classics of Medicine Library.

Guerrini A. 2000. *Obesity and Depression in the Enlightenment*. Norman, OK: University of Oklahoma Press.

Haller A. 1757. *Elementa physiologiae corporis humani*. Lausanne: Marci–Michael Boursquet & Sociorum.

Haller A. 1756. Corpulence ill cured; large cryptae of the stomach (etc). *Path Observ* 44–49.

Harington J. 1920. *The School of Salernum Regimen Sanitatis Salernitanum*. New York: Paul Hoeber.

Hartog P.J. 1941. The new views of Priestley and Lavoisier. *Ann Sci* 5:1–56.

Harvey W. 1872. *On Corpulence in Relation to Disease: With Some Remarks on Diet*. London: Henry Renshaw.

Harvey W. 1928. *The Anatomical Exercises of Dr. William Harvey. De Motu Cordis 1628: De circulatione sanguinis 1649: The first English text of 1653 now newly edited by Geoffrey Keynes*. London: Nonesuch Press.

Haslam D., Haslam F. 2009. *Fat, Gluttony and Sloth. Obesity in Literature, Art and Medicine*. Liverpool: Liverpool University Press.

Hassall A. 1849a. *The Microscopic Anatomy of the Human Body, in Health and Disease*. London: Samuel Highley.

Hassall A. 1849b. Observations on the development of the fat vesicle. *Lancet* i:63–64.

Hassall A.H. 1855. *Food and Its Adulterations; Comprising the Reports of the Analytical Sanitary Commission of The Lancet for the years 1851 to 1854 Inclusive, Revised and Extended*. London: Longman, Brown, Green, and Longmans.

Hassall A. 1893. *The Narrative of a Busy Life; An Autobiography*. London: Longman Green.

Helmholtz H.L.F. 1847. *Über die Erhaltung der Kraft, eine physikalische Abhandlung*. Berlin: G. Reimer.

Helmholtz, H. von. 1851. *Beschreibung eines Augen–spiegels zur untersuchung der netzhaut im lebenden auge*. Berlin: A. Forstner'sche Verlagsbuchhandlung.

Helmholtz, H. von. 1863. *Die Lehre von den Tonempfindungen als physiologische Grundlage fur die Theorie der Musik*. Braunschweig: Friedrich Vieweg und Sohn.

Helmholtz, H. von. 1867. *Handbuch der physiologischen Optik*. Leipzig: Leopold Voss.

Henle F.G.J. 1841. *Allgemeine Anatomie*. Leipzig: L. Voss.

Hippocrates. 1839–1861. *Oeuvres completes d'Hippocrate*, traduction nouvelle avec le texte Grec en regard, collationne sur les manuscrits et toutes les editions; Accompangnee d'une introduction de commentaires medicaux, de variantes et de notes philosophiques; suivie d'une table generale des matieres par E. Littre. Paris: J.B. Bailliere.

Hodgkin T. 1832. On some morbid appearances of the absorbent glands and spleen. *Med Chir Trans* 17:68–114.

Hoggan G., Hogan F.E. 1879. On the development and retrogression of the fat cell. *J R Microscop Soc* 2:353.

Holmes F.L. 1974. *Claude Bernard and Animal Chemistry. The Emergence of a Scientist*. Cambridge, MA: Harvard University Press.

Holmes F.L. 1985. *Lavoisier and the Chemistry of Life. An Exploration of Scientific Creativity*. Madison: University of Wisconsin Press.

Hooke R. 1665–67. *Micrographia, or Some Physiological Descriptions of Minute Bodies Made by Magnifying Glasses; With Observations and Inquiries Thereupon*. London: J. Martyn & J. Allestry.

Jenner E. 1801. *An Inquiry into the Causes and Effects of the Variolae Vaccinae, a Disease Discovered in Some of the Western Counties of England, Particularly Goucestershire, and Known by the Name of Cow Pox*. London: D.N. Shury.

Kirkland E.C. 1974. Scientific eating: New Englanders prepare and promote a reform. *Proc Mass Hist Soc* 86:28–52.

Koch R. 1884. Die Aetiologie der Tuberkulose. IN: *Mittheilungen aus dem Kaiserlichen Gesunheitsamte*. 2nd vol. Berlin: August Hirschwald.

Koenigsberger, L. 1906. *Hermann von Helmholtz*. Transl. Frances A. Welby. Oxford: At the Clarendon Press.

Kryger M.H. 1985. Fat, sleep, and Charles Dickens: Literary and medical contributions to the understanding of sleep apnea. *Clin Chest Med* 6:555–562.

Kryger M.H. 1983. Sleep apnea. From the needles of Dionysius to continuous positive airway pressure. *Arch Intern Med* 143:2301–2303.

Kuhn T.S. 1962. *The Structure of Scientific Revolutions*. Chicago: University of Chicago Press.

Laennec R.-T.-H. 1819. *De l'Auscultation Médiate, ou Traité du Diagnostic des Maladies des Poumons et du Coeur*. Paris: Brosson J.-A. et Chaude J.-S.

Lavoisier A.O. 1775. Memoire sur la nature du principe qui se combine avedc les metaux pendant leur calcinations, et qui en augment le poids. *Hist Acad roy Sci* 1778:520–526.

Lavoisier A.L. 1778. Sur la nature du principe qui se combine avec les metaux pendant leur calcination, & qui en augmente le poids. Mémoire de L'Academie Royale 1775 Published 520–526.

Lavoisier A.L., Laplace P.S. 1783. *Memoir on Heat*. Read to the Royal Academy of Sciences, 28 June. Trans. H Guerlac. New York: Neale Watson Academic Publications, Inc. 1982.

Lavoisier A.L. 1789. *Traité élémentaire de chimie, présenté dans un ordre nouveau et d'après les découvertes modernes*. Paris: Chez Cuchet.

Lavoisier A.L. LaPlace P.S. 1880. Memoire sur la chaleur. *Hist Acad roy Sci* (Paris) 1784:335–408.

Leeuwenhoek van A. 1800. *The select works of Antony van Leeuwenhoek, containing his microscopial discoveries in many of the works of nature, translated from the Dutch and Latin editions published by the author Samual Hoole*. London: G. Sidney.

Liebeg J. 1842. *Chemistry in Its Application to Agriculture and Physiology*. Transl. Lyon Playfair. London: Taylor and Walton.

Linnaeus C.V. 1753. *Species Plantarum*. Stockholm: Salvius.

Lister J.B. 1870. On the effects of the antiseptic system of treatment upon the salubrity of a surgical hospital. *Lancet* 1:4–6, 40–42.

Lister J.B. 1909. *The collected papers of Joseph, Baron Lister. Member of the order of merit, fellow and sometime president of the Royal Society, Knight Grand Cross of the Danish Order of the Danebrog Knight of the Prussian Order pour le Merite Associe Etranger de l'Institut de France*. Oxford: Clarendon Press.

Long C.W. 1849. An account of the first use of sulphuric ether by inhalation as an anaesthetic in surgical operations. *South Med Surg J* 5:705–713.

Loudon J., Loudon I. 1992. Medicine, politics and the medical periodical 1800–1850. In *Medical Journals and Medical Knowledge: Historical Essays*. W.F. Bynum, S. Lock, R. Porter, eds. New York: Routledge, pp 49–69.

Lower R. 1669. *Tractatus de corde. Item de motu & colore sanguinis et chyli in eum transitu*. Amstelodami: Daniele Webem Elzevirium.

Lower R. 1666. The method observed in transfusing the bloud out of one live animal into another. *Phil Trans* 1:353–358.

Maccary A. 1811. *Traité sur la polysarcie*. Paris: Gabon.

McCollum E.V. 1957. *A History of Nutrition. The Sequence of Ideas in Nutrition Investigations*. Boston: Houghton Mifflin.

McNaughton J. 1829. Cases of polysarcia adiposa in childhood. *New York Medical and Physical Journal* No. XXX, July. New Series – No II. New York: C.S. Francis.

Magendie F. 1828. *Formulary for the Preparation and Employment of Several New Remedies, Namely, Resin of Nux Vomica, Strychnine, Morphine, Hydrocyanic Acid, Preparations of Cinchona.* (Translated from the Formulaire of M. Magendie, published in Paris, October 1827). London: T. and G. Underwood.

Magendie F. 1816. *Precis elementaire de physiologie*. Paris: Mequignon-Marvis.

Major R. 1954. *A History of Medicine.* Springfield, IL: Charles C Thomas.

Malpighi M. 1686. *Opera omnia*. Londini: R. Scott.

Maynard L.A. 1962. Wilbur O. Atwater—A biographical sketch. *J Nutr* 1962 78:39–52.

Mayow J. 1674. *Tractatus quinque medico–physici. Quorum primus agit de salnitro, et spirtu nitro–aereo. Secundus de respiratione. Tertius de rspiratione foetus in uteret, et ovo. Quartus de motu musculari, et spiritubus animalibus, Ultimus de rachitide*. Oxford: Theatro Sheldoniano.

Mayer J. 1951. Claude Bernard. *J Nutr* 45:3–19.

Mayer J.R. von 1842. Remarks on the forces of inorganic nature. Transl. from Bermerkungen uber die krafte der unbelebten natur. *Ann der Chemie Pharm* 42:233–240.

Medvei V.C. *A History of Endocrinology.* Lancaster: MTP Press Limited.

Mettler C.C., Mettler F.A. 1947. *History of Medicine.* Philadelphia: Blakiston.

Morgagni G.B. 1761. *De sedibus, et causis morborum per anatomen indagatis libriquinque*. Venetiis: typog. Remordiniana.

Morton R. 1689. *Phthisologia seu excertitationes de Phthisi tribus libris comprehensae*. Londini: Samuel Smith.

Müller J. 1834. *Handbuch der Physiologie des Menschen*. Coblenz: Holscher J.

Munks. 1955. *Rolls: Lives of the fellows of the Royal College of Physicians of London, 1826–1925.* Compiled by Brown, O.H., Litt, M.A.B. London: Published by the College 4:48–49,1826,1925.

Osler W. 1904. The "Phthisologia" of Richard Morton, M.D. *Med Lib Hist J.*

Paracelsus. 1573. *Wunder artzney, vonn allerley leibs gebruchen, und zu fallende Krankheiten, ohn sondere Beschwerung, Unlust unnd Verdrusz, kurtzlich zu heilen, unnd die Gesundheit widerumb mit geringem Kosten zun Wegen zubringen* . . . . Basel: Sebastian Henricpetri.

Partington J.R. 1951. *A Short History of Chemistry*, 2nd ed. London: Macmillan and Co. Ltd.

Pasteur L. 1922–1939. *Oeuvres de Pasteur*. Reunies par Pasteur Vallery–Radot. Paris: Masson & Cie.

Pettenkofer M.J., Voit C. Untersuchuingen über die Respiration. *Ann Chem Pharm (Heidelberg).* 1862–63 (Suppl 2):52–70.

Popper Selections. 1985. D. Miller, ed. Princeton: Princeton University Press.

Potts D.B. 1992. *Wesleyan University 1831–1910. Collegiate Enterprise in New England*. New Haven: Yale University Press.

Power D.A. 1937–38. William Wadd (1776–1829). In *The Dictionary of National Biography*. L. Stephen, S. Lee eds. London: Oxford University Press, Vol XX.

Price D.J. Desolla. 1961. *Science since Babylon*. New Haven: Yale University Press.

Priestley J. 1775. *Experiments and Observation on Different Kinds of Air*. London: J. Johnson.

Quetelet A. 1835. *Sur l'homme et le développement de ses facultés, ou essai de physique sociale*. Paris: Bachelier.

Reamur R.A.F. 1756. Sur la digestion des oiseaux. *His Acad Roy Sci* 266–307, 461–495.

Regneller G.D. 1839. Traite complet de l'obesite et de la maigreur, de leurs causes et de leur guerison Paris: For Bohaire, Gosseline and Ledoyen.

Roentgen W. 1895. Eine neue art von Strahlen. *Sitz Wurz Physik Med Gesellschaft.*, pp 3–12.

Rony H.R. 1940. *Obesity and Leanness*. Philadelphia: Lea and Febiger.

Rubner M. 1902. *Die gesetze des Energieverbrauchs bei der Ernahrung*. Leipzig: Franz Deuticke.

Rubner M. 1982. *The Laws of Energy Consumption in Nutrition*. New York: Academic Press.

Russell J. 1866. A case of polysarka, in which death resulted from deficient arterialisation of the blood. *Br Med J* i:220–221.

Santorio S. 1624. Ars . . . de statica medicina aphorismorum sectionibus septem comprehensa. Accessit Statico Mastrix, sive ejusdem artis demolitio Hippolyti Obicii. Leipzig: Gregor Ritsch fur Zacharia Schurer und Matthias Gotzen.

Santorio S. 1676. *Medicina Statica: or, Rules of Health, in Eight Sections of Aphorisms. English'd by J.D.* London: John Starkey.

Santorio S. 1720. *Medicina Statica: Being the aphorisms of Sanctorius, translated into English with large explanations. The second edition. To which is added Dr. Keil's Medicina statica Britannica, with comparative remarks and explanations. As also medic–physical essays . . . by John Quincy*. London: W. and J. Newton, A. Bell, W. Taylor and J. Osborne.

Sauvages F.B. 1768. *Nosologia methodica sistens morborum classes juxta Sydenhami menten and botanicorum ordinem*. Amstelodami: Fratrum de Tournes.

Scheele C.W. 1777. *The discovery of Oxygen Part 2*. Edinburgh: William F. Clay; 1894. Alembic Club Reprint No. 8. From *Chemische Abhandlung von der Luft und dem Feuer*, Uppsala und Leipzig.

Schindler C.S. 1871. Monstrose Fettsucht. *Wiener Med Presse* 12:410–412; 436–439.

Schleiden M.J. 1839. Beitrage zur Phytogenesis. *Arch Anat Physiol Wiss Med* 137–176.

Schwann T. 1839. *Mikroscopische Untersuchungen über di Ubereinstimmung in der Struktur un dem Wachstum der Thiere und Pflanzen*. Berlin: Sander.

Short T. 1727. *A Discourse Concerning the Causes and Effects of Corpulency Together with the Method for Its Prevention and Cure*. London: J. Roberts.

Spallanzani L. 1776. *Opusculi di fisica animale e vegetabile*. Moedena: Soc. Tipografica.

Spallanzani L. 1796. *Dissertations relative to the natural history of animals and vegetables*. Transl. from the Italian. London: J. Murray and S. Highley.

Stahl G.E. 1708. *Theoria medica vera. Physiologiam & pathologiam*. Halae: Literis Ophanotrophei.

Sydenham T. 1676. *Observationes medicae circa morborum acutorum historiam et curationem*. Londini: G. Kettilby.

Talbot J.H. 1970. *A Biographical History of Medicine: Excerpts and Essays on the Men and Their Work*. New York: Grune & Stratton.

Taylor F.S. 1949. *A Short History of Science and Scientific Thought: With Readings from the Great Scientists from the Babylonians to Einstein*. New York: W.W. Norton & Company.

Tweedie J. 1799. *Hints on Temperence and Exercise, Shewing their Advantage in the Cure of Dyspepsia, Rheumatism, Polysarcia, and Certain States of Palsy*. London: T. Rickaby.

Uglow J. 2002. *Lunar Men. Five Friends Whose Curiosity Changed the World*. New York: Farrar, Straus and Giroux.

Vesalius A. 1543. *De humani corporis fabrica*. Basileae: Joannis Oporini.

Virchow R. 1858. *Die Cellularpathologie in inrer Begrundung auf physiologische and pathologische Gewebelehre*. Berlin: August Hirschwald.

Visscher N.B. 1971. *Dictionary of Scientific Biography* 3:68–70.

Voit C. 1860. *Untersuchungen uber den Einfluss des Kochsalzes, des Kaffee's und der Muskelbewegungen auf den Stoffwechsel*. Munchen: J.G. Cotta'schen.

Wadd W. 1810. *Cursory Remarks on Corpulence: By a Member of the Royal College of Surgeons*. London: J Callow.

Wadd W., F.L.S. 1829. *Surgeon Extraordinary to the King etc.etc.etc. Comments on Corpulence Lineaments of Leanness Mems on Diet and Dietetics*. London: John Ebers & Co.

Wangensteen O.H. and Wangensteen S.D. 1978. *The Rise of Surgery. From Empiric Craft to Scientific Discipline*. Minneapolis: University of Minnesota Press.

Warren E. 1847. *Some Account of the Letheon: Or, Who Is the Discoverer of Anesthesia*. Boston: Dutton and Wentworth.

Weissmann G. 1990. *The Doctor with Two Heads and Other Essays*. New York: Alfred A. Knopf.

Wells H. 1847. *A History of the Discovery of the Application of Nitrous Oxide Gas, Ether, and Other Vapors to Surgical Operations*. Hartford: J. Gaylord Wells.

Willis T. 1681. *Opera Omnia*. Leiden: Joannis Antonij Juguetan & Co.

Wood T. 1785. A sequel to the case of Mr. Thomas Wood, of Billericay, in the Country of Essex, by the same. *Med Trans (College of Physicians, London)* 3:309–318.

Worthington L.S. 1875. *De l'Obésité. Étiologie, Thérapeutique et Hygiene*. Paris: E Martinet.

Ziman J. 1976. *The Force of Knowledge. The Scientific Dimension of Society*. Cambridge: Cambridge University Press.

CHAPTER 2

Alberti K.G., Zimmet P., Shaw J. 2006. Metabolic syndrome—A new world-wide definition. A Consensus Statement from the International Diabetes Federation. *Diabet Med* 23:469–480.

Alberti K.G., Eckel R.H., Grundy S.M., Zimmet P.Z., Cleeman J.I., Donato K.A., Fruchart J.C., James W.P., Loria C.M., Smith S.C. Jr; International Diabetes Federation Task Force on Epidemiology and Prevention; National Heart, Lung, and Blood Institute; American Heart Association; World Heart Federation; International Atherosclerosis Society; International Association for the Study of Obesity.

2009. Harmonizing the metabolic syndrome: A joint interim statement of the International Diabetes Federation Task Force on Epidemiology and Prevention; National Heart, Lung, and Blood Institute; American Heart Association; World Heart Federation; International Atherosclerosis Society; and International Association for the Study of Obesity. *Circ* 120(16):1640–1645.

Anderson S.E., Whitaker R.C. 2009. Prevalence of obesity among US preschool children in different racial and ethnic groups. *Arch Pediatr Adolesc Med* 163(4):344–348.

Asia Pacific Cohort Studies Collaboration. 2004. Body mass index and cardiovascular disease in the Asia-Pacific Region: An overview of 33 cohorts involving 310,000 participants. *Int J Epidemiol* 33:751–758.

Actuarial Society of America. *Transactions, 1901–1903*. 7:492–497.

Actuarial Society of America and Association of Life Insurance Directors. *Medico-Actuarial Mortality Investigation*. New York, 1913.

Anderson S.E., Whitaker R.C. 2009. Prevalence of obesity among US preschool children in different racial and ethnic groups. *Arch Pediatr Adolesc Med* 163(4):344–348.

Baird J., Fisher D., et al. 2005. Being big or growing fast: Systematic review of size and growth in infancy and later obesity. *Br Med J* 331(7522): 929.

Baskin M.L., Ard J., Franklin F., Allison D.B. 2005. Prevalence of obesity in the United States. *Obes Rev* 6(1):5–7.

Baumgartner R.N., Wayne S.J., Waters D.L., Janssen I., Gallagher D., Morley J.E. 2004. Sarcopenic obesity predicts instrumental activities of daily living disability in the elderly. *Obes Res* 12:1995–2004.

Behnke A.R., Feen B.G., Welham W.C. 1942. The specific gravity of healthy men. *JAMA* 118:495–498.

Berghofer A., Pischon T., Reinhold T., Apovian C.M., Sharma A.M., Willich S.N. 2008. Obesity prevalence from a European perspective: a systematic review. *BMC Public Health* 8:200.

Björntorp P. 2001. Do stress reactions cause abdominal obesity and comorbidities? *Obes Rev* 2(2):73–86.

Bray G.A. 1976. *The Obese Patient: Major Problems in Internal Medicine*. Philadelphia: W.B. Saunders Co.

Bray G.A. 2002. Predicting obesity in adults from childhood and adolescent weight. *Am J Clin Nutr* 76(3): 497–498.

Bray G.A., DeLany J.P., et al. 2002. Prediction of body fat in 12-y-old African American and white children: Evaluation of methods. *Am J Clin Nutr* 76(5):980–990.

Bray G.A., Fujimoto W., Jablonski K., Barrett-Connor E., Haffner S., Hubbard V., Stamm E., Pi-Sunyer X.P. 2006. The relationship of body size and shape to the development of diabetes in the Diabetes Prevention Program. *Obesity* 14:2107–2117.

Bray G.A. 2007. *The Battle of the Bulge*. Pittsburgh: Dorrance Publishing Inc.

Bray G.A., Jablonski K.A., Fujimoto W.Y., Barrett-Connor E., Haffner S., Hanson R.L., Hill J.O., Hubbard V., Kriska A., Stamm E., Pi-Sunyer F.X. 2008. Diabetes Prevention Program Research Group. Relation of central adiposity and body mass index to the development of diabetes in the Diabetes Prevention Program. *Am J Clin Nutr* 87(5):1212–1218.

Browning L.M., Hsieh S.D., Ashwell M. 2010. A systematic review of waist-to-height ratio as a screening tool in the prediction of cardiovascular disease and diabetes. *Nutr Res Rev* 2010, in press.

Chen C.M. 2007. Overview of obesity in Mainland China. *Obes Rev* 9(Suppl 1):14–21.

Cushing, H.W. 1943. *A Bio-Bibliography of Andreas Vesalius*. New York: Schuman's.

DeLany J.P., Bray G.A., et al. 2002. Energy expenditure in preadolescent African American and white boys and girls: The Baton Rouge Children's Study. *Am J Clin Nutr* 75(4):705–713.

Dey D.K., Bosaeus I., Lissner L., Steen B. 2009. Changes in body composition and its relation to muscle strength in 75-year-old men and women: A 5-year prospective follow-up study of the NORA cohort in Göteborg, Sweden. *Nutrition*. Feb 9, 2010.

Directory of Medical Specialists. Evanston, IL: American Board of Medical Specialities, 1989–1990.

Ezzati M., Martin H., Skjold S., Hoorn S.V., Murray C.J.L. 2006. Trends in national and state-level obesity in the USA after correction for self-report bias: Analysis of health surveys. *J Royal Soc Med* 99:250–257.

Fakhrawi D.H., Beeson L., Libanati C., Feleke D., Kim H., Quansah A., Darnell A., Lammi-Keefe C.J., Cordero-Macintyre Z. 2009. Comparison of Body Composition by Bioelectrical Impedance and dual-energy X-ray absorptiometry in overweight/obese postmenopausal women. *J Clin Densitom*. March 12, 2009.

Fernandez J.R., Heo M., Heymsfield S.B., Pierson R.N. Jr, Pi-Sunyer F.X., Wang Z.M., Wang J., Hayes M., Allison D.B., Gallagher D. 2003. Is percentage body fat differentially related to body mass index in Hispanic Americans, African Americans, and European Americans? *Am J Clin Nutr* 77:71–75.

Finkelstein E.A., Fiebelkorn I.C., et al. 2004. State-.level estimates of annual medical expenditures attributable to obesity. *Obes Res* 12(1):18–24.

Flegal K.M., Carroll M.D., et al. 2002. Prevalence and trends in obesity among US adults, 1999–2000. *JAMA* 288(14):1723–1727.

Flegal K.M., Carroll M.D., Ogden C.L., Curtin L.R. 2010. Prevalence and trends in obesity among US adults, 1999–2008. *JAMA* 303:235–241.

Forbes G.B. 1987. *Human Body Composition: Growth, Aging, Nutrition, and Activity*. New York: Springer Verlag.

Ford E.S., Giles W.H., et al. 2002. Prevalence of the metabolic syndrome among US adults: Findings from the third National Health and Nutrition Examination Survey. *JAMA* 287(3):356–359.

Ford E.S., Giles W.H., et al. 2004. Increasing prevalence of the metabolic syndrome among U.S. Adults. *Diabetes Care* 27(10):2444–2449.

Ford E.S., Mokdad A.H., et al. 2003. Trends in waist circumference among U.S. adults. *Obes Res* 11(10):1223–1231.

Ford E.S., Mokdad A.H., et al. 2005. Geographic variation in the prevalence of obesity, diabetes, and obesity-related behaviors. *Obes Res* 13(1):118–122.

Freedman D.S., Khan L.K., et al. 2004. Inter-relationships among childhood BMI, childhood height, and adult obesity: The Bogalusa Heart Study. *Int J Obes Relat Metab Disord* 28(1):6–10.

Freudenthal H. 1975. Lamber-Adolphe-Jacques Quetelet. In C.C. Billespie, ed. *Dictionary of Scientific Biography.* New York: Charles Scribner's Sons.

Gallagher D., Heymsfield S.B., et al. 2000. Healthy percentage body fat ranges: An approach for developing guidelines based on body mass index. *Am J Clin Nutr* 72(3):694–701.

Gallagher D., Kuznia P., Heshka S., Albu J., Heymsfield S.B., Goodpaster B., Visser M., Harris T.B. 2005. Adipose tissue in muscle: A novel depos similar in size to visceral adipose tissue. *Am J Clin Nutr* 81:903–910.

Gallagher D., Song M.Y. 2003. Evaluation of body composition: practical considerations. *Prim Care* 30:249–265.

Garrison F.H. 1929. *History of Medicine*, 4th ed. Philadelphia: W.B. Saunders and Co.

Ginde S.R., Geliebter A., Rubiano F., Silva A.M., Wang J., Heshka S., Heymsfield S.B. 2005. Air displacement plethysmography: Validation in overweight and obese subjects. *Obes Res* 13:1232–1237.

Goel M.S., McCarthy E.P., et al. 2004. Obesity among US immigrant subgroups by duration of residence. *JAMA* 292(23):2860–2867.

Gordon C.C. and Chumlea W.C. 1988. Stature, recumbent length, and weight. *Anthropometric Standardization Reference Manual*. Champaign, Illinois: Human Kinetics Books, Vols 3–8.

Grundy S., et al. 2001. Executive Summary of The Third Report of The National Cholesterol Education Program (NCEP) Expert Panel on Detection, Evaluation, and Treatment of High Blood Cholesterol in Adults (Adult Treatment Panel III). *JAMA* 285(19):2486–2497.

Haslam D., Haslam F. 2009. *Fat, Gluttony and Sloth. Obesity in Literature, Art and Medicine*. Liverpool: Liverpool University Press.

He Q., Heo M., Heshka S., Wang J., Pierson R.N. Jr, Albu J., Wang Z., Heymsfield S.B., Gallagher D. 2003. Total body potassium differs by sex and race across the adult age span. *Am J Clin Nutr* 78:72–77.

Hedley A.A., Ogden C.L., et al. 2004. Prevalence of overweight and obesity among US children, adolescents, and adults, 1999–2002. *JAMA* 291(23):2847–2850.

Heymsfield S.B., Baumgartner R.N., Allison D.B., Shen W., Wang Z., Ross R. 2004. Evaluation of regional and total adiposity. In *Handbook of Obesity: Etiology and Pathophysiology*, 2nd ed. G.A. Bray and C. Bouchard, eds. New York: Marcel Dekker, pp 33–79.

Heymsfield S.B., Shen W., Wang Z., Baumgartner R.N., Allison D.B., Ross R. 2004. Evaluation of total and regional adiposity. In *Handbook of Obesity* GA Bray, C Bouchard, eds. New York: Marcel Dekker, pp 33–79.

Huxley B., James W.P.T., Barzi F., Patel J.V., Lear S.A., Suriyawongpaisal P., Janus E., Caterson I., Zimmet P., Prabhakaran D., Reddy S., Woodward M. 2007. Ethnic comparisons of the cross–sectional relationships between measures of body size with diabetes and hypertension. *Obes Rev* 9(Suppl 1):53–61.

Jaffiol C. 2004. de Jean Vague. *Bull Acad Nationale Med* 188:895.

James P.T. 2004. Obesity: The worldwide epidemic. *Clin Dermatol* 22(4):276–80. Review.

Janssen I., Katzmarzyk P.T., Boyce W.F., Vereecken C., Mulvihill C., Roberts C., Currie C., Pickett W. 2005. Health Behaviour in School Aged Children Obesity Working Group. *Obes Rev* 6:123–132.

Jolliffe D. 2004. Extent of overweight among US children and adolescents from 1971 to 2000. *Int J Obes Relat Metab Disord* 28(1):4–9.

Kinra S., Baumer J.H., et al. 2005. Early growth and childhood obesity: A historical cohort study. *Arch Dis Child* 90(11):1122–1127.

Kissebah A.H., Vydelingum N., et al. 1982. Relation of body fat distribution to metabolic complications of obesity. *J Clin Endocrinol Metab* 54(2):254–260.

Knowler W.C., Barrett-Connor E., et al. 2002. Reduction in the incidence of type 2 diabetes with lifestyle intervention or metformin. *N Engl J Med* 346(6):393–403.

Koenigsberger L. 1906. *Hermann von Helmholtz*. Transl. Frances A. Welby. Oxford: Clarendon Press.

Laforgia J., Dollman J., Dale M.J., Withers R.T., Hill A.M. 2009. Validation of DXA vody composition estimates in obese men and women. *Obesity* (Silver Spring) 17(4):821–826.

Lapidus L., Bengtsson C., et al. 1984. Distribution of adipose tissue and risk of cardiovascular disease and death: A 12 year follow up of participants in the population study of women in Gothenburg, Sweden. *BMJ* (*Clin Res Ed*) 289(6454):1257–1261.

Larsson B., Svardsudd K., et al. 1984. Abdominal adipose tissue distribution, obesity, and risk of cardiovascular disease and death: 13 year follow up of participants in the study of men born in 1913. *BMJ* (*Clin Res Ed*) 288(6428):1401–1404.

Levitt D.G., Heymsfield S.B., Pierson R.N. Jr, Shapses S.A., Kral J.G. 2007. Physiological models of body composition and human obesity. *Nutr Metab* 4:19.

Lee S.Y., Gallagher D. 2008. Assessment methods in human body composition. *Curr Opin Clin Nutr Metab Care* 11(5):566–572. Review.

Li L., Law C., Contle R.L., Powers C. 2009. Intergenerational influences on childhood body mass index: The effect of parental body mass index trajectories. *Am J Clin Nutr* 89:551–557.

Lohman T.G. 1992. *Advances in Body Composition Assessment*. Champaign, Illinois: Human Kinetics.

Mamun A.A., Hayatbakhsh M.R., O'Callaghan M., Williams G., Najman J. 2009. Early overweight and pubertal maturation—pathways of association with young adults' overweight: A longitudinal study. *Intern J Obes* 33:14–20.

Miech R.A., Kumanyika S.K., Stettler N., Link B.G., Phelan J.C., Chang V.W. 2006. Trends in the association of poverty with overweight among US adolescents, 1971–2004. *JAMA* 295:2385–2393.

National Institutes of Health. 1998. Clinical guidelines on the identification, evaluation, and treatment of overweight and obesity in adults: The evidence report. *Obes Rev* 6(Suppl. 2):51S–209S.

Ogden C.L., Yanovski S.Z., Carroll M.D., Flegal K.M. 2007. The epidemiology of obesity. *Gastroenterology* 132:2087–2102.

Ogden C.L., Carroll M.D., et al. 2006. Prevalence of overweight and obesity in the United States, 1999–2004. *JAMA* 295(13):1549–1555.

Ogden C.L., Flegal K.M., Carroll M.D., Johnson C.L. 2002. Prevalence and trends in overweight among US children and adolescents, 1999–2000. *JAMA* 288(14):1728–1732.

Ogden C.L., Carroll M.D., Flegal K.M. 2008. High body mass index for age among US children and adolescents 2003–2006. *JAMA* 299:2401–2405.

Ogden C.L., Carroll M.D., Curtin L.R., Lamb M.M., Flegal K.M. 2010. Prevalence of high body mass index in US children and adolescents, 2007–2008. *JAMA* 303(3):242–249.

Osler W. 1921. *The Evolution of Medicine*. New Haven: Yale University Press.

Parikh N.I., Pencina M.J., Wang T.J., Lanier K.J., Fox C.S., D'Agostin R.B., Vasan R.S. 2007. Increasing trends in incidence of overweight and obesity over 5 decades. *Am J Med* 120:242–252.

Pierce M.B., Leon A. 2005. Age at menarche and adult BMI in the Aberdeen children of the 1950s cohort study. *Am J Clin Nutr* 82(4):733–739.

Quetelet L.-J.-A. 1835. *Sur l'homme et le developpement de ses facultes, ou essai de physique sociale*. Paris: Bachelier, pp 10.

Quetelet L.-J.-A. 1869. *Physique sociale; ou, Essai sur le développement des facultés de l'homme*. Brussels: C. Marquardt.

Reaven G.M. 1988. Banting lecture 1988. Role of insulin resistance in human disease. *Diabetes* 37(12):1595–1607.

Romero-Corral A., Somers V.K., Sierra-Johnson J., Thomas R.J., Collazo-Clavell M.L., Korinek J., Allison T.G., Batsis J.A., Sert-Kuniyoshi F.H., Lopez-Jimenez F. 2008. Accuracy of body mass index in diagnosing obesity in the adult general population. *Intern J Obes* 32:959–966.

Rossner S. Per Bjorntorp (1931–2002). *Obes Rev* 2010, in press.

Saha C., Eckert G.J., et al. 2005. Onset of overweight during childhood and adolescence in relation to race and sex. *J Clin Endocrinol Metab* 90(5):2648–2652.

Salans L.B., Knittle J.L., Hirsch J. 1968. The role of adipose cell size and adipose tissue insulin sensitivity in the carbohydrate intolerance of human obesity. *J Clin Invest* 47(1):153–165.

Schlieden M.J. 1838. Beitrage zur phytogenesis. *Arch Anat Physiol wiss Med* 137–176.

Schwann T.H. 1839. *Mikroscopische Untersuchungen uber die Uebereinstimmung in der Struktur un dem Wachsthum der Thiere und Pflanzen*. Berlin: Sander.

Schwann T.H. 1847. *Microscopical Researches into the Accordance in the Structure and Growth of Animals and Plants*. Transl. H. Smith. London: Sydenham Society.

Seidell J.C., Rissanen A.M. 1997. Time trends in worldwide prevalence of obesity. In *Handbook of Obesity*. G.A. Bray, C. Bouchard, W.P. James, eds. New York: Marcel Dekker Inc., pp 79–91.

Shen W., Punyanitya M., Chen J., Gallagher D., Albu J., Pi-Sunyer X., Lewis C.E., Grunfeld C., Heshka S., Heymsfield S.B. 2006. Waist circumference correlated with metabolic syndrome indicators better than percentage fat. *Obesity* 14:727–736.

Shen W., Punyanitya M., Wang Z., Gallagher D., St-Onge M.P., Albu J., Heymsfield S.B., Heshka S. 2004. Visceral adipose tissue: Relations between single-slice areas and total volume. *Am J Clin Nutr* 80:271–278.

Sjostrom L., Kvist H., et al. 1986. Determination of total adipose tissue and body fat in women by computed tomography, 40K, and tritium. *Am J Physiol* 250(6 Pt 1):E736–E745.

Sjostrom L. 2004. Per Bjorntorp 1931–2002. *Intern J Obesity* 28:351.

Smith S.R., De Jonge L., et al. 2005. Effect of pioglitazone on body composition and energy expenditure: A randomized controlled trial. *Metabolism* 54(1):24–32.

Strauss R.S., Pollack H.A. 2001. Epidemic increase in childhood overweight, 1986–1998. *JAMA* 286(22): 2845–2848.

Talbot J.H. 1972. *A Biographic History of Medicine*. New York: Grune & Stratton.

Vague J. 1947. La differenciation sexuelle facteur determinant des formes de l'obésité. Transl. J Vague. *Presse Medicale* 55:339–340.

Vague J. 1956. The degree of masculine differentiation of obesities: A factor determining predisposition to diabetes, atherosclerosis, gout, and uric calculous disease. *Am J Clin Nutr* 4(1): 20–34.

Vasan R.S., Pencina M.J., Cobain M., Freibert M.S., D'Agostino R.B. 2005. Estimated risk for developing obesity in the Framingham Heart Study. *Ann Int Med* 143:473–480.

Veldhuis J.D., Roemmich J.N., et al. 2005. Endocrine control of body composition in infancy, childhood, and puberty. *Endocr Rev* 26(1):114–146.

Vesalius A. 1543. 2004. *De humani corporis fabrica*. Basileae: Joannis Oporini.

Völgyi E., Tylavsky F.A., Lyytikäinen A., Suominen H., Alén M., Cheng S. 2008. Assessing body composition with DXA and bioimpedance: Effects of obesity, physical activity, and age. *Obesity* (Silver Spring). 16(3):700–705

Wadden T.A., Butryn M.L. 2004. Efficacy of lifestyle modification for long-term weight control. *Obes Res* 12(Suppl):151S–162S.

Wadden T.A., Berkowitz R.I., Womble L.G., Sarwer D.B., Phelan S., Cato R.K., Hesson L.A., Osei S.Y., Kaplan R., Stunkard A.J. 2005. Randomized trial of lifestyle modification and pharmacotherapy for obesity. *N Engl J Med* 353(20):2111–2120.

Walker H. 1929. *Studies in the History of Statistical Method*. Baltimore: Williams and Wilkins Co.

Wang Z.M., Pierson R.N., Jr., et al. 1992. The five-level model: A new approach to organizing body-composition research. *Am J Clin Nutr* 56(1):19–28.

Weeks R.W. 1904. An experiment with the specialized investigation. In *Actuarial Society of America. Transactions* 8:17–23.

Weiss R., Dziura J., et al. 2004. Obesity and the metabolic syndrome in children and adolescents. *N Engl J Med* 350(23):2362–2374.

Whitaker R.C., Gooze R.A., Hughes C.C., Finkelstein D.M. 2009. A national survey of obesity prevention practices in head start. *Arch Pediatr Adolesc Med* 163(12):1144–1150.

WHO. 2000. Obesity: Preventing and managing the global epidemic. Report of a WHO consultation. *World Health Organ Tech Rep Ser* 894:i–xii;1–253.

CHAPTER 3

Abizaid A., Liu Z.W., Andrews Z.B., Shanabrough M., Borok E., Elsworth J.D., Roth R.H., Sleeman M.W., Picciotto M.R., Tschöp M.H., Gao X.B., Horvath T.L. 2006. Ghrelin modulates the activity and synaptic input organization of midbrain dopamine neurons while promotong appetite. *J Clin Invest* 116:3229–3239.

Adams A.K., Harvey H.E., Prince R.J. 2005. Association of material smoking with overweight at age 3 in American Indian Children. *Am J Clin Nutr* 82:393–398.

Agras W.S., Hammer L.D., McNichols F., Kraemer H.C. 2004. Risk factors for childhood overweight: A prospective study from birth to 9.5 years. *J Pediatr* 145:20–25.

Ailhaud G., Guesnet P. 2004. Fatty acid composition of fats is an early determinant of childhood obesity: A short review and an opinion. *Obes Rev* 5(1):21–26.

Al Mamun A., Lawlor D.A., Cramb S., O'Callaghean M., Williams G., Najman J. 2007. Do childhood sleeping problems predict obesity in young adulthood? Evidence from a prospective birth cohort study. *Am J Epidemiol* 166:1368–1373.

Allison D.B., Mentore J.L., Heo M., Chandler L.P., Cappelleri J.C., Infante M.C., Weiden P.J. 1999. Antipsychotic-induced weight gain: A comprehensive research synthesis. *Am J Psychiatry* 156(11):1686–1696.

Allison K.C., Ahima R.S., O'Reardon J.P., Dinges D.F., Sharma V., Cummings D.E., Heo M., Martino N.S., Stunkard A.J. 2005b. Neuroendocrine profiles associated with energy intake, sleep and stress in the night eating syndrome. *JCEM* 90:6214–6217.

Allison K.C., Grilo C.M., Masheb R.M., Stunkard A.J. 2005a. Binge-eating disorder and night-eating syndrome: A comparative study of disordered eating. *J Consult Clin Psychol* 73:1107–1115.

Allison K.C., Wadden T.A., Sarwer D.B., Fabricatore A.N., Crerand C.E., Gibbons L.M., Stack R.M., Stunkard A.J., Williams N.N. 2006. Night-eating syndrome and binge-eating disorder among persons seeking bariatric surgery: Prevalence and related features. *Obesity* Suppl 4:77S–82S.

Alonso-Alonso M., Pascual-Leone A. 2007. The right brain hypothesis for obesity. *JAMA* 297:1819–1822.

Arenz S., Rückerl R., Koletzko B., von Kries R. 2004. Breast-feeding and childhood obesity—A systematic review. *Int J Obes Relat Metab Disord* 28(10):1247–1256.

Astrup A., Grunwald G.K., Melanson E.L., Saris W.H., Hill J.O. 2000. The role of low-fat diets in body weight control: A meta-analysis of ad libitum dietary intervention studies. *Int J Obes Relat Metab Disord* 24(12):1545–1552.

Astrup A., Rossner S., Van Gaal L., Niskanen L., Al Hakim M., Madsen J., Rasmussen M.F., Lean M.E.J. on behalf of the NN8022-1807 Study Group. 2009. Effects of liraglutide in the treatment of obesity: A randomised, double-blind, placebo-controlled study. *Lancet* 374(9701):1606–1616.

Atkinson R.L. 2007. Viruses as an etiology of obesity. *Proc Mayo Clinic* 82:1192–1198.

Atlantis E., Baker M. 2008. Obesity effects on depression: Systematic review of epidemiological studies. *Intern J Obes* 32:881–889.

Attie A.D., Scherer P.E. 2009. Adipocyte metabolism and obesity. *J Lipid Res* 50(Suppl):S395–S399.

Atwater W.O., Rosa E.B. 1899. *Description of a New Respiration Calorimeter and Experiments on the Conservation of Energy in the Human Body*. USDA Bull. 63, Washington, D.C.: USDA Office of Experimental Station.

Backhed F., Ding H., Wang T., et al. 2004. The gut microbioata as an environmental factor that regulated fat storage. *Proc Natl Acad Sci USA* 101:15718–15723.

Backman L., Kolmodin-Hedman B. 1978. Concentration of DDT and DDE in plasma and subcutaneous adipose tissue before and after intestinal bypass operation for treatment of obesity. *Toxicol Appl Pharmacol* 46:663–669.

Baillie-Hamilton P.F. 2002. Chemical toxins: A hypothesis to explain the global obesity epidemic. *J Altern Complement Med* 8(2):185–192.

Barker, D.J., Hales, C.N., Fall, C.H., Osmond, C., Phipps, K., Clark, P.M. 1993. Type 2 (non-insulin-dependent) diabetes mellitus, hypertension and hyperlipidaemia (syndrome X): Relation to reduced fetal growth. *Diabetologia* 36(1):62–67.

Barker D.J., Eriksson J.G., Forsén T., Osmond C. 2002. Fetal origins of adult disease: Strength of effects and biological basis. *Int J Epidemiol* 31(6):1235–1239.

Barnes M.J., Holmes G., Primeaux S.D., York D.A., Bray G.A. 2006. Increased expression of mu-opioid receptors in animals susceptible to diet-induced obesity. *Peptides* 27:3292–3298.

Barnes M.J., Argyropoulos G., Bray G.A. 2010. Preference for a high fat diet, but not hyperphagia following activation of mu opioid receptors is blocked in AgRP knockout mice. *Brain Res* 1317C:100–107.

Barth S.W., Riediger T., Lutz T.A., Rechkemmer G. 2004. Peripheral amylin activates circumventricular organs expressing calcitonin receptor a/b subtypes and receptor-activity modifying proteins in the rat. *Brain Res* 997(1):97–102.

Bartke A. 2008. Growth hormone and aging: A challenging controversy. *Clin Interv Aging* 3(4):659–665.

Barton B.A., Eldridge A.L., Thompson D., Affenito S.G., Striegel-Moore R.H., Franko D.L., Albertson A.M., Crockett S.J. 2005. The relationship of breakfast and cereal consumption to nutrient intake and body mass index: The National Heart, Lung, and Blood Institute Growth and Health Study. *J Am Diet Assoc* 105(9):1383–1389.

Bazzano L.Y., Song Y., Bubes V., Good C.K., Manson J.E., Liu S. 2005. Dietary intake of whole and refined grain breakfast cereals and weight gain in men. *Obes Res* 13:1952–1960.

Beglinger C., Degen L. 2006. Gastrointestinal satiety signals in humans—Physiologic roles for GLP-1 and PYY? *Physiol Behav* 89:460–464.

Bell E.A., Castellanos V.H., Pelkman C.L., Thorwart M.L., Rolls B.J. 1998. Energy density of foods affects energy intake in normal-weight women. *Am J Clin Nutr* 67(3):412–420.

Benison S., Barger A.C., Wolfe E.L., Cannon W.B. 1987. *The Life and Time of a Young Scientist*. Cambridge: Belknap Press.

Berkey C.S., Rockett H.R., Field A.E., Gillman M.W., Colditz G.A. 2004. Sugar-added beverages and adolescent weight change. *Obes Res* 12(5):778–788.

Berthoud H.R., Morrison C. 2008. The brain, appetite, and obesity. *Annu Rev Psychol* 59:55–92.

Blair S.N., Brodney S. 1999. Effects of physical inactivity and obesity on morbidity and mortality: Current evidence and research issues. *Med Sci Sports Exerc* 31(11 Suppl):S646–S662.

Blundell J.E., MacDiarmid J.I. 1997. Fat as a risk factor for overconsumption: Satiation, satiety, and patterns of eating. *J Am Diet Assoc* 97(7 Suppl):S63–S69.

Bohlooly Y.M., Olsson B., Bruder C.E., Lindén D., Sjögren K., Bjursell M., Egecioglu E., Svensson L., Brodin P., Waterton J.C., Isaksson O.G., Sundler F., Ahrén B., Ohlsson C., Oscarsson J., Törnell J. 2005. Growth hormone overexpression in the central nervous system results in hyperphagia-induced obesity associated with insulin resistance and dyslipidemia. *Diabetes* 54(1):51–62. Erratum in *Diabetes* 54(4):1249. Bohlooly, Mohammad [corrected to Bohlooly-Y, Mohammad].

Bosy-Westphal A., Kossel E., Goele K., Later W., Hitze B., Settler U., Heller M., Glüer C.C., Heymsfield S.B., Müller M.J. 2009. Contribution of individual organ mass loss to weight loss-associated decline in resting energy expenditure. *Am J Clin Nutr* 90(4):993–1001.

Bouchard C., Tremblay A., Després J.P., Nadeau A., Lupien P.J., Thériault G., Dussault J., Moorjani S., Pinault S., Fournier G. 1990. The response to long-term overfeeding in identical twins. *N Engl J Med* 322(21):1477–1482.

Bowman S.A., Gortmaker S.L., Ebbeling C.B., Pereira M.A., Ludwig D.S. 2004. Effects of fast-food consumption on energy intake and diet quality among children in a national household survey. *Pediatrics* 113(1 Pt 1):112–118.

Bray G.A. 1972. Lipogenesis in human adipose tissue: Some effects of nibbling and gorging. *J Clin Invest* 51:537–548.

Bray G.A. 1976. *The Obese Patient: Major Problems in Internal Medicine*. Philadelphia: W.B. Saunders & Co.

Bray G.A, Popkin BM. 1998. Dietary fat intake does affect obesity! *Am J Clin Nutr* 68(6):1157–1173.

Bray G.A, Greenway F.L. 1999. Current and potential drugs for treatment of obesity. *Endocr Rev* 20(6):805–875.

Bray G.A., Nielsen S.J., Popkin B.M. 2004. Consumption of high-fructose corn syrup in beverages may play a role in the epidemic of obesity. *Am J Clin Nutr* 79(4):537–543. Erratum in *Am J Clin Nutr* 80(4):1090.

Bray G.A. 2007a. *The Metabolic Syndrome and Obesity*. Totowa, NJ: The Humana Press, Inc.

Bray G.A. 2007b. *The Battle of the Bulge*. Pittsburgh: Dorrance Publishing.

Bray G.A., Flatt J.P., Volaufova J., Delany J.P., Champagne C.M. 2008. Corrective responses in human food intake identified from an analysis of 7-d food-intake records. *Am J Clin Nutr* 88(6):1504–1510.

Bray G.A. 2009. The GI hormones and weight management: A commentary. *Lancet,* in press.

Briefel R.R., Crepinsek M.K., Cabili C., Wilson A., Gleason P.M. 2009. School food environments and practices affect dietary behaviors of US public school children. *J Am Diet Assoc* 109:S91–S107.

Buse J.B., Rosenstock J., Sesti G., Schmidt W.E., Montanya E., Brett J.H., Zychma M., Blonde L. 2009. LEAD-6 Study Group. Liraglutide once a day versus exenatide twice a day for type 2 diabetes: A 26-week randomised, parallel-group, multinational, open-label trial (LEAD-6). *Lancet* 374(9683):39–47.

Campfield L.A., Smith F.J. 2003. Blood glucose dynamics and control of meal initiation: A pattern detection and recognition theory. *Physiol Rev* 83(1):25–58.

Cannon W.B. 1911. *The Mechanical Factors in Digestion*. London: E. Arnold.

Cannon W.B., Washburn A.L. 1912. An explanation of hunger. *Am J Physiol* 29:441–454.

Cannon W.B. 1915. *Bodily Changes in Pain, Hunger, Fear, and Rage*. New York: D. Appleton & Co.

Cannon W.B. 1945. *The Way of an Investigator*. New York: W.W. Norton & Co.

Carlson A.J. 1912. Contributions to the physiology of the stomach. II. The relations between the concentration of the empty stomach and the sensation of hunger. *Am J Pyhysiol* 31:175–192.

CDC (Centers for Disease Control and Prevention) 2009. *MMWR* 52:80–82.

Cecil J.E., Tavendale R., Watt P., Hetherington M.M., Palmer C.N. 2008. An obesity-associated FTO gene variant and increased energy intake in children. *N Engl J Med* 359(24):2558–2566.

Champagne C.M., Bray G.A., Kurtz A.A., Monteiro J.B., Tucker E., Volaufova J., Delany J.P. 2002. Energy intake and energy expenditure: A controlled study comparing dietitians and non-dietitians. *J Am Diet Assoc* 102(10):1428–1432.

Choi H.K., Curhan G. 2008. Soft drinks, fructose consumption, and the risk of gout in men: Prospective cohort study. *BMJ* 336:309–312.

Christakis N.A., Fowler J.H. 2007. The spread of obesity in a large social network over 32 years. *N Engl J Med* 357:370–379.

Cleave T.L., Campbell G.D. 1966. *Diabetes, Coronary Thrombosis, and the Saccharine Disease*. Bristol: John Wright & Sons.

Cowley M.A., Pronchuk N., Fan W., Dinulescu D.M., Colmers W.F., Cone R.D. 1999. Integration of NPY, AGRP, and melanocortin signals in the hypothalamic paraventricular nucleus: Evidence of a cellular basis for the adipostat. *Neuron* 24(1):155–163.

Crawley H., Summerbell C. 1997. Feeding frequency and BMI among teenagers aged 16–17 years. *Int J Obes Relat Metab Disord* 21(2):159–161.

Crespo C.J., Smit E., Troiano R.P., Bartlett S.J., Macera C.A., Andersen R.E. 2001. Television watching, energy intake, and obesity in US children: Results from the third National Health and Nutrition Examination Survey, 1988–1994. *Arch Pediatr Adolesc Med* 155(3):360–365

Critser G. 2003. *Fat Land. How Americans Became the Fattest People in the World*. New York: Houghton Mifflin.

Cummings D.E. 2006. Ghrelin and the short- and long-term regulation of appetite and body weight. *Physiol Behav* 89:71–84.

Cutler D.M., Glaeser E.L., Shapiro J.M. 2003. Why have Americans become more obese? *J Economic Perspectives* 17:93–118.

Cypess A.M., Lehman S., Williams G., Tal I., Rodman D., Goldfine A.B., Kuo F.C., Palmer E.L., Tseng Y.H., Doria A., Kolodny G.M., Kahn C.R. 2009. Identification and importance of brown adipose tissue in adult humans. *N Engl J Med* 360:1509–1517.

Dabelea D., Pettitt D.J., Hanson R.L., Imperatore G., Bennett P.H., Knowler W.C. 1999. Birth weight, type 2 diabetes, and insulin resistance in Pima Indian children and young adults. *Diabetes Care* 22(6):944–950.

Davenport C.B. 1923. *Body-Build and Its Inheritance*. Washington, DC: Carnegie Institution of Washington.

Davies K.M., Heaney R.P., Recker R.R., Lappe J.M., Barger-Lux M.J., Rafferty K., Hinders S. 2000. Calcium intake and body weight. *J Clin Endocrinol Metab* 85(12):4635–4638.

Dhingra R., Sullivan L., Jacques R.F., Wang T.J., Fox C.S., Meigs J.B., D'Agostino R.B., Faziano J.M., Vasan R.S. 2007. Soft drink consumption and risk of developing cardiometabolic risk factors and the metabolic syndrome in middle-aged adults in the community. *Circ* 116(5):480–488. Erratum in *Circ* 116(23):e557.

Dietz W.H., Jr, Gortmaker S.L. 1985. Do we fatten our children at the television set? Obesity and television viewing in children and adolescents. *Pediatrics* 75(5):807–812.

Dietz W.H. 2006. Sugar-sweetened beverages, milk intake, and obesity in children and adolescents. *J Pediatr* 148(2):152–154.

Diliberti N., Bordi P.L., Conklin M.T., Roe L.S., Rolls B.J. 2004. Increased portion size leads to increased energy intake in a restaurant meal. *Obes Res* 12:562–568.

Dixon J.B., Dixon M.E., et al. 2003. Depression in association with severe obesity: Changes with weight loss. *Arch Intern Med* 163(17):2058–2065.

Dockray G.J. 2004. The expanding family of RFamide peptides and their effects on feeding behaviour. *Exp Physiol* 89(3):229–235.

Drewnowski A., Darmon N. 2005. The economics of obesity: Dietary energy density and energy cost. *Am J Clin Nutr* 82(1 Suppl):265S–273S.

Drewnowski A., Specter S.E. 2004. Poverty and obesity: The role of energy density and energy costs. *Am J Clin Nutr* Jan 79(1):6–16.

Dubois L., Farmer A., Girard M., Peterson K. 2007. Regular sugar-sweetened beverage consumption between meals increases risk of overweight among preschool-aged children. *J Am Diet Assn* 107:924–934.

Ebbeling C.B., Sinclair K.B., Pereira M.A., Garcia-Lago E., Feldman H.A., Ludwig D.S. 2004. Compensation for energy intake from fast food among overweight and lean adolescents. *JAMA* 291(23):2828–2833.

Edholm O.G., Fletcher J.G., Widdowson E.M., McCance R.A. 1955. The energy expenditure and food intake of individual men. *Br J Nutr* 9(3):286–300.

Epstein L.H., Roemmich J.N., Paluch R.A., Raynor H.A. 2005. Influence of changes in sedentary behavior on energy and macronutrient intake in youth. *Am J Clin Nutr* 81(2):361–366.

Farooqi I.S., Keogh J.M., Yeo G.S., Lank E.J., Cheetham T., O'Rahilly S. 2003. Clinical spectrum of obesity and mutations in the melanocortin 4 receptor gene. *N Engl J Med* 348(12):1085–1095.

Farooqi I.S., O'Rahilly S. 2008. Genetic evaluation of obese patients. In *Handbook of Obesity, Clinical Applications*, 3rd ed. G.A. Bray, C. Bouchard, eds. New York: Informa; pp 45–54.

Farshchi H.R., Taylor M.A., Macdonald I.A. 2005. Beneficial metabolic effects of regular meal frequency on dietary thermogenesis, insulin sensitivity, and fasting lipid profiles in healthy obese women. *Am J Clin Nutr* 81(1):16–24.

Fetita L.-A., Sobngwi E., Serradas P., Calvo F., Gautier J.-F. 2006. Review. Consequences of fetal exposure to material diabetes in offspring. *J Clin Endocrinol Metab* 91:3718–3724.

Field A.E., Willet W.C., Lissner L., Colditz G.A. 2007. Dietary fat and weight gain among women in the Nurses' Health Study. *Obesity* 15:967–976.

Filizof C., Fernandez Pinilla M.C., Fernandez-Crus A. 2004. Smoking cessation and weight gain. *Obes Rev* 5:95–103.

Finkelstein E.A., Ruhm C.J., Kosa K.M. 2005. Economic causes and consequences of obesity. *Annu Rev Public Health* 26:239–257.

Flatt J.P. 1995. Use and storage of carbohydrate and fat. *Am J Clin Nutr* 61(4 Suppl):952S–959S.

Flegal K.M., Troiano R.P., Pamuk E.R., Kuczmarski R.J., Campbell S.M. 1995. The influence of smoking cessation on the prevalence of overweight in the United States. *N Engl J Med* 333(18):1165–1170.

Forshee R.A., Anderson P.A., Storey M.L. 2008. Sugar-sweetened beverages and body mass index in children and adolescents: A meta-analysis. *Am J Clin Nutr* 67:1662–1671.

Franco M., Ordunez P., Caballero B., et al. 2007. Impact of energy intake, physical activity, and population-wide weight loss on cardiovascular disease and diabetes mortality in Cuba, 1980–2005. *Am J Epidemiol* 166:1374–1380.

Frazao E., Allshouse J. 2003. Strategies for intervention: Commentary and debate. *J Nutr* 133(3):844S–847S.

Fukuhara A., Matsuda M., Nishizawa M., Segawa K., Tanaka M., Kishimoto K., Matsuki Y., Murakami M., Ichisaka T., Murakami H., Watanabe E., Takagi T., Akiyoshi M., Ohtsubo T., Kihara S., Yamashita S., Makishima M., Funahashi T., Yamanaka S., Hiramatsu R., Matsuzawa Y., Shimomura I. 2005. Visfatin: a protein secreted by visceral fat that mimics the effects of insulin. *Science* Jan 21;307(5708):426–430. Retraction in: Fukuhara A., Matsuda M., Nishizawa M., Segawa K., Tanaka M., Kishimoto K., Matsuki Y., Murakami M., Ichisaka T., Murakami H., Watanabe E., Takagi T., Akiyoshi M., Ohtsubo T., Kihara S., Yamashita S., Makishima M., Funahashi T., Yamanaka S., Hiramatsu R., Matsuzawa Y., Shimomura I. 2007. *Science* 318(5850):565.

Gable S., Change Y., Kruss J.L. 2007. Television watching and frequency of family meals are predictive of overweight onset and persistence in a national sample of school-aged children. *J Am Diet Assn* 107:53–61.

Gallagher D., Belmonte D., Deurenberg P., et al. 1998. Organ-tissue mass measured allows modeling of REE and metabolically active tissue mass. *Am J Physiol* 275:E249–E258.

Gangwisch J.E., Malaspina D., Boden-Albala B., Heymsfield S.B. 2005. Inadequate sleep as a risk factor for obesity: Analyses of the NHANES I. *Sleep* 28(10):1289–1296.

Gilbertson T.A., Liu L., Kim I., Burks C.A., Hansen D.R. 2005. Fatty acid responses in taste cells from obesity-prone and -resistant rats. *Physiol Behav* 86(5):681–690.

Gillman M.W., Rifas-Shiman S.L., Berkey C.S., Frazier A.L., Rockett H.R., Camargo C.A. Jr, Field A.E., Colditz G.A. 2007. Breast-feeding and overweight in adolescence: Within-family analysis [corrected]. *Epidemiology* 2006 Jan17(1):112–114. Erratum in: *Epidemiology* 18(4):506.

Gluck M.E., Venti C.A., Salbe A.D., Krakoff J. 2009. Nighttime eating: Commonly observed and related to weight gain in an inpatient food intake study. *Am J Clin Nutr* 88:900–905.

Gortmaker S.L., Must A., Sobol A.M., Peterson K., Colditz G.A., Dietz W.H. 1996. Television viewing as a cause of increasing obesity among children in the United States, 1986–1990. *Arch Pediatr Adolesc Med* 150(4):356–362.

Graham K.A., Perkins D.O., Edwards L.J., Barrier Jr R.C., Lieberman J.A., Harp J.B. 1995. Effect of olanzapine on body composition and energy expenditure in adults with first-episode psychosis. *Am J Psychiatry* 162:118–123.

Green H., Meuth M. 1974. An established pre-adipose cell line and its differentiation in culture. *Cell* 3(2):127–133.

Gupta N.K., Mueller W.H., Chan W., Meininger J.C. 2002. Is obesity associated with poor sleep quality in adolescents? *Am J Hum Biol* 14(6):762–768.

Haines P.S., Hama M.Y., Guilkey D.K., Popkin B.M. 2003. Weekend eating in the United States is linked with greater energy, fat and alcohol intake. *Obesity* 11:945–949.

Halberg N., Wernstedt I., Scherer P.E. 2008. The adipocyte as an endocrine cell. *Endocrinol Metab Clin North Am* 37:753–764.

Halberg N., Khan T., Trujillo M.E., Wernstedt-Asterholm I., Attie A.D., Sherwani S., Wang Z.V., Landskroner-Eiger S., Dineen S., Magalang U.J., Brekken R.A., Scherer P.E. 2009. Hypoxia-inducible factor 1a induces fibrosis and insulin resistance in white adipose tissue. *Mol Cell Biol* 29:4467–4483.

Halford J.C., Harrold J.A., Lawton C.L., Blundell J.E. 2005. Serotonin (5-HT) drugs: Effects on appetite expression and use for the treatment of obesity. *Curr Drug Targets* 6(2):201–213.

Hallgreen C.E., Hall K.D. 2008. Allometric relationship between changes of visceral fat and total fat mass. *Int J Obes* (Lond) 32:845–852.

Hall K.D. 2006. Computational model of in vivo human energy metabolism during semistarvation and refeeding. *Am J Physiol Endocrinol Metab* 291(1):E23–E37.

Hamedani A., Akhavan T., Samra R.A., Anderson G.H. 2009. Reduced energy intake at breakfast is not compensated for at lunch if a high-insoluble-fiber cereal replaces a low-fiber cereal. *Am J Clin Nutr* 89:1343–1349.

Hancox R.J., Milne B.J., Poulton R. 2004. Association between child and adolescent television viewing and adult health: A longitudinal birth cohort study. *Lancet* 364(9430):257–262.

Harder T., Bergmann R., Kallischnigg G., Plagemann A. 2005. Duration of breastfeeding and risk of overweight: A meta-analysis. *Am J Epidemiol* 162(5):397–403.

Havel P.J. 2002. Control of energy homeostasis and insulin action by adipocyte hormones: Leptin, acylation stimulating protein, and adiponectin. *Curr Opin Lipidol* 13(1):51–59.

Heindel J.J. 2003. Endocrine disruptors and the obesity epidemic. *Toxicol Sci* 76(2):247–249.

Hellerstein M.K., Neese R.A., Schwarz J.M. 1993. Model for measuring absolute rates of hepatic de novo lipogenesis and reesterification of free fatty acids. *Am J Physiol* 265(5 Pt 1):E814–E820.

Helmholtz, H. von. 1847. Uber die Erhaltung der Kraft, ein physikalische Abhandlung, vorgetragen in der Sitzung der physicalischen Gesellschaft zu Berlin am 23sten Juli 1847. Berlin: G. Reimer.

HHS. 1996. *Physical Activity and Health: A Report of the Surgeon General.* Atlanta, GA: U.S. Department of Health and Human Services.

Hida K., Wada J., Eguchi J., Zhang H., Baba M., Seida A., Hashimoto I., Okada T., Yasuhara A., Nakatsuka A., Shikata K., Hourai S., Futami J., Watanabe E., Matsuki Y., Hiramatsu R., Akagi S., Makino H., Kanwar Y.S. 2005. Visceral adipose tissue-derived serine protease inhibitor: A unique insulin-sensitizing adipocytokine in obesity. *Proc Natl Acad Sci U S A* 102(30):10610–10615.

Hill J.O., Peters J.C. 1998. Environmental contributions to the obesity epidemic. *Science* 280(5368): 1371–1374.

Hill J.O., Wyatt H.R., Reed G.W., Peters J.C. Obesity and the environment: Where do we go from here? *Science* 299:853–855.

Himenez M., Leger B., Canola K., Lehr L., Arboit P., Seydoux J., Russell A.P., Giacobino J.-P., Muzzin P., Preitner F. 2002. B1/B2/B3 adrenoceptor knockout mice are obese and cold-sensitive but have normal lipolytic responses to fasting. *FEBS Lett* 530:37–40.

Howard A.D., Wang R., Pong S.S., Mellin T.N., Strack A., Guan X.M., Zeng Z., Williams D.L. Jr, Feighner S.D., Nunes C.N., Murphy B., Stair J.N., Yu H., Jiang Q., Clements M.K., Tan C.P., McKee K.K., Hreniuk D.L., McDonald T.P., Lynch K.R., Evans J.F., Austin C.P., Caskey C.T., Van der Ploeg L.H., Liu Q. 2000. Identification of receptors for neuromedin U and its role in feeding. *Nature* 406:70–74.

Hu F.B., Willett W.C., Li T., Stampfer M.J., Colditz G.A., Manson J.E. 2004. Adiposity as compared with physical activity in predicting mortality among women. *N Engl J Med* 351(26):2694–2703.

Hücking K., Hamilton-Wessler M., Ellmerer M., Bergman R.N. 2003. Burst-like control of lipolysis by the sympathetic nervous system in vivo. *J Clin Invest* 111(2):257–264.

Iglowinski I., Jenni O.G., Molinari L., Largo R.H. 2003. Sleep duration from infancy to adolescence: Reference values and generational trends. *Pediatrics* 111:302–307.

James J., Thomas P., Cavan D., Kerr D. 2004. Preventing childhood obesity by reducing consumption of carbonated drinks: Cluster randomised controlled trial. *BMJ* 328(7450):1237. Erratum in *BMJ* 328(7450):1236.

Jeffery R.W., Baxter J., McGuire M., Linde J. 2006. Are fast food restaurants an environmental risk factor for obesity? *Int J Behav Nutr Phys Act* 3:2.

Jeffery R.W., Gray C.W., French S.A., Hellerstedt W.L., Murray D., Luepker R.V., Blackburn H. 1995. Evaluation of weight reduction in a community intervention for cardiovascular disease risk: Changes in body mass index in the Minnesota Heart Health Program. *Int J Obes Relat Metab Disord* 19(1):30–39.

Johnson L., Mander A.P., Jones L.R., Emmett P.M., Jebb S.A. 2008. A prospective analysis of dietary energy density at age 5 and 7 years and fatness at 9 years among UK children. *Int J Obes (Lond)* 32(4):586–593.

Johnson R.J., Perez-Pozo S.E., Sautin Y.Y., Manitius J., Sanchez-Lozada L.G., Feig D.I., Shafiu M., Segal M., Glassock R.J., Shimada M., Roncal C., Nakagawa T. 2009. Hypothesis: Could excessive fructose intake and uric acid cause type 2 diabetes? *Endocr Rev* 30(1):96–116.

Kalliomaki M., Collado M.C., Salminen S., Isolauri E. 2008. Early differences in fecal microbiota composition in children may predict overweight. *Am J Clin Nutr* 87:534–538.

Kannisto K., Pietiläinen K.H., Ehrenborg E., Rissanen A., Kaprio J., Hamsten A, Yki-Järvinen H. 2004. Overexpression of 11beta-hydroxysteroid dehydrogenase-1 in adipose tissue is associated with acquired obesity and features of insulin resistance: Studies in young adult monozygotic twins. *J Clin Endocrinol Metab* 89(9):4414–4421.

Kershaw E.E., Flier J.S. 2004. Adipose tissue as an endocrine organ. *J Clin Endocrinol Metab* 89(6):2548–2556.

Khan T., Muise E.S., Iyengar P., Wang Z.V., Chandalia M., Abate N., Zhang B.B., Bonaldo P., Chua S., Scherer P.E. 2009. Metabolic dysregulation and adipose tissue fibrosis: Role of collagen VI. *Mol Cell Biol* 29:1575–1591.

Kim J.-Y. van de Wall E., Laplante M., Azzara A., Trujillo M.E., Hofmann S.M., Schraw T., Durand J.L., Li H., Li G., Jelicks L.A., Meher M.F., Hui D.Y., Deshaies Y., Shulman G.I., Schwartz G.J., Scherer P.E. 2007. Obesity-associated improvements in metabolic profile through expansion of adipose tissue. *J Clin Invest* 117:2621–2632.

Kimm S.Y. et al. 2002. Decline in physical activity in Black girls and White girls during adolescence. *N Engl J Med* 347(10):709–715.

Kirkland E.C. 1974. Scientific eating: New Englanders prepare and promote a reform. *Proc Mass Hist Soc* 86:28–52.

Koletzko B., von Kries R., Closa R., Escribano J., Scaglioni S., Giovannini M., Beyer J., Demmelmair H., Anton B., Gruszfeld D., Dobrzanska A., Sengier A., Langhendries J.P., Rolland-Cachera M.F., Grote V. 2009. Can infant feeding choices modulate later obesity risk? *Am J Clin Nutr* 89:1502S–1508S.

Konttinen H., Haukkala A., Sarlio-Lähteenkorva S., Silventoinen K., Jousilahti P. 2009. Eating styles, self-control and obesity indicators. The moderating role of obesity status and dieting history on restrained eating. *Appetite* 53(1):131–134.

Koupil I., Toivanen P. 2008. Social and early-life determinants of overweight and obesity in 18-year old Swedish men. *Int J Obes* 32:73–81.

Kral T.V., Roe L.S., Rolls B.J. 2004. Combined effects of energy density and portion size on energy intake in women. *Am J Clin Nutr* 79(6):962–968.

Kripke D.F., Garfinkel L., Wingard D.L., Klauber M.R., Marler M.R. 2002. Mortality associated with sleep duration and insomnia. *Arch Gen Psychiatry* 59(2):131–136.

Kromhout D. 1983. Body weight, diet, and serum cholesterol in 871 middle-aged men during 10 years of follow-up (the Zutphen Study). *Am J Clin Nutr* 38(4):591–598

Kromhout D., Bloemberg B., Seidell J.C., Nissinen A., Menotti A. 2001. Physical activity and dietary fiber determine population body fat levels: The Seven Countries Study. *Int J Obes Relat Metab Disord* 25:301–306.

Lakdawalla D., Philipson T. 2009. The growth of obesity and technological change: A theoretical and empirical examination. National Bureau of Economic Research Working Paper No W 8946, Washington, DC.

Lamerz A., Kuepper-Nybelen J., Bruning N., Wehle C., Trost-Brinkhues G., Brenner H., Hebebrand J., Herpertz-Dahlmann B. 2005. Prevalence of obesity, binge eating and night eating in a cross-sectional field survey of 6-year-old children and their parents in a German urban population. *J Child Psychol Psychiatry* 46:385–393.

Laugerette F., Passilly-Degrace P., Patris B., Niot I., Febbraio M., Montmayeur J.P., Besnard P. 2005. CD36 involvement in orosensory detection of dietary lipids, spontaneous fat preference, and digestive secretions. *J Clin Invest* 115(11):3177–3184.

Lawlor D.A., Smith G.D., O'Callaghan M., Alati R., Mamun A.A., Williams G.M., Najman J.M. 2006. Epidemiologic evidence for the fetal overnutrition hypothesis: Findings from the Mater-University Study of Pregnancy and Its Outcomes. *Am J Epidemiol* 165:418–424.

Ley R.E., Turnbaugh P.J., Klein S., Gordon J.I. 2006. Microbial ecology: Human gut microbes associated with obesity. *Nature* 444(7122):1022–1023.

Leary S.D., Smith G.D., Rogers I.S., Reilly J.J., Wells J.C.K., Ness A.R. 2006. Smoking during pregnancy and offspring fat and lean mass in childhood. *Obesity* 14:2284–2293.

Levin B.E., Dunn-Meynell A.A., Ricci M.R., Cummings D.E. 2003. Abnormalities of leptin and ghrelin regulation in obesity-prone juvenile rats. *Am J Physiol* 285:E949–E957.

Levine A.S., Winsky-Sommerer R., Huitron-Resendiz S., Grace M.K., de Lecea L. 2005. Injection of neuropeptide W into paraventricular nucleus of hypothalamus increases food intake. *Am J Physiol Regul Integr Comp Physiol*. 288(6):R1727–R1732.

Levitsky D.A., Obarzanek E., Mrkjenovic G., Strupp B.J. 2005. Imprecise control of energy intake; absence of a reduction in food intake following overfeeding in young adults. *Physiol Behav* 84:669–675.

Lieberman J.A., Stroup T.S., McEvoy J.P., Swartz M.S., Rosenheck R.A., Perkins D.O., Keefe R.S.E., Davis S.M., Davis C.E., Lebowitz B.D., Severe J., Jsiao J.K. Effectiveness of antipsychotic drugs in patients with chronic schizophrenia. *NEJM* 353:1209–1223.

Li M., Guo D., Isales C.M., Eizirik D.L., Atkinson M., She J.X., Wang C.Y. 2005. Sumo wrestling with type 1 diabetes. *J Mol Med* 83(7):504–513.

Liem E.T., Sauer P.J.J, Oldehinkel A.J., Stolk R.P. 2008. Association between depressive symptoms in childhood and adolescence and overweight in later life. *Arch Pediatr Adolesc Med* 162:981–988.

Locard E., Mamelle N., Billette A., Miginiac M., Munoz F., Rey S. 1992. Risk factors of obesity in a five year old population. Parental versus environmental factors. *Int J Obes Relat Metab Disord* 16(10):721–729.

Ludwig D.S., Peterson K.E., Gortmaker S.L. 2001. Relation between consumption of sugar-sweetened drinks and childhood obesity: A prospective, observational analysis. *Lancet* 357(9255):505–508.

Ludwig D.S., Tritos N.A., Mastaitis J.W., Kulkarni R., Kokkotou E., Elmquist J., Lowell B., Flier J.S., Maratos-Flier E. 2001. Melanin-concentrating hormone overexpression in transgenic mice leads to obesity and insulin resistance. *J Clin Invest* 107(3):379–386.

Lumey L.H., Stein A.D., Kahn H.S., Romijn J.A. 2009. Lipid profiles in middle-aged men and women after famine exposure during gestation: The Dutch Hunger Winter Families Study. *Am J Clin Nutr* 89:1737–1743.

Lundgren J.D., Allison K.C., Crow S., O'Reardon J.P., Berg K.C., Galbraight J., Martino N.S., Stunkard A.J. 2006. Prevalence of the night eating syndrome in a psychiatric population. *Am J Psychiatry* 163:156–158.

McDevitt R.M., Bott S.J., Harding M., Coward W.A., Bluck I.J., Prentice A.M. 2001. De novo lipogenesis during controlled overfeeding with sucrose or glucose in lean and obese women. *Am J Clin Nutr* 74:737–746.

MacDowell E.C. 1946. Charles Benedict Davenport, 1866–1944: A study of conflicting influences. *Bios* 17:3–50.

McLaren L. 2007. Socioeconomic status and obesity. *Epidemiol Rev* 29:29–48.

Malik V.S., Schulze F.B., Hu F. 2006. Intake of sugar-sweetened beverages and weight gain: A systematic review. *AJCN* 84(2):274–288.

Malik V.S., Popkin B.M., Bray G.A., Després J.P., Hu F.B. 2009. Sugar sweetened beverages and obesity and cardiometabolic risk: A systematic review and meta-analysis, in press.

Masaki T., Chiba S., Yasuda T., Noguchi H., Kakuma T., Watanabe T., Sakata T., Yoshimatsu H. 2004. Involvement of hypothalamic histamine H1 receptor in the regulation of feeding rhythm and obesity. *Diabetes* 53(9):2250–2260.

Mayer J.R. von. 1842. Bermerkungen uber die krafte der unbelebten natur. *Ann der Chemie Pharm* 42: 233–240.

Mayer J. 1965. Walter Bradford Cannon—A Biographical Sketch. *J Nutr* 87:3–8.

Maynard L.A. 1969. Francis Gano Benedict—A Biographical Sketch. *J Nutr* 98:1–8.

Mendel G.J. 1866. Versuch über Pflanzen-Hybriden. *Verb naturf Vereins Brunn* 4:3–47.

Merten M.J., Williams A.L., Shriver L.H. 2009. Breakfast consumption in adolescence and young adulthood: Parental presence, community context, and obesity. *J Am Dietetic Assn* 109:1384–1391.

Messerli F.J., Bell, D.S.H., Fonseca V., Katholi R.E., McGill J.B., Phillips R.A., Raskin P., Wright J.T., Jr, Bangalore S., Holdbrook F.K., Lukas M.A., Anderson K.M., Bakris G.L., for the GEMINI Investigators. 2007. *Am J Med* 120:610–615.

Mizutani T., Suzuki K., Kondo N., Yamagata Z. 2007. Association of material lifestyles including smoking during pregnancy with childhood obesity. *Obesity* 15:3133–3139.

Morens C., Nørregaard P., Receveur J.M., van Dijk G., Scheurink A.J. 2005. Effects of MCH and a MCH1-receptor antagonist on (palatable) food and water intake. *Brain Res* 1062(1–2):32–38.

Morton N.M., Seckl J.R. 2008. 11-beta-hydroxysteroid dehydrogenase type 1 and obesity. *Front Horm Res* 36:146–164.

Müller M.J., Bosy-Westphal A., Kutzner D., Heller M. 2002. Metabolically active components of fat-free mass and resting energy expenditure in humans: Recent lessons from imaging technologies. *Obes Rev* 3(2):113–122.

Nakagawa T., Hu H., Zharikov S., Tuttle K.R., Short R.A., Glushakova O., Ouyang X., Feig D.I., Block E.R., Herrera-Acosta J., Patel J.M., Johnson R.J. 2006. A causal role for uric acid in fructose-induced metabolic syndrome. *Am J Physiol Renal Physiol* 290(3):F625–F631.

Nedergaard J., Bengtsson T., Cannon B. 2007. Unexpected evidence for active brown adipose tissue in adult humans. *Am J Physiol* 293:E444–E452.

Newman C. 2004. Why are we so fat? The heavy cost of fat. *National Geographic* 206(2):46–61.

Newman H.H., Freeman F.N., Holzinger K.J. 1937. *Twins: A Study of Heredity and Environment.* Chicago: University of Chicago Press.

Nielsen S.J., Popkin B.M. 2003. Patterns and trends in food portion sizes, 1977–1998. *JAMA* 289(4):450–453.

Norman J.E., Bild D., Lewis C.E., Liu K., West D.S. 2003. CARDIA Study. The impact of weight change on cardiovascular disease risk factors in young black and white adults: The CARDIA study. *Int J Obes Relat Metab Disord* 27(3):369–376.

O'Reardon J.P., Allison K.C., Martino N.S., Lundgren J.D., Heb M., Stunkard A.J. 2006. A randomized placebo-controlled trial of sertraline in the treatment of the night eating syndrome. *Am J Psychiatry* 164: 893–898.

Olney J.W. 1969. Brain lesions, obesity, and other disturbances in mice treated with monosodium glutamate. *Science* 164(880):719–721.

Olsen N.J., Heitmann B.L. 2008. Intake of calorically sweetened beverages and obesity. *Obes Rev* 10:68–75.

Paeratakul S., Ferdinand D.P., Champagne C.M., Ryan D.H., Bray G.A. 2003. Fast-food consumption among US adults and children: Dietary and nutrient intake profile. *J Am Diet Assoc* 103(10):1332–1338.

Pagotto U., Marsicano G., Cota D., Lutz B., Pasquali R. 2006. The emerging role of the endocannabinoid system in endocrine regulation and energy balance. *Endocr Rev* 27:73–100.

Paras M.L., Murad M.H., Chen L.P., Goranson E.N., Sattler A.L., Colbenson K.M., Elamin M.B., Seime R.J., Prokop L.J., Zirakzadeh A. 2009. Sexual abuse and lifetime diagnosis of somatic disorders. A systematic review and meta-analysis. *JAMA* 302:550–561.

Park K.W., Halperin D.S., Tontonoz P. 2008. Before they were fat: Adipose progenitors. *Cell Metab* 8:454–457.

Pasacrica M., Sereda O.R., Redman L.M., Albarado D.C., Hymel D.T., Roan L.E., Rood J.C., Burk D.H., Smith S.R. 2009. Reduced adipose tissue oxygenation in human obesity. Evidence for rarefaction, macrophage chemotaxis, and inflammation with an angiogenic response. *Diabetes* 58:718–725.

Pasarica M., Gowronska-Kozak B., Burk D., Renedios I., Hymel D., Gimble J., Ravussin E., Bray G.A., Smith S.R. 2009. Adipose tissue collagen VI in obesity. *J Clin Endocrinol Metab* 94:5155–5162.

Pasquet P., Apfelbaum M. 1994. Recovery of initial body weight and composition after long-term massive overfeeding in men. *Am J Clin Nutr* 60:861–863.

Patel S.R., Hu F.B. 2008. Short sleep duration and weight gain: A systematic review. *Obesity* 16:643–653.

Patel S.R., Mjalhotra A., White D.P., Gottlieb D.J., Hu F.B. 2006. Association between reduced sleep and weight gain in women. *Am J Epidemiol* 164:947–954.

Patti M.E., Kahn B.B. 2004. Nutrient sensor links obesity with diabetes risk. *Nat Med* 10(10):1049–1050.

Pereira M.A., Jacobs D.R. Jr, Van Horn L., Slattery M.L., Kartashov A.I., Ludwig D.S. 2002. Dairy consumption, obesity, and the insulin resistance syndrome in young adults: The CARDIA Study. *JAMA* 287(16):2081–2089.

Pelchat M.L., Johnson A., Chan R., Valdez J., Ragland J.D. 2004. Images of desire: Food-craving activation during fMRI. *Neuroimage* 23(4):1486–1493.

Pereira M.A., Kartashov A.I., Ebbeling C.B., Van Horn L., Slattery M.L., Jacobs D.R. Jr, Ludwig D.S. 2005. Fast-food habits, weight gain, and insulin resistance (the CARDIA study): 15-year prospective analysis. *Lancet* 365(9453):36–42. Erratum in *Lancet* 365(9464):1030.

Pérusse L., Rankinen T., Zuberi A., Chagnon Y.C., Weisnagel S.J., Argyropoulos G., Walts B., Snyder E.E., Bouchard C. 2005. The human obesity gene map: The 2004 update. *Obes Res* 13(3):381–490.

Pijl H. 2003. Reduced dopaminergic tone in hypothalamic neural circuits: Expression of a "thrifty" genotype underlying the metabolic syndrome? *Eur J Pharmacol* 480(1–3):125–131.

Polivy J., Herman C.P. 2002. If at first you don't succeed. False hopes of self-change. *Am Psychol* 57(9):677–689.

Popkin B.M., Armstrong L.E., Bray G.M., Caballero B., Frei B., Willett W.C. 2007. A new proposed guidance system for beverage consumption in the United States. *Am J Clin Nutr* 2006 83(3):529–542. Erratum in *Am J Clin Nutr* 86(2):525.

Pospisilik J.A., Schramek D., Schnidar H., Cronin S.J., Nehme N.T., Zhang X., Knauf C., Cani P.D., Aumayr K., Todoric J., Bayer M., Haschemi A., Puviindran V., Tar K., Orthofer M., Neely G.G., Dietzl G., Manoukian A., Funovics M., Prager G., Wagner O., Ferrandon D., Aberger F., Hui C.C., Esterbauer H., Penninger J.M. 2010. Drosophila genome-wide obesity screen reveals hedgehog as a determinant of brown versus white adipose cell fate. *Cell* 140(1):148–160.

Potts D.B. 1992. *Wesleyan University 1831–1910. Collegiate Enterprise in New England.* New Haven: Yale University Press.

Power C., Jefferis B.J. 2002. Fetal environment and subsequent obesity: A study of maternal smoking. *Int J Epidemiol* 31(2):413–419.

Prentice A.M., Jebb S.A. 2003. Fast foods, energy density and obesity: A possible mechanistic link. *Obes Rev* 4(4):187–194.

Price T.O., Farr S.A., Yi X., Vinogradov S., Batrakova E.V., Banks W.A., Kabanov A.V. 2010. Transport across the blood-brain barrier of pluronic leptin. *J Pharmacol Exp Ther* Jan 6, 2010.

Primeaux S.D., Blackmon C., Barnes M.J., Braymer H.D., Bray G.A. 2008. Central administration of the RF peptides QRFP-26 and QRFP-43 increases high fat food intake. *Peptides* 29:1994–2000.

Putnam J., Allshouse J.E. 1999. *Food consumption, prices and expenditures, 1970–97*. Washington, DC: U.S. Department of Agriculture Economic Research Service.

Raben A., Christensen N.J., Madsen J., Holst J.J., Astrup A. 1994. Decreased postprandial thermogenesis and fat oxidation but increased fullness after a high-fiber meal compared with a low-fiber meal. *Am J Clin Nutr* 59(6):1386–1394.

Raben A., Agerholm-Larsen L., Flint A., Holst J.J., Astrup A. 2003. Meals with similar energy densities but rich in protein, fat, carbohydrate, or alcohol have different effects on energy expenditure and substrate metabolism but not on appetite and energy intake. *Am J Clin Nutr* 77(1):91–100.

Racette S.B., Weiss E.P., Schechtman K.B., Steger-May K., Villareal D.T., Obert K.A., Holloszy J.O. 2008. Influence of weekend lifestyle patterns on body weight. *Obesity* (Silver Spring) 16(8):1826–1830.

Ravelli A.C., van Der Meulen J.H., Osmond C., Barker D.J., Bleker O.P. 1999. Obesity at the age of 50 y in men and women exposed to famine prenatally. *Am J Clin Nutr* 70(5):811–816.

Ravussin E., Lillioja S., Anderson T.E., Christin L., Bogardus C. 1986. Determinants of 24-hour energy expenditure in man. Methods and results using a respiratory chamber. *J Clin Invest* 78(6):1568–1578.

Ravussin E., Smith S.R., Mitchell J.A., Shringarpure R., Shan K., Maier H., Koda J.E., Weyer C. 2009. Enhanced weight loss with pramlintide/metreleptin: An integrated neurohormonal approach to obesity pharmacotherapy. *Obesity* (Silver Spring). 17(9):1736–1743.

Redden D.T., Allison D.B. 2004. The Quebec Overfeeding Study: A catalyst for new hypothesis generation. *Obes Rev* 5:1–2.

Reilly J.J., Armstrong J., Dorosty A.R., Emmett P.M., Ness A., Rogers I., Steer C., Sherriff A. 2005. Avon Longitudinal Study of Parents and Children Study Team. Early life risk factors for obesity in childhood: Cohort study. *BMJ* 330(7504):1357.

Richard D., Guesdon B., Timofeeva E. 2009. The brain endocannabinoid system in the regulation of energy balance. *Best Pract Res Clin Endocrinol Metab* 23:17–32.

Roberts, S.B. 2000. High-glycemic index foods, hunger, and obesity: Is there a connection? *Nutr Rev* 58(6):163–169.

Rogers I. 2003. EURO-BLCS Study Group. The influence of birthweight and intrauterine environment on adiposity and fat distribution in later life. *Int J Obes Relat Metab Disord* 27(7):755–777.

Rolls B.J. 2009. The relationship beween dietary energy density and energy intake. *Physiol Behav* 97:609–615.

Rolls B.J., Morris E.L., Roe L.S. 2002. Portion size of food affects energy intake in normal-weight and overweight men and women. *Am J Clin Nutr* 76(6):1207–1213.

Rolls B.J., Roe L.S., Kral T.V., Meengs J.S., Wall D.E. 2004. Increasing the portion size of a packaged snack increases energy intake in men and women. *Appetite* 42(1):63–69.

Rosen E.D., MacDougald O.A. 2006. Adipocyte differentiation from the inside out. *Nature Rev Mol Cell Biol* 7:885–889.

Rosenbaum M., Goldsmith R., Bloomfield D., Magnano A., Weimer L., Heymsfield S., Gallagher D., Mayer L., Murphy E., Leibel R.L. 2005. Low-dose leptin reverses skeletal muscle, autonomic, and neuroendocrine adaptations to maintenance of reduced weight. *J Clin Invest* 115(12):3579–3586.

Rosenbaum M., Sy M., Pavlovich K., Leibel R.L., Hirsch J. 2008. Leptin reverses weight loss-induced change in regional neural activity responses to visual food stimuli. *J Clin Invest* 118:2583–2591.

Rosenbaum M., Hirsch J., Gallgher D.A., Leibel R.L. 2008. Long-term persistence of adaptive thermogenesis in subjects who have maintained a reduced body weight. *Am J Clin Nutr* 88:906–912.

Rossner S. 2009. Albert Stunkard (born 1922). *Obes Rev* 10(5):583–584.

Rutkowski J.M., David K.E., Scherer P.E. 2009. Mechanisms of obesity and related pathologies: The macro- and microcirculation of adipose tissue. *FEBS J* 276:5738–5746.

Saelens B.E., Sallis. J.F., Black J.B., Chen D. 2003. Neighborhood-based differences in physical activity: An environment scale evaluation. *Am J Public Health* 93(9):1552–1558.

Scholtens S., Brunekreef B., Smit H.A., Gast G.C., Hoekstra M.O., de Jongste J.C., Postma D.S., Gerritsen J., Seidell J.C., Wijga A.H. 2008. Do differences in childhood diet explain the reduced overweight risk in breastfed children? *Obesity* 16:2498–2503.

Scharoun-Lee M., Kaufman J.S., Popkin B.M., Gordon-Larsen P. 2009. Obesity, race/ethnicity and life course socioeconomic status across the transition from adolescence to adulthood. *J Epidemiol Community Health* 63(2):133–139.

Schulze M.B., Manson J.E., Ludwig D.S., Colditz G.A., Stampfer M.J., Willett W.C., Hu F.B. 2004. Sugar-sweetened beverages, weight gain, and incidence of type 2 diabetes in young and middle-aged women. *JAMA* 292(8):927–934.

Schutz Y. 2000. Human overfeeding experiments: Potentials and limitations in obesity research. *Br J Nutr* 84:135–137.

Schwann T. 1839. *Mikroscopische Untersuchungen uber die Uebereinstimmung in der Struktur un dem Wachsthum der Thiere und Pflanzen*. Berlin: Sander.

Schwann, T. 1847. *Microscopical researches into the accordance in the structure and growth of animals and plants. Transl. Henry Smith*. London: Sydenham Society.

Schwartz M.W. 2006. Central nervous system regulation of food intake. *Obesity* (Silver Spring) 14 (Suppl 1):1S–8S.

Seeley R.J., Matson C.A., Chavez M., Woods S.C., Dallman M.F., Schwartz M.W. 1996. Behavioral, endocrine, and hypothalamic responses to involuntary overfeeding. *Am J Physiol* 271(3 Pt 2):R819–R823.

Sekine M., Yamagami T., Handa K., Saito T., Nanri S., Kawaminami K., Tokui N., Yoshida K., Kagamimori S. 2002. A dose-response relationship between short sleeping hours and childhood obesity: Results of the Toyama Birth Cohort Study. *Child Care Health Dev* 28(2):163–170.

Sharma A.J., Cogeswell M.E., Li R. 2008. Dose-response association between maternal smoking during pregnancy and subsequent childhood obesity: Effect modification by material race/ethnicity in a low-income US cohort. *Am J Epidem* 168:995–1007.

Shimizu H., Oh-I S., Okada S., Mori M. 2009. Nesfatin-1: An overview and future clinical application. *Endocr J* 56(4):537–543.

Shimomura Y., Harada M., Goto M., Sugo T., Matsumoto Y., Abe M., Watanabe T., Asami T., Kitada C., Mori M., Onda H., Fujino M. 2002. Identification of neuropeptide was the endogenous ligand for orphan G-protein-coupled receptors GPR7 and GPR8. *J Biol Chem.* 277(39):35826–35832.

Simpson S.J., Raubenheimer D. 2005. Obesity: The protein leverage hypothesis. *Obes Rev* 6:133–142.

Sims E.A., Danforth E., Horton E.S., Bray G.A., Glennon J.A., Salans B. 1973. Endocrine and metabolic effects of experimental obesity in man. *Rec Prog Horm Res* 29:457–487.

Small C.J., Bloom S.R. 2004. Gut homones as peripheral antiobesity targets. *Current Drug Targets—CNS & Neurological Disorders* 3:379–388.

Smith S.R., de Jonge L., Zachwieja J.J., Roy H., Nguyen T., Rood J.C., Windhauser M.M., Bray G.A. 2000. Fat and carbohydrate balances during adaptation to a high-fat. *Am J Clin Nutr* 71(2):450–457.

Smith S.R., De Jonge L., Volaufova J., Li Y., Xie H., Bray G.A. 2005. Effect of pioglitazone on body composition and energy expenditure: A randomized controlled trial. *Metabolism* 54:24–32.

Soloveva V., Graves R.A., Rasenick M.M., Spiegelman B.M., Ross S.R. 1997. Transgenic mice overexpressing the b1 adrenergic receptor in adipose tissue are resistant to obesity. *Mol Endocrinol* 11:27–38.

Song Y., You N.-C., Hsu Y.-H., Howard B.V., Langer R.D., Manson J.E., Nathan L., Niu T., Tinker L.F., Liu. 2008. FTO polymorphisms are associated with obesity but not diabetes risk in postmenopausal women. *Obesity* 16:2472–2480.

Sørensen L.B., Raben A., Stender S., Astrup A. 2005. Effect of sucrose on inflammatory markers in overweight humans. *Am J Clin Nutr* 82(2):421–427.

Sparti A., Delany J.P., de la Bretonne J.A., Sander G.E., and Bray G.A. 1997a. Relationship between resting metabolic rate and the composition of the fat-free mass. *Metabolism* 46:1225–1230.

Sparti A., Windhauser M.M., Champagne C.M., and Bray G.A. 1997b. Effect of an acute reduction in carbohydrate intake on subsequent food intake in healthy men. *Am J Clin Nutr* 66:1144–1150.

Spiegel K., Tasali E., Penev P., Van Cauter E. 2004. Brief communication: Sleep curtailment in healthy young men is associated with decreased leptin levels, elevated ghrelin levels, and increased hunger and appetite. *Ann Intern Med* 141(11):846–850.

Stanworth R.D., Jones T.H. 2008. Testosterone for the aging male: Current evidence and recommended practice. *Clin Interv Aging* 3(1):25–44.

Stookey J.D., Barclay D., Arieff A., Popkin B.M. 2007a. The altered fluid distribution in obesity may reflect plasma hypertonicity. *Eur J Clin Nutr* 61(2):190–199.

Stookey J.D., Constant F., Gardner C.D., Popkin B.M. 2007b. Replacing sweetened caloric beverages with drinking water is associated with lower energy intake. *Obesity* (Silver Spring) 15(12):3013–3022.

Striegel-Moore R.H., Franko D.L., Thompson D., Affentito S., Kraemer H.C. 2006. Night eating: Prevalence and demographic correlated. *Obes Res* 14:139–147.

Striegel-Moore R.H., Thompson D., Affenito S.G., Franko D.L., Obarzanek E., Barton B.A., Schreiber G.B., Daniels S.R., Schmidt M., Crawford P.B. 2006. Correlates of beverage intake in adolescent girls: The National Heart, Lung, and Blood Institute Growth and Health Study. *J Pediatr* 148(2):183–187.

Stubbs R.J., Johnstone A.M., Harbron C.G., Reid C. 1998. Covert manipulation of energy density of high carbohydrate diets in 'pseudo free-living' humans. *Int J Obes Relat Metab Disord* 22(9):885–892.

Stunkard A.J. 1976. *The Pain of Obesity.* Palo Alto: Bull Publishing.

Stunkard A.J., Grace W.J., Wolff H.G. 1955. The night-eating syndrome: A pattern of food intake among certain obese patients. *Am J Med* 19(1):78–86.

Stunkard A.J., Sorensen T.I., Hanis C., et al. 1986. An adoption study of human obesity. *N Engl J Med* 314:193–198.

Stunkard A.J., Harris J.R., Pedersen N.L., et al. 1990. The body-mass index of twins who have been reared apart. *N Engl J Med* 322:1483–1487.

Sui X., LaMonte M.J., Laditka J.N., Hardin J.W., Chase N., Hooker S.P., Blair S.N. 2007. Cardiorespiratory fitness and adiposity as mortality predictors in older adults. *JAMA* 298(21):2507–2516.

Swinburn B.A., Sacks G., Lo S.K., Westerterp K.R., Rush E.C., Rosenbaum M., Luke A., Schoeller D.A., Delany J.P., Butte N.F., Ravussin E. 2009. Estimating the changes in energy flux that characterize the rise in obesity prevalence. *Am J Clin Nutr* 89:1723–1728.

Swinburn B., Sacks G., Ravussin E. 2009. Increased food energy supply is more than sufficient to explain the US epidemic of obesity. *Am J Clin Nutr* 90(6):1453–1456.

Tappy L. 2004. Metabolic consequences of overfeeding in humans. *Curr Opin Clin Nutr Metab Care* 7:623–628.

Taveras E.M., Rifas-Shiman S.L., Berkey C.S., Rockett H.R., Field A.E., Frazier A.L., Colditz G.A., Gillman M.W. 2005. Family dinner and adolescent overweight. *Obes Res* 13(5):900–906.

Teran-Garcia M., Despres J.P., Couillard C., Tremblay A., Bouchard C. 2004. Effects of long-term overfeeding on plasma lipoprotein levels in identical twins. *Atherosclerosis* 173:277–283.

The N.S., Gordon-Larsen P. 2009. Entry into romantic partnership is associated with obesity. *Obesity* doi:10.1038/oby.2009.97.

Theander-Carrillo C., Wiedmer P., Cettour-Rose P., Nogueiras R., Perez-Tilve D., Pfluger P., Castaneda T.R., Muzzin P., Schürmann A., Szanto I., Tschöp M.H., Rohner-Jeanrenaud F. 2006. Ghrelin action in the brain controls adipocyte metabolism *J Clin Invest* 116:1983–1993.

Tholin S., Lindroos A.K., Rynelius P., Akerstedt T., Stunkard A.J., Bulik C. 2009. Prevalence of night eating in obese and non-obese twins. *Obesity* In press.

Thomas D.M., Ciesla A., Levine J.A., Steven J.G., Martin C.K. 2009a. A mathematical model of weight change with adaptation. *Math Biosci Engin* 6:873–887.

Thomas D.M., Martin C.K., Heymsfield S., Redman L.M., Schoeller D.A., Levine J.A. 2009b. *J Bio Dynam* 1–21.

Tillotson J.E. 2005. Wal-Mart and our food. *Nutrition Today* 40:234–237.

Toschke A.M., Ehlin A.G., von Kries R., Ekbom A., Montgomery S.M. 2003. Maternal smoking during pregnancy and appetite control in offspring. *J Perinat Med* 31(3):251–256.

Travernier G., Jimenez M., Giacobino J.-P., Hulo N., Lafontan M., Muzzin P., Langin D. 2005. Norepinephrine induces lipolysis in B1/B2/B2 adrenoceptor knockout mice. *Mol Pharmaco l* 68:793–799.

Tremblay A., Pelletier C., Doucet E., Imbeault P. 2004. Thermogenesis and weight loss in obese individuals: A primary association with organochlorine pollution. *Int J Obes Relat Metab Disord* 28(7):936–939.

Tremblay A., St-Pierre S. 1996. The hyperphagic effect of a high-fat diet and alcohol intake persists after control for energy density. *Am J Clin Nutr* 63(4):479–482.

Tu Y., Thupari J.N., Kim E.K., Pinn M.L., Moran T.H., Ronnett G.V., Kuhajda F.P. 2005. C75 alters central and peripheral gene expression to reduce food intake and increase energy expenditure. *Endocrinology* 146(1):486–493.

Ukropcova B., McNeil M., Sereda O., de Jonge L., Xie H., Bray G.A., Smith S.R. 2005. Dynamic changes in fat oxidation in human primary myocytes mirror metabolic characteristics of the donor. *J Clin Invest* 115(7):1934–1941.

USDA. 2006. *ERS/USDA Data—Food Consumption (Per Capita) Data System*. Retrieved 13 April, 2006, from http://www.ers.usda.gov/Data/FoodConsumption/.

Van Ittersum K., Wansink B. 2007. Do children really prefer large portions? Viscual illusions bias their estimates and intake. *J Am Diet Assn* 107:1107–1110.

Vartanian L.R., Schwartz M.B., Brownell K.D. 2007. Effects of soft drink consumption on nutrition and health: A systematic review and meta-analysis. *Am J Public Health* 97(4):667–675.

Verdich C., Flint A., Gutzwiller J.P., Näslund E., Beglinger C., Hellström P.M., Long S.J., Morgan L.M., Holst J.J., Astrup A. 2001. A meta-analysis of the effect of glucagon-like peptide-1 (7-36) amide on ad libitum energy intake in humans. *J Clin Endocrinol Metab* 86(9):4382–4389.

Vioque J., Torres A., Quiles J. 2000. Time spent watching television, sleep duration and obesity in adults living in Valencia, Spain. *Int J Obes Relat Metab Disord* 24(12):1683–1688.

Virtanen K.A., Lidell M.E., Orava J., Heglind M., Westergren R., Niemi T., Taittonen M., Laine J., Savisto N.J., Enerbäck S., Nuutila P. 2009. Functional brown adipose tissue in healthy adults. *NEJM* 360:1518–1525.

von Kries R., Toschke A.M., Wurmser H., Sauerwald T., Koletzko B. 2002. Reduced risk for overweight and obesity in 5- and 6-y-old children by duration of sleep—A cross-sectional study. *Int J Obes Relat Metab Disord* 26(5):710–716.

von Verschuer O. 1927. Die Verebungsbiologische Zwillingsforschung. Ihre Biologischen Grundlagen. Mit 18 Abbildungen. *Ergebnisse der Inneren Medizin und Kinderheilkunde*. Berlin: Verlag Von Julius Springer.

Wang G.-J., Volkow N.D., Telang F., Jayne M., Ma Y., Pradhan K., Zhu W., Wong C.T., Thanos P.K., GEliebter A., Biegon A., Fowler J.S. 2009. Evidence of gender differences in the ability to inhibit brain activation elicited by food stimulation. *Proc Natl Acad Sci USA* 106:1249–1254.

Wang Y., Beydoun M.A. 2007. The obesity epidemic in the United States—Gender, age, socioeconomic, racial/ethnic, and geographic characteristics: a systematic review and meta-regression analysis. *Epidemiol Rev* 29:6–28.

Wang Y.C., Gortmaker S.L., Sobol A.M., Kuntz K.M. 2006. Estimating the energy gap among US children: A counterfactual approach. *Pediatrics* 118:1721–1733.

Wang Y., Reydoun M.A. 2009. Meat consumption is associated with obesity and central obesity among US adults. *Int J Obes* 33:621–628.

Wang Z., Heshka S., Heymsfield S.B., Shen W., Gallagher D. 2005. A cellular-level approach to predicting resting energy expenditure across the adult years 1–3. *Am J Clin Nutr* 81:799–806.

Wansink B., Painter J.E., Lee Y.K. 2006. The office candy dish: Proximity's influence on estimated and actual consumption. *Int J Obes (Lond)* 30(5):871–875.

Wansink B., van Ittersum K. 2007. Portion size me: Downsizing our consumption norms. *J Am Diet Assn* 1103–1106.

Wardle J., Carnell S., Haworth C.M.A., Plomin R. 2008. Evidence for a strong genetic influence on childhood adiposity despite the force of the obesogenic environment. *Am J Clin Nutr* 87:398–404.

Wellman P.J. 2005. Modulation of eating by central catecholamine systems. *Curr Drug Targets* 6(2):191–199.

Welsh J.A., Cogswell M.E., Rogers S., Rockett H., Mei Z., Grummer-Strawn L.M. 2005. Overweight among low-income preschool children associated with the consumption of sweet drinks: Missouri, 1999–2002. *Pediatrics* 115(2):e223–e229.

Westerterp K., Speakman J.R. 2008. Physical activity energy expenditure has not declined since the 1980s and matches energy expenditures of wild mammals. *Int J Obes (Lond)* 32(8):1256–1263.

Whincup P.H., Kay S.J., Owen C.C., et al. 2008. Birth weight and risk of type 2 diabetes. A systematic review. *JAMA* 300:2886–2897.

Wijers S.L., Saris W.H., van Marken Lichtenbelt W.D. 2009. Recent advances in adaptive thermogenesis: Potential implications for the treatment of obesity. *Obes Rev* 10(2):218–226.

Willer C.J., Speliotes E.K., Loos R.J., Li S., Lindgren C.M., Heid I.M., Berndt S.I., Elliott A.L., Jackson A.U., Lamina C., Lettre G., Lim N., Lyon H.N., McCarroll S.A., Papadakis K., Qi L., Randall J.C., Roccasecca R.M., Sanna S., Scheet P., Weedon M.N., Wheeler E., Zhao J.H., Jacobs L.C., Prokopenko I., Soranzo N., Tanaka T., Timpson N.J., Almgren P., Bennett A., Bergman R.N., Bingham S.A., Bonnycastle L.L., Brown M., Burtt N.P., Chines P., Coin L., Collins F.S., Connell J.M., Cooper C., Smith G.D., Dennison E.M., Deodhar P., Elliott P., Erdos M.R., Estrada K., Evans D.M., Gianniny L., Gieger C., Gillson C.J., Guiducci C., Hackett R., Hadley D., Hall A.S., Havulinna A.S., Hebebrand J., Hofman A., Isomaa B., Jacobs K.B., Johnson T., Jousilahti P., Jovanovic Z., Khaw K.T., Kraft P., Kuokkanen M., Kuusisto J., Laitinen J., Lakatta E.G., Luan J., Luben R.N., Mangino M., McArdle W.L., Meitinger T., Mulas A., Munroe P.B., Narisu N., Ness A.R., Northstone K., O'Rahilly S., Purmann C., Rees M.G., Ridderstråle M., Ring S.M., Rivadeneira F., Ruokonen A., Sandhu M.S., Saramies J., Scott L.J., Scuteri A., Silander K., Sims M.A., Song K., Stephens J., Stevens S., Stringham H.M., Tung Y.C., Valle T.T., Van Duijn C.M., Vimaleswaran K.S., Vollenweider P., Waeber G., Wallace C., Watanabe R.M., Waterworth D.M., Watkins N., Witteman J.C., Zeggini E., Zhai G., Zillikens M.C., Altshuler D., Caulfield M.J., Chanock S.J., Farooqi I.S., Ferrucci L., Guralnik J.M., Hattersley A.T., Hu F.B., Jarvelin M.R., Laakso M., Mooser V., Ong K.K., Ouwehand W.H., Salomaa V., Samani N.J., Spector T.D., Tuomi T., Tuomilehto J., Uda M., Uitterlinden A.G., Wareham N.J., Deloukas P., Frayling T.M., Groop L.C., Hayes R.B., Hunter D.J., Mohlke K.L., Peltonen L., Schlessinger D., Strachan D.P., Wichmann H.E., McCarthy M.I., Boehnke M., Barroso I., Abecasis G.R., Hirschhorn J.N. Genetic Investigation of ANthropometric Traits Consortium. 2008. Six new loci associated with body mass index highlight a neuronal influence on body weight regulation. *Nat Genet* 41:25–34.

Williamson D.F., Madans J., Anda R.F., Kleinman J.C., Giovino G.A., Byers T. 1991. Smoking cessation and severity of weight gain in a national cohort. *N Engl J Med* 324(11):739–745.

Woods S.C., Seeley R.J., Cota D. 2008. Regulation of food intake through hypothalamic signaling networks involving mTOR. *Annu Rev Nutr* 28:295–311.

Wrotniak B.H., Shuls J., Butts S., Stettler N. 2008. Gestational weight gain and risk of overweight in the offspring at age 7 y in a multicenter, multiethnic cohort study. *Am J Clin Nutr* 87:1818–1824.

Xue B., Kahn B.B. 2006. AMPK integrates nutrient and hormonal signals to regulate food intake and energy balance through effects in the hypothalamus and peripheral tissues. *J Physiol* 574(Pt 1):73–83.

Yanovski J.A., Parikh S.J., Yanoff L.B., Denkinger B.I., Calis K.A., Reynolds J.C., Sebring N.G., McHugh T. 2009. Effects of calcium supplementation on body weight and adiposity in overweight and obese adults: A randomized trial. *Ann Intern Med* 150(12):821–829.

Yudkin J. 1986. *Pure, White and Deadly*. London: Penguin Books,

Zemel M.B., Shi H., Greer B., Dirienzo D., Zemel P.C. 2000. Regulation of adiposity by dietary calcium. *FASEB J* 14(9):1132–1138.

Zhang H., Dibaise J.K., Zuccolo A., et al. 2009. Human gut microbiota in obesity and after gastric bypass. *Proc Natl Acad Sci USA* 106:2365–2370.

Zhang J.V., Ren P.G., Avsian-Kretchmer O., Luo C.W., Rauch R., Klein C., Hsueh A.J. 2005. Obestatin, a peptide encoded by the ghrelin gene, opposes ghrelin's effects on food intake. *Science* 310:996–999.

Zhang Y., Proenca R., Maffei M., Barone M., Leopold L., Friedman J.M. 1995. Positional cloning of the mouse obese gene and its human homologue. *Nature* 372(6505):425–432. Erratum in: *Nature* 374(6521):479.

Zheng H., Corkern M., Stoyanova I., Patterson L.M., Tian R., Berthoud H.R. 2003. Peptides that regulate food intake: Appetite-inducing accumbens manipulation activates hypothalamic orexin neurons and inhibits POMC neurons. *Am J Physiol Regul Integr Comp Physiol* 284(6):R1436–R1444.

Zurlo F., Lillioja S., Esposito-Del Puente A., Nyomba B.L., Raz I., Saad M.F., Swinburn B.A., Knowler W.C., Bogardus C., Ravussin E. 1990. Low ratio of fat to carbohydrate oxidation as predictor of weight gain: Study of 24-h RQ. *Am J Physiol* 259(5 Pt 1):E650–E657.

CHAPTER 4

Actuarial Society of America. *Transactions.* 1901–1903;7:492–497.

Actuarial Society of America and Association of Life Insurance Directors, 1913. *Medico-Actuarial Mortality Investigation*, Vol. 2, pp 5–9, 44–47. New York.

Adams K.F., Schatzkin A., Harris T.B., Kipnis V., Mouw T., Ballard-Barbash R., Hollenbeck A., Leitzmann M.F. 2006. Overweight, obesity and mortality in a large prospective cohort of persons 50–71 years old. *New Engl J Med* Aug 24;355(8):763–778.

Adams, T.D., Gress, R.E., et al. 2007. Long-term mortality after gastric bypass surgery. *New Engl J Med* 357:753–761.

Alberti K.G., Eckel R.H., Grundy S.M., Zimmet P.Z., Cleeman J.I., Donato K.A., Fruchart J.C., James W.P., Loria C.M., Smith S.C., Jr. 2009. Harmonizing the metabolic syndrome: A joint interim statement of the International Diabetes Federation Task Force on Epidemiology and Prevention; National Heart, Lung, and Blood Institute; American Heart Association; World Heart Federation; International Atherosclerosis Society; and International Association for the Study of Obesity. *Circ* 120(16):1640–1645.

Alley D.E., Chang V.W. 2007. The changing relationship of obesity and disability, 1988–2004. *JAMA* 298(17):2020–2027.

Allison D.B., Fontaine K.R., et al. 1999. Annual deaths attributable to obesity in the United States. *JAMA* 282(16): 1530–1538.

Allison D.B., Downey M., Atkinson R.L., Billington C.J., Bray G.A., Eckel R.H., Finkelstein E.A., Jensen M.D., Tremblay A. 2008. Obesity as a disease: A white paper on evidence and arguments commissioned by the Council of the Obesity Society. *Obesity* (Silver Spring) 16(6):1161–1177.

Angelico F., Del Ben M., et al. 2005. Insulin resistance, the metabolic syndrome, and nonalcoholic fatty liver disease. *J Clin Endocrinol Metab* 90(3):1578–1582.

Atlantis E., Baker M. 2008. Obesity effects on depression: Systematic review of epidemiological studies. *Intern J Obes* 32:881–889.

Bahrami H., Bluemke D., Kronmal R., et al. 2008. Novel metabolic risk factors for incident heart failure and their relationship with obesity: The MESA study. *J Am Coll Cardiol* 51:1775–1783.

Baik I., Curhan G.C., et al. 2000. A prospective study of age and lifestyle factors in relation to community-acquired pneumonia in US men and women. *Arch Intern Med* 160(20):3082–3088.

Bazzano L.A., Gu D., Whelton M.R., Wu X., Chen C.-S., Duan X., Chen J., Chen J., He J. 2010. Body mass index and risk of stroke among Chinese men and women. *Ann Neurol* 67:11–20.

Bellentani S., Saccoccio G., et al. 2000. Prevalence of and risk factors for hepatic steatosis in northern Italy. *Ann Intern Med* 132(2):112–117.

Benetos A., Thomas F., Pannier B., Bean K., Jego B., Guize L. 2008. All-cause and cardiovascular mortality using the different definitions of the metabolic syndrome. *Am J Cardiol* 102:188–191.

Berenson G.S., Srinivasan S.R., et al. 1998. Association between multiple cardiovascular risk factors and atherosclerosis in children and young adults. The Bogalusa Heart Study. *N Engl J Med* 338(23):1650–1656.

Bjorge T., Engeland A., Tverdal A., Smith G.D. 2008. Body mass index of adolescence in relation to cause-specific mortality: A follow-up of 230,000 Norwegian adolescents. *Am J Epidemiol* 168:30–37.

Björntorp P. 2001. Do stress reactions cause abdominal obesity and comorbidities? *Obes Rev* 2(2):73–86.

Black E., Holst C., et al. 2005. Long-term influences of body-weight changes, independent of the attained weight, on risk of impaired glucose tolerance and type 2 diabetes. *Diabet Med* 22(9):1199–1205.

Bogers R.P., Bemelmans W.J.E., Hoogenveen R.T., Boshuizen H.C., Woodward M., Knekt P., van Dam R.M., Hu F.B., Visscher T.L., Menotti A., Thorpe R.J. Jr, Jamrozik K., Calling S., Strand B.H., Shipley M.J.; for the BMI-CHD Collaboration Investigators. 2007. Association of overweight with increase risk of coronary heart disease partly independent of blood pressure and cholesterol levels: a meta-analysis of 21 cohort studies including more than 300,000 persons. *Arch Intern Med* 167:1720–1728.

Brawer R., Brisbon N., Plumb J. 2009. Obesity and cancer. *Prim Care* 36(3):509–531.

Bray G.A. 1978. Definition, measurement, and classification of the syndromes of obesity. *Int J Obes* 2(2):99–112.

Bray G.A. 2003. *Contemporary Diagnosis and Management of Obesity*. Newtown, PA: Handbooks in Health Care.

Bray G.A. 2004a. Medical consequences of obesity. *J Clin Endocrinol Metab* 89(6):2583–2589.

Bray G.A. 2004b. Obesity is a chronic, relapsing neurochemical disease. *Int J Obes Relat Metab Disord* 28(1):34–38.

Bray G.A., Champagne C.M. 2005. Beyond energy balance: There is more to obesity than kilocalories. *J Am Diet Assoc* 105(5 Pt 2):17–23.

Bray G.A. 2007a. *The Battle of the Bulge*. Pittsburgh: Dorrance Publishing.

Bray G.A. 2007b. *Metabolic Syndrome and Obesity*. Totowa, NJ: Humana Press.

Bray G.A, Jablonski K.A., Fujimoto W.Y., Barrett-Connor E., Haffner S., Hanson R.L., Hill J.O., Hubbard V., Kriska A., Stamm E., Pi-Sunyer F.X. 2008. Diabetes Prevention Program Research Group. Relation of central adiposity and body mass index to the development of diabetes in the Diabetes Prevention Program. *Am J Clin Nutr* 87(5):1212–1218.

Browning J.D., Szczepaniak L.S., Dobbins R., Nuremberg P., Horton J.D., Cohen J.C., Grundy S.M., Hobbs H.H. 2004. Prevalence of hepatic steatosis in an urban population in the United States: Impact of ethnicity. *Hepatology* 40(6):1387–1395.

Browning L.M., Hsieh S.D., Ashwell M. 2010. A systematic review of waist-to-height ratio as a screening tool in the prediction of cardiovascular disease and diabetes. *Nutr Res Rev,* in press.

Buchwald H., Estok R., Fahrbach K., Banel D., Jensen M.D., Pories W.J., Bantle J.P., Sledge I. 2009. Weight and type 2 diabetes after bariatric surgery: Systematic review and meta-analysis. *Am J Med* 122(3):248–256.

Burns T.L., Leutchy E.M., Paulos R., Witt J. 2009. Childhood predictors of the metabolic syndrome in middle-aged adults: The Muscatine Study. *J Pediatrics* 155:S5.e17–S5.e26.

Calle E.E., Kaaka R. 2004. Overweight, obesity and cancer: Epidemiological evidence and proposed mechanisms. *Nature Rev Cancer* 4:579–591.

Calle E.E., Rodriguez C., et al. 2003. Overweight, obesity, and mortality from cancer in a prospectively studied cohort of U.S. adults. *N Engl J Med* 348(17):1625–1638.

Calle E.E., Thun M.J., et al. 1999. Body-mass index and mortality in a prospective cohort of U.S. adults. *N Engl J Med* 341(15):1097–1105.

Caroli-Bosc F.X., Pugliese P., et al. 1999. Gallbladder volume in adults and its relationship to age, sex, body mass index, body surface area and gallstones. An epidemiologic study in a nonselected population in France. *Digestion* 60(4):344–348.

Carpenter K.M., Hasin D.S., et al. 2000. Relationships between obesity and DSM-IV major depressive disorder, suicide ideation, and suicide attempts: Results from a general population study. *Am J Public Health* 90(2):251–257.

CDC (Centers for Disease Control and Prevention). 2004. Prevalence of overweight and obesity among adults with diagnosed diabetes—United States, 1988–1994 and 1999–2000. *MMWR CDC Surveillance Summaries* 53:1066–1068.

CDC. 2005. National Center for Health Statistics. Retrieved March, 2005 from http://www.cdc.gov/nchs/.

Chan J.M., Rimm E.B., et al. 1994. Obesity, fat distribution, and weight gain as risk factors for clinical diabetes in men. *Diabetes Care* 17(9):961–969.

Chirinos J.A., Franklin S.S., Townsend R.R., Raij L. 2009. Body mass index and hypertension hemodynamic subtypes in the adult US population. *Arch Int Med* 169:580–586.

Choban P.S., Onyejekwe J., et al. 1999. A health status assessment of the impact of weight loss following Roux-en-Y gastric bypass for clinically severe obesity. *J Am Coll Surg* 188(5):491–497.

Clinton Smith J. 2004.The current epidemic of childhood obesity and its implications for future coronary heart disease. *Pediatric Clin North Am* 51(6):1679–1695.

Coccagna G., Pollini A., Provini F. 2006. Cardiovascular disorders and obstructive sleep apnea syndrome. *Clin Exp Hypertens* 28:217–224.

Colditz G.A., Willett W.C., et al. 1995. Weight gain as a risk factor for clinical diabetes mellitus in women. *Ann Intern Med* 122(7):481–486.

Colman R.J., Anderson R.M., Johnson S.C., Kastman E.K., Kosmatka K.J., Beasley T.M., Allison D.B., Cruzen C., Simmons H.A., Kemnitz J.W., Weindruch R. 2009. Caloric restriction delays disease onset and mortality in rhesus monkeys. *Science* 325(5937):201–204.

Custis B., Sierra-Johnson J., Tynan A. 2009. Diabetes, depression and obesity: A complex relationship. Findings from NHANES 2005–06. *Diabetes ABS* 958-P.

Da Silva A.A., do Carmo J., Dubinion J., Hall J.E. 2009. The role of the sympathetic nervous system in obesity-related hypertension. *Curr Hypertens Rep* 11(3):206–211.

Daviglus M.L., Liu K., et al. 2004. Relation of body mass index in young adulthood and middle age to Medicare expenditures in older age. *JAMA* 292(22):2743–2749.

Denison F.C., Price J., Graham C., Wild S., Liston W.A. 2008. Maternal obesity, length of gestation, risk of post-dates pregnancy and spontaneous onset of labor at term. *Brit J Obstet Gyn* 115:720–725.

Despres J.P., Krauss R.M. 2002. Obesity and lipoprotein metabolism. In *Handbook of Obesity*. G.A. Bray, C. Bouchard, eds. New York: Marcel Dekker.

Dixon J.B., Dixon M.E., et al. 2003. Depression in association with severe obesity: Changes with weight loss. *Arch Intern Med* 163(17):2058–2065.

Douketis J.D., Macie C., et al. 2005. Systematic review of long-term weight loss studies in obese adults: Clinical significance and applicability to clinical practice. *Int J Obes* (London) 29(10): 1153–1167.

Dublin, L. 1930. The influence of weight on certain causes of death. *Hum Biol* 2:159–184.

Eliassen A.H., Colditz G.A., Rosner B., Willett W.C., Hankinson S.E. 2006. Adult weight change and risk of postmonopausal breast cancer. *JAMA* 296:193–201.

Elsayed E.F., Sarnak M.J., Tighiouart H., Griffith J.L., et al. 2008. Waist-to-hip ratio, body mass index, and subsequent kidney disease and death. *Am J Kid Dis* 52:29–38.

Emberson J.R., Whincup P.H., et al. 2005. Lifestyle and cardiovascular disease in middle–aged British men: The effect of adjusting for within-person variation. *Eur Heart J* 26(17):1774–1782.

Engeland A., Bjørge T., Søgaard A.J., Tverdal A. 2003. Body mass index in adolescence in relation to total mortality: 32-year follow-up of 227,000 Norwegian boys and girls. *Am J Epidemiol* 157(6):517–523.

Engeland A., Bjørge T., Tverdal A., Søgaard A.J. 2004. Obesity in adolescence and adulthood and the risk of adult mortality. *Epidemiology* 15(1):79–85.

Ensrud K.E., Fullman R.L., et al. 2005. Voluntary weight reduction in older men increases hip bone loss: The osteoporotic fractures in men study. *J Clin Endocrinol Metab* 90(4):1998–2004.

Escalante A., Haas R.W., et al. 2005. Paradoxical effect of body mass index on survival in rheumatoid arthritis: Role of comorbidity and systemic inflammation. *Arch Intern Med* 165(14):1624–1629.

Fabbini E., Magkos F., Mohammed B.S., Pietka T., Abumrad N.A., Patterson B.W., Okunade A., Klein S. 2009. Intrahepatic fat, not visceral fat, is linked with metabolic complications of obesity. *Proc Natl Acad Sci USA*.

Felson D.T., Anderson J.J., et al. 1988. Obesity and knee osteoarthritis. The Framingham Study. *Ann Intern Med* 109(1):18–24.

Finkelstein E.A., Fiebelkorn I.C., et al. 2004. State-level estimates of annual medical expenditures attributable to obesity. *Obes Res* 12(1):18–24.

Finkelstein E.A., Trogdon J.G., Brown D.S., Allaire B.T., Dellea P.S., Kamal-Bahl S.J. 2008. The lifetime medical cost burden of overweight and obesity: Implications for obesity prevention. *Obesity* (Silver Spring). 16(8):1843–1848.

Finkelstein E.A., Trogdon J.G., Cohen J.W., Dietz W. 2009. Annual medical spending attributable to obesity: Payer- and service-specific estimates. *Health Aff* (Millwood) 28(5):w822–w831.

Flegal K.M., Graubard B.I., et al. 2005. Excess deaths associated with underweight, overweight, and obesity. *JAMA* 293(15):1861–1867.

Flemyng M. 1760. A discourse on the nature, causes, and cure of corpulency. Illustrated by a remarkable case. Read before the Royal Society November 1757. London: L. Davis and C. Reymers.

Flint A.J., Hu F.B., Glynn R.J., Caspard H., Manson J.E., Willett W.C., Rimm E.B. 2009. Excess weight and the risk of incident coronary heart disease among men and women. *Obesity* (Silver Spring) 18(6):1069.

Flum D.R., Dellinger E.P. 2004. Impact of gastric bypass operation on survival: A population-based analysis. *J Am Coll Surg* 199(4): 543–551.

Folmann N.B., Bossen K.S., Willaing I., Sørensen J., Andersen J.S., Ladelund S. 2007. Obesity, hospital services use and costs. *Adv Health Econ Health Serv Res* 17:319–332.

Fontaine K.R., Cheskin L.J., et al. 1996. Health-related quality of life in obese persons seeking treatment. *J Fam Pract* 43(3):265–270.

Fontaine K.R., Redden D.T., et al. 2003. Years of life lost due to obesity. *JAMA* 289(2):187–193.

Fontaine K.R., Barofsky I., Bartlett S.J., Franckowiak S.C., Andersen R.E. 2004. Weight loss and health-related quality of life: Results at 1-year follow-up. *Eat Behav* 5(1):85–88.

Fontaine K.R., Barofsky I. 2001. Obesity and health-related quality of life. *Obes Rev* 2(3):173–182.

Ford E.S., Li C., Sattar N. 2008. Metabolic syndrome and incident diabetes. Current state of the evidence. *Diabetes Care* 31:1898–1904.

Foster G.D., Sanders M.H., Millman R., Zammit G., Borradaile K.E., Newman A.B., Wadden T.A., Kelley D., Wing R.R., Sunyer F.X., Darcey V., Kuna S.T. Sleep AHEAD Research Group. 2009. Obstructive sleep apnea among obese patients with type 2 diabetes. *Diabetes Care* 32:1017–1019.

Foster M.D., Hwang S.-J., Larson M.G., et al. 2008. Overweight, obesity, and the development of stage 3 CKD: The Framingham Heart Study. *Am J Kid Dis* 52:39–48.

Franssen R., Monajemi H., Stroes E.S., Kastelein J.J. 2008. Obesity and dyslipidemia. *Endocrinol Metab Clin North Am* 37(3):623–633.

Freedman D.M., Ron E., Ballard-Barbash R., Doody M.M., Linet M. 2006. Body mass index and all-cause mortality in a nationwide US cohort. *Intern J Obes* 30:822–829.

Freedman D.S. 2002. *Risk of CVD Complications. Child and Adolescent Obesity*. Cambridge: Cambridge University Press, pp 221–239.

Freedman D.S., Dietz W.H., et al. 2004. The relation of obesity throughout life to carotid intima-media thickness in adulthood: The Bogalusa Heart Study. *Int J Obes Relat Metab Disord* 28(1):159–166.

Freemantle N., Holmes J., Hockey A., Kumar S. 2008. How strong is the association between abdominal obesity and the incidence of type 2 diabetes? *Int J Clin Pract* 62:1391–1396.

Frisch R.E. 1978. Menarche and fatness: Reexamination of the critical body composition hypothesis. *Science* 200(4349):1509–1513.

Garcia Hidalgo, L. 2002. Dermatological complications of obesity. *Am J Clin Dermatol* 3(7):497–506.

Garg A. 2004. Acquired and inherited lipodystrophies. *N Engl J Med* 350(12):1220–1234.

Gelber R.P, Kurth T., Kausz A.T., Manson J.E., Buring J.E., Levey A.S., Gaziano J.M. 2005. Association between body mass index and CKD in apparently healthy men. *Am J Kidney Dis* 46(5):871–880.

Goodman N., Dornbusch S.M., et al. 1963. Variant reactions to physical disabilities. *American Sociological Review* 28:429–435.

Gorospe E.C., Davie J.K. 2007. The risk of dementia with increased body mass index. *Age and Aging* 36:23–29.

Gortmaker S.L., Must A., et al. 1993. Social and economic consequences of overweight in adolescence and young adulthood. *N Engl J Med* 329(14):1008–1012.

Gregg E.W., Cheng Y.J., et al. 2005. Secular trends in cardiovascular disease risk factors according to body mass index in US adults. *JAMA* 293(15):1868–1874.

Gregg E.W., Gerzoff R.B., et al. 2003. Intentional weight loss and death in overweight and obese U.S. adults 35 years of age and older. *Ann Intern Med* 138(5):383–389.

Greenburg D.L., Lettieri C.J., Eliasson A.H. 2009. Effects of surgical weight loss on measures of obstructive sleep apnea: A meta-analysis. *Am J Med* 122:535–542.

Griffin F.M., Scuderi G.R., Insall J.N., Colizza W. 1998. Total knee arthroplasty in patients who were obese with 10 years follow-up. *Clin Orthopedics Rel Res* 356:28–33.

Grodstein F., Goldman M.B., et al. 1994. Body mass index and ovulatory infertility. *Epidemiology* 5(2):247–250.

Grotle M., Hagen K.B., Natvig B., Dahl F.A., Kvien T.K. 2008. Obesity and osteoarthritis in knee, hip and/or hand: An epidemiological study in the general population with 10 years follow-up. *BMC Musculoskelet Disord* 9:132.

Gu D., He J., et al. 2006. Body weight and mortality among men and women in China. *JAMA* 295(7): 776–783.

Gunderson E.P., Jacobs D.R. Jr, Chiang V., Lewis C.E., Tsai A., Quesenberry C.P. Jr, Sidney S. 2009. Childbearing is associated with higher incidence of the metabolic syndrome among women of reproductive age controlling for measurements before pregnancy: The CARDIA Study. *Am J Ob Gyn* 201:177–179.

Gunnell D.J., Frankel S.J., et al. 1998. Childhood obesity and adult cardiovascular mortality: A 57-y follow-up study based on the Boyd Orr cohort. *Am J Clin Nutr* 67(6):1111–1118.

Hamaguchi M., Kojima T., et al. 2005. The metabolic syndrome as a predictor of nonalcoholic fatty liver disease. *Ann Intern Med* 143(10):722–728.

Hampel H., Abraham N.S., et al. 2005. Meta-analysis: Obesity and the risk for gastroesophageal reflux disease and its complications. *Ann Intern Med* 143(3):199–211.

Hansen B.C., Bodkin N.L., et al. 1999. Calorie restriction in nonhuman primates: Mechanisms of reduced morbidity and mortality. *Toxicol Sci* 52(2 Suppl):56–60.

Haslam D. 2007. Obesity: A medical history. *Obes Rev* 8(Suppl. 1):31–36.

Haslam D., Haslam F. 2009. *Fat, Gluttony and Sloth. Obesity in Literature, Art and Medicine*. Liverpool: Liverpool University Press.

Hauger M.S., Gibbons L., Vik T., Belizan J.M. 2008. Prepregnancy weight status and the risk of adverse pregnancy outcome. *Acta Obstet et Gynecol* 87:953–959.

Heitmann B.L., Frederiksen P. 2009. Thigh circumference and risk of heart disease and premature death: Prospective cohort study. *BMJ* 339:b3292. doi: 10.1136/bmj.b3292.

Hjelmesaeth J., Hofso D., Aasheim E.T., Jenssen T., Moan J., Hager H., Roislien J., Bollerslev J. 2009. Parathyroid hormone, but not vitamin D, is associated with the metabolic syndrome in morbidly obese women and men: A cross-sectional study. *Cardiovasc Diabetol* 8:7.

Ho J.S., Cannaday J.J., Barlow M.E., Mitchell T.L., Cooper K.H., FitzGerald S.J. 2008. Relation of the number of metabolic syndrome factors with all-cause and cardiovascular mortality. *Am J Cardiol* 102:689–692.

Hsu C.Y., McCulloch C.E., et al. 2006. Body mass index and risk for end-stage renal disease. *Ann Intern Med* 144(1):21–28.

Istvan, J., Zavela K., et al. 1992. Body weight and psychological distress in NHANES I. *Int J Obes Relat Metab Disord* 16(12):999–1003.

Jaffiol C. 2004. de Jean Vague. *Bull Acaddemie Nationale Medicine* 188:895.

Janssen I., Mark A.E. 2007. Elevated body mass index and mortality risk in the elderly. *Obes Res* 8:41–59.

Janssen I., Katzmarzyk P.T., et al. 2004. Waist circumference and not body mass index explains obesity-related health risk. *Am J Clin Nutr* 79(3):379–384.

Jee S.H., Sull J.W., Park J., et al. 2006. Body-mass index and mortality in Korean men and women. *N Engl J Med* 355:779–787.

Jensen M.K., Chiuve S.E., Rimm E.B., et al. 2008. Obesity, behavioral lifestyle factors, and risk of acute coronary events. *Circ* 117:3062–3069.

Jin R., Grunkemeier G.L., et al. 2005. Is obesity a risk factor for mortality in coronary artery bypass surgery? *Circ* 111(25):3359–3365.

Jood T., Jern C., Wilhelmsen L., Rosengren A. 2004. Body mass index in mid-life is associated with a first stroke in men: A prospective population study over 28 years. *Stroke* 35:2764–2769.

Kambham N., Markowitz G.S., et al. 2001. Obesity-related glomerulopathy: An emerging epidemic. *Kidney Int* 59(4):1498–1509.

Kenchaiah S., Evans J.C., et al. 2002. Obesity and the risk of heart failure. *N Engl J Med* 347(5):305–313.

Khong S.Y., Jackson S. 2008. Obesity and urinary incontinence. *Menopause Int* 14(2):53–56. Review.

Knowler W.C., Barrett-Connor E., et al. 2002. Reduction in the incidence of type 2 diabetes with lifestyle intervention or metformin. *N Engl J Med* 346(6):393–403.

Ko C.W., Lee S.P. 2002. Obesity and gallbladder disease. In *Handbook of Obesity: Etiology and Pathophysiology*. GA Bray, C. Bouchard, eds. New York: Marcel Dekker, pp 919–934.

Koch, D. 2010. Waaler revisited: The anthropometrics of mortality. *Econ Hum Biol*.

Koster A., Leitzmann M.F., Schatzkin A., Mouw T., Adams K.F., van Eijk J.T.M., Hollenbeck A.R., Harris T.B. 2008. Waist circumference and mortality. *Am J Epidemiol* 167:1465–1475.

Kotronen A., Peltonen M., Hakkarainen A., Sevastianova K., Bergholm R., Johansson L.M., Lundbom N., Rissanen A., Ridderstrale M., Groop L., Orho-Melander M., Yki-Jarvinen H. 2009. Prediction of non-alcoholic fatty liver disease and liver fat using metabolic and genetic factors. *Gastroenterology* 137:865–872.

Kurth T., Gaziano J.M., Rexrode K.M., et al. 2005. Prospective study of body mass index and risk of stroke in apparently healthy women. *Circulation* 111:1992–1998.

Lakdawalla D.N., et al. 2004. *Health Aff* (Millwood) 23:168–176.

Landbo V., Prescott E., Lange P., Vestbo J., Almdal T.P. 1999. Prognostic value of nutritional status in chronic obstructive pulmonary disease. *Am J Respir Crit Care Med* 160:1856–1861.

Lang I.A., Llewellyn D.J., Alexander K. Melzer D. 2008. Obesity, physical function and mortality in older adults. *J Am Geriatric Soc* 56:1474–1478.

Latner J.D., Stunkard A.J. 2003. Getting worse: The stigmatization of obese children. *Obes Res* 11(3):452–456.

Lavie C.J., Milani R.V., Ventura H.O., Cardenas G.A., Mehra M.R., Messerli F.H. 2007. Disparate effects of left ventricular geometry and obesity on mortality in patients with preserved left ventricular ejection fraction. *Am J Cardiol* 100(9):1460–1464.

Lawlor D.A., Hart C.L., Hole D.J., Smith G.D. 2006. Reverse causality and confounding and the associations of overweight and obesity with mortality. *Obesity* 12:2294–2304.

Lee C.M., Huxley R.R., Wildman R.P., Woodward M. 2008. Indices of abdominal obesity are better discriminators of cardiovascular risk factors than BMI: A meta-analysis. *J Clin Epidemiol* 61:646–653.

Lee E.S., Kim Y.H., et al. 2005. Depressive mood and abdominal fat distribution in overweight premenopausal women. *Obes Res* 13(2):320–325.

Lementowski P.W., Zelicof S.B. 2008. Obesity and osteoarthritis. *Am J Orthop* 37(3):148–151.

Leung T.Y., Leung T.N., Sahota D.S., Chan O.K., Chan L.W., Fung T.Y., Lau T.K. 2008. Trends in maternal obesity and associated risks of adverse pregnancy outcomes in a population of Chinese women. *BJOG* 115:1529–1537.

Lew E., End J.A., et al. 1979. The new build and blood pressure study. *Trans Assoc Life Insur Med Dir Am* 62:154–174.

Lew E.A. 1985. Mortality and weight: Insured lives and the American Cancer Society studies. *Ann Intern Med* 103(6 Pt 2):1024–1029.

Lewis C.E., McTigue K.M., Burke L.E., Poirier P., Eckel R.H., Howard B.V., Allison D.B., Kumanyika S., Pi-Sunyer F.X. 2009. *Circ* 119:3263–3271.

Li G., Zhang P., Wang J., Gregg E.W., Yang W., Gong Q., Li H., Li H., Jiang Y., An Y., Shuai Y., Zhang B., Zhang J., Thompson T.J., Gerzoff R.B., Roglic G., Hu Y., Bennett P.H. 2008. The long-term effect of lifestyle interventions to prevent diabetes in the China Da Qing Diabetes Prevention Study: A 20-year follow-up study. *Lancet* 371(9626):1783–1789.

Li T.Y., Rana J.S., Manson J.E., Willett W.C., Stampfer M.J., Colditz G.A., Rexrode K.M., Hu FB. 2006. Obesity as compared with physical activity in predicting risk of coronary heart disase in women. *Circulation* 113:499–506.

Liem E.T., Sauer P.J.J., Oldehinkel A.J., Stolk R.P. 2008. Association between depressive symptoms in childhood and adolescence and overweight in later life. *Arch Pediatr Adolesc Med* 162:981–988.

Luchsinger J.A., Gustafson D.R. 2009. Adiposity, type 2 diabetes, and Alzheimer's disease. *J Alzheimers Dis* 16(4):693–704.

Magnusson P.K., Rasmussen F., Lawlor D., Tynelius P., Gunnell D. 2006. Association of body mass index with suicide mortality: a prospective cohort study of more than one million men. *Am J Epidemiol* 163(1):1–8. Epub 2005 Nov 3.

Mahoney L.T., Burns T.L., et al. 1996. Coronary risk factors measured in childhood and young adult life are associated with coronary artery calcification in young adults: The Muscatine Study. *J Am Coll Cardiol* 27(2):277–284.

Mannisto S., Smith-Warner S.A. 2006. Body mass index, height and risk of renal cell cancer in a pooled analysis of 13 cohort studies. *Obes Rev* 7(Suppl 2):106.

Manson J.E., Willett W.C., et al. 1995. Body weight and mortality among women. *N Engl J Med* 333(11):677–685.

Mason C., Craig C.L., Katzmarzyk P.T. 2008. Influence of central and extremity circumferences on all-cause mortality in men and women. *Obesity* 16:2690–2696.

Matsuo T., Sairenchi T., Iso H., Irie F., Tanaka K., Fukasawa N., Ota H., Muto T. 2008. Age- and gender-specific BMI in terms of the lowest mortality in Japanese general population. *Obesity* 16:2348–55. Epub 2008 Jul 24.

Matteoni C.A., Younossi Z.M., et al. 1999. Nonalcoholic fatty liver disease: A spectrum of clinical and pathological severity. *Gastroenterology* 116(6):1413–1419.

McTigue K., Larson J.C., VAloski A., Burke G., Kotchen J., Lewis C.E., Stefanick M.L., Horn L.V., Kuller L. 2006. Mortality and cardiac and vascular outcomes in extremely obese women. *JAMA* 296:79–86

Meigs J.B., D'Agostino R.B. Sr, et al. 1997. Risk variable clustering in the insulin resistance syndrome. The Framingham Offspring Study. *Diabetes* 46(10):1594–1600.

Messier S.P. 2009. Obesity and osteoarthritis: Disease genesis and nonpharmacologic weight management. *Med Clin North Am* 93(1):145–159.

Meyer H.E., Sogaard A.J., Tverdal A., Selmer R.M. 2002. Body mass index and mortality: The influence of physical activity and smoking. *Med Sci Sports Exerc* 34:1065–1070.

Moore L.L., Visioni A.J., et al. 2005. Weight loss in overweight adults and the long-term risk of hypertension: The Framingham study. *Arch Intern Med* 165(11):1298–1303.

Moore S.C., Mayne S.T., Graubaud B.I., Schatzkin A., et al. 2008. Past body mass index and risk of mortality among women. *Intern J Obes* 32:730–739.

Must A., Jacques P.F., et al. 1992. Long-term morbidity and mortality of overweight adolescents. A follow-up of the Harvard Growth Study of 1922 to 1935. *N Engl J Med* 327(19):1350–1355.

Mosen D.M., Schatz M., Magid D.J., Camargo C.A. Jr. 2008. The relationship between obesity and asthma severity and control in adults. *J Allergy Clin Immunol* 122(3):507–511.e6.

Must A. 2003. Does overweight in childhood have an impact on adult health? *Nutr Rev.* 61(4):139–142.

Naal F.D., Neuerburg C., Salzmann G.M., Kriner M., von Knoch F., Preiss S., Drobny T., Munzinger U. 2009. Association of body mass index and clinical outcomes 2 years after unicompartmental knee arthroplasty. *Arch Orthop Trauma Surg* 129:463–468.

National Institutes of Health. 1998. Clinical guidelines on the identification, evaluation, and treatment of overweight and obesity in adults—The evidence report. *Obes Res* 6(Suppl 2):51S–209S.

Neovius K., Johansson K., Rössner S., Neovius M. 2008. Disability pension, employment and obesity status: A systematic review. *Obes Rev* 9(6):572–581.

Ness R.B., Zhang J., Bass D., Klebanoff M.A. 2008. Interacions between smoking and weight in pregnancies complicated by preeclampsia and small-for-gestational-age birth. *Am J Epidem* 168:427–433.

Neter J.E., Stam B.E., Kok F.J., Grobbee D.E., Geleijnse J.M. 2003. Influence of weight reduction on blood pressure: A meta-analysis of randomized controlled trials. *Hypertension* 42:878–884.

Nguyen N.T., Magno C.P., Lane K.T., Hinojosa M.W., Lane J.S. 2008. Association of hypertension, diabetes, dyslipidemia, and metabolic syndrome with obesity: Findings from the National Health and Nutrition Examination Survey, 1999–2004. *J Am Coll Surg* 207:928–934.

Ni Mhurchu C., Rodgers A., Pan W.H., Gu D.F., Woodward M., Asia Pacific Cohort Studies Collaboration. 2004. Body mass index and cardiovascular disease in the Asia-Pacific Region: An overview of 33 cohorts involving 310,000 participants. *Int J Epidemiol* 33:751–758.

Nohr E.A., Vaeth M., Baker J.L., et al. 2008. Combined associations of prepregnancy body mass index and gestational weight gain with the outcome of pregnancy. *Am J Clin Nutr* 87:1750–1759.

Okoro C.A., Hootman J.M., et al. 2004. Disability, arthritis, and body weight among adults 45 years and older. *Obes Res* 12(5):854–861.

Oliveros H., Villamor E. 2008. Obesity and mortality in critically ill adults: A systematic review and meta-analysis. *Obesity* 16:515–552.

Olshansky S.J, Passaro D.J, et al. 2005. A potential decline in life expectancy in the United States in the 21st century. *N Engl J Med* 352(11):1138–1145.

Ostbye T., Dement J.M., Krause K.M. 2007. Obesity and workers' compensation: Results from the Duke Health and Safety Surveillance System. *Arch Inter Med* 23(167):766–773.

Park J.W., Lee W.Y., Kim S.Y., Che H., Jee S.H. 2008. BMI and stroke risk in Korean women. *Obesity* 16:396–401.

Peeters A., Barendregt J.J., et al. 2003. Obesity in adulthood and its consequences for life expectancy: A life-table analysis. *Ann Intern Med* 138(1):24–32.

Peppard P.E., Young T., et al. 2000. Longitudinal study of moderate weight change and sleep-disordered breathing. *JAMA* 284(23):3015–3021.

Peters D., Chen C., Markson L.E., Allen-Ramey F.C., Vollmer W.M. 2006. Using an asthma control questionnaire and administrative data to predict health-care utilization. *Chest* 129(4):918–924.

Pischon T., et al. 2008. General and abdominal adiposity and risk of death in Europe. *N Engl J Med* 359:2105–2120.

Price G.M., Uauy R., Breeze E., Bulpitt C.J., Fletcher A.E. 2006. Weight, shape and mortality risk in older persons: Elevated waist-hip ratio, not high body mass index is associated with a greater risk of death. *Am J Clin Nutr* 84:449–460.

Porter S.A., Massaro J.M., Hoffmann U., Vasan R.S., O'Donnell C.J., Fox C.S. 2009. Abdominal subcutaneous adipose tissue: A protective fat depot? *Diabetes Care* 32:1068–1075.

Prospective Studies Collaboration (Whitclock G., Lewington S., Sherlicker P., Clarke R., Emberson J., Halsey J., Qizilbash N., Collins R., Peto R.). 2009. Body-mass index and cause specific mortality in 900,000 adults: Collaborative analyses of 57 prospective studies. *Lancet* 373(9669):1083–1096.

Puhl R.M., Lattner J.D. 2007. Stigma, obesity, and the health of the nation's children. *Psychol Bull* 133(4):557–580.

Quesenberry C.P. Jr, Caan B., et al. 1998. Obesity, health services use, and health care costs among members of a health maintenance organization. *Arch Intern Med* 158(5):466–472.

Rasmussen S.A., Chu S.Y., Kim S.Y., Schmid C.H., Lau J. 2008. Maternal obesity and risk of neural tube defects: A metaanalysis. *Am J Obstet Gyn* June, 2008:611–619.

Ravaud P., Flipo R.M.., Boutron I., Roy C., Mahmoudi A., Giraudeau B., Pham T. 2009. ARTIST (osteoarthritis intervention standardized) study of standardized consultation versus usual care for patients with osteoarthritis of the knee in primary care in France: Pragmatic randomized controlled trial. *BMJ* 338:421 doi:10.1136/bmj.b421.

Ray K.K., Seshasai S.R., Wijesuriya S., Sivakumaran R., Nethercott S., Preiss D., Erqou S., Sattar N. 2009. Effect of intensive control of glucose on cardiovascular outcomes and death in patients with diabetes mellitus: A meta-analysis of randomised controlled trials. *Lancet* 373(9677):1765–1772.

Reeves G.K., Pirie K., Beral V. 2007. Cancer incidence and mortality in relation to body mjass index in the Million Women Study: Cohort study. *BMJ* 335:1134–1139.

Rexrode K.M., Carey V.J., Hennekens C.H., Walters E.E., Colditz G.A., Stampfer M.J., Willett W.C., Manson J.E. 1998. Abdominal adiposity and coronary heart disease in women. *JAMA* 280:1843–1848.

Rexrode K.M, Hennekens C.H., Willett W.C., Colditz G.A., Stampfer M.J., Rich-Edwards J.W., Speizer F.E., Manson J.E. 1997. A prospective study of body mass index, weight change, and risk of stroke in women. *JAMA* 277:1539–1545.

Rich-Edwards J.W., Goldman M.B., et al. 1994. Adolescent body mass index and infertility caused by ovulatory disorder. *Am J Obstet Gynecol* 171(1):171–177.

Richardson S.A., Goodman N., et al. 1961. Cultural uniformity in reaction of physical disabilities. *American Sociological Review* 26:241–247.

Ridker P.M., Rifai N., et al. 2002. Comparison of C-reactive protein and low-density lipoprotein cholesterol levels in the prediction of first cardiovascular events. *N Engl J Med* 347(20):1557–1565.

Rocchini A.P. 2004. Obesity and blood pressure regulation. In *Handbook of Obesity*. G.A. Bray and C. Bouchard. New York: Marcel Dekker.

Rosenberg T.J., Garbers S., et al. 2005. Maternal obesity and diabetes as risk factors for adverse pregnancy outcomes: Differences among 4 racial/ethnic groups. *Am J Public Health* 95(9):1545–1551.

Ryo S., Change Y., Woo H.-Y., Kin S.-G., Kim D.-I., Kim W.S., Suh B.-S., Choi N.-K., Lee J.-T. 2008. Changes in body weight predict CKD in healthy men. *J Am Soc Nephrol* 19:1798–1805.

Salihu H.M., Lynch L'.N., Alio A.P., Liu J. 2008. Obesity subtypes and risk of spontaneous versus medically indicated preterm births in singletons and twins. *Am J Epidemiol* 168:13–20.

Schapira D.V., Clark R.A., et al. 1994. Visceral obesity and breast cancer risk. *Cancer* 74(2):632–639.

Schwimmer J.B., Burwinkle T.M., et al. 2003. Health-related quality of life of severely obese children and adolescents. *JAMA* 289(14):1813–1819.

Silventoinen K., Magnusson K.E., Neovius M., Sundstrom J., Batty G.D., Tynelius P., Rasmussen F. 2008. Does obesity modify the effect of blood pressure on the risk of cardiovascular disease? A population-based cohort study of more than one million Swedish men. *Circ* 118:1637–1642.

Simpson J.A., MacInnis R.J., Peeters A., Hopper J.L., Giles G.G., English D.R. 2007. A comparison of adiposity measures as predictors of all-cause mortality: The Melbourne Collaborative Cohort Study. *Obesity* 15(4):994–1003.

Sin D.D., Sutherland E.R. 2008. Obesity and the lung: Obesity and asthma. *Thorax* 63(11):1018–1023.

Sjostrom C.D., Lissner L., et al. 1997. Relationships between changes in body composition and changes in cardiovascular risk factors: The SOS Intervention Study. Swedish Obese Subjects. *Obes Res* 5(6):519–530.

Sjostrom L., Lindroos A.K., et al. 2004. Lifestyle, diabetes, and cardiovascular risk factors 10 years after bariatric surgery. *N Engl J Med* 351(26):2683–2693.

Sjostrom L.V. 1992. Mortality of severely obese subjects. *Am J Clin Nutr* 55(2 Suppl):516S–523S.

Sjöström L., Gummesson A., Sjöström C.D., Narbro K., Peltonen M., Wedel H., Bengtsson C., Bouchard C., Carlsson B., Dahlgren S., Jacobson P., Karason K., Karlsson J., Larsson B., Lindroos A.K., Lönroth H., Näslund I., Olbers T., Stenlöf K., Torgerson J., Carlsson L.M. 2009. Effects of bariatric surgery on cancer incidence in obese patients in Sweden (Swedish Obese Subjects Study): A prospective, controlled intervention trial. Swedish Obese Subjects Study. *Lancet Oncol* 10(7):653–662.

Sjostrom L., Jacobson P., Peltonen M., Karason K., Narbro K., Sjostrom C.D., Carlsson L.M. 2009. Bariactic sugery and myocardial infarction: Effect-modification of baseline fasting glucose in the prospective, controlled intervention trial Swedish Obese Subjects. *Obesity Society Late Breaking Abstracts*.

Smith G.C.S., Shah I., Pell J.P., Crossley J.A., Dobbie R. 2007. Maternal obesity in early pregnancy and risk of spontaneous and elective preterm deliveries: A retrospective cohort study. *Am J Pub Health* 97:157–162.

Smith S.R., De Jonge L., et al. 2005. Effect of pioglitazone on body composition and energy expenditure: A randomized controlled trial. *Metabolism* 54(1):24–32.

Smith M., Zhou M., Whitlock G., Yang G., Offer A., Hui G., Peto R., Huang Z., Chen Z. 2008. Esophageal cancer and body mass index: Results from a prospective study of 220,000 men in China and a meta-analysis of published studies. *Int J Cancer* 122:1604–1610.

Song Y., Smith G.D., Sung J. 2003. Adult height and cause-specific mortality: A large prospective study of South Korean men. *Am J Epidemiol* 158:479–485.

Song Y.-M., Sung J., Ha M. 2008. Obesity and risk of cancer in postmenopausal Korean women. *Am J Oncol* 26:3395–3402.

Spalding K.L., Arner E., Westermark P.O., Bernard S., Buchholz B.A., Bergmann O., Blomqvist L., Hoffstedt J., Näslund E., Britton T., Concha H., Hassan M., Rydén M., Frisén J., Arner P. 2008. Dynamics of fat cell turnover in humans. *Nature* 453(7196):783–787.

Stampfer M.J., Maclure K.M., et al. 1992. Risk of symptomatic gallstones in women with severe obesity. *Am J Clin Nutr* 55(3):652–658.

Stevens J., Cai J., et al. 1998. The effect of age on the association between body-mass index and mortality. *N Engl J Med* 338(1):1–7.

Stevens V.J., Obarzanek E., et al. 2001. Long-term weight loss and changes in blood pressure: Results of the Trials of Hypertension Prevention, phase II. *Ann Intern Med* 134(1):1–11.

Stothard K.J., Tennant P.W.G., Bell R., Rankin J. 2009. Maternal overweight and obesity and the risk of congenital anomalies. A systematic review and meta-analysis. *JAMA* 301(6):636–650.

Strauss R.S., Pollack H.A. 2003. Social marginalization of overweight children. *Arch Pediatr Adolesc Med* 157(8):746–752.

Strohl K.P., Strobel R.J., et al. 2004. Obesity and pulmonary function. In *Handbook of Obesity*. G.A. Bray, C. Bouchard, eds. New York: Marcel Dekker.

Sturm R. 2002. The effects of obesity, smoking, and drinking on medical problems and costs. *Health Aff* (Millwood) 21(2):245–253.

Sturm R. 2004. *Health Aff* (Millwood) 23:199–205.

Subak L.L., Wing R., West D.S., Franklin F., Vittinghoff E., Creasman J.M., Richter H.E., Myers D., Burgio K.L., Gorin A.A., Macer J., Kusek J.W., Grady D. 2009. PRIDE investigators weight loss to treat urinary incontinence in overweight and obese women. *N Engl J Med* 360(5):481–490.

Sweeney C., Blair C.K., et al. 2004. Risk factors for breast cancer in elderly women. *Am J Epidemiol* 160(9):868–875.

Taveras, E.M., Rifas-Shiman, S.L., Camargo, C.A., Jr, Gold, D.R., Litonjua, A.A., Oken, E., Weiss, S.T., Gillman, M.W. 2008. Higher adiposity in infancy associated with recurrent wheeze in a prospective cohort of children. *J Allergy Clin Immunol* 121(5):1161–1166.

Taylor E.N., Stampfer M.J., et al. 2005. Obesity, weight gain, and the risk of kidney stones. *JAMA* 293(4):455–462.

Tetri L.H., Basaranoglu M., Brunt E.M., Yerian L.M., Neuschwander-Tetri B.A. 2008. Severe NAFLD with hepatic necroinflammatory changes in mice fed trans fats and a high-fructose corn syrup equivalent. *Am J Physiol Gastrointest Liver Physiol* 295:G987–G995.

Thompson D., Brown J.B., et al. 2001. Body mass index and future healthcare costs: A retrospective cohort study. *Obes Res* 9(3):210–218.

Thompson D., Wolf A.M. 2001. The medical-care cost burden of obesity. *Obes Rev* 2(3):189–197.

Thompson D., Edelsberg J., et al. 1999. Lifetime health and economic consequences of obesity. *Arch Intern Med* 159(18):2177–2183.

Trasande L., Liu Y., Fryer G., Weitzman M. 2009. Effects of childhood obesity on hospital care and costs, 1999–2005. *Health Aff* (Millwood) 28(4):w751–w760.

Trogdon J.G., Finkelstein E.A., Hylands T., Dellea P.S., Kamal-Bahl S.J. 2008. Indirect costs of obesity: A review of the current literature. *Obes Rev* 9(5):489–500.

Tsang T.S.M., Barnes M.E., Miyasaka Y., Cha S.S., Bailey K.R., Verzosa G.C., Seward J.B., Gersh B.J. 2008. Obesity as a risk factor for the progression of paroxysmal to permanent atrial fibrillation: A longitudinal cohort study of 21 years. *Eur Heart* J 29:2227–2233.

Uneli I.U., Skybo T., Camargo C.A. Jr. 2008. Weight loss and asthma: A systematic review. *Thorax* 63:671–676.

Usha Kiran T.S., Hemmadi S., et al. 2005. Outcome of pregnancy in a woman with an increased body mass index. *BJOG* 112(6):768–772.

Utzschneider K.M., Kahn S.E. 2006. Review. The role of insulin resistance in nonalcoholic fatty liver disease. *JCEM* 91:4753–4761.

Vague J. 1947. La differenciation sexuelle facteur determinant des formes de l'obésité. Transl. J Vague. *Presse Medicale* 55:339–340.

Vague J. 1956. The degree of masculine differentiation of obesities: A factor determining predisposition to diabetes, atherosclerosis, gout, and uric calculous disease. *Am J Clin Nutr* 4:20–34.

van Dam R.M., Willet W.C., Manson J.E., Hu F.B. 2006. The relationship between overweight in adolescence and premature death in women. *Ann Intern Med* 145:91–97.

van Kruijsdijk R.C., van der Wall E., Visseren F.L. 2009. Obesity and cancer: The role of dysfunctional adipose tissue. *Cancer Epidemiol Biomarkers Prev* 18(10):2569–2578.

Visscher T.L., Rissanen A., et al. 2004. Obesity and unhealthy life-years in adult Finns: An empirical approach. *Arch Intern Med* 164(13):1413–1420.

Visscher T.L., Seidell J.C. 2001. The public health impact of obesity. *Annu Rev Public Health* 22:355–375.

Waaler, H. 1984. Height, weight and mortality. The Norwegian experience. *Acta Med Scand Suppl* 679:1–56.

Waaler H.T., Lund E. 1983. Association between body height and death from breast cancer. *Br J Cancer* 48(1):149–150.

Wadd, W. 1810. *Cursory Remarks on Corpulence: By a Member of the Royal College of Surgeons*. London: J. Callow.

Wanahita N., Messerli F.H., Bangalore S., Gami A.S., Somers V.K., Steinberg J.S. 2008. Atrial fibrillation and obesity—results of a meta-analysis. *Am Heart J* 155(2):310–315.

Wang T.J., Parise H., et al. 2004. Obesity and the risk of new-onset atrial fibrillation. *JAMA* 292(20):2471–2477.

Weaver J.U. 2008. Classical endocrine diseases causing obesity. *Front Horm Res* 36:212–228.

Weeks R.W. 1904. An experiment with the specialized investigation. In *Actuarial Society of America Transactions* 8:17–23.

Weinstein A.R., Sesso H.D., et al. 2004. Relationship of physical activity vs body mass index with type 2 diabetes in women. *JAMA* 292(10):1188–1194.

Whitlock G., Lewington S., Sherlicker P., Clarke R., Emberson J., Halsey J., Qizilbash N., Collins R., Peto R. 2009. Body-mass index and cause specific mortality in 900,000 adults: Collaborative analyses of 57 prospective studies. *Lancet* 373(9669):1083–1096.

Whitmer R.A., Gunderson E.P., Barrett-Connor E., Quesenberry C.P. Jr, Yaffe K. 2005. Obesity in middle age and future risk of dementia: A 27 year longitudinal population based study. *BMJ* 330(7504):1360.

WHO. 2000. Obesity: Preventing and managing the global epidemic. Report of a WHO consultation. *World Health Organ Tech Rep Ser* 894:i–xii, 1–253.

Williams J., Wake M., et al. 2005. Health-related quality of life of overweight and obese children. *JAMA* 293(1):70–76.

Williamson D.A., O'Neil P.M. 1998. Obesity and quality of life. In *Handbook of Obesity*. G.A. Bray, C. Bouchard. New York: Marcel Dekker Inc.

Williamson D.F., Pamuk E., et al. 1995. Prospective study of intentional weight loss and mortality in never-smoking overweight US white women aged 40–64 years. *Am J Epidemiol* 141(12):1128–1141.

Williamson D.F., Thompson T.J., et al. 2000. Intentional weight loss and mortality among overweight individuals with diabetes. *Diabetes Care* 23(10):1499–1504.

Withrow D., Alter D.A. 2010. The economic burden of obesity worldwide: A systematic review of the direct costs of obesity. *Obes Rev.* Jan 27. [Epub ahead of print].

Wolf A.M., Colditz G.A. 1994. The cost of obesity: The US perspective. *Pharmacoeconomics* 5(Suppl 1):34–37.

Wolf A.M., Colditz G.A. 1998. Current estimates of the economic cost of obesity in the United States. *Obes Res* 6(2):97–106.

Yamagata K., Ishida K., Sairenchi T., Takahashi H., Ohba S., Shigai T., Narita M., Koyama A. 2007. Risk factors for chronic kidney disease in a community-based population: A 10-year follow-up study. *Nephrology* 71:159–166.

Yan L.L., Daviglus M.L., et al. 2006. Midlife body mass index and hospitalization and mortality in older age. *JAMA* 295(2):190–198.

Yan L.L., Daviglus M.L., Liu K., Stamler J., Wang R., Pirzada A., Garside D.B., Dyer A.R., Van Horn L., Liao Y., Fries J.F., Greenland P. 2006. Midlife body mass index and hospitalization and mortality in older age. *JAMA*. 295(2):190–198.

Yen S.S.C. 1999. Chronic anovluation due to CNS-hypothalamic-pituitary dysfunction. In *Reproductive Endocrinology: Physiology, Pathophysiology and Clinical Management*. S.S.C. Yen, R.B. Jaffee, R.L. Barbieri, eds. Philadelphia: Saunders, pp 516.

Young T., Peppard P.E., et al. 2005. Excess weight and sleep-disordered breathing. *J Appl Physiol* 99(4):1592–1599.

Yusuf S., Hawken S., Ounpuu S., Dans T., Avezum A., Lanas F., McQueen M., Budaj A., Pais P., Varigos J., Lisheng L.; INTERHEART Study Investigators. 2004. Effect of potentially modifiable risk factors associated with myocardial infarction in 52 countries (the INTERHEART study): A case-control study. *Lancet* 364(9438):937–952.

Yusuf S., Hawken S., et al. 2005. Obesity and the risk of myocardial infarction in 27,000 participants from 52 countries: A case-control study. *Lancet* 366(9497):1640–1649.

Zeve D., Suh J.M., Bosnakovski D., Kyba M., Hammer R.E., Tallquist M.D., Graff J.M. 2008. White fat progenitor cells reside in the adipose vasculature. *Science* 322(5901):542–543.

Zhou M., Offer A., Yang G., Smith M., Hui G., Whitlock G., Collins R., Huang Z., Peto R., Chen Z. 2008. Body mass index, blood pressure and mortality from stroke: A nationally representative prospective study of 212,000 Chinese men. *Stroke* 39:753–759.

CHAPTER 5

AAFP Recommendations for clinical preventives services. Obesity. http//:www.aafp.org/online/en/home/clinical/exam/k-o.html.

Alberti K.G., Eckel R.H., Grundy S.M., Zimmet P.Z., Cleeman J.I., Donato K.A., Fruchart J.C., James W.P., Loria C.M., Smith S.C. Jr; International Diabetes Federation Task Force on Epidemiology and Prevention; National Heart, Lung, and Blood Institute; American Heart Association; World Heart Federation; International Atherosclerosis Society; International Association for the Study of Obesity. 2009. Harmonizing the metabolic syndrome: A joint interim statement of the International Diabetes Federation Task Force on Epidemiology and Prevention; National Heart, Lung, and Blood Institute; American Heart Association; World Heart Federation; International Atherosclerosis Society; and International Association for the Study of Obesity. *Circ* 120(16):1640–1645.

Allison D.B., Mentore J.L., Heo M., et al. 1999. Antipsychotic-induced weight gain: A comprehensive research synthesis. *Am J Psychiatry* 156:1686–1696.

Al Mamun A., Lawlor D.A., Cramb S., O'Callaghan M., Williams G., Najman J. 2007. Do childhood sleeping problems predict obesity in young adulthood? Evidence from a prospective birth cohort study. *Am J Epidemiol* 166(12):1368–1373.

Aloia J.F., Vaswani A., Russo L., Sheehan M., Flaster E. 1995. The influence of menopause and hormonal replacement therapy on body cell mass and body fat mass. *Am J Obstet Gynecol* 172:896–900.

American Dietetic Association. 2006. Position of the American Dietetic Association: Individual, family, school, and community-based interventions for pediatric overweight. *J Am Diet Assoc* 106:925–945.

Anderson L.M., Quinn T.A., Glanz K., Ramirez G., Kahwati L.C., Johnson D.B., Buchanan L.R., Archer W.R., Chattopadhyay S., Kalra G.P., Katz D.L. 2009. Task Force on Community Preventive Services. The effectiveness of worksite nutrition and physical activity interventions for controlling employee overweight and obesity: A systematic review. *Am J Prev Med* 37(4):340–357.

Apovian C.M., Baker C., Ludwig D.S., Hoppin A.G., Hsu G., Lenders C., Pratt J.S., Forse R.A., O'Brien A., Tarnoff M. 2005. Best practice guidelines in pediatric/adolescent weight loss surgery. *Obes Res* 13:1274–1282.

Appel L.J., Moore T.J., Obarzanek E., Vollmer W.M., Svetkey L.P., Sacks F.M., Bray G.A., Vogt T.M., Cutler J.A., Windhauser M.M., Lin P.H., Karanja N. 1997. A clinical trial of the effects of dietary patterns on blood pressure. DASH Collaborative Research Group. *N Engl J Med* 336(16):1117–1124.

Arnaldi G., et al. 2003. Diagnosis and complications of Cushing's syndrome: A consensus statement. *JCEM.* 88:5593–5602.

Astrup A., Ryan L., Grunwald G.K., et al. 2000. The role of dietary fat in body fatness: Evidence from a preliminary meta-analysis of ad libitum low-fat dietary intervention studies. *Br J Nutr* 83 Suppl 1:S25–S32.

August G.P., Caprio S., Fennoy I., Freemark M., Kaufman F.R., Lustig R.H., Silverstein J.H., Speiser P.W., Styne D.M., Montori V.M. 2008. Prevention and treatment of pediatic obesity. An Endocrine Society clinical practice guideline based on expert opinion. *J Clin Endocrinol Metab* 93:4576–4599.

Babinski J.F.F. 1900. Tumeur du corps pituitaire sans acromégalie et avec arrêt de développement des organes génitaux. *Rev Neurol* 8:531–533.

Balikova I., Katzaki E., Pescucci C., Uliana V., Papa F.T., Ariani F., Meloni I., Priolo M., Selicorni A., Milani D., Fischetto R., Celle M.E., Grasso R., Dallapiccola B., Brancati F., Bordignon M., Tenconi R., Federico A., Mari F., Renieri A., Longo I., Balikova I. *J Hum Genet.* 52(12):1011–1017.

Balikova I., Lehesjoki A.E., de Ravel T.J., Thienpont B., Chandler K.E., Clayton-Smith J., Träskelin A.L., Fryns J.P., Vermeesch J.R. 2009. Deletions in the VPS13B (COH1) gene as a cause of Cohen syndrome. *Hum Mutat* 30(9):E845–E854.

Barker D.J., Hales C.N., Fall C.H., Osmond C., Phipps K., Clark P.M. 1993. Type 2 (non-insulin-dependent) diabetes mellitus, hypertension and hyperlipidaemia (syndrome X): Relation to reduced fetal growth. *Diabetologia.* 36:62–67.

Beauregard C., Dickstein G., Lacroix A. 2002. Classic and recent etiologies of Cushing's syndrome: Diagnosis and therapy. *Treat Endocrinol* 1(2):79–94.

Beauregard C., Utz A.L., Schaub A.E., Nachtigall L., Biller B.M., Miller K.K., Klibanski A. 2008. Growth hormone decreases visceral fat and improves cardiovascular risk markers in women with hypopituitarism: A randomized, placebo-controlled study. *J Clin Endocrinol Metab* 93(6):2063–2071.

Bergmann K.E., Bergmann R.L., von Kries G., Bohm O., Richter R., Dudenhausen J.W., Wahn U. 2003. Early deminants of childhood overweight and adiposity in a birth cohort study. The role of breast-feeding. Rogers I and the EURO-BLCS study group. Influence of birthweight and intrauterine environment on adiposity and fat distribution in later life. *Intern J Obese* 27:755–777.

Berkowitz R.I., Moore R.H., Faith M.S., Stallings V.A., Kral T.V., Stunkard A.J. 2009. Identification of an obese eating style in 4-year-old children born at high and low risk for obesity. *Obesity* (Silver Spring) 18(3):505–512.

Bhargava S.K., Sachdev H.S., Fall C.H., et al. 2004. Relation of serial changes in childhood body-mass index to impaired glucose tolerance in young adulthood. *N Engl J Med* 350:865–875.

Birdsall K.M., Vyas S., Khazaezadeh N., Oten-Ntim E. 2009. Material obesity: A review of interventions. *Int J Clin Prac* 63:494–507.

Bonny A.E., Ziegler J., Harvey R., Debanne S.M., Secic M., Cromer B.A. 2006. Weight gain in obese and nonobese adolescent girls initiating depot medroxyprogesterone, oral contraceptive pills, or no hormonal contraceptive method. *Arch Pediatr Adolesc Med* 160(1):40–45.

Bolland M.J., Grey A.B., Gamble G.D., Reid I.R. 2005. Association between primary hyperparathyroidism and increased body weight: A meta-analysis. *J Clin Endocrinol Metab* 90(3):1525–1530.

Bonaglia M.C., Ciccone R., Gimelli G., Gimelli S., Marelli S., Verheij J., Giorda R., Grasso R., Borgatti R., Pagone F., Rodrìguez L., Martinez-Frias M.L., van Ravenswaaij C., Zuffardi O. 2008. Detailed phenotype-genotype study in five patients with chromosome 6q16 deletion: Narrowing the critical region for Prader-Willi-like phenotype. *Eur J Hum Genet* 16(12):1443–1449.

Boosalis M.G., Gemayel N., Lee A., Bray G.A., Laine L., Cohen H. 1992. Cholecystokinin and satiety: Effect of hypothalamic obesity and gastric bubble insertion. *Am J Physiol* 262(2 Pt 2):R241–R244.

Bouchard C., Tremblay A., Despres J.P., et al. 1990. The response to long-term overfeeding in identical twins. *N Engl J Med* 322:1477–1482.

Bougneres P., Panalone L., Linglart A., Rothenbuhler A., Le Stunff C. 2008. Endocrine manifestation of the rapid-onset obesity with hypoventilation, hypothalamic, autonomic dysregulation, and neural tumor syndrome in childhood. *JCEM* 93:3971–3980.

Bourgeois J.A., Coffey S.M., Rivera S.M., Hessl D., Gane L.W., Tassone F., Greco C., Finucane B., Nelson L., Berry-Kravis E., Grigsby J., Hagerman P.J., Hagerman R.J. 2009. A review of fragile X premutation disorders: Expanding the psychiatric perspective. *J Clin Psychiatry* 70(6):852–862.

Bray G.A., Gallagher T.F., Jr. 1975. Manifestations of hypothalamic obesity in man: A comprehensive investigation of eight patients and a reveiw of the literature. *Medicine* (Baltimore) 54:301–330.

Bray G.A., ed. 1976. *Obesity in Perspective. Fogarty International Center Series on Preventive Med.* Vol 2, parts 1 and 2, Washington, DC: U.S. Government Printing Office, DHEW Publication #75-708.

Bray G.A. 1976. *The Obese Patient: Major Problems in Internal Medicine*. Philadelphia: W.B. Saunders.

Bray G.A. 1978. Definitions, measurements and classification of the syndromes of obesity. *Int J Obes* 2(2):99–112.

Bray G.A., York D.A. 1979. Hypothalamic and genetic obesity in experimental animals: An autonomic and endocrine hypothesis. *Physiol Rev* 59(3):719–809.

Bray G.A., Dahms W.T., Swerdloff R.S., Fiser R.H., Atkinson R.L., Carrel R.E. 1983. The Prader-Willi Syndrome: A study of 40 patients and a review of the literature. *Medicine* 62(2):59–80.

Bray G.A., Popkin B.M. 1998. Dietary fat intake does affect obesity. *Am J Clin Nutr* 68:1157–1173.

Bray G.A., York D.A. 1998. The MONA LISA hypothesis in the time of leptin. *Recent Prog Horm Res* 53:95–117; discussion 117–8.

Bray G.A., Nielsen S.J., Popkin B.M. 2004. High fructose corn syrup and the epidemic of obesity. *Am J Clin Nutr* 79:537–544.

Bray G.A. 2007. *Metabolic Syndrome and Obesity*. Totowa, NJ: Humana Press.

Bray G.A. 2008. Are non-prescription medications needed for weight control? *Obesity* 17:566–571.

Bray G.A, Bouchard C., Church T.S., Cefalu W.T., Greenway F.L., Gupta A.K., Kaplan L.M., Ravussin E., Smith S.R., Ryan D.H. 2009. Is it time to change the way we report and discuss weight loss? *Obesity* 17:619–621.

Bray G.A. 1998. Obesity: A time bomb to be defused. *Lancet* 352(9123):160–161.

Brobeck J.R., Tepperman J., Long C.N.H. 1943. Experimental hypothalamic hyperphagia in the albino rat. *Yale J Biol Med* 15:831–853.

Brownell K. 1990. Dieting readiness. *Weight Control Digest* 1:1–9.

Brownell K.D., Farley T., Willett W.C., Popkin B.M., Chaloupka F.J., Thompson J.W., Ludwig D.S. 2009. The public health and economic benefits of taxing sugar-sweetened beverages. *N Engl J Med* 361(16):1599–1605.

Browning L.M., Hsieh S.D., Ashwell M. 2010. A systematic review of the evidence for the use for waist-to-height ratio as a screening tool in the prediction of CVD and diabetes: Superiority of waist-to-height ratio over BMI and waist circumference for health promotion. *Nutr Res Rev,* in press.

Bruch H. 1939. The Frohlich Syndrome: Report of the original case. *Am J Dis Child* 58:1281–1289.

Buell J.L., Calland D., Hanks F., Johnston B., Pester B., Sweeney R., Thorne R. 2008. Presence of metabolic syndrome in football linemen. *J Athl Train*. Oct–Dec;43(6):608–616.

Butler M.G., Lee P.D.K., Whitman V.Y., eds. 2006. *Management of Prader-Willi syndrome,* 3rd ed. New York: Springer.

Buzby J.C., Guthrie J.F., Kantor L.S. 2003. *Evaluation of the USDA Fruit and Vegetable Pilot Program: Report to Congress*. Washington, DC: U.S. Department of Agriculture, Economic Research Service. E-FAN-03-006 (www.ers.usda.gov/publications/efan03006).

CDC. 1996. Surgeon General's Report on Physical Activity and Health. From the Centers for Disease Control and Prevention. *JAMA* 276:522.

Cagnacci A., Zanin R., Cannoletta M., Generali M., Caretto S., Volpe A. 2007. Menopause, estrogens, progestins, or their combination on body weight and anthropometric measures. *Fertil Steril* 88(6):1603–1608.

Calton M.A., Ersoy B.A., Zhang S., Kane J.P., Malloy M.J., Pullinger C.R., Bromberg Y., Pennacchio L.A., Dent R., McPherson R., Ahituv N., Vaisse C. 2009. Association of functionally significant Melanocortin-4 but not Melanocortin-3 receptor mutations with severe adult obesity in a large North American case-control study. *Hum Mol Genet* 18(6):1140–1147.

Carpenter G. 1901. Two sisters showing malformations of the skull and other congenital abnormalities. *Rep Soc Study Dis Child Lond* 1:110–118.

Carrel A.L., Clark R.R., Peterson S.E., Nemeth B.A., Sullivan J., Allen D.B. 2005. Improvement of fitness, body composition, and insulin sensitivity in overweight children in a school-based exercise program: A randomized, controlled study. *Arch Pediatr Adolesc Med* 159(10):963–968.

Cassidy S.B., Driscoll D.J. 2009. Prader-Willi Syndrome. *Eur J Hum Genetics* 17:3–13.

Clement K., Vaisse C., Lahlou N., et al. 1998. A mutation in the human leptin receptor gene causes obesity and pituitary dysfunction. *Nature* 392:398–401.

Collin G.B., Marshall J.D., Ikeda A., So W.V., Russell-Eggitt I., Maffei, Beck S., Boerkoel C.F., Sicolo N., Martin M., Nishina P.M., Naggart J.K. 2002. Mutations in ALMS1 cause obesity, type 2 diabetes and neursensory degeneration in Alstrom syndrome. *Nat Gen* 31:74–78.

Coutant R., Maurey H., Rouleau S., Mathieu E., Mercier P., Limal J.M., et al. 2003. Defect in epinephrine production in children with craniopharyngioma: Functional or organic origin. *JCEM* 88:5969–5975.

Coviello A.D., Legro R.S., Dunaif A. 2006. Adolescent girls with polycystic ovary syndrome have an increased risk of the metabolic syndrome associated with increasing androgen levels independent of obesity and insulin resistance. *J Clin Endocrinol Metab* 91(2):492–497.

Crane J.M., White J., Murphy P., Burrage L., Hutchens D. 2009. The effect of gestational weight gain by body mass index on maternal and neonatal outcomes. *J Obstet Gynaecol Can* 31(1):28–35.

Crespo C.J., Smit E., Troiano R.P., Bartlett S.J., Macera C.A., Andersen R.E. 2001. Television watching, energy intake, and obesity in US children: From the third National Health and Nutrition Examination Survey, 1988–1994. *Arch Pediatr Adolesc Med* 155:360–365.

Croft L.B., Belanger A., Miller M.A., Roberts A., Goldman M.E. 2008. Comparison of National Football League linemen versus nonlinemen of left ventricular mass and left atrial size. *Am J Cardiol* 102(3):343–347.

Cuenot L. 1906. Pure strains and their combinations in the mouse. *Arch Zoo Exptl Gen Ser* 4(3):122–123; *Bull Soc Med Paris* 23:1310.

Cummings D., Clement K., Purnell J., Vaisse C., Foster K.E., Frayo S., Schwarz M., Basdevant A., Weigle D. 2002. Elevated plasma ghrelin levels in Prader-Willi syndrome. *Nat Med* 643–644.

Cushing H. 1912. *The Pituitary Body and Its Disorders*. Philadelphia: JB Lippincott.

Cushing H. 1925. *The Life of Sir William Osler.* Oxford: Clarendon Press.

Cushing H. 1928. The emancipator. In *Consecratio Medici and Other Papers*. Boston: Little, Brown, and Company, pp 271–276.

Cushing H. 1936. *From a Surgeon's Journal, 1915–1918*. Boston: Little, Brown and Co.

Cushing H. 1943. *A Bio-bibliography of Andreas Vesalius*. New York: Schuman's.

Cutler D.M., Glaeser E.L., Shapiro J.M. 2003. Why have Americans become more obese? *Journal of Economic Perspectives* 17(3):93–118.

Daniels S.R., Arnett D.K., Eckel R.H., Gidding S.S., Hayman L.L., Kumanyika S., Robinson T.N., Scott B.J., St Jeor S., Williams C.L. 2005. Overweight in children and adolescents: Pathophysiology, consequences, prevention, and treatment. *Circ* 111:1999–2012.

Danielsson P., Harson A., Norgren S., Marcus C. 2007. Impact of sibutramine therapy in children with hypothalamic obesity or obesity with aggravating syndromes. *JCEM* 92:4101–4106.

Danielzik S., Czerwinski-Mast M., Langnäse K., Dilba B., Müller M.J. 2004. Parental overweight, socioeconomic status and high birth weight are the major determinants of overweight and obesity in 5–7 y-old children: Baseline data of the Kiel Obesity Prevention Study (KOPS). *Int J Obes Relat Metab Disord* 28(11):1494–1502.

Daousi C., MacFarlane I.A., English P.J., Wilding J.P., Paterson M., Dovery T.M., et al. 2005. Is there a role for ghrelin and peptide-YY in the pathogenesis of obesity in adults with acquired structural hypothalamic damage? *JCEM* 90:5025–5030.

Dardeno T.A., Sharon H., Chou S.H., Moon H.-S., Chamberland J.P., Mantzoros C.S. 2010. Leptin in human physiology and therapeutics. *Frontiers in Neuroendocrinology* 31(3):377–393.

Davies K.M., Heaney R.P., Recker R.R., et al. 2000. Calcium intake and body weight. *J Clin Endocrinol Metab* 85:4635–4638.

Diabetes Prevention Program Research Group (Knowler W.C., Barrett-Connor E., Fowler S.E., Hamman R.F., Lachin J.M., Walker E.A., Nathan D.M.). 2002. Reduction in the incidence of type 2 diabetes with lifestyle intervention or metformin. *NEJM* 346:393–403.

Diabetes Prevention Program Research Group (Knowler W.C., Fowler S.E., Hamman R.F., Christophi C.A., Hoffman H.J., Brenneman A.T., Brown-Friday J.O., Goldberg R., Venditti E., Nathan D.M.). 2009. 10-year follow-up of diabetes incidence and weight loss in the Diabetes Prevention Program Outcomes Study. *Lancet* 374(9702):1677–1686.

Douketis J.D., Macie C., Thabane L., Williamson D.F. 2005. Systematic review of long-term weight loss studies in obese adults: Clinical significance and applicability to clinical practice. *Int J Obes (London)* 29(10):1153–1167.

Dowda M., James F., Sallis J.F., McKenzie T.L., Rosengard P., Kohl H.W. 3rd. 2005. Evaluating the sustainability of SPARK physical education: A case study of translating research into practice. *Res Q Exerc Sport* 76(1):11–19.

Drewnowski A., Darmon N. 2005. The economics of obesity: Dietary energy density and energy cost. *Am J Clin Nutr* 82(Suppl. 1):S265–S273.

Ekelund U., Ong K.K., Linne Y., Neovius M., Brage S., Dunger D.B., Wareham N.J., Rossner S. 2007. Association of weight gain in infancy and early childhood with metabolic risk in young adults. *JCEM* 92:98–103.

Epstein L.H., Valoski A., Wing R.R., McCurley J. 1990. Ten-year follow-up of behavioral, family-based treatment for obese children. *JAMA* 264(19):2519–2523.

Faith M.S., Fontaine K.R., Baskin M.L., Allison D.B. 2007. Toward the reduction of population obesity: Macrolevel environmental approaches to the problems of food, eating, and obesity. *Psychol Bull* 133(2):205–226.

Farooqi I.S., Bullmore E., Keogh J., Gillard J., O'Rahilly S., Fletcher P.C. 2007. Leptin regulates striatal regions and human eating behavior. *Science* 317(5843):1355.

Farooi I.S., Matarese G., Lord B.M., Keogh J.M., Lawrence E., Agwu C., Sanna V., Jebb S.A., Perna F., Fontant S., Lechler R.I., DePaoli A.M., O'Rahilly S. 2002. Beneficial effects of leptin on obesity, T cell hyporesponsiveness, and neurendocrine/metabolic dysfunction of human congenital leptin deficiency. *J Clin Invest* 110:1093–1103.

Farooqi I.S., Wangensteen T., Collins S., Kimber W., Matarese G., Keogh J.M., Lank E., Bottomley B., Lopez-Fernandez J., Ferraz-Amaro I., Dattani M.T., Ercan O., Myhre A.G., Retterstol L., Stanhope R., Edge J.A., McKenzie S., Lessa N., Ghodsi M., De Rosa V., Perna F., Fontana S., Barroso I., Undlien D.E., O'Rahilly S. 2007. Clinical and molecular genetic spectrum of congenital deficiency of the leptin receptor. *NEJM* 356:237–247.

Farooqi I.S., Keogh J.M., Kamath S., Jones S., Gibson W.T., Trussell R., Jebb S.A., Lip G.Y.H., O'Rahilly S. 2001. Partial leptin deficiency and human adiposity. *Nature* 414:34–35.

Farooqi I.S., Keogh J.M., Yeo G.S., Lank E.J., Cheetham T., O'Rahilly S. 2003. Clinical spectrum of obesity and mutations in the melanocortin 4 receptor gene. *N Engl J Med* 348(12):1085–1095.

Farooqi I.S., O'Rahilly S. 2005. Monogenic obesity in humans. *Annu Rev Med* 56:443–458.

Farooqi I.S., O'Rahilly S. 2006. Genetics of obesity in humans. *Endocr Rev* 27(7):710–718.

Festen D.A.M., et al. 2006. Sleep-related breathing disorders in prepubertal children with Prader-Willi Syndrome and effects of growth hormone treatment. *JCEM* 91:4911–4915.

Field A.E., Malspeis S., Willett W.C. 2009. Weight cycling and mortality among middle-aged or older women. *Arch Intern Med* 169(9):881–886.

Findling J.W., Raff H., eds. 2005. Screening and diagnosis of Cushing's syndrome. *Endocrinol Metab Clin North Am* 34(2):385–402.

Findling J.W., Raff H. 2006. Clinical review: Cushing's syndrome: Important issues in diagnosis and management. *JCEM* 91:3746–3753.

Fischbach B.V., Trout K.L., Lewis J., Luis C.A., Sika M. 2005. WAGR syndrome: A clinical review of 54 cases. *Pediatrics* 116:984–988.

Flegal K.M., Carroll M.D., Ogden C.L., Johnson C.L. 2002. Prevalence and trends in obesity among US adults, 1999–2000. *JAMA* 288:1723–1727.

Flegal K.M., Troiano R.P., Pamuk E.R., Kuczmarski R.J., Campbell S.M. 1995. The influence of smoking cessation on the prevalence of overweight in the United States. *N Engl J Med* 333:1165–1170.

Flegal K.M., Carroll M.D., Ogden C.L., Curtin L.R. 2010. Prevalence and trends in obesity among US adults, 1999–2008. *JAMA* 303(3):235–241.

Fleisch A.F., Agarwal N., Roberts M.D., Han J.C., Theim K.R., Vexler A., Troendle J., Yanovski S.Z., Yanovski J.A. 2007. Influence of serum leptin on weight and body fat growth in children at high risk for adult obesity. *J Clin Endocrinol Metab* 92(3):948–954.

Fonkalsrud E.W., Bray G.A. 1981. Vagotomy for treatment of obesity in childhood due to Prader-Willi syndrome. *J Ped Surg* 16:888–889.

Food and Agricultural Organization/World Health Organization Report. 2005.

Forbes C., Shirran L., Bagnall A.M., Duffy S., ter Riet G. 2001. A rapid and systematic review of the clinical effectiveness and cost-effectiveness of topotecan for ovarian cancer. *Health Technol Assess* 5(28):1–110.

Foster G.D., Wadden T.A., Vogt R.A., Brewer G. 1997. What is a reasonable weight loss? Patients' expectations and evaluations of obesity treatment outcomes. *J Consult Clin Psychol* 65(1):79–85.

Franco C., Koranyi J., Brandberg J., Lönn L., Bengtsson B.K., Svensson J., Johannsson G. 2009. The reduction in visceral fat mass in response to growth hormone is more marked in men than in oestrogen-deficient women. *Growth Horm IGF Res* 19(2):112–120.

Franklin R.M., Ploutz-Snyder L., Kanaley J.A. 2009. Longitudinal changes in abdominal fat distribution with menopause. *Metabolism* 58(3):311–315.

French S.A., Wechsler H. 2004. School-based research and initiatives: Fruit and vegetable environment, policy and pricing workshop. *Prev Med* 39(Suppl 2):S101–S107.

Frohlich A. 1901. Ein Fall von Tumor der Hypophysis cerebri ohne Akromegalie. *Wien klin Rundschau* 15:883–886, 906–908.

Frohman L.A., Bernardis L.L., Schnatz J.D., Burek L. 1969. Plasma insulin and triglyceride levels after hypothalamic lesions in weanling rats. *Am J Physiol* 216(6):1496–1501.

Fulton J. 1946. *Harvey Cushing: A Biography.* Springfield, IL: Charles C. Thomas.

Gallo S. 1994. Short biographies of Mabel Giddings Wilkin, MD, and Hilde Bruch, MD. *Texas Med* 10:60–70.

Garfinkel P.E. 1986. Hilde Bruch, M.D.: A seeker of truth. In *Women Physicians in Leadership Roles.* Arlington, VA: American Psychiatric Press.

Gallagher D., Heymsfield S.B., Heo M., Jebb S.A., Murgatroyd P.R., Sakamoto Y. 2000. Healthy percentage body fat ranges: An approach for developing guidelines based on body mass index. *Am J Clin Nutr* 72(3):694–701.

Gambineri A., Patton L., Vaccina A., Cacciari M., Morselli-Labate A.M., Cavazza C., Pagotto U., Pasquali R. 2006. Treatment with flutamide, metformin, and their combination added to a hypocaloric diet in overweight-obese women with polycystic ovary syndrome: A randomized, 12-month, placebo-controlled study. *J Clin Endocrinol Metab* 91(10):3970–3980.

Gillman M.W., Rifas-Shiman S.L., Camargo C.A., Jr., et al. 2001. Risk of overweight among adolescents who were breastfed as infants. *JAMA* 285:2461–2467.

Gillman M.W., Rifas-Shiman S., Berkey C.S., Field A.E., Colditz G.A. 2003. Maternal gestational diabetes, birth weight, and adolescent obesity. *Pediatrics* 111(3):e221–e226.

Gillman M.W., Rifas-Shiman S.L., Kleinman K., Oken E., Rich-Edwards J.W., Taveras E.M. 2008. Developmental origins of childhood overweight: Potential public health impact. *Obesity* (Silver Spring) 16(7):1651–1656.

Glanz K., Hoelscher D. 2004. Increasing fruit and vegetable intake by changing environments, policy and pricing: Restaurant-based research, strategies, and recommendations. *Prev Med* 39(Suppl 2):S88–S93.

Glanz K., Yaroch A.L. 2004. Strategies for increasing fruit and vegetable intake in grocery stores and communities: Policy, pricing, and environmental change. *Prev Med* 39(Suppl 2):S75–S80.

Goldstone A.P. 2004. Prader-Willi syndrome: Advances in its genetics, pathophysiology and treatment. *Trends Endocrinol Metab* 15:12–20.

Goldstone A.P., Holland A.J., Hauffa B.P., Hokken-Koelega A.C., Tauber M. 2008. Recommendations for the diagnosis and management of Prader-Willi syndrome. *J Clin Endo Metab* 93:4183–4197.

Gortmaker S.L., Peterson K., Wiecha J., Sobol A.M., Dixit S., Fox M.K., Laird N. 1999. Reducing obesity via a school-based interdisciplinary intervention among youth. Planet Health. *Arch Ped Adol Med* 153:409–418.

Grace C., Beales P., Summerbell C., Kopelman P. 2001. The effect of Bardet-Biedl syndrome in the components on energy balance. *International Journal of Obesity and Related Metabolic Disorders* 25(Suppl 2):S42.

Gray J., Yeo G.S., Cox J.J., Morton J., Adlam A.L., Keogh J.M., Yanovski J.A., El Gharbawy A., Han J.C., Tung Y.C., Hodges J.R., Raymond F.L., O'Rahilly S., Farooqi I.S. 2006. Hyperphagia, severe obesity, impaired cognitive function, and hyperactivity associated with functional loss of one copy of the brain-derived neurotrophic factor (BDNF) gene. *Diabetes* 55(12):3366–3371.

Greenway F.L., Bray G.A. 2008. Treatment of hypothalamic obesity with caffeine and ephedrine. *Endocr Pract* 14:697–703.

Gunay-Aygun M., Cassidy S.B., Nicholls R.D. 1997. Prader-Willi and other syndromes associated with obesity and mental retardation. *Behav Genet* 27:307–324.

Haarbo J., Christiansen C. 1992. Treatment-induced cyclic variations in serum lipids, lipoproteins, and apolipoproteins after 2 years of combined hormone replacement therapy: Exaggerated cyclic variations in smokers. *Obstet Gynecol* 80:639–644.

Han J.C., Liu Q.R., Jones M., et al. 2008. Brain-derived neurotrophic factor and obesity in the WAGR syndrome. *N Engl J Med* 359:918–927.

Han P., Frohman L.A. 1970. Hyperinsulinemia in tube-fed hypophysectomized rats bearing hypothalamic lesions. *Am J Physiol* 219(6):1632–1636.

Harris K.C., Kuramoto L.K., Schulzer M., Retallack J.E. 2009. Effect of a school-based physical activity interventions on body mass index in children: A meta-analyhsis. *CMAJ* 180:719–726.

Hediger M.L., Overpeck M.D., Kuczmarski R.J., Ruan W.J. 2001. Association between infant breast-feeding and overweight in young children. *JAMA* 285:2453–2460.

Herring S.J., Oken E., Haines J., Rich-Edwards J.W., Rifas-Shiman S.L., Kleinman ScD K.P., Gillman M.W. 2008. Misperceived pre-pregnancy body weight status predicts excessive gestational weight gain: Findings from a US cohort study. *BMC Pregnancy Childbirth* 8:54.

Hetherington A.W., Ranson S.W. 1940. Hypothalamic lesions and adiposity in the rat. *Anat Rec* 78:149–172.

Hidestrand P., Vasconez H., Cottrill C. 2009. Carpenter syndrome. *J Craniofac Surg* 20(1):254–256.

Hill J.O., Peters J.C. 1998. Environmental contributions to the obesity epidemic. *Science* 280(5368): 1371–1374.

Hinney A., Schmidt A., Nottebom K., et al. 1999. Several mutations in the melanocortin-4 receptor gene including a nonsense and a frameshift mutation associated with dominantly inherited obesity in humans. *J Clin Endocrinol Metab* 84:1483–1486.

Hochberg I., Hochberg Z. 2010. Expanding the definition of hypothalamic obesity. *Obes Rev*; in press.

Inge T.H., Pfluger P., Zeller M., Rose S.R., Burget L., Sundararajan S., et al. 2007. Gastric bypass surgery for treatment of hypothalamic obesity after craniopharyngioma therapy. *Nat Clin Pract Endoctrinol Metab* 3606–3609.

Institute for Clinical Systems Improvement (ICSI). 2005. *Prevention and Management of Obesity (Mature Adolescents and Adults)*. Bloomington, MN: ICSI.

Ismail D., O'Connell M.A., Zacharin M.R. 2006. Dexamphetamine use for management of obesity and hypersomnolence following hypothalamic injury. *J Pediatr Endocrinol Metab* 19:129–134.

Ize-Ludlow D., Gray J.A., Sperling M.A., Berry-Kravis E.M., Milunsky J.M., Farooqi I.S., et al. 2007. Rapid-onset obesity with hypothalamic dysfunction, hypoventilation and autonomic dysregulation presenting in childhood. *Pediatrics* 120:179–188.

Jackson R.S., Creemers J.W., Ohagi S., et al. 1997. Obesity and impaired prohormone processing associated with mutations in the human prohormone convertase 1 gene. *Nat Genet* 16:303–306.

James W.P.T., Gill T.P. 2008. Prevention of obesity. In *Handbook of Obesity: Clinical Applications*. GA Bray and C Bouchard, eds. New York: Informa Healthcare, pp 157–175.

Jeffrey R.W., Summerbell C.D., Waters E., Edmunds L.D., Kelly S., Brown T., Campbell K.J., et al. 2005. Interventions for preventing obesity in children. The Cochran Collaboration (Review). *The Cochrane Library* Issue 3 (see PIER folders).

Jeffery R.W., Forster J.L., Folsom A.R., Luepker R.V., Jacobs D.R. Jr., Blackburn H. 1989. The relationship between social status and body mass index in the Minnesota Heart Health Program. *Int J Obes* 13:59–67.

Jeffery R.W., French S.A. 1999. Preventing weight gain in adults: The pound of prevention study. *Am J Public Health* 89:747–751.

Jenkins D., Seelow D., Jehee F.S., Perlyn C.A., Alonso L.G., Bueno D.F., Donnai D., Josifiova D., Mathijssen I.M.J., Morton J.E.V., Ørstavik K.H., Sweeney E., Wall S.A., Marsh J.L., Nürnberg P., Passos-Bueno M.R., Wilkie A.O.M. 2007. *RAB23* mutations in Carpenter syndrome imply an unexpected role for hedgehog signaling in cranial-suture development and obesity. *Am J Hum Genet* 80(6):1162–1170.

Jenkins D.J., Wolever T.M., Vuksan V., et al. 1989. Nibbling versus gorging: Metabolic advantages of increased meal frequency. *N Engl J Med* 321:929–934.

Kanumakala S., Greaves R., Pedreira C.C., Donath S., Warne G.L., Zacharin M.R., Harris M. 2005. Fasting ghrelin levels are not elevated in children with hypothalamic obesity. *J Clin Endocrinol Metab* 90(5):2691–2695.

Katsanis N., Beales P.L., Woods M.O., et al. 2000. Mutations in MKKS cause obesity, retinal dystrophy and renal malformations associated with Bardet-Biedl syndrome. *Nat Genet* 26:67–70.

Katz D.L., O'Connell M., Yeh M.C., Nawaz H., Njike V., Anderson L.M., Cory S., Dietz W. 2005. Task Force on Community Preventive Services. Public health strategies for preventing and controlling overweight and obesity in school and worksite settings: A report on recommendations of the Task Force on Community Preventive Services. *MMWR Recomm Rep* 54(RR–10):1–12. Review.

Kennedy B.M., Paeratakul S., Ryan D.H., Bray G.A. 2007. Socioeconomic status and health disparity in the United States. *J Human Behav Soc Envir* 15(2/3):13–23.

Kim J.C., Badano J.L., Sibold S., Esmail M.A., et al. 2004. The Bardet-Biedl protein BBS-4 targets cargo to the pericentriolar region and is required for microtubule anchoring and cell cycle progression. *Nat Genetics* 36:462–470.

King B.M. 2006. The rise, fall, and resurrection of the ventromedial hypothalamus in the regulation of feeding behavior and body weight. *Physiol Behav* 87(2):221–244.

Koplan J.P., Liverman C.T., Kraak V.I., eds. 2005. *Preventing Childhood Obesity. Health in the Balance*. Committee on Prevention of Obesity in Children in Youth. Food and Nutrition Board and Board of Health Promotion and Disease Prevention. Institute of Medicine. Washington, DC: National Academy Press.

Kramer M.S., Matus L., Vanilovich I., Platt R.W., Bogdanovich N., Sevkovskaya Z., Dzikovich I., Shishko G., Collet H.-P., Martin R.M., Smith G.D., Gillman M.W., Chalmers B., Hodnett E., Shapiro S. 2007. Effects of prolonged and exclusive breast feeding on child height, weight, adiposity, and blood pressure at age 6.5 y: Evidence from a large randomized clinical trial. *Am J Clin Nutr* 86:1717–1721.

Kromhout D., Bloemberg B., Seidell J.C., Nissinen A., Menotti A. 2001. Physical activity and dietary fiber determine population body fat levels: The Seven Countries Study. *Int J Obes Relat Metab Disord* 25:301–306.

Kromhout D. 1983. Changes in energy and macronutrients in 871 middle-aged men during 10 years of follow-up (the Zutphen study). *Am J Clin Nutr* 37:287–294.

Krude H., Biebermann H., Luck W., Horn R., Brabant G., Gruters A. 1998. Severe early-onset obesity, adrenal insufficiency and red hair pigmentation caused by POMC mutations in humans. *Nat Genet* 19:155–157.

Kuller L.H., Simkin-Silverman L.R., Wing R.R., Meilahn E.N., Ives D.G. 2001. Women's Healthy Lifestyle Project: A randomized clinical trial. Results at 54 months. *Circ* 103:32–37.

Kumanyika S.K., Daniels S.R. 2006. Obesity Endo in *Overweight and the Metabolic Syndrome: From Bench to Bedside*, G.A. Bray and D.H. Ryan (eds.), Endocrine Updates, pp 233–253.

Kumanyika S.K., Obarzanek E., Stettler N., Bell R., Field A.E., Fortmann S.P., Franklin B.A., Gillman M.W., Lewis C.E., Poston W.C. 2nd, Stevens J., Hong Y. 2008. American Heart Association Council on Epidemiology and Prevention, Interdisciplinary Committee for Prevention. Population-based prevention of obesity: The need for comprehensive promotion of healthful eating, physical activity, and energy balance: A scientific statement from American Heart Association Council on Epidemiology and Prevention, Interdisciplinary Committee for Prevention (formerly the expert panel on population and prevention science). *Circ* 118(4):428–464.

Landon M.B., Spong Cy., Thom E., Carpeter M.W., Ramin S.M., Casey B., Wapner R.J., Varner M.W., Rouse D.J., Thorp J.M. Jr, Sciscione A., Catalano P., Harper M., Saade G., Lain K.Y., Sorokin Y., Peaceman A.M., Tolosa J.E., Anderson G.B., For the Eunice Kennedy Shriver National Institute of Child Health and Human Development Maternal-Fetal Medicine Unites Network. 2009. A multicenter, randomized trial of treatment for mild gestational diabetes. *N Engl J Med* 361:1339–1348.

Lawson O.J., Williamson D.A., Champagne C.M., et al. 1995. The association of body weight, dietary intake, and energy expenditure with dietary restraint and disinhibition. *Obes Res* 3:153–161.

Leibel R.L. 2008. Molecular physiology of weight regulation in mice and humans. *Int J Obes* (London) 32(Suppl 7):S98–S108.

Licinio J., Caglayan S., Ozata M., Yildiz B.O., de Miranda P.B., O'Kirwan F., et al. 2004. Phenotypic effects of leptin replacement on morbid obesity, diabetes mellitus, hypogonadism, and behavior in leptin-deficient adults. *Proc Natl Acad Sci USA* 101:4531–4536.

Lindgren A.C., Lindberg A. 2008. Growth hormone treatment completely normalizes adult height and improves body composition in Prader-Willi syndrome: Experience from KIGS (Pfizer International Growth Database). *Horm Res* 70(3):182–187.

Lonn L., Johansson G., Sjostrom L., Kvist H., Oden A., Bengtsson B.A. 1996. Body composition and tissue distributions in growth hormone deficient adults before and after growth hormone treatment. *Obes Res* 4:45–54.

Loriaux D.L. 1992. Harvey Williams Cushing 1869–1939. *The Endocrinologist* 2(l):2–5.

Ludwig D.S., Peterson K.E., Gortmaker S.L. 2001. Relation between consumption of sugar-sweetened drinks and childhood obesity: A prospective, observational analysis. *Lancet* 357:505–508.

Lustig R.H., Rose S.R., Burghen G.A., Velasquez–Mieyer P., Broome D.C., Smith K., Li H., Hudson M.M., Heideman R.L., Kun L.E. 1999. Hypothalamic obesity caused by cranial insult in children: Altered glucose and insulin dynamics and reversal by a somatostatin agonist. *J Pediatr* 135:162–168.

Lustig R.H., Hinds P.S., Ringwald-Smith K., Christensen R.K., Kaste S.C., Schreiber R.E., Rai S.N., Lensing S.Y., Wu S., Xiong X. 2003. Octreotide therapy of pediatric hypothalamic obesity: A double-blind, placebo-controlled trial. *J Clin Endocrinol Metab* 88(6):2586–2592.

McCarron D.A., Morris C.D., Henry H.J., Stanton J.L. 1984. Blood pressure and nutrient intake in the United States. *Science* 224:1392–1398.

McGavock J.M., Torrance B.D., McGuire A., Wozny P.D., Lewanczuk R.Z. 2009. Cardiorespiratory fitness and the risk of overweight in youth: The Health Hearts Longitudinal Study of Cardiometabolic Health. *Obesity* 17:1802–1807.

Mamun A.A., Lawlor D.A., O'Callaghan M.J., Williams G.M., Najman J.M. 2005. Family and early life factors associated with changes in overweight status between ages 5 and 14 years: Findings from the Mater University Study of Pregnancy and its outcomes. *Intern J Obes* 29(5):475–482.

Mangelsdorf M., Chevrier E., Mustonen A., Picketts D.J. 2009. Börjeson-Forssman-Lehmann Syndrome due to a novel plant homeodomain zinc finger mutation in the PHF6 gene. *J Child Neurol* 24(5):610–614.

Marion V., Stoetzel C., Schlicht D., Messaddeq N., Koch M., Flori E., Danse J.M., Mandel J.L., Dollfus H. 2009. Transient ciliogenesis involving Bardet-Biedl syndrome proteins is a fundamental characteristic of adipogenic differentiation. *Proc Natl Acad Sci U S A* 106(6):1820–1825.

Marshall J.D., Bronson R.T., Collin G.B., Nortstrom A.D., Maffei P., Paisey R.B., Carey C., MacDermott S., Russell-Eggit I., Shea S.E., Davis J., Beck S., Shatirishvili G., Mihai C.M., Hoeltzenbein M., Pozzan G.B., Hopkinson I., Sicolo N., Naggarat J.K., Nishina P.M. 2005. New Alstrom syndrome phenotypes based on the evaluation of 182 cases. *Arch Intern Med* 165:675–683.

Mason P.W., Krawiecki N., Meacham L.R. 2002. The use of dextroamphetamine to treat obesity and hyperphagia in children treated for craniopharyngioma. *Arch Pediatr Adolesc Med* 156:887–892.

MCR MSS on frequency of BMI measurements in advance of HEDIS.

Medvei V.C. 1982. *A History of Endocrinology.* Lancaster: MTP Press, pp 598.

Mogul H.R., Lee P.D., Whitman B.Y., Zipf W.B., Frey M., Myers S., Cahan M., Pinyerd B., Southren A.L. 2008. Growth hormone treatment of adults with Prader-Willi syndrome and growth hormone deficiency improves lean body mass, fractional body fat, and serum triiodothyronine without glucose impairment: Results from the United States multicenter trial. *J Clin Endocrinol Metab* 93(4):1238–1245.

Mokdad A.H., Ford E.S., Bowman B.A., et al. 2003. Prevalence of obesity, diabetes, and obesity-related health risk factors, 2001. *JAMA* 289:76–79.

Monda K.L., Adair L.S., Zhai F., Popkin B.M. 2008. Longitudinal relationships between occupational and domestic physical activity patterns and body weight in China. *Eur J Clin Nutr* 62(11):1318–1325.

Montague C.T., Farooqi I.S., Whitehead J.P., et al. 1997. Congenital leptin deficiency is associated with severe early-onset obesity in humans. *Nature* 387:903–908.

Muller H.L., Bueb K., Bartels U., Roth C., Harz K., Graf N., Korinthenbom R., Bettendorf M., Kuhl J., Gutjahr P., Sorensen N., Calaminus G. 2001. Obesity after childhood craniopharyngioms—German multicenter study on pre-operative risk factors and quality of life. *Klin Pediatr* 213:244–249.

Must A., Jacques P.F., Dallal G.E., Bajema C.J., Dietz W.H. 1992. Long-term morbidity and mortality of overweight adolescents. A follow-up of the Harvard Growth Study of 1922 to 1935. *N Engl J Med* 327:1350–1355.

National Task Force on the Prevention and Treatment of Obesity, Atkinson R.L., Dietz W.H., Foreyt J.P., Goodwin N.J., Hill J.O., Hirsch J., Pi-Sunyer F.X., Weinsier R.L., Wing R., Hoofnagle J.H., Everhart J., Hubbard V.S., Zelitch Yanovski S. 1994. Weight cycling. *JAMA* 272:1196–1202.

Newell-Price J., Trainer P., Besser M., Grossman A. 1998. The diagnosis and differential diagnosis of Cushing's syndrome and pseudo-Cushing's states. *Endocr Rev* 19(5):647–672.

NHLBI Obesity Education Initiative Expert Panel on the Identification, Evaluation, and Treatment of Overweight and Obesity in Adults. 1998. Clinical guidelines on the identification, evaluation and treatment of overweight and obesity in adults—The evidence report. *Obes Res* 6(Suppl 2):51S–209S.

Nieman L.K. 2002. Medical therapy of Cushing's disease. *Pituitary* 5(2):77–82.

Nishizawa T., Akaoka I., Nishida Y., Kawaguchi Y., Hayashi E. 1976. Some factors related to obesity in the Japanese sumo wrestler. *Am J Clin Nutr* 29:1167–1174.

Obarzanek E., Schreiber G.B., Crawford P.B., et al. 1994. Energy intake and physical activity in relation to indexes of body fat: The National Heart, Lung, and Blood Institute Growth and Health Study. *Am J Clin Nutr* 60:15–22.

O'Dea D., Parfrey P.S., Harnett J.D., Hefferton D., Cramer B.C., Green J. 1996. The importance of renal impairment in the natural history of Bardet-Biedl syndrome. *Am J Kidney Dis* 27:776–783.

Ogden C.L., Flegal K.M., Carroll M.D., Johnson C.L. 2002. Prevalence and trends in overweight among US children and adolescents, 1999–2000. *JAMA* 288:1728–1732.

Oken E., Taveras E.M., Kleinman K.P., Rich-Edwards J.W., Gillman M.W. 2007. Gestational weight gain and child adiposity at age 3 years. *Am J Obstet Gynecol* 196(4):322.

Olson C.M. 2008. Achieving a healthy weight gain during pregnancy. *Annu Rev Nutr* 28:411–423.

Orth D.N. 1995. Cushing's syndrome. *N Engl J Med* 332:791–803.

Ozata M., Ozdemir I.C., Licinio J. 1999. Human leptin deficiency caused by a missense mutation: Multiple endocrine defects, decreased sympathetic tone, and immune system dysfunction indicate new targets for leptin action, greater central than peripheral resistance to the effects of leptin, and spontaneous correction of leptin-mediated defects. *J Clin Endocrinol Metab* 84:3686–3695.

Panagiotakos D.B., Papadimitriou A., Anthracopoulos M.B., Konstantinidou M., Antonogeorgos G., Fretzayas A., Priftis K.N. 2008. Birthweight, breast-feeding, parental weight and prevalence of obesity in schoolchildren aged 10–12 years, in Greece: The Physical Activity, Nutrition and Allergies in Children Examined in Athens (PANACEA) study. *Pediatr Int* 50(4):563–568.

Papas M.A., Alberg A.J., Ewing R., Helzlsouer K.J., Gary T.L., Klassen A.C. 2007. The built environment and obesity. *Epidemiol Rev* 29:129–143.

Park W.J., Oh Y.J., Kim G.Y., Kim S.E., Paik K.-H., Han S.J., Kim A.H., Chu S.H., Kwon E.K., Kim S.W., Jin D.-K. 2007. Obestatin is not elevated or correlated with insulin in children with the Prader-Willi Syndrome. *JCEM* 92:229–234.

Parker M., Rifas-Shiman S.L., Belfort M.B., Taveras E.M., Oken E., Mantzoros C., Gillman M.W. 2010. Gestational glucose tolerance and cord blood leptin levels predict slower weight gain in early infancy. *J Pediatr* [Epub ahead of print].

Partonen T., Lonnqvist J. 1998. Seasonal affective disorder. *Lancet* 352:1369–1374.

Perri M.G., Limacher M.C., Durning P.E., Janicke D.M., Lutes L.D., Bobroff L.B., Dale M.S., Daniels M.J., Radcliff T.A., Martin A.D. 2008. Extended-care programs for weight management in rural communities: The treatment of obesity in underserved rural settings (TOURS) randomized trial. *Arch Intern Med* 168(21):2347–2354.

Plotz C.M., Knowlton A.I., Ragan C. 1952. The natural history of Cushing's syndrome. *Am J Med* 13:597–614.

Pollan M. 2008. Farmer in chief. What the next president can and should do to remake the way we grow and eat our food. *New York Times Magazine* 62–68.

Prader A., Labhart A., Willi H. 1956. Ein syndrome von adipositas, kleinwuchs, kryptorchismus und oligophrenie nach myotonieartigem zustand im neugeborenenalter. *Schweiz Med Wochenschr* 86:1260–1261.

Prentice A.M., Jebb S.A. 1995. Obesity in Britain: Gluttony or sloth? *BMJ* 311:437–439.

Prospective Studies Collaboration, Whitlock G., Lewington S., Sherliker P., et al. 2009. Body-mass index and cause-specific mortality in 900,000 adults: Collaborative analyses of 57 prospective studies. *Lancet* 373(9669):1083–1096. Epub 2009 Mar 18.

Rasmussen K.M., Yaktine A.L. 2009. *Weight Gain during Pregnancy: Reexamining the Guidelines*. Washington, DC: The National Academies Press.

Reilly J.J., Armstrong J., Dorosty A.R., Emmett P.M., Ness A., Rogers I., Steer C., Sherriff A. 2005. Avon longitudinal study of parents and children study team. Early life risk factors for obesity in childhood: Cohort study. *BMJ* 330(7504):1357.

Reubinoff B.E., Grubstein A., Meirow D., Berry E., Schenker J.G., Brzezinski A. 1995. Effects of low-dose estrogen oral contraceptives on weight, body composition, and fat distribution in young women. *Fertil Steril* 63:516–521.

Rijpert M., Evers I.M., de Vroede M.A.M.J., de Valk H.W., Heijnen C.J., Visser G.H.A. 2009. Risk factors for childhood overweight in offspring of Type 1 diabetic women with adequate glycemic control during pregnancy. *Diab Care* 32:2099–2104.

Ristow M., Muller-Wieland D., Pfeiffer A., Krone W., Kahn C.R. 1998. Obesity associated with a mutation in a genetic regulator of adipocyte differentiation. *N Engl J Med* 339:953–959.

Roberts S.B., Pi-Sunyer F.X., Dreher M., et al. 1998. Physiology of fat replacement and fat reduction: Effects of dietary fat and fat substitutes on energy regulation. *Nutr Rev* 56:S29–S41; discussion S41–S49.

Rodekamp E., Harder T., Kohlhoff R., Franke K., Dudenhausen J.W., Plagemann A. 2005. Long-term impact of breast-feeding on body weight and glucose tolerance in children of diabetic mothers. *Diabetes Care* 28:1457–1462.

Roth C.L., Hunneman D.H., Gebhardt U., Stoffel-Wagner B., Reinehr R., Muller H.L. 2007. Reduced sympathetic metabolites in urine of obese patients with craniopharyngioma. *Ped Res* 61:496–501.

Sacher P.M., Chadwick P., Wells J.C., Williams J.E., Cole T.J., Lawson M.S. 2005. Assessing the acceptability and feasibility of the MEND Programme in a small group of obese 7–11-year-old children. *J Hum Nutr Diet* 18(1):3–5.

Sacks F.M., Svetkey L.P., Vollmer W.M., Appel L.J., Bray G.A., Harsha D., Obarzanek E., Conlin P.R., Miller E.R. 3rd, Simons-Morton D.G., Karanja N., Lin P.H. 2001. DASH-Sodium Collaborative Research Group. Effects on blood pressure of reduced dietary sodium and the Dietary Approaches to Stop Hypertension (DASH) diet. DASH-Sodium Collaborative Research Group. *N Engl J Med* 344(1):3–10.

Sallis J.F., Glanz K. 2009. Physical activity and food environments: Solutions to the obesity epidemic. *Milbank Q* 87(1):123–154.

Salmeron J., Manson J.E., Stampfer M.J., Colditz G.A., Wing A.L., Willett W.C. 1997. Dietary fiber, glycemic load, and risk of non-insulin-dependent diabetes mellitus in women. *JAMA* 277:472–477.

Savastano D.M., Tanofsky-Kraff M., Han J.C., Ning C., Sorg R.A., Roza C.A., Wolkoff L.E., Anandalingam K., Jefferson-George K.S., Figueroa R.E., Sanford E.L., Brady S., Kozlosky M., Schoeller D.A., Yanovski J.A. 2009. Energy intake and energy expenditure among children with polymorphisms of the melanocortin-3 receptor. *Am J Clin Nutr* 90(4):912–920.

Schack-Nielsen L., Michaelsen K.F., Gamborg M., Mortensen E.L., Sorensen T.I.A. 2010. Gestational weight gain in relation to offspring body mass index and obesity from infancy through adulthood. *Intern J Obes* 34:67–74.

Scheimann A.O., Butler M.G., Gourash L., Cuffari C., Klish W. 2008. Critical analysis of bariatric procedures in Prader-Willi syndrome. *J Pediatr Gastroenterol Nutr* 46(1):80–83.

Scholtens S., Brunekreef B., Smit H.A., Gast G.C., Hoekstra M.O., de Jongste J.C., Postma D.S., Gerritsen J., Seidell J.C., Wijga A.H. 2008. Do differences in childhood diet explain the reduced overweight risk in breastfed children? *Obesity* 16:2498–2503.

Schultes B., Ernest B., Schmid F., Thurneheer M. 2009. Distal gastric bypass surgery for the treatment of hypothalamic obesity after childhood craniopharyngioma. *Eur J Endocrinol* 161:201–206.

Seidell J.C., Nooyens A.J., Visscher T.L. 2005. Cost-effective measures to prevent obesity: Epidemiological basis and appropriate target groups. *Proc Nutr Soc* 64:1–5.

Shaikh M.G., Grundy R.G., Kirk J.M. 2008. Hyperliptinaemia rather than fasting hyperinsulinaemia is associated with obesity following hypothalamic damage in children. *Eur J Endocrinol* 159:791–797.

Sherwood N.E., Jeffery R.W., French S.A., Hannan P.J., Murray D.M. 2000. Predictors of weight gain in the Pound of Prevention study. *Int J Obes Relat Metab Disord* 24:395–403.

Simkin-Silverman L.R., Wing R.R., Boraz M.A., Kuller L.H. 2003. Lifestyle intervention can prevent weight gain during menopause: Results from a 5-year randomized clinical trial. *Ann Behav Med* 26:212–220.

Smed S., Denver S. 2005a. Taxing as Economic Tools in Health Policy. Presented at 97th EAAE Seminar, University of Reading, April 21–22, 2005.

Smed S., Jensen J.D., Denver S. 2005. Differentiated Food Taxes as a Tool in Health and Nutrition Policy. Presented at XIth Congress of the European Association of Agricultural Economists, Copenhagen, DK, August 24–27, 2005.

Smith D.E., Lewis C.E., Caveny J.L., Perkins L.L., Burke G.L., Bild D.E. 1994. Longitudinal changes in adiposity associated with pregnancy. The CARDIA Study. Coronary Artery Risk Development in Young Adults Study. *JAMA* 271:1747–1751.

Smith P.E. 1927. The disabilities caused by hypophysectomy and their repair. The tuberal (hypothalamic) syndrome in the rat. *JAMA* 88:159–161.

Smith D.K., Sarfeh J., Howard L. 1983. Truncal vagotomy in hypothalamic obesity. *Lancet* 1:1330–1331.

Snow V., Barry P., Fitterman N., Qaseem A., Weiss K. 2005. Pharmacologic and surgical management of obesity in primary care: A clinical practice guideline from the American College of Physicians. *Ann Intern Med* 142:525–531.

Snyder E.E., Walts B., Perusse L., et al. 2004. The human obesity gene map: The 2003 update. *Obes Res* 12:369–439.

Srinivasan S., Ogle G.D., Garnett S.P., Briody J.N., Lee J.W., Cowell C.T. 2004. Features of the metabolic syndrome after childhood craniopharyngioma. *J Clin Endocrinol Metab* 89:81–86.

Stables G.J., Subar A.F., Patterson B.H., Dodd K., Heimendinger J., Van Duyn M.A., Nebeling L. 2002. Changes in vegetable and fruit consumption and awareness among US adults: Results of the 1991 and 1997 5-a-Day for Better Health Program surveys. *J Am Diet Assoc* 102:809–817.

Stein I.F., Leventhal M.L. 1935. Amenorrhea associated with bilateral polycystic ovaries. *Am J Obstet Gynecol* 29:181–191.

Stettler N., Kumanyika S.K., Katz S.H., Zemel B.S., Stallings V.A. 2003. Rapid weight gain during infancy and obesity in young adulthood in a cohort of African Americans. *Am J Clin Nutr* 77(6):1374–1378.

Strobel A., Issad T., Camoin L., Ozata M., Strosberg A.D. 1998. A leptin missense mutation associated with hypogonadism and morbid obesity. *Nat Genet* 18:213–215.

Stunkard A. 2000. Two eating disorders: Binge eating disorder and the night eating syndrome. *Appetite* 34:333–334.

Stunkard A.J. 1955. The night eating syndrome: A pattern of food intake among certain obese patients. *American Journal of Medicine* 19:78–86.

Swinburn B.A., Caterson I., Seidell J.C., James W.P. 2004. Diet, nutrition and the prevention of excess weight gain and obesity. *Public Health Nutr* 7(1A):123–146.

Talbott J.H. 1970. *A Biographical History of Medicine: Excerpts and Essays on the Men and Their Work*. New York: Grune & Stratton.

Tanofsky-Kraff M., Han J.C., Anandalingam K., Shomaker L.B., Columbo K.M., Wolkoff L.E., Kozlosky M., Elliott C., Ranzenhofer L.M., Roza C.A., Yanovski S.Z., Yanovski J.A. 2009. The FTO gene rs9939609 obesity-risk allele and loss of control over eating. *Am J Clin Nutr* 90(6):1483–1488.

Taveras E.M., Rifas-Shiman S.L., Belfort M.B., Kleinman K.P., Oken E., Gillman M.W. 2009 Weight status in the first 6 months of life and obesity at 3 years of age. *Pediatrics* 123(4):1177–1183.

Theodoro M.F., Talebizadeh Z., Butler M.G. 2006. Body composition and fatness patterns in Prader-Willi syndrome: Comparison with simple obesity. *Obesity* 14:1685–1690.

Thomson E.H. 1950. *Harvey Cushing. Surgeon, Author, Artist*. New York: Schuman.

Toschke A.M., Beyerlein A., von Kries R. 2005. Children at high risk for overweight. A classification and regression trees analysis approach. *Obes Res* 13:1270–1274.

Trasande L., Cronk C., Durkin M., Weiss M., Schoeller D.A., Gall E.A., Hewitt J.B., Carrel A.L., Landrigan P.J., Gillman M.W. 2009. Environment and obesity in the National Children's Study. *Environ Health Perspect* 117(2):159–166.

Tuomilehto J., Lindström J., Eriksson J.G., Valle T.T., Hämäläinen H., Ilanne-Parikka P., Keinänen-Kiukaanniemi S., Laakso M., Louheranta A., Rastas M., Salminen V., Uusitupa M. 2001. Finnish Diabetes Prevention Study Group. Prevention of type 2 diabetes mellitus by changes in lifestyle among subjects with impaired glucose tolerance. *N Engl J Med* 344(18):1343–1350.

Turner G., Lower K.M., White S.M., Delatycki M., Lampe A.K., Wright M., Smith J.C., Kerr B., Schelley S., Hoyme H.E., De Vries B.B., Kleefstra T., Grompe M., Cox B., Gecz J., Partington M. 2004. The clinical picture of the Börjeson-Forssman-Lehmann syndrome in males and heterozygous females with PHF6 mutations. *Clin Genet* 65(3):226–232.

Urbanek M., Woodroffe A., Ewens K.G., Diamanti-Kandarakis E., Legro R.S., Strauss J.F. 3rd, Dunaif A., Spielman R.S. 2005. Candidate gene region for polycystic ovary syndrome on chromosome 19p13.2. *J Clin Endocrinol Metab* 90(12):6623–6629.

U.S. Preventive Task Force. 2003. Screening for obesity in adults: Recommendations and rationale. *Ann Intern Med* 139:930–932.

Vaisse C., Clement K., Guy-Grand B., Froguel P. 1998. A frameshift mutation in human MC4R is associated with a dominant form of obesity. *Nat Genet* 20:113–114.

Van Dam R.M., Willett W.C., Manson J.E., Hu F.B. 2006. The relationship between overweight in adolescence and premature death in women. *Ann Intern Med* 145(2):91–97.

Venditti E.M., Bray G.A., Carrion-Petersen M.L., Delahanty L.M., Edelstein S.L., Hamman R.F., Hoskin M.A., Knowler W.C., Ma Y. 2008. Diabetes Prevention Program Research Group. First versus repeat treatment with a lifestyle intervention program: Attendance and weight loss outcomes. *Int J Obes (Lond)* 32(10):1537–1544.

Von Kries R., Koletzko B., Sauerwald T., et al. 1999. Breast feeding and obesity: Cross sectional study. *BMJ* 319:147–150.

Weidemann H.-R. 1984. Andrea Prader: On the occasion of his 65th birthday. *Eur J Ped* 143:80–81.

Welt C.K., et al. 2006. Characterizing discrete subsets of polycystic ovary syndrome as defined by the Rotterdam Criteria: The impact of weight on phenotype and metabolic features. *JCEM* 91:4842–4848.

Westerterp K., Speakman J. 2008. Physical activity energy expenditure has not declined since the 1980s and matches energy expenditures of wild mammals. *Int J Obes* (London) 32(8):1256–1263.

Whitaker R.C., Pepe M.S., Wright J.A., Seidel K.D., Dietz W.H. 1998. Early adiposity rebound and the risk of adult obesity. *Pediatrics* 101:E5.

Whitaker R.C., Wright J.A., Pepe M.S., Seidel K.D., Dietz W.H. 1997. Predicting obesity in young adulthood from childhood and parental obesity. *N Engl J Med* 337:869–873.

Whitlock E.P., Williams S.B., Gold R., Smith P.R., Shipman S.A. 2005. Screening and interventions for childhood overweight: A summary of evidence for the US Preventive Services Task Force. *Pediatrics* 116(1):e125–e144.

Whitlock E.A., O'Connor E.P., Williams S.B., Beil T.L., Lutz K.W. 2008. Effectiveness of weight management programs in children and adolescents. *Evid Rep Technol Assess* (Full Rep). 170:1–308.

WHO. 2000. Obesity: Preventing and managing the global epidemic. Report of a WHO consultation. *World Health Organ Tech Rep Ser* 894:i–xii, 1–253.

WHO/FAO Joint Expert Consultation on Diet, Nutrition and the Prevention of Chronic Disease. 2002. Geneva: WHO Technical Series. Report #916.

Williamson D.A., Lawson O.J., Brooks E.R., et al. 1995. Association of body mass with dietary restraint and disinhibition. *Appetite* 25:31–41.

Williamson D.F., Madans J., Pamuk E., Flegal K.M., Kendrick J.S., Serdula M.K. 1994. A prospective study of childbearing and 10-year weight gain in US white women 25 to 45 years of age. *Int J Obes Relat Metab Disord* 18:561–569.

Wilson L.C., Hall C.M. 2002. Albright's hereditary osteodystrophy and pseudohypoparathyroidism. *Semin Musculoskelet Radiol* 6(4):273–283.

Wolk A., Manson J.E., Stampfer M.J., et al. 2004. 1999. Long-term intake of dietary fiber and decreased risk of coronary heart disease among women. *JAMA* 281:1998.

Wong F., Huhman M., Heitzler C., Asbury L., Bretthauer-Mueller R., McCarthy S., Londe P. 2004. VERB—a social marketing campaign to increase physical activity among youth. *Prev Chronic Dis* 1:A10.

Wright C.S., Rifas–Shiman S.L., Rich-Edwards J.W., Taveras E.M., Gillman M.W., Oken E. 2009. Intrauterine exposure to gestational diabetes, child adiposity, and blood pressure. *Am J Hypertens* 22(2):215–220.

Yanovski S.Z. 1994. Binge eating disorder affects outcome of comprehensive very-low-calorie diet treatment. *Obes Res* 2:205–212.

Yeo G.S., Farooqi I.S., Aminian S., Halsall D.J., Stanhope R.G., O'Rahilly S. 1998. A frameshift mutation in MC4R associated with dominantly inherited human obesity. *Nat Genet* 20:111–112.

Yu-Poth S., Zhao G., Etherton T., Naglak M., Jonnalagadda S., Kris-Etherton P.M. 1999. Effects of the National Cholesterol Education Program's Step I and Step II dietary intervention programs on cardiovascular disease risk factors: A meta-analysis. *Am J Clin Nutr* 69:632–646.

Zaghloul N.A., Katsanis N. 2009. Mechanistic insights into Bardet-Biedl syndrome, a model ciliopathy. *J Clin Invest* 119(3):428–437.

Zemel M.B., Shi H., Greer B., Dirienzo D., Zemel P.C. 2000. Regulation of adiposity by dietary calcium. *Faseb J* 14:1132–1138.

Zhai F., Wang H., Du S., He Y., Wang Z., Ge K., Popkin B.M. 2009. Prospective study on nutrition transition in China. *Nutr Rev* 67(Suppl 1):S56–S61.

CHAPTER 6

Alhassan S., Kim S., Bersamin A., King A.C., Gardner C.D. 2008. Dietary adherence and weight loss success among overweight women: Results from the A to Z weight loss study. *Intern J Obes* 32:985–991.

Andersen R.E., Wadden T.A., et al. 1999. Effects of lifestyle activity vs. structured aerobic exercise in obese women: A randomized trial. *JAMA* 281(4):335–340.

Anderson J.W., Konz E.C., et al. 2001. Long-term weight-loss maintenance: A meta-analysis of US studies. *Am J Clin Nutr* 74(5):579–584.

Appel L.J., Moore T.J., et al. 1997. A clinical trial of the effects of dietary patterns on blood pressure. DASH Collaborative Research Group. *N Engl J Med* 336(16):1117–1124.

Ashley J.M., Herzog H., Clodfelder S., Bovee V., Schrage J., Pritsos C. 2007. Nutrient adequacy during weight loss interventions: A randomized study in women comparing the dietary intake in a meal replacement group with a traditional food group. *Nutr J* 25:6–12.

Astrup A. 2001. The role of dietary fat in the prevention and treatment of obesity. Efficacy and safety of low fat diets. *Int J Obes Relat Metab Disord* 25(Suppl 1):S46–S50.

Astrup A., Grunwald G.K., et al. 2000. The role of low-fat diets in body weight control: A meta-analysis of ad libitum dietary intervention studies. *Int J Obes Relat Metab Disord* 24(12):1545–1552.

Atkins R.C. 2002. *Dr. Atkins's New Diet Revolution*. New York: Avon.

Atwater W.O., Rosa E.B. 1899. *Description of a New Respiration Calorimeter and Experiments on the Conservation of Energy in the Human Body*. U.S. Department of Agriculture Bull No 63, pp 1–94. Washington, DC: U.S. Government Printing Office.

Avenell A., Broom J., et al. 2004. Systematic review of the long-term effects and economic consequences of treatments for obesity and implications for health improvement. *Health Technol Assess* 8(21):iii–iv; 1–182.

Avenell A., Brown T.J., McGee M.A., Campbell M.K., Grant A.M., Broom J., Jung R.T., Smith W.C. 2004. What interventions should we add to weight reducing diets in adults with obesity? A systematic review of randomized controlled trials of adding drug therapy, exercise, behaviour therapy or combinations of these interventions. *J Hum Nutr Diet* 17(4):293–316.

Bandura A., Simon K.M. 1977. The role of proximal intentions in self-regulation of refractory behavior. *Cognitive Therapy Research* 1:177–193.

Banting W. 1863. *A Letter on Corpulence Addressed to the Public*. London: Harrison and Sons.

Baranowski T., Baranowski J.C., et al. 2003. The Fun, Food, and Fitness Project (FFFP): The Baylor GEMS pilot study. *Ethn Dis* 13(1 Suppl 1):S30–S39.

Benedict F.G. 1915. *A Study of Prolonged Fasting*. Report No. 203. Washington, DC: Carnegie Institution of Washington.

Benedict F.G., Miles W.R., Roth P., Smith H.M. 1919. *Human Vitality and Efficiency under Prolonged Restricted Diet*. Washington, DC: Carnegie Institution of Washington.

Bennett G.G., Herring S.J., Puleo E., Stein E.K., Emmons K.M., Gillman M.W. 2009. Web-based weight loss in primary care: A randomized controlled trial. *Obesity* (Silver Spring) 18:308–313.

Berkowitz R.I., Wadden T.A., et al. 2003. Behavior therapy and sibutramine for the treatment of adolescent obesity: A randomized controlled trial. *JAMA* 289(14):1805–1812.

Blackburn G.L., Bray G.A. 1985. *Management of Obesity by Severe Caloric Restriction.* Littleton, MA: PSG Publishing.

Blair S.N., Kampert J.B., et al. 1996. Influences of cardiorespiratory fitness and other precursors on cardiovascular disease and all-cause mortality in men and women. *JAMA* 276(3):205–210.

Bloom W.L. 1959. Fasting as an introduction to the treatment of obesity. *Metabolism* 8:214–220.

Bond D.S., Phelan S., Leahey T.M., Hill J.O., Wing R.R. 2009. Weight-loss maintenance in successful weight losers: Surgical vs. non-surgical methods. *Int J Obes* (London) 33(1):173–180.

Bonomi, A.G., Goris, A.H., Yin, B., Westerterp, K.R. 2009. Detection of type, duration, and intensity of physical activity using an accelerometer. *Med Sci Sports Exerc* 41(9):1770–1777.

Bouchard C., Tremblay A., et al. 1990. The response to long-term overfeeding in identical twins. *N Engl J Med* 322(21):1477–1482.

Bouché C., Rizkalla S.W., Luo J., Vidal H., Veronese A., Pacher N., Fouquet C., Lang V., Slama G. 2002. Five-week, low-glycemic index diet decreases total fat mass and improves plasma lipid profile in moderately overweight nondiabetic men. *Diabetes Care* 25(5):822–828.

Boule N.G., Weisnagel S.J., et al. 2005. Effects of exercise training on glucose homeostasis: The HERITAGE Family Study. *Diabetes Care* 28(1):108–114.

Brand-Miller J., Wolever T.M., Foster-Powell K., Colagiuri S. 2003. *The New Glucose Revolution: The Glycemic Index Solution for a Healthier Future*. New York: Avalon Publishing Group.

Bravata D.M., Sanders L., et al. 2003. Efficacy and safety of low-carbohydrate diets: A systematic review. *JAMA* 289(14):1837–1850.

Bravata D.M., Smith-Spangler D., Sundaram V., Gienger A.L., Lin N., Lewis R., Stave C.D., Olkin I., Sirard J.R. 2007. Using pedometers to increase physical activity and improve health: A systematic review *JAMA* 298(19):2296–2304.

Bray G.A. 2009. *The Low-Fructose Approach to Weight Loss.* Pittsburgh: Dorrance Publishing.

Bray G.A., Popkin B.M. 1998. Dietary fat intake does affect obesity! *Am J Clin Nutr* 68(6):1157–1173.

Bray G.A., Vollmer W.M., Sacks F.M., Obarzanek E., Svetkey L., Appel L.J., for the DASH Collaborative Research Group. 2004. A further subgroup analysis of the effects of the DASH diet and three dietary sodium levels on blood pressure: Results of the DASH–Sodium Trial. *Am J Cardiol* 94:222–227.

Brehm B.J., Seeley R.J., et al. 2003. A randomized trial comparing a very low carbohydrate diet and a calorie-restricted low fat diet on body weight and cardiovascular risk factors in healthy women. *J Clin Endocrinol Metab* 88(4):1617–1623.

Brehm B.J., Spang S.E., et al. 2005. The role of energy expenditure in the differential weight loss in obese women on low-fat and low-carbohydrate diets. *J Clin Endocrinol Metab* 90(3):1475–1482.

Brinkworth G.D., Noakes M., Buckley J.D., Keogh J.B., Clifton P.M. 2009. Long-term effects of a very-low-carbohydrate weight loss diet compared with an isocaloric low-fat diet after 12 mo. *Am J Clin Nutr* 90:23–32.

Brownell, K. 1991. *The LEARN Program for Weight Control: Lifestyle, Exercise, Attitudes, Relationships, Nutrition.* Dallas: American Health Pub.

Burnett K.F., Taylor C.B., et al. 1985. Ambulatory computer-assisted therapy for obesity: A new frontier for behavior therapy. *J Consult Clin Psychol* 53(5):698–703.

Butryn M.L., Phelan S., Hill J.O., Wing R.R. 2007. Consistent self-monitoring of weight: A key component of successful weight loss maintenance. *Obesity* (Silver Spring) 15(12):3091–3096.

Cahill G.F. Jr. 1976. Starvation in man. *Clin Endocrinol Metab* 5(2):397–415.

Campbell W.W., Haub M.D., Wolfe R.R., Ferrando A.A., Sullivan D.H., Apolzan J.W., Iglay H.B. 2009. Resistance training preserves fat-free mass without impacting changes in protein metabolism after weight loss in older women. *Obesity* 17:1332–1339.

Carpenter K.F. 1994. *Protein and Energy: A Study of Changing Ideas in Nutrition*. Cambridge: Cambridge University Press.

Champagne C.M., Bray G.A., et al. 2002. Energy intake and energy expenditure: A controlled study comparing dietitians and non-dietitians. *J Am Diet Assoc* 102(10):1428–1432.

Chomitz V.R., McGowan R.J., Wendel J.M., Williams S.A., Cabral H.J., King S.E., Olcott D.B., Cappello M., Breen S., Hacker K.A. 2010. Healthy living Cambridge kids: A community-based participatory effort to promote healthy weight and fitness. *Obesity* 18(Suppl 1):S45–S53.

Church T.S., Earnest C.P., Skinner J.S., Blair S.N. 2007. Effects of different doses of physical activity on cardiorespiratory fitness among sedentary, overweight or obese postmenopausal women with elevated blood pressure. *JAMA* 2081–2091.

Church T.S., Cheng Y.J., et al. 2004. Exercise capacity and body composition as predictors of mortality among men with diabetes. *Diabetes Care* 27(1):83–88.

Church T.S., Martin C.K., Thompson A.M., Earnest C.P., Mikus C.R., Blair S.N. 2009. Changes in weight, waist circumference and compensatory responses with different doses of exercise among sedentary, overweight postmenopausal women. *PLoS One* 4(2):e4515.

Cordain L., Eaton S.B., et al. 2005. Origins and evolution of the Western diet: Health implications for the 21st century. *Am J Clin Nutr* 81(2):341–354.

Cox K.L., Burke V., et al. 2003. The independent and combined effects of 16 weeks of vigorous exercise and energy restriction on body mass and composition in free-living overweight men—A randomized controlled trial. *Metabolism* 52(1):107–115.

Craddick S.R., Elmer P.J., et al. 2003. The DASH diet and blood pressure. *Curr Atheroscler Rep* 5(6):484–491.

Crespo C.J., Smit E., et al. 2001. Television watching, energy intake, and obesity in US children: Results from the third National Health and Nutrition Examination Survey, 1988–1994. *Arch Pediatr Adolesc Med* 155(3):360–365.

Daniels M.C., Popkin B.M. 2010. The impact of water intake on energy intake and weight status: A review. *Nutr Rev*, in press.

Dansinger M.L., Gleason J.A., et al. 2005. Comparison of the Atkins, Ornish, Weight Watchers, and Zone diets for weight loss and heart disease risk reduction: A randomized trial. *JAMA* 293(1):43–53.

Dansinger M.L., Tatsioni A., Wong J.B., Chung M., Balk E.M. 2007. Meta-analysis: The effect of dietary counseling for weight loss. *Ann Int Med* 147:41–50.

Davidson L.E., Hudson R., Kilpatrick K., Kuk J.L., McMillan K., Janiszewski P.M., Lee S., Lam M., Ross R. 2009. Effects of exercise modality on insulin resistance and functional limitation in older adults. *Arch Int Med* 169:122–131.

Davis N.J., Tomuta N., Schechter C., Isasi C.R., Segal-Isaacson C.J., Stein D., Zonszein J., Wylie-Rosett J. 2009. Comparative study of the effects of a 1-year dietary intervention of a low-carbohydrate diet versus a low-fat diet on weight and glycemic control in type 2 diabetics. *Diabetes Care* 32:1147–1152.

Dawson-Hughes B., Harris S.S., et al. 2004. Effect of dietary protein supplements on calcium excretion in healthy older men and women. *J Clin Endocrinol Metab* 89(3):1169–1173.

De Jonge L., Bray G.A. 1997. The thermic effect of food and obesity: A critical review. *Obes Res* 5:622–631.

DeLany J.P., Bray G.A., et al. 2004. Energy expenditure in African American and white boys and girls in a 2-y follow-up of the Baton Rouge Children's Study. *Am J Clin Nutr* 79(2):268–273.

Despres J.P., Pouliot M.C., et al. 1991. Loss of abdominal fat and metabolic response to exercise training in obese women. *Am J Physiol* 261(2 Pt 1):E159–E167.

Diabetes Prevention Program Research Group. (Wing R.R., Hamman R.F., Bray G.A., Delahanty L., Edelstein S.L., Hill J.O., Horton E.S., Hoskin M.A., Kriska A., Lachin J., Mayer-Davis E.J., Pi-Sunyer X., Regensteiner J.G., Venditti B., Wylie-Rosett J.). 2004. Achieving weight and activity goals among Diabetes Prevention Program lifestyle participants. *Obes Res* 12:1426–1434.

Diabetes Prevention Program Research Group. 2009. 10-year follow-up of diabetes incidence and weight loss in the Diabetes Prevention Program Outcomes Study. *Lancet* 374:1677–1686.

Digenio A.G., Mancuso J.P., Gerer R.A., Dvorak R.V. 2009. Comparison of methods for delivering a lifestyle modification program for obese patients. A randomized trial. *Ann Intern Med* 150:255–262.

Donnelly J.E., Hill J.O., et al. 2003. Effects of a 16-month randomized controlled exercise trial on body weight and composition in young, overweight men and women: The Midwest Exercise Trial. *Arch Intern Med* 163(11):1343–1350.

Donnelly J.E., Blair S.N., Jakicic J.M., Manore M.M., Rankin J.W., Smith B.K. 2009. American College of Sports Medicine. American College of Sports Medicine Position Stand. Appropriate physical activity intervention strategies for weight loss and prevention of weight regain for adults. *Med Sci Sports Exerc* 41(2):459–471.

Dorland W.A.N. 2003. *Dorland's Illustrated Medical Dictionary.* Philadelphia: W.B. Saunders Company.

Douketis J.D., Macie C., Thabane L., Williamson D.F. 2005. Systematic review of long-term weight loss studies in obese adults: Clinical significance and applicability to clinical practice. *Int J Obes* (London) 29(10):1153–1167.

Drewnowski A. 2005. Concept of a nutritious food: Toward a nutrient density score. *Am J Clin Nutr* 82(4):721–732.

Dubois L., Farmer A., Girard M., Peterson K. 2008. Social factors and television use during meals and snacks is associated with higher BMI among pre-school children. *Public Health Nutr* 11:1267–1279.

Due A., Larsen T.M., Mu H., Hermansen K., Stender S., Astrup A. 2008. Comparison of 3 ad libitum diets for weight-loss maintenance, risk of cardiovascular disease, and diabetes: A 6-mo randomized controlled trial. *Am J Clin Nutr* 88:1232–1241.

Due A., Toubro S., et al. 2004. Effect of normal-fat diets, either medium or high in protein, on body weight in overweight subjects: A randomised 1-year trial. *Int J Obes Relat Metab Disord* 28(10):1283–1290.

Due A., Tourbro S., Slender S., Skov A.R., Astrup A. 2005. The effect of diets high in protein or carbohydrate on inflammatory markers in overweight subjects. *Diab Obes Metabol* 7:223–229.

Ebbeling C.B., Leidig M.M., Sinclair K.B., Hangen J.P., Ludwig D.S. 2003. A reduced-glycemic load diet in the treatment of adolescent obesity. *Arch Pediatr Adolesc Med* 157(8):773–779.

Ebbeling C.B., Leidig M.M., Sinclair K.B., Seger-Shippee L.G., Feldman H.A., Ludwig D.S. 2005. Effects of an ad libitum low-glycemic load diet on cardiovascular disease risk factors in obese young adults. *Am J Clin Nutr* 81(5):976–982.

Ebbeling C.B., Leidig M.M., Fedlman H.A., Lovesky M.M., Ludwig D.S. 2007. Effect of a low-glycemic load vs. low-fat diet in obese young adults. *JAMA* 297:1092–2102.

Edholm O.G., Fletcher J.G., et al. 1955. The energy expenditure and food intake of individual men. *Br J Nutr* 9(3):286–300.

Epstein L.H., Valoski A., et al. 1990. Ten-year follow-up of behavioral, family-based treatment for obese children. *JAMA* 264(19):2519–2523.

Esposito K., Pontillo A., et al. 2003. Effect of weight loss and lifestyle changes on vascular inflammatory markers in obese women: A randomized trial. *JAMA* 289(14):1799–1804.

Evans F.A. 1926. A radical cure of simple obesity by dietary measures alone. *Atlantic Med J* 30:140–141.

Ferster C.B., Nurenberger J.I., Levitt E.B. 1962. The control of eating. *J Math* 1:87–109.

Field A.E., Wing R.R., et al. 2001. Relationship of a large weight loss to long-term weight change among young and middle-aged US women. *Int J Obes Relat Metab Disord* 25(8):1113–1121.

Fisler J.S., Drenick E.J. 1987. Starvation and semistarvation diets in the management of obesity. *Annu Rev Nutr* 7:465–484.

Flechtner-Mors M., Ditschuneit H.H., et al. 2000. Metabolic and weight loss effects of long-term dietary intervention in obese patients: Four-year results. *Obes Res* 8(5): 399–402.

Fogelholm M. 2010. Physical activity, fitness and fatness: Relations to mortality, morbidity and disease risk factors. A systematic review. *Obes Rev* 11(3):202–221.

Foreyt J.P., Goodrick G.K. 1991. Factors common to successful therapy for the obese patient. *Med Sci Sports Exerc* 23(3):292–297.

Foster G.D., Wyatt H.R., et al. 2003. A randomized trial of a low-carbohydrate diet for obesity. *N Engl J Med* 348(21):2082–2090.

Foster G.D., Makris A.P., Bailer B.A. 2005. Behavioral treatment of obesity. *Am J Clin Nutr* 82(Suppl 1): 230S–234S.

Foster G.D., Sherman S., Borradaile K.E., Grundy K.M., Vander Veur S.S., Nachmani J., Karpyn A., Kumanyika S., Shults J. 2008. A policy-based school intervention to prevent overweight and obesity. *Pediatrics* 121:794–802.

Fraser A., Abel R., Lawlor D.A., Fraser D., Ethayany A. 2008. A modified Mediterranean diet is associated with the greatest reduction in alanine aminotransferase levels in obese type 2 diabetes ptients: Results of a quasi-randomised controlled trial. *Diabetologia* 51:1616–1622.

Freedman M.R., King J., et al. 2001. Popular diets: A scientific review. *Obes Res* 9(Suppl 1):1S–40S.
Freud S. 1901. *Uber den Traum* Wiesbaden: Verlag von J.F. Bergmann.
Freud S. 1913. *The Interpretation of Dreams.* New York: Macmillan.
Gardner C.D., Kiazand A., Alhassan S., Kim S., Stafford R.S., Balise R.R., Kraemer H.C., King A.C. 2007. Comparison of the Atkins, Zone, Ornish, and LEARN Diets for change in weight and related risk factors among overweight premenopausal women. *JAMA* 297:969–977.
Garrow J.S. 1974. *Energy Balance and Obesity in Man.* Amsterdam: North Holland Publishing Co.
Garrow J.S. 1981. *Treat Obesity Seriously: A Clinical Manual.* New York: Churchill Livingston.
Gibbons R.J., Balady G.J., et al. 1997. ACC/AHA Guidelines for Exercise Testing. A report of the American College of Cardiology/American Heart Association Task Force on Practice Guidelines (Committee on Exercise Testing). *J Am Coll Cardiol* 30(1):260–311.
Gibbons R.J., Balady G.J., et al. 2002. ACC/AHA 2002 Guideline Update for Exercise Testing: Summary article: A report of the American College of Cardiology/American Heart Association Task Force on Practice. *Circ* 106(14):1883–1892.
Gold E.C., Burke S., et al. 2004. Weight loss on the web: A pilot study comparing a commercial website to a structured online behavioral intervention. *Obes Res* 12:A24.
Gorin A.A., Wing R.R., Fava J.L., Jakicic J.M., Jeffrey R., West D.S., Brelje K., DiLillo V.G. 2008. Weight loss treatment influences untreated spouses and the home environment: Evidence of a ripple effect. *Intern J Obes* 32:1678–1684.
Grundy S.M., Blackburn G., et al. 1999. Physical activity in the prevention and treatment of obesity and its comorbidities. *Med Sci Sports Exerc* 31(11 Suppl):S502–S508.
Guare J.C., Wing R.R., et al. 1989. Analysis of changes in eating behavior and weight loss in type II diabetic patients. Which behaviors to change. *Diabetes Care* 12(7):500–503.
Gulick A. 1922. A study of weight regulation in the adult human body during over-nutrition. *Am J Physiol* 60:371–395.
Gutin B., Yin Z., et al. 2005. Relations of moderate and vigorous physical activity to fitness and fatness in adolescents. *Am J Clin Nutr* 81(4):746–750.
Harvey-Berino J., Pintauro S.J., et al. 2002. The feasibility of using Internet support for the maintenance of weight loss. *Behav Modif* 26(1):103–116.
Harvey-Berino J., Pintauro S.J., et al. 2002. Does using the Internet facilitate the maintenance of weight loss? *Int J Obes Relat Metab Disord* 26(9):1254–1260.
Harvey-Berino J., Pintauro S.J., et al. 2004. Effect of internet support on the long-term maintenance of weight loss. *Obes Res* 12(2):320–329.
Hays J.H., DiSabatino et al. 2003. Effect of a high saturated fat and no-starch diet on serum lipid subfractions in patients with documented atherosclerotic cardiovascular disease. *Mayo Clin Proc* 78(11):1331–1336.
Heilbronn L.K., De Jonge L., Frisard M.I., DeLany J.P., Larson-Meyer D.E., Rood J., Nguyen T., Martin C.K., Volaufova J., Most M.M., Greenway F.L., Smith S.R., Deutsch W.A., Williamson D.A., Ravussin E. 2006. Pennington CALERIE Team. Effect of 6-month calorie restriction on biomarkers of longevity, metabolic adaptation, and oxidative stress in overweight individuals: A randomized controlled trial. *JAMA*. 295(13):1539–1548.
Heller R.F. 1993. *The Carbohydrate Addict's Diet: The Lifelong Solution to Yo-Yo Dieting*. New York: Signet.
Heshka S., Anderson J.W., et al. 2003. Weight loss with self-help compared with a structured commercial program: A randomized trial. *JAMA* 289(14):1792–1798.
Heymsfield S.B., Van Mierlo C.A., Knaap H.C., Heo M., Frier H.I. 2003. Weight management using a meal replacement strategy: Meta and pooling analysis from six studies. *Int J Obes* 27:537–549.
Heymsfield S.B., Harp J.B., Reitman M.L., Beetsch J.W., Schoeller D.A., Erondu N., Pietrobelli A. 2007. Why do obese patients not lose more weight when treated with low-calorie diets? A mechanistic perspective. *Am J Clin Nutr* 85:346–354.
HHS. 1996. Physical activity and health: A report of the Surgeon General. Atlanta, GA: U.S. Department of Health and Human Services.
HHS. 2005. *Dietary Guidelines for Americans* 2005. Washington, D.C.: U.S. Department of Health and Human Services. Retrieved 7 April, 2006 from http://www.healthierus.gov/dietaryguidelines.
Hoelscher D.M., Springer A.E., Ranjit N., Perry C.L., Evans A.E., Stigler M., Helder S.H. 2010. Reductions in child obesity among disadvantaged school children with community involvement: The Travis Country CATCH Trial. *Obesity* 18(Suppl 1):S36–S44.
Howard B.V., Manson J.E., et al. 2006. Low-fat dietary pattern and weight change over 7 years: The Women's Health Initiative Dietary Modification Trial. *JAMA* 295(1):39–49.

Hu F.B. 2005. Protein, body weight, and cardiovascular health. *Am J Clin Nutr* 82(1 Suppl):242S–247S.

Hu F.B., Willett W.C., et al. 2004. Adiposity as compared with physical activity in predicting mortality among women. *N Engl J Med* 351(26):2694–2703.

Hu G., Rico-Sanz J., Lakka T.A., Tuomilehto J. 2006. Exercise, genetics and prevention of type 2 diabetes. *Essays Biochem* 42:177–192.

Hunter G.R., Brock D.W., Byrne N.M., Chandler-Laney P.C., Del Corral P., Gower B.A. 2009. Exercise training prevents regain of visceral fat for 1 year following weight loss. *Obesity* (Silver Spring) 18(4):690–695.

Irwin M.L., Yasui Y., et al. 2003. Effect of exercise on total and intra-abdominal body fat in postmenopausal women: A randomized controlled trial. *JAMA* 289(3):323–330.

Jackson D.M., Djafarian K., Stewart J., Speakman J.R. 2009. Increased television viewing is associated with elevated body fatness but not with lower total energy expenditure in children. *Am J Clin Nutr* 89:1031–1036.

Jacobs D.R. Jr, Sluik D., Tokling-Andersen M.H., Anderssen S.A., Drevon C.A. 2009. Association of 1-y changes in diet pattern with cardiovascular disease risk factors and adipokines: Results from 1-y randomized Oslo Diet and Exercise Study. *Am J Clin Nutr* 89:509–517.

Jakicic J.M., Marcus B.H., Gallagher K.I., Napolitano M., Lang W. 2003. Effect of exercise duration and intensity on weight loss in overweight, sedentary women: A randomized trial. *JAMA* 290(10):1323–1330.

Jakicic J.M., Winters C., Lang W., Wing R.R. 1999. Effects of intermittent exercise and use of home exercise equipment on adherence, weight loss, and fitness in overweight women: A randomized trial. *JAMA* 282(16):1554–1560.

Jakicic J.M., Marcus B.H., Lang W., Janney C. 2008. Effect of exercise on 24-month weight loss maintenance in overweight women. *Arch Intern Med* 168(14):1550–1559.

Janssen I., Fortier A., Hudson R., Ross R. 2002. Effects of an energy-restrictive diet with or without exercise on abdominal fat, intermuscular fat, and metabolic risk factors in obese women. *Diabetes Care* 25(3):431–438.

Jeffery R.W., Drewnowski A., et al. 2000. Long-term maintenance of weight loss: Current status. *Health Psychol* 19(1 Suppl):5–16.

Jenkinson C.M., Doherty M., Avery A.J., Read A., Taylor M.A., Sach T.H., Silcocks P., Muir K.R. 2009. Effects of dietary intervention and quadriceps strengthening exercises on pain and function in overeweight people with knee pain: Randomized controlled trial. *BMJ* 339:b3170.

Katzmarzyk P.T., Church T.S., Craig C.L., Bouchard C. 2009. Sitting time and mortality from all causes, cardiovascular disease, and cancer. *Med Sci Sports Exerc* 41(5):998–1005.

Keys A., Brozek J., et al. 1950. *The Biology of Human Starvation*, Vols 1 and 2. Minneapolis: University of Minnesota Press.

Kimm S.Y., Glynn N.W., et al. 2000. Longitudinal changes in physical activity in a biracial cohort during adolescence. *Med Sci Sports Exerc* 32(8):1445–1454.

Kimm S.Y., Glynn N.W., et al. 2002. Decline in physical activity in black girls and white girls during adolescence. *N Engl J Med* 347(10):709–715.

Kinsell L.W., Gunning B., et al. 1964. Calories do count. *Metabolism* 13:195–204.

Klem M.L., Wing R.R., et al. 1997. A descriptive study of individuals successful at long-term maintenance of substantial weight loss. *Am J Clin Nutr* 66(2):239–246.

Knowler W.C., Barrett-Connor E., et al. 2002. Reduction in the incidence of type 2 diabetes with lifestyle intervention or metformin. *N Engl J Med* 346(6):393–403.

Kodama S., Saito K., Tanaka S., Maki M., Yachi Y., Asumi M., Sugawara A., Totsuka K., Shimano H., Ohashi Y., Yamada N., Sone H. 2009. Cardiorespiratory fitness as a quantitative predictor of all-cause mortality and cardiovascular events in healthy men and women: A meta-analysis. *JAMA* 301(19):2024–2035.

Krebs-Smith S.M., Kris-Etherton P. 2007. How does MyPyramid compare to other population-based recommendations for controlling chronic disease? *J Am Diet Assn* 107:830–837.

Kris-Etherton P.M., Pearson T.A., et al. 1999. High-monounsaturated fatty acid diets lower both plasma cholesterol and triacylglycerol concentrations. *Am J Clin Nutr* 70(6):1009–1015.

Kushner R.F., Doerfler B. 2008. Low-carbohydrate, high-protein diets revisited. *Curr Opin Gastroenterol* 24(2):198–203.

Lavoisier A.L. 1789. *Traite elementaire de chemie, presente dan un order nouveau et d'apres les couvertes modernes*. Paris: Chez Cuchet.

Layman D.K., Evans E., et al. 2005. Dietary protein and exercise have additive effects on body composition during weight loss in adult women. *J Nutr* 135(8):1903–1910.

Lee D.-C., Lee I.-M., Sui X., Blair S.N., Church T.S. 2009. Associations of cardiorespiratory fitness and obesity with risks of impaired fasting glucose and type 2 diabetes in men. *Diabetes Care* 32:257–262.

Lee C.D., Blair S.N., et al. 1999. Cardiorespiratory fitness, body composition, and all-cause and cardiovascular disease mortality in men. *Am J Clin Nutr* 69(3):373–380.

Lee L., Kumar S., et al. 1994. The impact of five-month basic military training on the body weight and body fat of 197 moderately to severely obese Singaporean males aged 17 to 19 years. *Int J Obes Relat Metab Disord* 18(2):105–109.

Lee S., Kuk J.L., Davidson L.E., Hudson R., Kilpatrick K., Graham T.E., Ross R. 2005. Exercise without weight loss is an effective strategy for obesity reduction in obese individuals with and without Type 2 diabetes. *J Appl Physiol* 99(3):1220–1225.

Levine J.A., McCrady S.K., Lanningham-Foster L.M., Kane P.H., Foster R.C., Manohar C.U. 2008. The role of free-living daily walking in human weight gain and obesity. *Diabetes* 57:548–554.

Lifson N., Gordon G.B., et al. 1949. The fate of utilized molecular oxygen and the source of the oxygen of respiratory carbon dioxide studied with the aid of heavy oxygen. *J Bio Chem* 180:803–811.

Lin, P.H., Proschan M.A., et al. 2003. Estimation of energy requirements in a controlled feeding trial. *Am J Clin Nutr* 77(3):639–645.

Linde J.A., Jeffery R.W., French S.A., Pronk N.P., Boyle R.G. 2005. Self-weighing in weight gain prevention and weight loss trials. *Ann Behav Med* 30(3):210–216.

Ludwig D.S. 2002. The glycemic index: Physiological mechanisms relating to obesity, diabetes, and cardiovascular disease. *JAMA* 287(18):2414–2423.

Luscombe-Marsh N.D., Noakes M., et al. 2005. Carbohydrate-restricted diets high in either monounsaturated fat or protein are equally effective at promoting fat loss and improving blood lipids. *Am J Clin Nutr* 81(4):762–772.

Lyerly F.W., Sui X., Lavie C.J., Church T.S., Hand G.A., Blair S.N. 2009. The association between cardiorespiratory fitness and risk of all-cause mortality among women with impaired fasting glucose or undiagnosed diaetes mellitus. *Mayo Clin Proc* 84:780–786.

Lyon X.H., Di Vetta V., et al. 1995. Compliance to dietary advice directed towards increasing the carbohydrate to fat ratio of the everyday diet. *Int J Obes Relat Metab Disord* 19(4):260–269.

Magendie F. 1841. Rapport fait á l'Academie des Sciences au nom de la Commission dite "de la gelatine." *C R Acad Sci (Paris)*:237–283.

Manios Y., Kourlaba G., Kondaki K., Grammatikaki E., Anatasiadou A., Roma-Giannikou E. 2009. Obesity and television watching in preschoolers in Greece: The GENESIS Study. *Obesity* 168(7):801–808.

Maynard L.A. 1969. Francis Gano Benedict—A biographical sketch. *J Nutr* 98:1–8.

McCollum E.V. 1957. *A History of Nutrition. The Sequence of Ideas in Nutrition Investigations*. Boston: Houghton Mifflin Co.

McLean N., Griffin S., et al. 2003. Family involvement in weight control, weight maintenance and weight-loss interventions: A systematic review of randomised trials. *Int J Obes Relat Metab Disord* 27(9):987–1005.

McMillan-Price J., Petocz P., Atkinson F., O'Neill K., Samman S., Steinbeck K., Caterson I., Brand-Miller J. 2006. Comparison of 4 diets of varying glycemic load on weight loss and cardiovascular risk reduction in overweight and obese young adults: A randomized controlled trial. *Arch Intern Med* 166(14):1466–1475.

Mekary R.A., Feskanich D., Hu F.B., Willett W.C., Field A.E. 2009. Physical activity in relation to long-term weight maintenance after intentional weight loss in premenopausal women. *Obesity* (Silver Spring) 18(1):167–174.

Micco M., Gold E.C., et al. 2004. Internet weight loss: Stand-alone intervention or adjunct to traditional behavioral treatment? *Obes Res* 12:A24.

Miller W.C., Koceja D.M., et al. 1997. A meta-analysis of the past 25 years of weight loss research using diet, exercise or diet plus exercise intervention. *Int J Obes Relat Metab Disord* 21(10):941–947.

Mintz S.W. 1986. *Sweetness and Power: The Place of Sugar in Modern History*. New York: Penguin.

Mitchell H.S. 1966. Ivan Petrovich Pavlov—A biographical sketch. *J Nutr* 88:3–8.

Moore M.E., Stunkard A.J., Srole L. 1962. Obesity, social class, and mental illness. *JAMA* 181:962–966.

Moore T., Svetkey L.P., et al. 2003. *The DASH Diet for Hypertension*. New York: Simon & Schuster.

Napolitano M.A., Fotheringham M., et al. 2003. Evaluation of an internet-based physical activity intervention: A preliminary investigation. *Ann Behav Med* 25(2):92–99.

National Institutes of Health, National Heart, and Blood Institute, et al. 2000. *Practical Guide in Identification, Evaluation and Treatment of Overweight and Obesity in Adults.* Washington, DC: National Institutes of Health.

Neumann R.O. 1902. Experimentel Beitrage zur Lehre von dem taglichen Nahrungsbedarf des Menschen unter besonderer Berucksichtigung der notwendigen Eiweifsmenge. *Arch Hyg* 45:1–87.

NLM. 2005. *Dietary Fats*. Bethesda, MD: U.S. National Library of Medicine. Retrieved 10 April, 2006 from http://www.nlm.nih.gov/medlineplus/dietaryfats.html.

Noakes M., Keogh J.B., et al. 2005. Effect of an energy-restricted, high-protein, low-fat diet relative to a conventional high-carbohydrate, low-fat diet on weight loss, body composition, nutritional status, and markers of cardiovascular health in obese women. *Am J Clin Nutr* 81(6):1298–1306.

Nordmann A.J., Nordmann A., et al. 2006. Effects of low-carbohydrate vs low-fat diets on weight loss and cardiovascular risk factors: A meta-analysis of randomized controlled trials. *Arch Intern Med* 166(3):285–293.

Norris S.L., Zhang X., et al. 2004. Long-term effectiveness of lifestyle and behavioral weight loss interventions in adults with type 2 diabetes: A meta-analysis. *Am J Med* 117(10):762–774.

Ornish D. 1993. *Eat More, Weigh Less: Dr. Dean Ornish's Life Choice Program for Losing Weight Safely while Eating Abundantly*. New York: HarperCollins.

Ostman M., Britton E., Jonsson E. 2004. *Physical Exercise. Treating and Preventing Obesity*. Weinheim, Germany: Wiley-VCH Verlag GmbH & Co. KgaA, pp 142–143.

Paffenbarger R.S. Jr, Hyde R.T., et al. 1993. The association of changes in physical-activity level and other lifestyle characteristics with mortality among men. *N Engl J Med* 328(8):538–545.

Parsons A.C., Shraim M., Inglis J., Aveyard P., Hajek P. 2009. Interventions for prevening weight gain after smoking cessation. Cochrane Database of Systematic Reviews, Issue 1. Art. No.: CD006219. DOI:10.1002/14651858.CD006219.pub2.

Pavlov I.P. 1902. *The Work of the Digestive Glands*. Transl. W.H. Thompson. London: Charles Griffin & Company, Ltd.

Pavlov I.P. 1927. *Conditioned Reflexes: An Investigation of the Physiological Activity of the Cerebral Cortex*. London: Oxford University Press.

Pereira M.A., Swain J., et al. 2004. Effects of a low-glycemic load diet on resting energy expenditure and heart disease risk factors during weight loss. *JAMA* 292(20):2482–2490.

Perri M.G., Nezu A.M., Viegener B.J. 1992. *Improving the Long-Term Management of Obesity: Theory, Research, and Clinical Guidelines*. New York: Wiley.

Perri M.G. 1998. The maintenance of treatment effects in the long-term management of obesity. *Clinical Psychology: Science and Practice* 5:526–543.

Perri M.G, Limacher M.C., Durning P.E., Janicke D.M., Lutes L.D., Bobroff L.B., Dale M.S., Daniels M.J., Radcliff T.A., Marton A.D. 2008. Extended-care programs for weight management in rural communities. *Arch Intern Med* 168:2347–2354.

Phelan S., Liu T., Gorin A., Lowe M., Hogan J., Fava J., Wing R.R. 2009. What distinguishes weight-loss maintainers from the treatment-seeking obese? Analysis of environmental, behavioral, and psychosocial variables in diverse populations. *Ann Behav Med* 38(2):94–104.

Phelan S., Lang W., Jordan D., Wing R.R. 2009. Use of artificial sweeteners and fat-modified foods in weight loss maintainers and always-normal weight individuals. *Int J Obes* (London) 33(10):1183–1190.

Phillips M.M., Raczynski J.M., West D.S., Pulley L.V., Bursac Z., Gauss C.H., Walker J.F. 2010. Changes in school environments with implementation of Arkansas Act 1220 of 2003. *Obesity* 18(Suppl 1): S54–S61.

Pirozzo S., Summerbell C., et al. 2003. Should we recommend low-fat diets for obesity? *Obes Rev* 4(2):83–90.

Pi-Sunyer X., Blackburn G., Brancati F.L., Bray G.A., Bright R., Clark J.M., Curtis J.M., Espeland M.A., Foreyt J.P., Graves K., Haffner S.M., Harrison B., Hill J.O., Horton E.S., Jakicic J., Jeffery R.W., Johnson K.C., Kahn S., Kelley D.E., Kitabchi A.E., Knowler W.C., Lewis C.E., Maschak-Carey B.J., Montgomery B., Nathan D.M., Patricio J., Peters A., Redmon J.B., Reeves R.S., Ryan D.H., Safford M., Van Dorsten B., Wadden T.A., Wagenknecht L., Wesche–Thorbaben J., Wing R.R., Yanovski S.Z. 2007. Reduction in weight and cardiovascular disease (CVD) risk factors in individuals with Type 2 Diabetes: One year results of Look AHEAD Trial. *Diabetes Care* 30:1374–1383.

Polivy J., Herman C.P. 2002. If at first you don't succeed. False hopes of self-change. *Am Psychol* 57(9):677–689.

Popkin B.M., Armstrong L.E., et al. 2006. A new proposed guidance system for beverage consumption in the United States. *Am J Clin Nutr* 83(3):529–542.

Popkin B.M., D'Ancie K.E., Rosenberg I.H. 2010. Water, hydration and health. *Nutr Rev* in press.

Popper H. 1962. *Conjectures and Refutations: The Growth of Scientific Knowledge*. New York: Basic Books.

Pritchard J.E., Nowson C.A., et al. 1997. A worksite program for overweight middle-aged men achieves lesser weight loss with exercise than with dietary change. *J Am Diet Assoc* 97(1):37–42.

Pritikin R. 1991. *The New Pritikin Program: The Easy and Delicious Way to Shed Fat, Lower Your Cholesterol, and Stay Fit*. New York: Pocket Books.

Rankinen T., Bouchard C. 2008. Gene-physical activity interactions: Overview of human studies. *Obesity* 16 (Suppl 1):S47–S50.

Reddy S.T., Wang C.Y., et al. 2002. Effect of low-carbohydrate high-protein diets on acid-base balance, stone-forming propensity, and calcium metabolism. *Am J Kidney Dis* 40(2):265–274.

Robinson T.N. 1999. Reducing children's television viewing to prevent obesity: A randomized controlled trial. *JAMA* 282(16):1561–1567.

Rock C.L., Piaz B., Flatt S.W., Quintana E.L. 2007. Randomized trial of a multifaceted commercial weight loss program. *Obesity* 15:939–949.

Rolls B.J., Barnett R.A. 2000. *Volumetrics: Feel Full on Fewer Calories*. New York, NY: HarperCollins.

Ross R., Dagnone D., Jones P.J., et al. 2000. Reduction in obesity and related comorbid conditions after diet-induced weight loss or exercise-induced weight loss in men. A randomized, controlled trial. *Ann Intern Med* 133:92.

Ross R., Janssen I., Dawson J., Kungl A.M., Kuk J.L., Wong S.L., Nguyen-Duy T.B., Lee S., Kilpatrick K., Hudson R. 2004. Exercise-induced reduction in obesity and insulin resistance in women: A randomized controlled trial. *Obes Res* 12(5):789–798.

Sacher P.M., Kolotourou M., Chadwick P.M., Cole T.J., Lawson M.S., Lucas A., Singhal A. 2010. Randomized controlled trial of the MEND program: A family-based community intervention for childhood obesity. *Obesity* 18(Suppl 1):S62–S74.

Sacks F.M., Bray G.A., Carey V., Smith S.R., Ryan D.H., Anton S., McManus K., Champagne C.M., Bishop L.N., Laranjo N., Leboff M.S., Rood J.C., Levitan L.D., Greenway F.L., Loria C.M., Obarzanek E., Williamson D.A. 2009. Comparison of weight-loss diets with different compositions of fat, carbohydrate and protein. *N Engl J Med* 360(9):859–873.

Sacks F.M., Svetkey L.P., et al. 2001. Effects on blood pressure of reduced dietary sodium and the Dietary Approaches to Stop Hypertension (DASH) diet. DASH–Sodium Collaborative Research Group. *N Engl J Med* 344(1):3–10.

Saelens B.E., Sallis J.F., et al. 2003. Neighborhood-based differences in physical activity: An environment scale evaluation. *Am J Public Health* 93(9):1552–1558.

Samaha F.F., Iqbal N., et al. 2003. A low-carbohydrate as compared with a low-fat diet in severe obesity. *N Engl J Med* 348(21):2074–2081.

Samaras K., Kelly P.J., et al. 1999. Genetic and environmental influences on total-body and central abdominal fat: The effect of physical activity in female twins. *Ann Intern Med* 130(11):873–882.

Schoeller D.A. 2003. But how much physical activity? *Am J Clin Nutr* 78:669–670.

Schoeller D.A., Field C.R. 1991. Human energy metabolism: What have we learned from the doubly labeled water method? *Annu Rev Nutr* 11:355–373.

Schoeller D.A., Shay K., et al. 1997. How much physical activity is needed to minimize weight gain in previously obese women? *Am J Clin Nutr* 66(3):551–556.

Schoeller D.A., Buchholz A.C. 2005. Energetics of obesity and weight control: Does diet composition matter? *J Am Dietet Assoc* 105:S24–S28.

Shai I., Schwarzfuchs D., Henkin Y., Shahar D.R., Witkow S., Greenberg I., Golan R., Fraser D., Bolotin A., Vardi H., Tangi-Rozental O., Zuk-Ramot R., Sarusi B., Brickner D., Schwartz Z., Sheiner E., Marko R., Katorza E., Thiery J., Fiedler G.M., Blüher M., Stumvoll M., Stampfer M.J. 2008. Dietary intervention randomized controlled trial (DIRECT) group. Weight loss with a low-carbohydrate, Mediterranean, or low-fat diet. *N Engl J Med* 359(3):229–241.

Skinner B.F. 1953. *Science and Human Behavior*. New York: Macmillan.

Skinner B.F. 1988. The operant side of behavior therapy. *J Behav Ther Exp Psychiatry* 19:171.

Skov A.R., Toubro S., et al. 1999. Randomized trial on protein vs carbohydrate in ad libitum fat reduced diet for the treatment of obesity. *Int J Obes Relat Metab Disord* 23(5):528–536.

Slabber M., Barnard H.C., Kuyl J.M., Dannhauser A., Schall R. 1994. Effects of a low-insulin-response, energy-restricted diet on weight loss and plasma insulin concentrations in hyperinsulinemic obese females. *Am J Clin Nutr* 60(1):48–53.

Slentz C.A., Duscha B.D., et al. 2004. Effects of the amount of exercise on body weight, body composition, and measures of central obesity: STRRIDE—A randomized controlled study. *Arch Intern Med* 164(1):31–39.

Sloth B., Krog-Mikkelsen I., Flint A., Tetens I., Björck I., Vinoy S., Elmståhl H., Astrup A., Lang V., Raben A. 2004. No difference in body weight decrease between a low-glycemic-index and a high-glycemic-index diet but reduced LDL cholesterol after 10-wk ad libitum intake of the low-glycemic-index diet. *Am J Clin Nutr* 80(2):337–347.

Sours H.E., Frattali V.P., Brand C.D., Feldman R.A., Forbes A.L., Swanson R.C., Paris A.L. 1981. Sudden death associated with very low calorie weight reduction regimens. *Am J Clin Nutr* 34:453–461.

Stern L., Iqbal N., et al. 2004. The effects of low-carbohydrate versus conventional weight loss diets in severely obese adults: One-year follow-up of a randomized trial. *Ann Intern Med* 140(10):778–785.

Stevens J., Evenson K.R., et al. 2004. Associations of fitness and fatness with mortality in Russian and American men in the lipids research clinics study. *Int J Obes Relat Metab Disord* 28(11):1463–1470.

Stevenson L.G. 1953. *Nobel Prize Winners in Medicine & Physiology 1901–1950*. New York: Henry Schuman.

Steward H.L., Bethea M.C., Andrew S.S., Balart L.A. 2002. *The New Sugar Busters! Cut Sugar to Trim Fat*. New York: Ballantine.

Stolley M.R., Fitzgibbon M.L., Schiffer L., Sharp L.K., Singh V., van Horn L., Dyer A. 2009. Obesity Reduction Black Intervention Trial (ORBIT): Six-month results. *Obesity* 17:100–106.

Stookey J.D., Constant F., Gardner C.D., Popkin B.M. 2007. Replacing sweetened caloric beverages with drinking water is associated with lower energy intake. *Obesity* (Silver Spring) 15(12):3013–3022.

Stookey J.D., Constant F., Popkin B.M., Gardner C.D. 2008. Drinking water is associated with weight loss in overweight dieting women independent of diet and activity. *Obesity* (Silver Spring) 16(11):2481–2488.

Stuart R.B. 1967. Behavioral control of overeating. *Behav Res Ther* 5:357–365.

Stuart R.B., Davis B. 1972. *Slim Chance in a Fat World*. Champaign, IL: Research Press Co.

Stubbe J.H., Boomsma D.I., et al. 2005. Sports participation during adolescence: A shift from environmental to genetic factors. *Med Sci Sports Exerc* 37(4):563–570.

Stunkard A.J., Mendelson M. 1967. Obesity and the body image. I. Characteristics of disturbances in the body image of some obese persons. *Am J Psychiatr* 123:1296–1300.

Sui X., LaMonte M.J., Laditka J.N., Hardin J.W., Chase N., Hooker S.P., Blair S.N. 2007. Cardiorespiratory fitness and adiposity as mortality predictors in older adults. *JAMA* 298(21):2507–2516.

Svetkey L.P., Stevens V.J., Brantley P.J., et al. 2008. Comparison of strategies for sustaining weight loss. The Weight Loss Maintenance Randomized Controlled Trial. *JAMA* 299:1139–1148.

Swinburn B., Shelly A. 2008. Effects of TV time and other sedentary pursuits. *Int J Obes* (London) 32(Suppl 7): S132–S136.

Swinburn B.A., Sacks G., Lo S.K., Westerterp K.R., Rush E.C., Rosenbaum M., Luke A., Schoeller D.A., DeLany J.P., Butte N.F., Ravussin E. 2009. *Am J Clin Nutr* 89(6):1723–1728.

Swinburn B., Sacks G., Ravussin E. 2009. Increased food energy supply is more than sufficient to explain the US epidemic of obesity. *Am J Clin Nutr* 90(6):1453–1456.

Talbott J.H. 1970. *A Biographical History of Medicine. Excerpts and Essays on the Men and Their Work*. New York: Grune & Stratton, p 903.

Tate D.F., Jackvony E.H., et al. 2003. Effects of Internet behavioral counseling on weight loss in adults at risk for type 2 diabetes: A randomized trial. *JAMA* 289(14):1833–1836.

Tate D.F., Wing R.R., et al. 2001. Using Internet technology to deliver a behavioral weight loss program. *JAMA* 285(9):1172–1177.

Thomas D.E., Elliott E.J., Baur L. 2007. Low glycemic index or low glycemic load diets for overweight and obesity (Review). *Cochrane Database of Systematic Reviews* Issue 3 Art No.: CD005105. DOI: 10.1002/14651858.CD005105.pub2.

Tinker L.F., Bonds D.E., Margolis K.L., et al. 2008. Low-fat dietary pattern and risk of treatment diabetes mellitus in postmenopausal women. *Arch Intern Med* 168:1500–1511.

Tooze J.A., Schoeller D.A., Subar A.F., Kipnis V., Schatzkin A., Troiano R.P. 2007. Total daily energy expenditure among middle-aged men and women: The OPEN Study. *Am J Clin Nutr* 86:382–387.

Treyzon L., Chen S., Hong K., Yan E., Carpenter C.L., Thames G., Bowerman S., Wang H.-J., Elashoff R., Li Z. 2008. A controlled trial of protein enrichment of meal replacements for weight reduction with retention of lean body mass. *Nutr J* 7:23–28.

Tsai A.G., Wadden T.A. 2005. Systematic review: An evaluation of major commercial weight loss programs in the United States. *Ann Intern Med* 142(1):56–66.

Tsai A.G., Wadden T.A. 2006. The evolution of very-low-calorie diets: An update and meta-analysis. *Obesity* (Silver Spring) 14(8):1283–1293.

Tsai A.M., Wadden T.A. 2009. Treatment of obesity in primary care practice in the United States: A systematic review. *J Gen Intern Med* 24:1072–1079.

Turk M.W., Yang K., Hravnak M., Sereika S.M., Ewing L.J., Burke L.E. 2009. Randomized clinical trials of weight loss maintenance: A review. *J Cardiovasc Nurs* 24(1):58–80.

Venditti E.M., Bray G.A., Carrion-Peterson M.L., Delahanty L.M., Edelstein S.L., Hamman R.F., Hoskin M.A., Knowler W.C., Ma Y., for the Diabetes Prevention Research Group. 2008. First versus repeat treatment with a lifestyle intervention program: Attendance and weight loss outcomes. *Intern J Obes* 32:1537–1664.

Villareal D.T., Fondata F., Weiss E.P., Racette S.B., Steger-May K., Schechtman K.B., Klein S., Holloszy J.O. 2006. Bone mineral density response to calorie restriction-induced weight loss or exericise-induced weight loss. *Arch Int Med* 166:2502–2510.

Volpp K.G., John L.K., Troxel A.B., Norton L., Fassbender J., Lowenstein G. 2008. Financial incentive-based approaches for weight loss. A randomized trial. *JAMA* 300:2631–2637.

Wadden T.A., Foster G.D., et al. 1992. A multicenter evaluation of a proprietary weight reduction program for the treatment of marked obesity. *Arch Intern Med* 200152(5):961–966.

Wadden T.A., Vogt R.A., et al. 1997. Exercise in the treatment of obesity: Effects of four interventions on body composition, resting energy expenditure, appetite, and mood. *J Consult Clin Psychol* 65(2):269–277.

Wadden T.A., Berkowitz R.I., Womble L.G., Sarwer D.B., Phelan S., Cato R.K., Hesson L.A., Osei S.Y., Kaplan R., Stunkard A.J. 2005. Randomized trial of lifestyle modification and pharmacotherapy for obesity. *N Engl J Med* 353(20):2111–2120.

Wadden T.A., Butryn M.L., Wilson C. 2007. Lifestyle modification for the management of obesity. *Gastroenterology* 132(6):2226–2238.

Wadden T.A., West D.S., Neiberg R.H., Wing R.R., Ryan D.H., Johnson K.C., Foreyt J.P., Hill J.O., Trence D.L., Vitolins M.Z., Look AHEAD Research Group. 2009. One-year weight losses in the Look AHEAD study: Factors associated with success. *Obesity* (Silver Spring) 17(4):713–722.

Wagner A., Simon C., et al. 2001. Leisure-time physical activity and regular walking or cycling to work are associated with adiposity and 5-y weight gain in middle-aged men: The PRIME Study. *Int J Obes Relat Metab Disord* 25(7):940–948.

Walsh M.F., Flynn T.J. 1995. A 54-month evaluation of a popular very low calorie diet program. *J Fam Pract* 41(3):231–236.

Wansink B., Van Ittersum K. 2007. Portion size me: Downsizing our consumption norms. *J Am Diet Assn* 1103–1106.

Wei M., Kampert J.B., et al. 1999. Relationship between low cardiorespiratory fitness and mortality in normal-weight, overweight, and obese men. *JAMA* 282(16):1547–1553.

Weiss E.P., Racette S.B., Villareal D.T., Fontana L., Steger-May K., Schechtman K.B., Klein S., Ehsani A.A., Holloszy J.O. 2007. Lower extremity muscle size and strength and aerobic capacity decrease with caloric restriction but not with exercise-induced weight loss. *J Appl Physiol* 102:634–640.

Westerterp K.R. 2009. Assessment of physical activity: A critical appraisal. *Eur J Appl Physiol* 105(6):823–828.

Westerterp K.R., Plasqui G. 2009. Physically active lifestyle does not decrease the risk of fattening. *PLoS One* 4(3):e4745.

Westerterp K.R., Speakman J.R. 2008. Physical activity energy expenditure has not declined since the 1980s and matches energy expenditures of wild mammals. *Int J Obes* (London) 32(8):1256–1263.

Westerterp-Plantenga M.S., Lejeune M.P., et al. 2004. High protein intake sustains weight maintenance after body weight loss in humans. *Int J Obes Relat Metab Disord* 28(1):57–64.

Westerterp-Plantenga M.S., Nieuwenhuizen A., Tomé D., Soenen S., Westerterp K.R. 2009. Dietary protein, weight loss, and weight maintenance. *Annu Rev Nutr* 29:21–41.

Willett W.C. 2004. Reduced-carbohydrate diets: No roll in weight management? *Ann Intern Med* 140(10):836–837.

Williamson D.A., Rejeski J., Lang W., Dorsten B.V., Fabricatore A.N., Toledo K. 2009. Impact of a weight management program on health-related quality of life in overweight adults with type 2 diabetes. *Arch Int Med* 169:163–171.

Williamson D.A., Walden H.M., White M.A., York-Crow E., Newton R.L. Jr, Alfonso A., Gordon S., Ryan D. 2006. Two-year internet-based randomized controlled trial for weight loss in African-American girls. *Obesity* 14:1231–1243.

Williamson D.A., Martin C.K., et al. 2006. Behavioral strategies for controlling obesity. In *Overweight and the Metabolic Syndrome: From Bench to Bedside*, G.A. Bray, D.H. Ryan, eds. Boston: Springer, pp 219–232.

Williamson D.A., Martin P.D., et al. 2005. Efficacy of an internet-based behavioral weight loss program for overweight adolescent African-American girls. *Eat Weight Disord* 10(3):193–203.

Williamson D.A., Anton S.D., Han H., Champagne C.M., Allen R., Leblanc E., Ryan D.H., McManus K., Laranjo N., Carey V.J., Loria C.M., Bray G.A., Sacks F.M. 2009. Adherence is a multi-dimensional construct in the POUNDS LOST trial. *J Behav Med* (33)1:35–46.

Williamson D., Ryan D.H., Harsha D., Martin C.K., Newton R., Stewart T., Han H. *Louisiana Health Study* (LA Health).

Williamson D.F., Madans J., et al. 1993. Recreational physical activity and ten-year weight change in a US national cohort. *Int J Obes Relat Metab Disord* 17(5):279–286.

Wiley F.H., Newburgh L.H. 1931. The doubtful nature of "Luxuskonsumption." *J Clin Invest* 10:733–744.

Winett R.A., Tate D.F., et al. 2005. Long-term weight gain prevention: A theoretically based Internet approach. *Prev Med* 41(2):629–641.

Wing R.R. 2004. Behavioral approaches to the treatment of obesity. *Handbook of Obesity: Clinical Applications*. G. Bray and C. Bouchard. New York: Marcel Dekker, Inc., pp 147–167.

Wing R.R., Hamman R.F., et al. 2004. Achieving weight and activity goals among diabetes prevention program lifestyle participants. *Obes Res* 12(9):1426–1434.

Wing R.R., Phelan S. 2005. Long-term weight loss maintenance. *Am J Clin Nutr* 82(1 Suppl): 222S–225S.

Wing R.R., Tate D.F., Gorin A.A., Raynor H.A., Fava J.L. 2006. A self-regulation program for maintenance of weight loss. *N Engl J Med* 355:1563–1571.

Wing R.R., Papandonatos G., Fava J.L., Gorin A.A., Phelan S., McCaffery J., Tate D.F. 2008. Maintaining large weight losses: The role of behavioral and psychological factors. *J Consult Clin Psychol* 76(6):1015–1021.

Wing R.R., Tate D.F., Gorin A.A., Raynor H.A., Fava J.L., Machan J. 2007. STOP regain: Are there negative effects of daily weighing? *J Consult Clin Psychol* 75(4):652–656.

Wing R.R., Papandonatos G., Fava J.L., Gorin A.A., Phelan S., McCaffery J., Tate D.F. 2008. Maintaining large weight losses: The role of behavioral and psychological factors. *J Consult Clin Psychol* 76(6):1015–1021.

Womble L.G., Wadden T.A., et al. 2004. A randomized controlled trial of a commercial internet weight loss program. *Obes Res* 12(6):1011–1018.

Wood P.D., Stefanick M.L., et al. 1988. Changes in plasma lipids and lipoproteins in overweight men during weight loss through dieting as compared with exercise. *N Engl J Med* 319(18):1173–1179.

Wood P.D., Stefanick M.L., et al. 1991. The effects on plasma lipoproteins of a prudent weight-reducing diet, with or without exercise, in overweight men and women. *N Engl J Med* 325(7): 461–466.

Yancy W.S. Jr, Olsen M.K., et al. 2004. A low-carbohydrate, ketogenic diet versus a low-fat diet to treat obesity and hyperlipidemia: A randomized, controlled trial. *Ann Intern Med* 140(10): 769–777.

CHAPTER 7

Alemany M., Fernandez-Lopez J.A., et al. 2003. Weight loss in a patient with morbid obesity under treatment with oleoyl-estrone. *Med Clin* (Barc) 121(13):496–499.

Amori R.E., Lau J., Pittas A.G. 2007. Efficacy and safety of incretin therapy in type 2 diabetes: Systematic review and meta-analysis. *JAMA* 298:194–206.

Anderson J.W., Greenway F.L., et al. 2002. Bupropion SR enhances weight loss: A 48-week double-blind, placebo-controlled trial. *Obes Res* 10(7):633–641.

Anderson J.W., Schwartz S.M., Hauptman J., Boldrin M., Rossi M., Bansal V., Hale C.A. 2006. Low-dose orlistat effects on body weight of mildly to moderately overweight individuals: A 16-week, double-blind, placebo-controlled trial. *Ann Pharmacother* 40(10):1717–1723.

Anderson K.D., Lambert P.D., et al. 2003. Activation of the hypothalamic arcuate nucleus predicts the anorectic actions of ciliary neurotrophic factor and leptin in intact and gold thioglucose-lesioned mice. *J Neuroendocrinol* 15(7):649–660.

Andersson C., Weeke P., Fosbøl E.L., Brendorp B., Køber L., Coutinho W., Sharma A.M., Van Gaal L., Finer N., James W.P., Caterson I.D., Rode R.A., Torp-Pedersen C., on behalf of the SCOUT Executive Steering Committee and the SCOUT investigators. 2009. Acute effect of weight loss on levels of total bilirubin in obese, cardiovascular high-risk patients: An analysis from the lead-in period of the Sibutramine Cardiovascular Outcome trial. *Metabolism* 58(8):1109–1115.

Anonymous. 1996. Dexfenfluramine for obesity. *Med Lett Drugs Ther* 38(979):64–65.

Apfelbaum M., Vague P., et al. 1999. Long-term maintenance of weight loss after a very-low-calorie diet: A randomized blinded trial of the efficacy and tolerability of sibutramine. *Am J Med* 106(2):179–184.

Apovian C., Bergenstal R., Cuddihy R., Qu Y., Lenox S., Lewis M., Glass L. 2009. Effect of exenatide versus placebo on weight loss in patients with type 2 diabetes participating in an intensive lifestyle modification program. *Diabetes Care*.

Arena Pharmaceuticals. 2005. Safety and efficacy of APD356 in the treatment of obesity. ClinicalTrials.gov Identifier: NCT00104507.

Aronne L.J., Halseth A.E., Burns C.M., Miller S., Shen L.Z. 2010. Enhanced weight loss following coadministration of pramlintide with sibutramine or phentermine in a multicenter trial. *Obesity* (Silver Spring) 18(9):1739–1746. Epub 2010 Jan 21.

Astrand A., Bohlooly Y.M., et al. 2004. Mice lacking melanin-concentrating hormone receptor 1 demonstrate increased heart rate associated with altered autonomic activity. *Am J Physiol Regul Integr Comp Physiol* 287(4):R749–R758.

Astrup A., Breum L., et al. 1992. The effect and safety of an ephedrine/caffeine compound compared to ephedrine, caffeine and placebo in obese subjects on an energy restricted diet. A double blind trial. *Int J Obes Relat Metab Disord* 16(4):269–277.

Astrup A., Caterson I., et al. 2004. Topiramate: Long-term maintenance of weight loss induced by a low-calorie diet in obese subjects. *Obes Res* 12(10):1658–1669.

Astrup A., Greenway F.L., Ling W., Pedicone L., Lachowicz J., Strader C.D., Kwan R., for the Ecopipam Obesity Study Group. 2007. Randomized controlled trials of the D1/D5 antagonist ecopipam for weight loss in obese subjects. *Obesity* 15:1717–1731.

Astrup A., Madsbad S., Breum L., Jensen T.J., Kroustrup J.P., Larsen T.M. 2008. Effect of tesofensine on bodyweight loss, body composition, and quality of life in obese patients: A randomised, double-blind, placebo-controlled trial. *Lancet* 372(9653):1906–1913.

Astrup A., Meier D.H., Mikkelsen B.O., Villumsen J.S., Larsen T.M. 2008. Weight loss produced by tesofensine in patients with Parkinson's or Alzheimer's disease. *Obesity* (Silver Spring) 16(6):1363–1369.

Astrup A., Rössner S., Van Gaal L., Rissanen A., Niskanen L., Al Hakim M., Madsen J., Rasmussen M.F., Lean M.E. 2009. NN8022-1807 Study Group. Effects of liraglutide in the treatment of obesity: A randomised, double-blind, placebo-controlled study. *Lancet* 374(9701):1606–1616.

Astrup A., Toubro S. 2004. Topiramate: A new potential pharmacological treatment for obesity. *Obes Res* 12(Suppl):167S–173S.

Avenell A., Brown T.J., et al. 2004. What interventions should we add to weight reducing diets in adults with obesity? A systematic review of randomized controlled trials of adding drug therapy, exercise, behaviour therapy or combinations of these interventions. *J Hum Nutr Diet* 17(4):293–316.

Avenell A., Broom J., Brown T.J., Poobalan A., Aucott L., Stearns S.C., Smith W.C.S., Jung R.T., Campbell M.K., Grant A.M. 2004. Systematic review of the long-term effects and economic consequences of treatments for obesity and implication for health improvement. *Health Technol Assess* 8(21):i–x; 1–458.

Barak N., Greenway F.L., Fujioka K., Aronne L.J., Kushner R.F. 2008. Effect of histaminergic manipulation on weight in obese adults: A randomized placebo controlled trial. *Intern J Obes* 32:1559–1565.

Barkeling B., Elfhag K., et al. 2003. Short-term effects of sibutramine (Reductil) on appetite and eating behaviour and the long-term therapeutic outcome. *Int J Obes Relat Metab Disord* 27(6):693–700.

Baranowska B., Wolinska-Witort E., Martynska L., et al. 2005. Sibutramine therapy in obese women—Effects on plasma neuropeptide Y (NPY), insulin, leptin and beta-endorphin concentrations. *Neuro Endocrinol Lett* 26:675–679.

Barr S.I. 2003. Increased dairy product or calcium intake: Is body weight or composition affected in humans? *J Nutr* 133(1):245S–248S.

Batterham R.L., Cohen M.A., et al. 2003. Inhibition of food intake in obese subjects by peptide YY3–36. *N Engl J Med* 349(10):941–948.

Bays H., Dujovne C. 2002. Anti-obesity drug development. *Expert Opin Investig Drugs* 11(9):1189–1204.

Belza A., Frandsen E., Kondrug J. 2007. Body fat loss achieved by stimulation of thermogenesis by a combination of bioactive food ingredients: A placebo-controlled, double-blind 8-week intervention in obese subjects. *Intern J Obes* 31:121–130.

Belza A., Toubro S., Astrup A. 2006. The acute effect of tyrosine and green tea on appetite and thermogenesis. *Obes Rev* 7(Suppl 2):Abs.

Ben-Menachem E., Axelsen M., et al. 2003. Predictors of weight loss in adults with topiramate-treated epilepsy. *Obes Res* 11(4):556–562.

Bensaid M., Gary-Bobo M., et al. 2003. The cannabinoid CB1 receptor antagonist SR141716 increases Acrp30 mRNA expression in adipose tissue of obese fa/fa rats and in cultured adipocyte cells. *Mol Pharmacol* 63(4):908–914.

Bent S., Padula A., et al. 2004. Safety and efficacy of citrus aurantium for weight loss. *Am J Cardiol* 94(10):1359–1361.

Berkowitz R., Fujioka K., et al. 2006. Weight loss in adolescents treated with sibutramine: A randomized, placebo-controlled trial. *Annals of Internal Medicine,* in press.

Berkowitz R.I., Wadden T.A., et al. 2003. Behavior therapy and sibutramine for the treatment of adolescent obesity: A randomized controlled trial. *JAMA* 289(14):1805–1812.

Birkenfeld A.L., Schroeder C., Boschmann M., Tank J., Franke G., Luft F.C., Biaggioni I., Sharma A.M., Jordan J. 2002. Paradoxical effect of sibutramine on autonomic cardiovascular regulation. *Circ* 106:2459–2465.

Birkenfeld A.L., Schroeder C., Pischon T., Tank J., Luft F.C., Sharma A.M., Jordan J. 2005. Paradoxical effect of sibutramine on autonomic cardiovascular regulation in obese hypertensive patients—Sibutramine and blood pressure. *Clin Auton Res* 15:200–206.

Boeles S., Williams C., et al. 1997. Sumatriptan decreases food intake and increases plasma growth hormone in healthy women. *Psychopharmacology* (Berlin) 129(2):179–182.

Bonetus T. 1700. *Sepulchretum, sive anatomia practica, ex cadaveribus morbo denatis, proponens historias omnium humani corporis affectum*. Genevae: Sumptibus Cramer & Perachon.

Bonet Theophile. 1684. *A Guide to the Practical Physician: Shewing, From the most Approved Authors, both Ancient and Modern, The Truest and safest way of Curing all Diseases, Internal and External, Whether by Medicine, Surgery or Diet*. London: Thomas Flesher.

Boozer C.N., JANasser, et al. 2001. An herbal supplement containing Ma Huang-Guarana for weight loss: A randomized, double-blind trial. *Int J Obes Relat Metab Disord* 25(3):316–324.

Borowsky B., Durkin M.M., et al. 2002. Antidepressant, anxiolytic and anorectic effects of a melanin-concentrating hormone-1 receptor antagonist. *Nat Med* 8(8):825–830.

Brakenhielm E., Cao R., et al. 2004. Angiogenesis inhibitor, TNP-470, prevents diet-induced and genetic obesity in mice. *Circ Res* 94(12):1579–1588.

Bray G.A., Blackburn G.L., et al. 1999. Sibutramine produces dose-related weight loss. *Obes Res* 7(2): 189–198.

Bray G.A., Gallagher T.F., Jr. 1975. Manifestations of hypothalamic obesity in man: A comprehensive investigation of eight patients and a reveiw of the literature. *Medicine* (Baltimore) 54(4):301–330.

Bray G.A., Greenway F.L. 1999. Current and potential drugs for treatment of obesity. *Endocr Rev* 20(6): 805–875.

Bray G.A., Greenway F.L. 2007. Pharmacological treatment of the overweight patient. *Pharmacol Rev* 59(2): 151–184.

Bray G.A., Hollander P., et al. 2003. A 6-month randomized, placebo-controlled, dose-ranging trial of topiramate for weight loss in obesity. *Obes Res* 11(6):722–733.

Broom I., Wilding J., et al. 2002. Randomised trial of the effect of orlistat on body weight and cardiovascular disease risk profile in obese patients: UK Multimorbidity Study. *Int J Clin Pract* 56(7):494–499.

Bryson A., de la Motte S., Dunk C. 2009. Reduction of dietary fat absorption by the novel gastrointestinal lipase inhibitor cetilistat in healthy volunteers. *Br J Clin Pharmacol* 67(3):309–315.

Buse J.B., Henry R.R., et al. 2004. Effects of exenatide (exendin-4) on glycemic control over 30 weeks in sulfonylurea-treated patients with type 2 diabetes. *Diabetes Care* 27(11):2628–2635.

Buse J.B., Rosenstock J., Sesti G., Schmidt W.E., Montanya E., Brett J.H., Zychma M., Blonde L. 2009. LEAD-6 Study Group Liraglutide once a day versus exenatide twice a day for type 2 diabetes: A 26-week randomised, parallel-group, multinational, open-label trial (LEAD-6). *Lancet* 374(9683):39–47.

Cangiano C., Ceci F., et al. 1992. Eating behavior and adherence to dietary prescriptions in obese adult subjects treated with 5-hydroxytryptophan. *Am J Clin Nutr* 56(5):863–867.

Cangiano C., Laviano A., et al. 1998. Effects of oral 5-hydroxy-tryptophan on energy intake and macronutrient selection in non-insulin dependent diabetic patients. *Int J Obes Relat Metab Disord* 22(7):648–654.

Cefalu W.T., Wang Z.Q., et al. 2002. Oral chromium picolinate improves carbohydrate and lipid metabolism and enhances skeletal muscle Glut-4 translocation in obese, hyperinsulinemic (JCR-LA corpulent) rats. *J Nutr* 132(6):1107–1114.

Chakrabarti R. 2009. Pharmacotherapy of obesity: Emerging drugs and targets. *Expert Opin Ther Targets* 13:195–207 (paper in Curr Opin Lipidology Fructose Folder).

Chan P., Tomlinson B., et al. 2000. A double-blind placebo-controlled study of the effectiveness and tolerability of oral stevioside in human hypertension. *Br J Clin Pharmacol* 50(3):215–220.

Chanoine J.P., Hampl S., et al. 2005. Effect of orlistat on weight and body composition in obese adolescents: A randomized controlled trial. *JAMA* 293(23):2873–2883.

Chanoine J.-P., Hauptman J., Boldin M. 2006. Weight reduction in overweight adolescents achieving early response to orlistat. *Obes Rev* 7(Suppl 2).

Chapman I., Parker B., Doran S., et al. 2005. Effect of pramlintide on satiety and food intake in obese subjects and subjects with type 2 diabetes. *Diabetologia* 48:838–848.

Chapman I., Parker B., Doran S., et al. 2007. Low-dose pramlintide reduced food intake and meal duration in healthy, normal-weight subjects. *Obesity* 15:1179–1186.

Chiba S., Itateyama E., Sakata T., Yoshimatsu H. 2009. Acute central administration of immepip, a histamine H3 receptor agonist, suppresses hypothalamic histamine release and elicits feeding behavior in rats. *Brain Res Bul* 79(1):37–40.

Cho S.-H., Lee J.-S., Thabane L., Lee J. 2009. Acupuncture for obesity: A systematic review and meta-analysis. *Intern J Obes* 33:183–196.

Chong A.Y., Lupsa B.C., Cochran E.K., Gorden P. 2010. Efficacy of leptin therapy in the different forms of human lipodystrophy. *Diabetologia* 53(1):27–35.

Cincotta A.H., Meier A.H. 1996. Bromocriptine (Ergoset) reduces body weight and improves glucose tolerance in obese subjects. *Diabetes Care* 19(6):667–670.

Colman, E. 2005. Anorectics on trial: A half century of federal regulation of prescription appetite suppressants. *Ann Intern Med* 143(5): 380–385.

Colman E. 2007. Dinitrophenol and obesity: An early twentieth-century regulatory dilemma. *Regul Toxicol Pharmacol* 48(2):115–117

Connelly H.M., Crary J.L., McGoon M.D. et al. 1997. Valvular heart disease associated with fenfluramine-phentermine *NEHM* 337:581–588.

Cowen P.J., Sargent P.A., et al. 1995. Hypophagic, endocrine and subjective responses to m-chlorophenyl-piperazine in healthy men and women. *Human Psychopharmacology* 10:385–391.

Davidoff R., McTierman A., Constantine G., et al. 2001. Echocardiographic examination of women previously treated with fenfluramine. *Arch Intern Med* 161:1429–1436.

Davidson M.H., Hauptman J., et al. 1999. Weight control and risk factor reduction in obese subjects treated for 2 years with orlistat: A randomized controlled trial. *JAMA* 281(3):235–242.

Davies K.M., Heaney R.P., et al. 2000. Calcium intake and body weight. *J Clin Endocrinol Metab* 85(12):4635–4638.

De Souza C.J., Burkey B.F. 2001. Beta 3-adrenoceptor agonists as anti-diabetic and anti-obesity drugs in humans. *Curr Pharm Des* 7(14):1433–1449.

DeFronzo R.A., Ratner R. E., et al. 2005. Effects of exenatide (exendin-4) on glycemic control and weight over 30 weeks in metformin-treated patients with type 2 diabetes. *Diabetes Care* 28(5):1092–1100.

Despres J.P., Golay, A. et al. 2005. Effects of rimonabant on metabolic risk factors in overweight patients with dyslipidemia. *N Engl J Med* 353(20):2121–2134.

Devinsky O., Vuong A., et al. 2000. Stable weight during lamotrigine therapy: A review of 32 studies. *Neurology* 54(4):973–975.

Drent M.L., Zelissen P.M., et al. 1995. The effect of dexfenfluramine on eating habits in a Dutch ambulatory android overweight population with an overconsumption of snacks. *Int J Obes Relat Metab Disord* 19(5):299–304.

Dunk C., Enunwa M., et al. 2002. Increased fecal fat excretion in normal volunteers treated with lipase inhibitor ATL-962. *Int J Obes Relat Metab Disord* 26(suppl):S135.

Dwyer J.T., Allison D.B., et al. 2005. Dietary supplements in weight reduction. *J Am Diet Assoc* 105(5 Suppl 1):S80–S86.

Edwards C.M., Stanley S.A., et al. 2001. Exendin-4 reduces fasting and postprandial glucose and decreases energy intake in healthy volunteers. *Am J Physiol Endocrinol Metab* 281(1):E155–E161.

Elfhag K., Finer N., Rössner S. 2008. Who will lose weight on sibutramine and orlistat? Psychological correlates for treatment success. *Diabetes Obes Metab* 10(6):498–505. Epub 2007 Jun 26.

Erondu N., Wadden T., Gantz I., et al. 2007. Effect of NPY5R antagonist MK-0557 on weight regain after very-low-calorie diet-induced weight loss. *Obesity* 15:895–905.

Ettinger M.P., Littlejohn T.W., et al. 2003. Recombinant variant of ciliary neurotrophic factor for weight loss in obese adults: A randomized, dose-ranging study. *JAMA* 289(14):1826–1832.

Fabricatore A.N., Wadden T.A., Moore R.H., Butryn M.L., Gravallese E.A., Erondu N.E., Heymsfield S.B., Nguyen A.M. 2009. Attrition from randomized controlled trials of pharmacological weight loss agents: a systematic review and analysis. *Obes Rev* 10(3):333–341. Epub 2009 Mar 6.

Fehm H.L., Smolnik R., Kern W., McGregor G.P., Bickel U., Born J. 2001. The melanocortin melanocyte-stimulating hormone/adrenocorticotrophin (4–10) decreased body fat in humans. *JCEM* 86:1144–1148.

Fineman M.S., Shen L.Z., et al. 2004. Effectiveness of progressive dose-escalation of exenatide (exendin-4) in reducing dose-limiting side effects in subjects with type 2 diabetes. *Diabetes Metab Res Rev* 20(5): 411–417.

Finer N., Ryan D.H., Renz C.L., Hewkin A.C. 2006. Prediction of response to sibutramine therapy in obese non-diabetic and diabetic patients. *Diab Obes Metab* 8:206–213.

Flemyng M. 1760. *A discourse on the nature, causes, and cure of corpulency. Illustrated by a remarkable case. Read before the Royal Society November 1757*. London: L. Davis and C. Reymers.

Foltin R.W., Haney M., et al. 1996. Effect of fenfluramine on food intake, mood, and performance of humans living in a residential laboratory. *Physiol Behav* 59(2):295–305.

Fontbonne A., Charles M.A., et al. 1996. The effect of metformin on the metabolic abnormalities associated with upper-body fat distribution. BIGPRO Study Group. *Diabetes Care* 19(9):920–926.

Foster G.D., Wadden T.A., Vogt R.A., Brewer G. 1997. What is a reasonable weight loss? Patients' expectations and evaluations of obesity treatment outcomes. *J Consult Clin Psychol* 65(1):79–85.

Foxx-Orenstein A., Camilleri M., et al. 2003. Effect of a somatostatin analogue on gastric motor and sensory functions in healthy humans. *Gut* 52(11):1555–1561.

Franco C., Brandberg J., et al. 2005. Growth hormone treatment reduces abdominal visceral fat in postmenopausal women with abdominal obesity: A 12-month placebo-controlled trial. *J Clin Endocrinol Metab* 90(3):1466–1474.

Fujioka K., Seaton T.B., et al. 2000. Weight loss with sibutramine improves glycaemic control and other metabolic parameters in obese patients with type 2 diabetes mellitus. *Diabetes Obes Metab* 2(3):175–187.

Gadde K.M., Franciscy D.M., et al. 2003. Zonisamide for weight loss in obese adults: A randomized controlled trial. *JAMA* 289(14):1820–1825.

Gadde K.M., Yonish G.M., Wagner H.R. II, Foust M.S., Allison D.B. 2006. *Int J Obes* (London) 30:1138–1142.

Gadde K.M., Parker C.B., et al. 2001. Bupropion for weight loss: An investigation of efficacy and tolerability in overweight and obese women. *Obes Res* 9(9):544–551.

Galgani J.E., Ryan D.H., Ravussin E. 2009. Effect of capsinoids on energy metabolism in human subjects. *Br J Nutr* 12:1–5.

Gardin J.M., Schumacher D., Constantine F., et al. 2000. Valvular abnormalities and cardiovascular status following exposure to dexfenfluramine or phentermine/fenfuramine. *JAMA* 283:1703–1709.

Garrison F.H. 1914. *An Introduction to the History of Medicine with Medical Chronology Bibliographic Data and Test Questions*. Philadelphia: W.B. Saunders.

Gedulin B.R., Nikoulina S.E., et al. 2005. Exenatide (exendin-4) improves insulin sensitivity and {beta}-cell mass in insulin-resistant obese fa/fa Zucker rats independent of glycemia and body weight. *Endocrinology* 146(4):2069–2076.

Gibson W.T., Ebersole B.J., et al. 2004. Mutational analysis of the serotonin receptor 5HT2c in severe early-onset human obesity. *Can J Physiol Pharmacol* 82(6):426–429.

Godoy-Matos A., Carraro L., et al. 2005. Treatment of obese adolescents with sibutramine: A randomized, double-blind, controlled study. *J Clin Endocrinol Metab* 90(3):1460–1465.

Gokcel A., Gumurdulu Y., Karakose H., Melek Ertorer E., Tanaci N., BascilTutuncu N., Guvener N. 2002. Evaluation of the safety and efficacy of sibutramine, orlistat and metformin in the treatment of obesity. *Diabetes Obes Metab* 4(1):49–55.

Goldstein D.J., Rampey A.H. Jr, et al. 1995. Efficacy and safety of long-term fluoxetine treatment of obesity-maximizing success. *Obes Res* 3(Suppl 4): 481S–490S.

Goudie A.J., Halford J.C., Dovey T.M., Cooper G.D., Neill J.C. 2003. H(1)-histamine receptor affinity predicts short-term weight gain for typical and atypical antipsychotic drugs. *Neuropsychopharmacology* 28(12):2209; author reply 2210–2211.

Gougeon R., Harrigan K., Tremblay J.-F., Hedrei P., Lamarche M., and Morais J.A. 2005. Increase in the thermic effect of food in women with adrenergic amines extracted from Citrum aurantium. *Obes Res* 13:1187–1194.

Greenway F.L. 1992. Clinical studies with phenylpropanolamine: A metaanalysis. *Am J Clin Nutr* 55(1 Suppl):203S–205S.

Greenway F.L. 2001. The safety and efficacy of pharmaceutical and herbal caffeine and ephedrine use as a weight loss agent. *Obes Rev* 2(3):199–211.

Greenway F.L., Bray G.A. 2010. *Combination Drug Therapy*. in press.

Greenway F.L., Dunayvich E., Tollefson G., Erickson J., Guttadauria M., Fujioks K., Cowley M.A., for the NB-201 Study Group. 2009. Comparison of combined bupropion and naltrexone therapy for obesity with monotherapy and placebo. *J Clin Endocrinol Metab* 94:1350–1358.

Greenway, S.E., Greenway F.L. III, et al. 2002. Effects of obesity surgery on non-insulin-dependent diabetes mellitus. *Arch Surg* 137(10):1109–1117.

Greenway F.L., Whitehouse M.J., Guttadauria M., Anderson J.W., Atkinson R.L., Fujioka K., Gadde K.M., Gupta A.K., O'Neil P., Schumacher D., Smith D., Dunayevich E., Tollefson G.D., Weber E., Cowley M.A. 2009. Rational design of a combination medication for the treatment of obesity. *Obesity* (Silver Spring) 17(1):30–39.

Gregersen S., Jeppesen P.B., et al. 2004. Antihyperglycemic effects of stevioside in type 2 diabetic subjects. *Metabolism* 53(1):73–76.

Guy-Grand B., Apfelbaum M., Crepaldi G., Gries A., Lefebvre P., Turner P. 1989. International trial of long-term dexfenfluramine in obesity. *Lancet* 2(8672):1142–1145.

Haddock C.K., Poston W.S., et al. 2002. Pharmacotherapy for obesity: A quantitative analysis of four decades of published randomized clinical trials. *Int J Obes Relat Metab Disord* 26(2):262–273.

Hainer V., Kunesova M., Bellisle F., Hill M., Braunerova R., Wagenknecht M. 2005. Psychobehavioral and nutritional predictors of weight loss in obese women treated with sibutramine. *Int J Obes* (Lond) 29(2):208–216.

Halaas J.L., Gajiwala K.S., et al. 1995. Weight-reducing effects of the plasma protein encoded by the obese gene. *Science* 269(5223):543–546.

Handlon A., Zhou H. 2005. Melanin-concentrating hormone-1 receptor antagonists. *J Med Chem* (in press).

Hansen D.L., Toubro S., et al. 1998. Thermogenic effects of sibutramine in humans. *Am J Clin Nutr* 68(6):1180–1186.

Harris S.C., Ivy A.C., Searle L.M. 1947. The mechamnism of phaetamine-induced loss of weight. A correlation of the theory of hunger and appetite. *JAMA* 134:1468–1474.

Hauptman, J. 2000. Orlistat: Selective inhibition of caloric absorption can affect long-term body weight. *Endocrine* 13(2):201–206.

He L., Sabet A., Djedjos S., Miller R., Sun X., Hussain M.A., Radovick S., Wondisford F.E. 2009. Metformin and insulin suppress hepatic gluconeogenesis through phosphorylation of CREB binding protein. *Cell* 137:635–646.

Heine R.J., Van Gaal L.F., et al. 2005. Exenatide versus insulin glargine in patients with suboptimally controlled type 2 diabetes: A randomized trial. *Ann Intern Med* 143(8):559–569.

Henderson D.C., Copeland P.M., Daley T.B., Borba C.P., Cather C., Nguyen D.D., Louie P.M., Evins A.E., Freudenreich O., Hayden D., Goff D.C. 2005. A double-blind, placebo-controlled trial of sibutramine for olanzapine-associated weight gain. *Am J Psychiatry* 162(5):954–962.

Heymsfield S.B., Allison D.B., et al. 1998. Garcinia cambogia (hydroxycitric acid) as a potential antiobesity agent: A randomized controlled trial. *JAMA* 280(18):1596–1600.

Heymsfield S.B., Greenberg A.S., et al. 1999. Recombinant leptin for weight loss in obese and lean adults: A randomized, controlled, dose-escalation trial. *JAMA* 282(16):1568–1575.

Heymsfield S.B., Segal K.R., et al. 2000. Effects of weight loss with orlistat on glucose tolerance and progression to type 2 diabetes in obese adults. *Arch Intern Med* 160(9):1321–1326.

Hill J.O., Hauptman J., et al. 1999. Orlistat, a lipase inhibitor, for weight maintenance after conventional dieting: A 1-y study. *Am J Clin Nutr* 69(6):1108–1116.

Hoffman A.R., Kuntze J.E., et al. 2004. Growth hormone (GH) replacement therapy in adult-onset gh deficiency: Effects on body composition in men and women in a double-blind, randomized, placebo-controlled trial. *J Clin Endocrinol Metab* 89(5):2048–2056.

Hollander P.A., Elbein S.C., et al. 1998. Role of orlistat in the treatment of obese patients with type 2 diabetes. A 1-year randomized double-blind study. *Diabetes Care* 21(8):1288–1294.

Hopkins K.D., Lehmann E.D. 1995. Successful medical treatment of obesity in 10th century Spain. *Lancet* 346:452.

Hsieh M.H., Chan P., et al. 2003. Efficacy and tolerability of oral stevioside in patients with mild essential hypertension: A two-year, randomized, placebo-controlled study. *Clin Ther* 25(11):2797–2808.

Huda M.S.B., Wilding J.P.H., Pinkney J.H. 2006. Appetite regulatory peptides. Gut peptides and the regulation of appetite. *Obes Rev* 7:163–182.

Hughes K.A., Webster S.P., Walker B.R. 2008. 11-Beta-hydroxysteroid dehydrogenase type 1 (11beta-HSD1) inhibitors in type 2 diabetes mellitus and obesity. *Expert Opin Investig Drugs* 17(4):481–496.

Hukshorn C.J., Saris W.H., et al. 2000. Weekly subcutaneous pegylated recombinant native human leptin (PEG-OB) administration in obese men. *J Clin Endocrinol Metab* 85(11):4003–4009.

Hukshorn C.J., Westerterp-Plantenga M.S., et al. 2003. Pegylated human recombinant leptin (PEG-OB) causes additional weight loss in severely energy-restricted, overweight men. *Am J Clin Nutr* 77(4):771–776.

Hutton B., Fergusson D. 2004. Changes in body weight and serum lipid profile in obese patients treated with orlistat in addition to a hypocaloric diet: A systematic review of randomized clinical trials. *Am J Clin Nutr* 80:1461–1468.

Jain A.K., Kaplan R.A., et al. 2002. Bupropion SR vs. placebo for weight loss in obese patients with depressive symptoms. *Obes Res* 10(10):1049–1056.

James W.P., Astrup A., et al. 2000. Effect of sibutramine on weight maintenance after weight loss: A randomised trial. STORM Study Group. Sibutramine Trial of Obesity Reduction and Maintenance. *Lancet* 356(9248):2119–2125.

Jollis J.G., Landotlfo C.F., Kisslo J., et al. 2000. Fenfluramine and phentermine and cardiovascular findings: Effect of treatment duration on prevalence of valve abnormalities. *Circ* 2000 101:2071–2077.

Jordan J., Scholze J., et al. 2005. Influence of ibutramine on blood pressure: Evidence from placebo-controlled trials. *Int J Obes* (London) 29(5):509–516.

Juan-Pico P., Fuentes E., et al. 2006. Cannabinoid receptors regulate Ca(2+) signals and insulin secretion in pancreatic beta-cell. *Cell Calcium* 39(2):155–162.

Jull A.B., Mihurchu C.N., Bennett D.A., Cunshea-Mooij C.A.E., Rodgers A. 2008. Chitosan for overweight or obesisty. *Cochrane Database of Systematic Reviews* Issue 3 Art No: CD003892.

Kamath V., Jones C.N., et al. 1997. Effects of a quick-release form of bromocriptine (Ergoset) on fasting and postprandial plasma glucose, insulin, lipid, and lipoprotein concentrations in obese nondiabetic hyperinsulinemic women. *Diabetes Care* 20(11):1697–1701.

Kamel E.G., McNeill G., Van Wijk M.C. 2000. Change in ingtraabdominal adipose tissue volume during weight loss in obese men and women: Correlation between magnetic resonance imaging and anthropometric measurements *Intern J Obes* 24:607–613.

Kanatani A., Hata M., et al. 2001. A typical Y1 receptor regulates feeding behaviors: Effects of a potent and selective Y1 antagonist, J-115814. *Mol Pharmacol* 59(3):501–505.

Kastin A.J., Akerstrom V. 2003. Entry of exendin-4 into brain is rapid but may be limited at high doses. *Int J Obes Relat Metab Disord* 27(3):313–318.

Kaya A., Aydin N., et al. 2004. Efficacy of sibutramine, orlistat and combination therapy on short-term weight management in obese patients. *Biomed Pharmacother* 58(10):582–587.

Kelley D.E., Bray G.A., et al. 2002. Clinical efficacy of orlistat therapy in overweight and obese patients with insulin-treated type 2 diabetes: A 1-year randomized controlled trial. *Diabetes Care* 25(6):1033–1041.

Kendall D.M., Riddle M.C., et al. 2005. Effects of exenatide (exendin-4) on glycemic control over 30 weeks in patients with type 2 diabetes treated with metformin and a sulfonylurea. *Diabetes Care* 28(5):1083–1091.

Kernan W.N., Viscoli C.M., et al. 2000. Phenylpropanolamine and the risk of hemorrhagic stroke. *N Engl J Med* 343(25):1826–1832.

Kim S.F., Huang A.S., Snowman A.M., Teuscher C., Snyder S.H. 2007. Antipsychotic drug-induced weight gain mediated by histamine H1 receptor-linked activation of hypothalamic AMP-kinase. *Proc Natl Acad Sci U S A* 104(9):3456–3459.

Kim S.H., Lee Y.M., et al. 2003. Effect of sibutramine on weight loss and blood pressure: A meta-analysis of controlled trials. *Obes Res* 11(9):1116–1123.

Kiortsis D.N., Tsouli S., Filippatos T.D., Konitsiotis S., Elisaf M.S. 2008. Effects of sibutramine and orlistat on mood in obese and overweight subjects: A randomised study. *Nutr Metab Cardiovasc Dis* 18(3):207–210.

Kirkham T.C. 2005. Endocannabinoids in the regulation of appetite and body weight. *Behav Pharmacol* 16(5–6):297–313.

Knowler W.C., Barrett-Connor E., et al. 2002. Reduction in the incidence of type 2 diabetes with lifestyle intervention or metformin. *N Engl J Med* 346(6):393–403.

Kopelman P., Bryson A., Hickling R., Rissanen A., Rossner S., Toubro S., Valensi P. 2007. Cetilistat (ATL-962), a novel lipase inhibitor: A 12-week randomized, placebo-controlled study of weight reduction in obese patients. *Int J Obes* (London) 31(3):494–499.

Kopelman P., De H Groot G., Rissanen A., Rossner S., Toubro S., Palmer R., Hallam R., Bryson A., Hickling R.I. 2009. Weight loss, HbA(1c) reduction, and tolerability of cetilistat in a randomized, placebo-controlled phase 2 trial in obese diabetics: Comparison with orlistat (Xenical). *Obesity* (Silver Spring) 18:108–115.

Kowalski T.J., Farley C., et al. 2004. Melanin-concentrating hormone-1 receptor antagonism decreases feeding by reducing meal size. *Eur J Pharmacol* 497(1):41–47.

Krishna R., Gumbiner B., Stevens C., Bret Musser B., Mallick M., Suryawanshi S., Maganti L., Zhu H., Scherer L., Simpson B., Cosgrove D., Gottesdiener K., Amatruda J., Rolls B.J., Blundell J., Bray G.A., Fujioka K., Heymsfield S.B., Wagner J.A., Herman G.A. 2009. Effect of MK-0493, a melanocortin receptor 4 agonist, on energy intake and weight loss in human volunteers. *Clin Pharmacol Ther* 86(6):659–666.

Kromhout D., Bloemberg B., et al. 2001. Physical activity and dietary fiber determine population body fat levels: The Seven Countries Study. *Int J Obes Relat Metab Disord* 25(3):301–306.

Kubota N., Yano W., Kubota T., Yamauchi T., Itoh S., Kumagai H., Kozono H., Takamoto I., Okamoto S., Shiuchi T., Suzuki R., Satoh H., Tsuchida A., Moroi M., Sugi K., Noda T., Ebinuma H., Ueta Y., Kondo T., Araki E., Ezaki O., Nagai R., Tobe K., Terauchi Y., Ueki K., Minokoshi Y., Kadowaki T. 2007. Adiponectin stimulates AMP-activated protein kinase in the hypothalamus and increases food intake. *Cell Metab* 6(1):55–68.

Kurt T.L., Anderson R., Petty C., Bost R., Reed G., Holland J. 1986. Dinitrophenol in weight loss: The poison center and public health safety. *Vet Hum Toxicol* 28(6):574–575.

Laferrere B., Abraham C., et al. 2005. Growth hormone releasing peptide-2 (GHRP-2), like ghrelin, increases food intake in healthy men. *J Clin Endocrinol Metab* 90(2):611–614.

Lagouge M., Argmann C., Gerhart-Hines Z., et al. 2006. Resveratrol improves mitochondrial function and protects against metabolic disease by activating SIRT-1 and PGC-1alpha. *Cell* 127:1109–1122.

Larsen T.M., Toubro S., et al. 2003. Efficacy and safety of dietary supplements containing CLA for the treatment of obesity: evidence from animal and human studies. *J Lipid Res* 44(12):2234–2241.

Larsen T.M., Toubro S., et al. 2002. Effect of a 28-d treatment with L-796568, a novel beta(3)-adrenergic receptor agonist, on energy expenditure and body composition in obese men. *Am J Clin Nutr* 76(4):780–788.

Lawton C.L., Wales J.K., et al. 1995. Serotoninergic manipulation, meal-induced satiety and eating pattern: Effect of fluoxetine in obese female subjects. *Obes Res* 3(4):345–356.

Leonhardt M., Langhans W. 2004. Fatty acid oxidation and control of food intake. *Physiol Behav* 83(4): 645–651.

Lesses M.F., Myerson A. 1938. Human autonomic pharmacology. XVI. Benzedrine sulfate as an aid in the treatment of obesity. *N Engl J Med* 218:119–124.

Leurs R., Bakker R.A., Timmerman H., de Esch I.J. 2005. The Histamine H-3 receptor: From gene cloning to H-3 receptor drugs. *Nat Rev Drug Discovery* 4:107–120.

Levens N.R., Della-Zuana O. 2003. Neuropeptide Y Y5 receptor antagonists as anti-obesity drugs. *Curr Opin Investig Drugs* 4(10):1198–1204.

Levin B.E., Dunn-Meynell A.A. 2000. Sibutramine alters the central mechanisms regulating the defended body weight in diet-induced obese rats. *Am J Physiol* 279:R2222–R2228.

Li Z., Maglione M., et al. 2005. Meta-analysis: Pharmacologic treatment of obesity. *Ann Intern Med* 142(7):532–546.

Lindgarde F. 2000. The effect of orlistat on body weight and coronary heart disease risk profile in obese patients: The Swedish Multimorbidity Study. *J Intern Med* 248(3):245–254.

Lindholm A., Bixo M., Björn I., Wölner-Hanssen P., Eliasson M., Larsson A., Johnson O., Poromaa I.S. 2008. Effect of sibutramine on weight reduction in women with polycystic ovary syndrome: A randomized, double-blind, placebo-controlled trial. *Fertil Steril* 89(5):1221–1228.

Lloret-Linares C., Greenfield J.R., Czernichow S. 2008. Effect of weight-reducing agents on glycemic parameters and progression to Type 2 diabetes: A review. *Diab Med* 25:1142–1150.

Ludwig D.S., Mountjoy K.G., et al. 1998. Melanin-concentrating hormone: A functional melanocortin antagonist in the hypothalamus. *Am J Physiol* 274(4 Pt 1):E627–E633.

Lugari R., Dei Cas A., et al. 2004. Glucagon-like peptide 1 (GLP–1) secretion and plasma dipeptidyl peptidase IV (DPP-IV) activity in morbidly obese patients undergoing biliopancreatic diversion. *Horm Metab Res* 36(2):111–115.

Lustig R., Greenway F., et al. 2003. Weight loss in obese adults with insulin hypersecretion treated with Sandostatin LAR Depot. *Obes Res* 11(Suppl.):A25.

Lustig R.H., Greenway F., et al. 2006. A multicenter, randomized, double-blind, placebo-controlled, dose-finding trial of a long-acting formulation of octreotide in promoting weight loss in obese adults with insulin hypersecretion. *Int J Obes* (London) 30(2):331–341.

Lustig R.H., Hinds P.S., et al. 2003. Octreotide therapy of pediatric hypothalamic obesity: A double-blind, placebo-controlled trial. *J Clin Endocrinol Metab* 88(6):2586–2592.

Lustig R.H., Rose S.R., et al. 1999. Hypothalamic obesity caused by cranial insult in children: Altered glucose and insulin dynamics and reversal by a somatostatin agonist. *J Pediatr* 135(2 Pt 1):162–168.

Maahs D., de Serna D.G., et al. 2006. Randomized, double-blind, placebo-controlled trial of orlistat for weight loss in adolescents. *Endocr Pract* 12(1):18–28.

Maffei M., Fei H., et al. 1995. Increased expression in adipocytes of ob RNA in mice with lesions of the hypothalamus and with mutations at the db locus. *Proc Natl Acad Sci USA* 92(15):6957–6960.

Maggs D., Shen L., et al. 2003. Effect of pramlintide on A1C and body weight in insulin-treated African Americans and Hispanics with type 2 diabetes: A pooled post hoc analysis. *Metabolism* 52(12):1638–1642.

Maggioni A.P., Caterson I., Coutinho W., Finer N., Gaal L.V., Sharma A.M., Torp-Pedersen C., Bacher P., Shepherd G., Sun R., James P., SCOUT Investigators. 2008. Tolerability of sibutramine during a 6 week treatment period in high-risk patients with cardiovascular disease and/or diabetes: A preliminary analysis of the Sibutramine Cardiovascular Outcomes (SCOUT) Trial. *J Cardiovasc Pharmacol* 52:393–402.

Mathus-Vliegen E.M. 2005. Long-term maintenance of weight loss with sibutramine in a GP setting following a specialist guided very-low-calorie diet: A double-blind, placebo-controlled, parallel group study. *Eur J Clin Nutr* 59(Suppl 1):S31–S38; discussion S39.

McCarron D.A., Morris C.D., et al. 1984. Blood pressure and nutrient intake in the United States. *Science* 224(4656):1392–1398.

McElroy S.L., Arnold L.M., et al. 2003. Topiramate in the treatment of binge eating disorder associated with obesity: A randomized, placebo-controlled trial. *Am J Psychiatry* 160(2):255–261.

McElroy S.L., Kotwal R., et al. 2004. Zonisamide in the treatment of binge-eating disorder: An open-label, prospective trial. *J Clin Psychiatry* 65(1):50–56.

McElroy S.L., Shapira N.A., et al. 2004. Topiramate in the long-term treatment of binge-eating disorder associated with obesity. *J Clin Psychiatry* 65(11):1463–1469.

McGovern L., Johnson J.N., Paulo R., et al. 2008. Treatment of pediatric obesity. A systematic review and meta-analysis of randomized trials. *J Clin Endocrinol Metab* 93:4600–4605.

McMahon F.G., Fujioka K., et al. 2000. Efficacy and safety of sibutramine in obese white and African American patients with hypertension: A 1-year, double-blind, placebo-controlled, multicenter trial. *Arch Intern Med* 160(14):2185–2191.

McNulty S.J., Ur E., et al. 2003. A randomized trial of sibutramine in the management of obese type 2 diabetic patients treated with metformin. *Diabetes Care* 26(1):125–131.

Makimura H., Mizuno T.M., Yang X.J., Silverstein J., Beasley J., Mobbs C.V. 2001. Cerulenin mimics effects of leptin on metabolic rate, food intake, and body weight independent of the melanocortin system, but unlike leptin, cerulenin fails to block neuroendocrine effects of fasting. *Diabetes* 50(4):733–739.

Meier A.H., Cincotta A.H., et al. 1992. Timed bromocriptine administration reduces body fat stores in obese subjects and hyperglycemia in type II diabetics. *Experientia* 48(3):248–253.

Meguid M.M., Fetissov S.O., Varma M., Sato T., Zhang L., Laviano A., Rossi-Fanelli F. 2000. Hypothalamic dopamine and serotonin in the regulation of food intake. *Nutrition* 16(10):843–857.

Merideth C., Southard C.K. 2005. A double-blind, placebo-controlled, evaluation of lamotrigine for obesity. *Obes Res.*

Mhurchu C.N., Dunshea-Mooij C., et al. 2005. Effect of chitosan on weight loss in overweight and obese individuals: A systematic review of randomized controlled trials. *Obes Rev* 6(1):35–42.

Miller L.J. 2009. Management of atypical antipsychotic drug-induced weight gain: Focus on metformin. *Pharmacotherapy* 29:725–735.

Miles J.M., Leiter L., et al. 2002. Effect of orlistat in overweight and obese patients with type 2 diabetes treated with metformin. *Diabetes Care* 25(7):1123–1128.

Mittendorfer, B., Ostlund R.E. Jr, et al. 2001. Orlistat inhibits dietary cholesterol absorption. *Obes Res* 9(10):599–604.

Morton N.M., Seckl J.R. 2008. 11beta-hydroxysteroid dehydrogenase type 1 and obesity. *Front Horm Res* 36:146–164.

Munro J., MacCuish A., et al. 1968. Comparison of continuous and intermittent anorectic therapy in obesity. *BMJ* 1:352–354.

Nam S.Y., Kim K.R., et al. 2001. Low-dose growth hormone treatment combined with diet restriction decreases insulin resistance by reducing visceral fat and increasing muscle mass in obese type 2 diabetic patients. *Int J Obes Relat Metab Disord* 25(8):1101–1107.

Nann-Vernotica E., Donny E.C., et al. 2001. Repeated administration of the D1/5 antagonist ecopipam fails to attenuate the subjective effects of cocaine. *Psychopharmacology* (Berlin) 155(4):338–347.

Nargund R.P., Strack A.M., Fong T.M. 2006. Melanocortin-4 receptor (MC4R) agonists for the treatment of obesity. *J Med Chem* 49:4035–4043.

Nasir J.M., Durning S.J., et al. 2004. Exercise-induced syncope associated with QT prolongation and ephedra-free Xenadrine. *Mayo Clin Proc* 79(8):1059–1062.

Nass R., Pezzoli S.S., Oliveri M.C., Patrie J.T., Harrell F.E. Jr, Clasey J.L., Heymsfield S.B., Bach M.A., Vance M.L., Thorner M.O. 2008. Effects of an oral ghrelin mimetic on body composition and clinical outcomes in healthy older adults. *Ann Int Med* 149:601–611.

National Heart and Blood Institute, et al. 2000. *Practical Guide in Identification, Evaluation and Treatment of Overweight and Obesity in Adults*. Bethesda: National Institutes of Health.

National Institutes of Health. 1985. NIH consensus development conference statement. Health implications of obesity. *Ann Intern Med* 103:1073–1077.

Nauck M.A., Ratner R.E., Kapitza C., Berria R., Boldrin M., Balena R. 2009. Treatment with the human once-weekly glucagon-like peptide-1 analog taspoglutide in combination with metformin improves glycemic control and lowers body weight in patients with type 2 diabetes inadequately controlled with metformin alone. *Diabetes Care* 32:1237–1243.

Neff L.M., Kushner R.G. 2010. Emerging role of GLP-1 receptor agonists in the treatment of obesity. *Diabetes Metab Syndr Obes* 3:263–273.

Neovius M., Johansson K., Rössner S. 2008. Head-to-head studies evaluating efficacy of pharmaco-therapy for obesity: A systematic review and meta-analysis. *Obes Rev* 9(5):420–427.

Nilsson B.M. 2005. 5-Hydroxytryptamine 2C (5-HT2C) receptor agonists as potential antiobesity agents. *J Med Chem* 49:4023–4034.

Norris S.L., Zhang X., et al. 2004. Efficacy of pharmacotherapy for weight loss in adults with type 2 diabetes mellitus: A meta-analysis. *Arch Intern Med* 164(13):1395–1404.

Nykamp D.L., Fackih M.N., et al. 2004. Possible association of acute lateral-wall myocardial infarction and bitter orange supplement. *Ann Pharmacother* 38(5):812–816.

Oral E.A., Simha V., et al. 2002. Leptin-replacement therapy for lipodystrophy. *N Engl J Med* 346(8): 570–578.

Ortega-Gonzalez C., Luna S., et al. 2005. Responses of serum androgen and insulin resistance to metformin and pioglitazone in obese, insulin-resistant women with polycystic ovary syndrome. *J Clin Endocrinol Metab* 90(3):1360–1365.

Padwal R., Li S.K., et al. 2004. Long-term pharmacotherapy for obesity and overweight. *Cochrane Database of Systematic Reviews* Issue 3: CD004094.

Padwal R., Majumdar S.R., et al. 2005. A systematic review of drug therapy to delay or prevent type 2 diabetes. *Diabetes Care* 28(3):736–744.

Pagotto U., Marsicano G., et al. 2006. The emerging role of the endocannabinoid system in endocrine regulation and energy balance. *Endocr Rev* 27(1):73–100.

Paranjpe P., Patki P., et al. 1990. Ayurvedic treatment of obesity: A randomised double-blind, placebo-controlled clinical trial. *J Ethnopharmacol* 29(1):1–11.

Park M.H., Kinra S., Ward K.J., White B., Viner R.M. 2009. Metformin for obesity in children and adolescents: A systematic review. *Diabetes Care* 32:1743–1745.

Parker E., Van Heek M., et al. 2002. Neuropeptide Y receptors as targets for anti-obesity drug development: Perspective and current status. *Eur J Pharmacol* 440(2–3):173–187.

Patriti A., Facchiano E., et al. 2004. The enteroinsular axis and the recovery from type 2 diabetes after bariatric surgery. *Obes Surg* 14(6):840–848.

Phytopharm. 2001. Successful completion of proof of principle clinical study of P57 for obesity [Dec 5 press release]. Available from URL: http://www.phytopharm.co.uk/press/P57%20Third%20Stage%20final.htm.

Pillitteria J.L., Burton S.L., Shiffman S., Rohay J.M., Harkins A.M., Pettinco G. 2006. Consumers' use and beliefs about dietary supplements for weight loss. *Obes Rev* 7(Suppl 2): Abs.

Pi-Sunyer F.X., Aronne L.J., et al. 2006. Effect of rimonabant, a cannabinoid-1 receptor blocker, on weight and cardiometabolic risk factors in overweight or obese patients: RIO-North America: Q randomized controlled trial. *JAMA* 295(7):761–775.

Pi-Sunyer X., Kissileff H.R., et al. 1982. C-terminal octapeptide of cholecystokinin decreases food intake in obese men. *Physiol Behav* 29(4):627–630.

Pijl H., Ohashi S., et al. 2000. Bromocriptine: A novel approach to the treatment of type 2 diabetes. *Diabetes Care* 23(8):1154–1161.

Pittler M.H., Ernst E. 2004. Dietary supplements for body-weight reduction: A systematic review. *Am J Clin Nutr* 79(4):529–536.

Pittler M.H., Ernst E. 2005. Complementary therapies for reducing body weight: A systematic review. *Int J Obes* (London) 29(9):1030–1038.

Poindexter G.S., Bruce M.A., et al. 2002. Dihydropyridine neuropeptide Y Y(1) receptor antagonists. *Bioorg Med Chem Lett* 12(3):379–382.

Poston W.S., Haddock C.K., et al. 2001. Lifestyle treatments in randomized clinical trials of pharmacotherapies for obesity. *Obes Res* 9(9):552–563.

Puhl R.M., Brownell K.D. 2003. Psychosocial origins of obesity stigma: Toward changing a powerful and pervasive bias. *Obes Rev* 4(4):213–227.

Putnam J. 1893. Cases of myxedema and acromegalia treated with benefit by sheep's thyroids: Recent observations respecting the pathology of the cachexias following disease of the thyroid: Clinical relationships of grave's disease and acromegalia. *Am J Med Sci* 106:125–148.

Ratner R.E., Dickey R., et al. 2004. Amylin replacement with pramlintide as an adjunct to insulin therapy improves long-term glycaemic and weight control in Type 1 diabetes mellitus: A 1-year, randomized controlled trial. *Diabet Med* 21(11):1204–1212.

Ravussin E., Smith S.R., Mitchell J.A., Shringarpure R., Shan K., Maier H., Koda J.E., Weyer C. 2009. Enhanced weight loss with pramlintide/metreleptin: An integrated neurohormonal approach to obesity pharmacotherapy. *Obesity* (Silver Spring) 17(9):1736–1743.

Reaven G., Segal K., et al. 2001. Effect of orlistat-assisted weight loss in decreasing coronary heart disease risk in patients with syndrome X. *Am J Cardiol* 87(7):827–831.

Redman L.M., De Jonge L., Fang X., Gamlin B., Recker D., Geenway F.L., Smith S.R., Ravussin E. 2007. Lack of an effect of a novel b3-adrenoceptor agonists, TAK-677, on energy metabolism in obese individuals: A double-blind, placebo-controlled randomized tudy. *J Clin Endocrinol Metab* 92:527–531.

Richelsen B., Niskanen L., Tonstad S., Madsbad S., Rossner S., Mustajoki P., Tourbro S., Rissanen A. 2007. Effect of orlistat on weight regain and cardiovascular risk factors following a very-low energy diet in abdominally obese patients. *Diabetes Care* 30:27–32.

Riddle M.C., Drucker D.J. 2006. Emerging therapies mimicking the effects of amylin and glucagon-like peptide 1. *Diabetes Care* 29(2):435–449.

Riserus U., Smedman A., et al. 2004. Metabolic effects of conjugated linoleic acid in humans: The Swedish experience. *Am J Clin Nutr* 79(6 Suppl):1146S–1148S.

Rissanen A., Lean M., Rossner S., Segal K., Sjostrom L. 2003. Predictive values of early weight loss in obesity management with orlistat: An evidence-based assessment of prescribing guidelines. *Int J Obes* 27:103–109.

Rodriquez de Fonseca F., Navarro M., et al. 2000. Peripheral versus central effects of glucagon-like peptide-1 receptor agonists on satiety and body weight loss in Zucker obese rats. *Metabolism* 49(6):709–717.

Rogers P.J., Blundell J.E. 1979. Effect of anorexic drugs on food intake and the micro-structure of eating in human subjects. *Psychopharmacology* (Berlin) 66(2):159–165.

Rolls B.J., Shide D.J., et al. 1998. Sibutramine reduces food intake in non-dieting women with obesity. *Obes Res* 6(1):1–11.

Rosenbaum M., Murphy E.M., et al. 2002. Low dose leptin administration reverses effects of sustained weight-reduction on energy expenditure and circulating concentrations of thyroid hormones. *J Clin Endocrinol Metab* 87(5):2391–2394.

Rosenbaum M., Sy M., Pavlovich K., Leibel R.L., Hirsch J. 2008. Leptin reverses weight-loss-induced changes in regional neural activity responses to visual food stimuli. *J Clin Invest* 118:2583–2591.

Rosenstock J., Hollander P., Gadde K.M., et al. 2007. A randomized, double-blind, placebo-controlled multicenter study to assess the efficacy and safety of topiramate controlled-release in the treatment of obese, type 2 diabetic patients. *Diabetes* 30:1480–1486.

Rossner S., Sjostrom L., et al. 2000. Weight loss, weight maintenance, and improved cardiovascular risk factors after 2 years treatment with orlistat for obesity. European Orlistat Obesity Study Group. *Obes Res* 8(1):49–61.

Rupnick M.A., Panigrahy D., et al. 2002. Adipose tissue mass can be regulated through the vasculature. *Proc Natl Acad Sci USA* 99(16):10730–10735.

Rucker D., Padwal R., Li S.K., Curioni C., Lau D.C. 2007. Long term pharmacotherapy for obesity and overweight: Updated meta-analysis. *BMJ* 335(7631):1194–1199.

Ryan D.H. 2008. Sibutramine in the management of obesity. In *Handbook of Obesity: Clinical Applications*, 3rd ed. G.A. Bray, C. Bouchard, eds. New York: Informa Inc, pp 303–315.

Ryan D.H., Johnson W.D., Myers V.H., Prather T.L., McGlone M.M., Rood J., Brantley P.J., Bray G.A., Gupta A.K., Broussard A.P., Barootes B.G., Elkins B.L., Gaudin D.E., Savory R.L., Brock R.D., Datz G., Pothakamuri S.R., McKnight G.T., Stenlof K., Sjöström L.V. 2010. Non-surgical weight loss for extreme obesity in primary care settings: Results of the Louisiana Obese Subjects Study. *Arch Int Med* 170(2):146–154.

Sajous C.E. de M. 1916. *The Internal Secretion and the Principles of Medicine,* 7th ed. Philadelphia: F.A. Davis Co.

Salmeron J., Manson J.E., et al. 1997. Dietary fiber, glycemic load, and risk of non-insulin-dependent diabetes mellitus in women. *JAMA* 277(6):472–477.

Sari R., Balci M.K., Cakir M., Altunbas H., Karayalcin U. 2004. Comparison of efficacy of sibutramine or orlistat versus their combination in obese women. *Endocr Res* 30(2):159–167.

Schteingart D.E. 1992. Effectiveness of phenylpropanolamine in the management of moderate obesity. *Int J Obes Relat Metab Disord* 16(7):487–493.

Setter S.M., Iltz J.L., Thams J., Campbell R.K. 2003. Metformin hydrochloride in the treatment of type 2 diabetes mellitus: A clinical review with a focus on dual therapy. *Clin Ther* 25(12):2991–3026.

Shapira N.A., Goldsmith T.D., et al. 2000. Treatment of binge-eating disorder with topiramate: A clinical case series. *J Clin Psychiatry* 61(5):368–372.

Shapira N.A., Lessig M.C., et al. 2004. Effects of topiramate in adults with Prader-Willi syndrome. *Am J Ment Retard* 109(4):301–309.

Shapira N.A., Lessig M.C., et al. 2002. Topiramate attenuates self-injurious behaviour in Prader-Willi syndrome. *Int J Neuropsychopharmacol* 5(2):141–145.

Shapses S.A., Heshka S., et al. 2004. Effect of calcium supplementation on weight and fat loss in women. *J Clin Endocrinol Metab* 89(2):632–637.

Shapses S.A., Von Thun N.L., et al. 2001. Bone turnover and density in obese premenopausal women during moderate weight loss and calcium supplementation. *J Bone Miner Res* 16(7):1329–1336.

Shearman L.P., Camacho R.E., et al. 2003. Chronic MCH-1 receptor modulation alters appetite, body weight and adiposity in rats. *Eur J Pharmacol* 475(1–3):37–47.

Shekelle P.G., Hardy M.L., et al. 2003. Efficacy and safety of ephedra and ephedrine for weight loss and athletic performance: A meta-analysis. *JAMA* 289(12):1537–1545.

Short T. 1727. *A Discourse Concerning the Causes and Effects of Corpulency Together with the Method for its Prevention and Cure*. London: J. Roberts.

Sjostrom L., Lindroos A.K., et al. 2004. Lifestyle, diabetes, and cardiovascular risk factors 10 years after bariatric surgery. *N Engl J Med* 351(26):2683–2693.

Sjostrom L., Rissanen A., et al. 1998. Randomised placebo-controlled trial of orlistat for weight loss and prevention of weight regain in obese patients. European Multicentre Orlistat Study Group. *Lancet* 352(9123):167–172.

Small C.J., Bloom S.R. 2004. Gut hormones as peripheral antiobesity targets. *Curr Drug Targets CNS Neurol Disord* 3(5):379–388.

Smathers S.A., Wilson J.G., et al. 2003. Topiramate effectiveness in Prader-Willi syndrome. *Pediatr Neurol* 28(2):130–133.

Smith I.G., Goulder M.A., on behalf of the members of the Sibutamine Clinical Study 1047 team. 2001. Randomized placebo-controlled trial of long-term treatment with sibutramine in mild to moderate obesity. *J Fam Pract* 50:505–512.

Smith S.R., Prosser W.A., Donahue D.J., Morgan M.E., Anderson C.M., Shanahan W.R. 2009. APD356–004 Study Group. Lorcaserin (APD356), a selective 5–HT(2C) agonist, reduces body weight in obese men and women. *Obesity* (Silver Spring) 17(3):494–503.

Smith, S.R., Weissman, N.J., Anderson, C.M., Sanchez M., Chuang E., Stubbe S., Bays H., Shanahan W.R., and the Behavioral Modification and Lorcaserin for Overweight Obesity and Management (BLOOM) Study Group. 2010. Multicenter, placebo-controlled trial of lorcaserin for weight management. *N Engl J Med* 363:245–256.

Snow V., Barry P., et al. 2005. Pharmacologic and surgical management of obesity in primary care: A clinical practice guideline from the American College of Physicians. *Ann Intern Med* 142(7): 525–531.

Sood N., Baker W.L., Coleman C.I. 2008. Effect of glucomannan on plasma lipid and glucose concentrations, body weight, and blood pressure: A systematic review and meta-analysis. *Am J Clin Nutr* 88:1167–1175.

Souers A.J., Gao J., et al. 2005. Identification of 2-(4-benzyloxyphenyl)-N-[1-(2-pyrrolidin-1-yl-ethyl)-1H-indazol-6-yl]acetamide, an orally efficacious melanin-concentrating hormone receptor 1 antagonist for the treatment of obesity. *J Med Chem* 48(5):1318–1321.

Stafford R.S., Radley D.C. 2003. National trends in antiobesity medication use. *Arch Intern Med* 163(9): 1046–1050.

Stenlof K., Rossner S., Vercruysse F., et al. 2007. Topiramate in the treamtent of obese subjects with drug naïve type 2 diabetes. *Diabetes Obes Metab* 9:360–368.

Stevenson L.G. 1953. *Nobel Prize Winners in Medicine & Physiology 1901–1950*. New York: Henry Schuman.

Sullivan C., Triscari J. 1977. Metabolic regulation as a control for lipid disorders. I. Influence of (—)-hydroxycitrate on experimentally induced obesity in the rodent. *Am J Clin Nutr* 30(5):767–776.

Suozzi J.C., Rancont C.M., McFee R.B. 2005. DNP 2,4-dinitrophenol: A deadly way to lose weight. *JEMS* 30(1):82–89, quiz 90–91.

Szayna M., Doyle M.E., et al. 2000. Exendin-4 decelerates food intake, weight gain, and fat deposition in Zucker rats. *Endocrinology* 141(6):1936–1941.

Tainter M. (see Colman 2007 for discussion of Tainter).

Tan K.C.B., Tso A.W.K., Tam S.C.F., Pang R.W.C., Lam K.S.L. 2002. Acute effect of orlistat on post-prandial lipaemia and free fatty acids in overweight patients with type 2 diabetes mellitus. *Diab Med* 19:944–948.

Tan T.M., Vanderpump M., et al. 2004. Somatostatin infusion lowers plasma ghrelin without reducing appetite in adults with Prader-Willi syndrome. *J Clin Endocrinol Metab* 89(8):4162–4165.

Toplak H., Hamann R., Moore R., Masson E., Gorska M., Vercruysse F., Sun X., Fitchet M., for the OBDM-002 Study Group. 2007. Efficacy and safety of topiramate in combination with metformin in the treatment of obese subjects with type 2 diabetes: A randomized, double-blind placebo-controlled study. *Intern J Obes* 31:138–146.

Toplak H., Ziegler O., Keller U., Hamann A., Godin C., Sittert G., Zanella M.-T., Zuniga-Guajardo S., Van Gaal L. 2006. X-PERT: Weight reduction with orlistat in obese subjects receiving a mildly or moderately reduced-energy diet. Early response to treatment predicts weight maintenance. *Diab Obes Metab* 7:699–708.

Torgerson J.S., Hauptman J., et al. 2004. XENical in the prevention of diabetes in obese subjects (XENDOS) study: A randomized study of orlistat as an adjunct to lifestyle changes for the prevention of type 2 diabetes in obese patients. *Diabetes Care* 27(1): 155–161.

Torp-Pedersen C., Caterson I., Coutinho W., et al. SCOUT investigators. 2007. Cardiovascular response to weight management and sibutramine in high-risk subjects: An analysis from the SCOUT trial. *Eur Heart J* 28:2915–2923.

Tziomalos K., Krassas G.E., Tzotas T. 2009. The use of sibutramine in the management of obesity and related disorders: An update. *Vasc Health Risk Manag* 5:441–452.

Van Baak M.A., Hul G.B., et al. 2002. Acute effect of L-796568, a novel beta 3-adrenergic receptor agonist, on energy expenditure in obese men. *Clin Pharmacol Ther* 71(4):272–279.

Van Gaal L.F., Rissanen A.M., et al. 2005. Effects of the cannabinoid-1 receptor blocker rimonabant on weight reduction and cardiovascular risk factors in overweight patients: 1-year experience from the RIO-Europe study. *Lancet* 365(9468):1389–1397.

Brandt G.A.S., Quay S., et al. 2004. Intranasal peptide YY 3-36: Phase 1 dose ranging and dose sequencing studies. *Obes Res* 12 (Suppl):A28.

Velasquez-Mieyer P.A., Cowan P.A., et al. 2003. Suppression of insulin secretion is associated with weight loss and altered macronutrient intake and preference in a subset of obese adults. *Int J Obes Relat Metab Disord* 27(2):219–226.

Vettor R., Serra R., et al. 2005. Effect of sibutramine on weight management and metabolic control in type 2 diabetes: A meta-analysis of clinical studies. *Diabetes Care* 28(4):942–949.

Vray M., Joubert J.M., Eschwage E., Liard F., Fagnani F., Montestruc F., Fages S., Bagaud B. 2005. [Results from the observations study EIGRAM: Management of excess weight in general practice and follow–up of patients treated with orlistat]. *Therapie* 60:17–24.

Wadden T.A., Berkowitz R.I., et al. 2001. Benefits of lifestyle modification in the pharmacologic treatment of obesity: A randomized trial. *Arch Intern Med* 161(2):218–227.

Wadden T.A., Berkowitz R.I., et al. 2000. Effects of sibutramine plus orlistat in obese women following 1 year of treatment by sibutramine alone: A placebo-controlled trial. *Obes Res* 8(6):431–437.

Wadden T.A., Berkowitz R.I., et al. 2005. Randomized trial of lifestyle modification and pharmacotherapy for obesity. *N Engl J Med* 353(20):2111–2120.

Weintraub M., Sundaresan P.R., Schuster B., et al. 1992. Long term weight control: The National Heart, Lung and Blood Institute funded multimodal intervention study. I-VII. *Clin Pharmacol Ther* 51:581–646.

Westerterp-Plantenga M.S., Lejeune M.P.G.M., Kovacs E.M.R. 2005. Body weight loss and weight maintenance in relation to habitual caffeine intake and green tea supplementation. *Obes Res* 13:1195–1204.

Wilding J., Van Gaal L., et al. 2004. A randomized double-blind placebo-controlled study of the long-term efficacy and safety of topiramate in the treatment of obese subjects. *Int J Obes Relat Metab Disord* 28(11):1399–1410.

Wilfley D.E., Crow S.J., Hudson J.I., Mitchell J.E., Berkowitz R.I., Blakesley V., Walsh B.T. 2008. Sibutramine Binge Eating Disorder Research Group. Efficacy of sibutramine for the treatment of binge eating disorder: A randomized multicenter placebo-controlled double-blind study. *Am J Psychiatry* 165(1):51–58.

Winkelman J.W. 2003. Treatment of nocturnal eating syndrome and sleep-related eating disorder with topiramate. *Sleep Med* 4(3):243–246.

Wirth A., Krause J. 2001. Long-term weight loss with sibutramine: A randomized controlled trial. *JAMA* 286(11):1331–1339.

Wolk A., Manson J.E., et al. 1999. Long-term intake of dietary fiber and decreased risk of coronary heart disease among women. *JAMA* 281(21):1998–2004.

Wynne K., Park A.J., et al. 2005. Subcutaneous oxyntomodulin reduces body weight in overweight and obese subjects: A double-blind, randomized, controlled trial. *Diabetes* 54(8):2390–2395.

Xue B., Kahn B.B. 2006. AMPK integrates nutrient and hormonal signals to regulate food intake and energy balance through effects in the hypothalamus and peripheral tissues. *J Physiol* 574(Pt 1):73–83.

Yanovski S.Z., Yanovski J.A. 2002. Obesity. *N Engl J Med* 346(8):591–602.

Yanovski J.A., Parikh S.J., Yanoff L.B., Denkinger B.I., Calis K.A., Reynolds J.C., Sebring N.G., McHugh T. 2009. Effects of calcium supplementation on body weight and adiposity in overweight and obese adults: A randomized trial. *Ann Intern Med* 150(12):821–829.

Zahorska-Markiewicz B., Obuchowicz E., et al. 2001. Neuropeptide Y in obese women during treatment with adrenergic modulation drugs. *Med Sci Monit* 7(3):403–408.

Zemel M.B., Richards J., et al. 2005. Dairy augmentation of total and central fat loss in obese subjects. *Int J Obes* (London) 29(4):391–397.

Zemel M.B., Richards J., et al. 2005. Effects of calcium and dairy on body composition and weight loss in African-American adults. *Obes Res* 13(7):1218–1225.

Zemel M.B., Shi H., et al. 2000. Regulation of adiposity by dietary calcium. *FASEB J* 14(9):1132–1138.

Zemel M.B., Thompson W., et al. 2004. Calcium and dairy acceleration of weight and fat loss during energy restriction in obese adults. *Obes Res* 12(4):582–590.

Zhi J., Mulligan T.E., et al. 1999. Long-term systemic exposure of orlistat, a lipase inhibitor, and its metabolites in obese patients. *J Clin Pharmacol* 39(1):41–46.

CHAPTER 8

Adams T.D., Hunt S.C. 2009. Cancer and obesity: Effect of bariatric surgery. *World J Surg* 33(10): 2028–2033.

Agren G., Narbro K., et al. 2002. Long-term effects of weight loss on pharmaceutical costs in obese subjects. A report from the SOS intervention study. *Int J Obes Relat Metab Disord* 26(2):184–192.

Andersen T., Backer O.G., et al. 1984. Randomized trial of diet and gastroplasty compared with diet alone in morbid obesity. *N Engl J Med* 310(6):352–356.

Andersen T., Stokholm K.H., et al. 1988. Long-term (5-year) results after either horizontal gastroplasty or very-low-calorie diet for morbid obesity. *Int J Obes* 12(4):277–284.

Angrisani L., Furbetta F., et al. 2003. Lap Band adjustable gastric banding system: The Italian experience with 1863 patients operated on 6 years. *Surg Endosc* 17(3):409–412.

Arterburn D., Livingston E.H., Schifftner T., Kahwati L.C., Henderson W.G., Maciejewski M.L. 2009. Predictors of long-term mortality after bariatric surgery performed in Veterans Affairs medical centers. *Arch Surg* 144(10):914–920.

ASBS. 2003. Bariatric centers of excellence. *ASBS Newsletter*. (American Society for Bariatric Surgery) Spring: 4.

Bajardi G., Ricevuto G., et al. 2000. Surgical treatment of morbid obesity with biliopancreatic diversion and gastric banding: Report on an 8-year experience involving 235 cases. *Ann Chir* 125(2):155–162.

Balsiger B.M., Murr M.M., et al. 2000. Gastroesophageal reflux after intact vertical banded gastroplasty: Correction by conversion to Roux-en-Y gastric bypass. *J Gastrointest Surg* 4(3):276–281.

Balsiger B.M., Murr M.M., et al. 2000. Bariatric surgery. Surgery for weight control in patients with morbid obesity. *Med Clin North Am* 84(2):477–489.

Batsis J.A., Lopez-Jimenez F., Collazo-Clavell M.L., Clark M.M., Somers V.K., Sarr M.G. 2009. Quality of life after bariatric surgery: A population-based cohort study. *Am J Med* 122(11):1055.e1–1055.e10.

Bigelow H.J. 1846. Insensibility during surgical operations produced by inhalation. *Boston Med Surg J* 35: 309–317.

Billroth C.A.T. 1881. Offenes Schreiben an Herrn Dr. L Wittelshofer. *Wien med Wschr* 31:161–165.

Bray G.A. 1976. *The Obese Patient: Major Problems in Internal Medicine*. Philadelphia: W.B. Saunders Company.

Bruno C., Fulford A.D., Potts J.R., McClintock R., Jones R., Cacucci B.M., Gupta C.E., Peacock M., Considine R.V. 2009. Serum markers of bone turnover are increased at six and 18 months after Roux-en-Y bariatric surgery: Correlation with the reduction in Leptin. *J Clin Endocrinol Metab* 95(1):159–166.

Buchwald H., Avidor Y., et al. 2004. Bariatric surgery: A systematic review and meta-analysis. *JAMA* 292(14):1724–1737.

Buchwald H., Estok R., Fahrbach K., Banel D., Sledge I. 2007. Trends in mortality in bariatric surgery: A systematic review and meta-analysis. *Surgery* 142(4):621–632.

Buchwald H., Estok R., Fahrbach K., Banel D., Jensen M.D., Pories W.J., Bantle J.P., Sledge I. 2009. Weight and type 2 diabetes after bariatric surgery: Systematic review and meta-analysis. *Am J Med* 122(3):248–256.

Burguera B., Agusti A., Arner P., Baltasar A., Barbe F., Barcelo A., Breton I., Cabanes T., Casanueva F.F., Couce M.E., Dieguez C., Fiol M., Fernandez Real J.M., Formiguera X., Fruhbeck G., Garcia Romero M., Garcia Sanz M., Ghigo E., Gomis R., Higa K., Ibarra O., Lacy A., Larrad A., Masmiquel L., Moizé V., Moreno

B., Moreiro J., Ricart W., Riesco M., Salinas R., Salvador J., Pi-Sunyer F.X., Scopinaro N., Sjostrom L., Pagan A., Pereg V., Sánchez Pernaute A., Torres A., Urgeles J.R., Vidal-Puig A., Vidal J., Vila M. 2007. Critical assessment of the current guidelines for the management and treatment of morbidly obese patients. *J Endocrinol Invest* 30(10):844–852.

Champion J.K., Williams M. 2003. Small bowel obstruction and internal hernias after laparoscopic Roux-en-Y gastric bypass. *Obes Surg* 13(4):596–600.

Christou N.V., Sampalis J.S., et al. 2004. Surgery decreases long-term mortality, morbidity, and health care use in morbidly obese patients. *Ann Surg* 240(3):416–423; discussion 423–424.

Christou N.V., Lieberman M., Sampalis F., Sampalis J.S. 2008. Bariatric surgery reduces cancer risk in morbidly obese patients. *Surg Obes Relat Dis* 4(6):691–695.

Colquitt J., Clegg A., et al. 2005. Surgery for morbid obesity. *Cochrane Database Syst Review* Issue 4: CD003641.

Cremieux P.Y., Buchwald H., Shikora S.A., Ghosh A., Yang H.E., Buessing M. 2008. A study on the economic impact of bariatric surgery. *Am J Manag Care* 14(9):589–596.

Csendes A., Maluenda F., Burgos A.M. 2009. A prospective randomized study comparing patients with morbid obesity submitted to laparotomic gastric bypass with or without omentectomy. *Obes Surg* 19:490–494.

Cummings D.E., Weigle D.S., et al. 2002. Plasma ghrelin levels after diet-induced weight loss or gastric bypass surgery. *N Engl J Med* 346(21):1623–1630.

Danish Obesity Project. 1979. Randomised trial of jejunoileal bypass versus medical treatment in morbid obesity. The Danish Obesity Project. *Lancet* 2(8155):1255–1258.

DeMaria E.J., Sugerman H.J., et al. 2001. High failure rate after laparoscopic adjustable silicone gastric banding for treatment of morbid obesity. *Ann Surg* 233(6):809–818.

DeMaria E.J., Portenier D., Wolfe L. 2007. Obesity surgery mortality risk score: Proposal for a clinically useful score to predict mortality risk in patients undergoing gastric bypass. *Surg Obes Relat Dis* 3(2):134–140.

DeWind L.T., Payne J.H. 1976. Intestinal bypass surgery for morbid obesity. Long-term results. *JAMA* 236(20):2298–2301.

Dixon A.F., Dixon J.B., et al. 2005. Laparoscopic adjustable gastric banding induces prolonged satiety: a randomized blind crossover study. *J Clin Endocrinol Metab* 90(2):813–819.

Dixon J.B., Schachter L.M., et al. 2001. Sleep disturbance and obesity: Changes following surgically induced weight loss. *Arch Intern Med* 161(1):102–106.

Dixon J.B., O'Brien P.E., Playfair J., Chapman L., Schachter L.M., Skinner S., Proietto J., Bailey M., Anderson M. 2008. Adjustable gastric banding and conventional therapy for type 2 diabetes. A randomized controlled trial. *JAMA* 299:316–323.

Dumonceau J.-M. 2008. Evidence-based review of Bioenterics intragastric balloon for weight loss. *Obes Surg* 18:1611–1617.

Flum D.R., Dellinger E.P. 2004. Impact of gastric bypass operation on survival: A population-based analysis. *J Am Coll Surg* 199(4):543–551.

Flum D.R., Salem L., et al. 2005. Early mortality among Medicare beneficiaries undergoing bariatric surgical procedures. *JAMA* 294(15):1903–1908.

Flum D.R., Khan T.V., Dellinger E.P. 2007. Toward the rational and equitable use of bariatric surgery. *JAMA* 298:1442–1444.

Flum D.R., Belle S.H., King W.C., Wahed A.S., Berk P., Chapman W., Pories W., Courcoulas A., McCloskey C., Mitchell J., Patterson E., Pomp A., Staten M.A., Yanovski S.Z., Thirlby R., Wolfe B. 2009. Longitudinal Assessment of Bariatric Surgery (LABS) Consortium. Perioperative safety in the longitudinal assessment of bariatric surgery. *N Engl J Med* 361(5):445–454.

Frachetti K.J., Goldfine A.B. 2009. Bariatric surgery for diabetes management. *Curr Opin Endocrinol Diabetes Obes* 16(2):119–124.

Friedman M.N., Sancetta A.J., Magovern G.J. 1955. The amelioration of diabetes mellitus following subtotal gastrectomy. *Surg Gynecol Obstet* 100(2):201–204.

Fritscher L.G., Mottin C.C., Canani S., Chatkin J.M. 2007. Obesity and obstructive sleep apnea-hypopnea syndrome: The impact of bariatric surgery. *Obes Surg* 17(1):95–99.

Fulop-Muller R. 1938. *Triumph over Pain.* (transl. Eden and Cedar Paul). New York: The Literary Guild of America.

Garb J., Welch G., Zagarins S., Kuhn J., Romanelli J. 2009. Bariatric surgery for the treatment of morbid obesity: A meta-analysis of weight loss outcomes for laparoscopic adjustable gastric banding and laparoscopic gastric bypass. *Obes Surg* 19(10):1447–1455.

Garrison, F. 1914. *An Introduction to the History of Medicine.* Philadelphia: W.B. Saunders Company.

Grunstein R.R., Stenlöf K., Hedner J.A., Peltonen M., Karason K., Sjöström L. 2007. Two year reduction in sleep apnea symptoms and associated diabetes incidence after weight loss in severe obesity. *Sleep* 30(6):703–710.

Haines K.L., Nelson L.G., Gonzalez R., Torrella T., Martin T., Kandil A., Dragotti R., Anderson W.M., Gallagher S.F., Murr M.M. 2007. Objective evidence that bariatric surgery improves obesity-related obstructive sleep apnea. *Surgery* 141(3):354–358.

Hamilton E.C., Sims T.L., et al. 2003. Clinical predictors of leak after laparoscopic Roux-en-Y gastric bypass for morbid obesity. *Surg Endosc* 17(5):679–684.

Hauer E. 1884. Darmresektion und Enterorhaphieen 1878–1883. *Z. Heilk* 5:83–108.

Higa K.D., Boone K.B., et al. 2000. Complications of the laparoscopic Roux-en-Y gastric bypass: 1,040 patients–what have we learned? *Obes Surg* 10(6):509–513.

Inge T.H., Krebs N.F., et al. 2004. Bariatric surgery for severely overweight adolescents: Concerns and recommendations. *Pediatrics* 114(1):217–223.

Inge T.H., Miyano G., Bean J., Helmrath M., Courcoulas A., Harmon C.M., Chen M.K., Wilson K., Daniels S.R., Garcia V.F., Brandt M.L., Dolan L.M. 2009. Reversal of type 2 diabetes mellitus and improvements in cardiovascular risk factors after surgical weight loss in adolescents. *Pediatrics* 123(1):214–222.

Jones S.B., Jones D.B. 2009. *Obesity Surgery. Patient Safety and Best Practices.*Woodbury CT: Cine-Med, Inc.

Karlsson J., Taft C., Rydén A., Sjöström L., Sullivan M. 2007. Ten-year trends in health-related quality of life after surgical and conventional treatment for severe obesity: The SOS intervention study. Effects of bariatric surgery on mortality in Swedish obese subjects. *Int J Obes* (London) 31(8):1248–1261.

Klein S., Fontana L., et al. 2004. Absence of an effect of liposuction on insulin action and risk factors for coronary heart disease. *N Engl J Med* 350(25):2549–2557.

Ko C.W., Lee S.P. 2004. Obesity and gallbladder disease In *Handbook of Obesity: Etiology and Pathophysiology,* G.A. Bray and C Bouchard, eds. New York: Marcel Dekker, Inc. pp 919–934.

Kothari S.N., DeMaria E.J., et al. 2002. Lap-band failures: Conversion to gastric bypass and their preliminary outcomes. *Surgery* 131(6):625–629.

Kremen A.J., Linner J.H., Nelson C.H. 1954. Experimental evaluation of nutritional importance of proximal and distal small intestine. *Ann Surg* 140:439–448.

Lee W.J., Yu P.J., et al. 2005. Laparoscopic Roux-en-Y versus mini-gastric bypass for the treatment of morbid obesity: A prospective randomized controlled clinical trial. *Ann Surg* 242(1):20–28.

Long S.D., O'Brien K., MacDonald K.G., Leggett-Frazier N., Swanson M.S., Pories W.J., Caro J.F. 1994. Weight loss in severely obese subjects prevents the progress of impaired glucose tolerance to Type II diabetes. *Diabetes Care* 17:372–375.

Longitudinal Assessment of Bariatric Surgery (LABS) Consortium, Flum D.R., Belle S.H., King W.C., Wahed A.S., Berk P., Chapman W., Pories W., Courcoulas A., McCloskey C., Mitchell J., Patterson E., Pomp A., Staten M.A., Yanovski S.Z., Thirlby R., Wolfe B. 2009. Perioperative safety in the longitudinal assessment of bariatric surgery. *N Engl J Med* 361(5):445–454.

Lottati M., Kolka C.M., Stefanovski D., Kirkman E., Bergman R.N. 2009. Greater omentectomy improves insulin sensitivity in nonobese dogs. *Obesity* 17:674–680.

Loux T.J., Haricharan R.N., Clements R.H., Kolotkin R.L., Bledsoe S.E., Haynes B., Leath T., Harmon C.M. 2008. Health-related quality of life before and after bariatric surgery in adolescents. *J Pediatr Surg* 43(7):1275–1279.

McCawley G.M., Ferriss J.S., Geffel D., Northup C.J., Modesitt S.C. 2009. Cancer in obese women: Potential protective impact of bariatric surgery. *J Am Coll Surg* 208(6):1093–1098.

Maggard M.A., Shugarman L.R., Suttorp M., Maglione M., Sugerman H.J., Livingston E.H., Nguyen N.T., Li Z., Mojica W.A., Hilton L., Rhodes S., Morton S.C., Shekelle P.G. 2005. Meta-analysis: Surgical treatment of obesity. *Ann Intern Med* 142(7):547–559.

Mari A., Manco M., Guidone C., Nanni G., Castagneto M., Mingrone G., Ferrannini E. 2006. Restoration of normal glucose tolerance in severely obese patients after bilio-pancreatic diversion: Role of insulin sensitivity and beta cell function. *Diabetologia* 49:2136–2143.

Mason E.E. 1982. Vertical banded gastroplasty for obesity. *Arch Surg* 117(5):701–706.

Mason E.E., Ito C. 1967. Gastric bypass in obesity. *Surg Clin North Am* 47(6):1345–1351.

Mason E.E., Ito C. 1970. Gastric bypass. *Ann Surg* 170:329–339.

Mechanick J.I., Kushner R.F., Sugerman H.J., Gonzalez-Campoy J.M., Collazo-Clavell M.L., Guven S., Spitz A.F., Apovian C.M., Livingston E.H., Brolin R., Sarwer D.B., Anderson W.A., Dixon J. 2008. American Association of Clinical Endocrinologists, The Obesity Society, and American Society for Metabolic & Bariatric Surgery Medical guidelines for clinical practice for the perioperative nutritional, metabolic, and nonsurgical support of the bariatric surgery patient. *Endocr Pract.* 14(Suppl 1):1–83.

Melinek J., Livingston E., et al. 2002. Autopsy findings following gastric bypass surgery for morbid obesity. *Arch Pathol Lab Med* 126(9):1091–1095.

Müller M.K., Wenger C., Schiesser M., Clavien P.A., Weber M. 2008. Quality of life after bariatric surgery—A comparative study of laparoscopic banding vs. bypass. *Obes Surg* 18(12):1551–1557.

Murr M.M., Balsiger B.M., et al. 1999. Malabsorptive procedures for severe obesity: Comparison of pancreaticobiliary bypass and very very long limb Roux-en-Y gastric bypass. *J Gastrointest Surg* 3(6):607–612.

Narbro K., Agren G., et al. 2002. Pharmaceutical costs in obese individuals: Comparison with a randomly selected population sample and long-term changes after conventional and surgical treatment: The SOS intervention study. *Arch Intern Med* 162(18):2061–2069.

National Institutes of Health. 1991. NIH conference. Gastrointestinal surgery for severe obesity. Consensus Development Conference Panel. *Ann Intern Med* 115(12):956–961.

Nguyen N.T., Goldman C., et al. 2001. Laparoscopic versus open gastric bypass: A randomized study of outcomes, quality of life, and costs. *Ann Surg* 234(3):279–89; discussion 289–291.

Nguyen N.T., Ho H.S., et al. 2000. A comparison study of laparoscopic versus open gastric bypass for morbid obesity. *J Am Coll Surg* 191(2):149–155; discussion 155–157.

Nguyen N.T., et al. 2009. A prospective randomized trial of laparoscopic gastric by-pass versus laparoscopic adjustable gastric banding for the treatment of morbid obesity: Outcomes, quality of life, and costs. *Ann Surg PMID* 19730234.

Nguyen N.T., Paya M., Stevens C.M., Mavandadi S., Zainabadi K., Wilson S.E. 2004. The relationship between hospital volume and outcome in bariatric surgery at academic medical centers. *Ann Surg* 240:586–593.

O'Brien P.E., Dixon J.B. 2003. Lap-band: Outcomes and results. *J Laparoendosc Adv Surg Tech A* 13(4): 265–270.

O'Brien P.E., Dixon J.B., et al. 2006. Treatment of mild to moderate obesity with laparoscopic adjustable gastric banding or an intensive medical program: A randomized trial. *Ann Intern Med* 144(9):625–633.

Payne J.H., Dewind L.T., et al. 1963. Metabolic observations in patients with jejunocolic shunts. *Am J Surg* 106:273–289.

Peterli R., Wölnerhanssen B., Peters T., Devaux N., Kern B., Christoffel-Courtin C., Drewe J., von Flüe M., Beglinger C. 2009. Improvement in glucose metabolism after bariatric surgery: Comparison of laparoscopic Roux-en-Y gastric bypass and laparoscopic sleeve gastrectomy: A prospective randomized trial. *Ann Surg* 250(2):234–241.

Picot J., Jones J., Colquitt J.L., Gospodarevskaya E., Loveman E., Baxter L., Clegg A.J. 2009. The clinical effectiveness and cost-effectiveness of bariatric (weight loss) surgery for obesity: A systematic review and economic evaluation. *Health Technol Assess* 13(41):1–190, 215–357.

Pories W.J., MacDonald K.G. Jr, Flickinger E.G., Dohm G.L., Sinha M.K., Barakat H.A., May H.J., Khazanie P., Swanson M.S., Morgan E., Leggett-Frazier N., Long S.D., Brown B.M., O'Brien K., Carol J.F. 1992a Is type II diabetes mellitus (NIDDM) a surgical disease? *Ann Surg* 215(6):633–642; discussion 643.

Pories W.J., Macdonald K.G., Morgan E.J., Sinha M.K., Dohm G.L., Swanson M.S., Barakat H.A., Khazanie P.G., Leggett-Frazier N., Long S.D., O'Brien K.F., Caro J.F. 1992b. Surgical treatment of obesity and its effect on diabetes: 10-yr follow-up. *Am J Clin Nutr* 55:582S–585S.

Pories W.J., Swanson M.S., MacDonald K.G., Long S.B., Morris P.G., Brow B.M., Barakat H.A., deRamon R.A., Israel G., Dolezal J.M., Dohn L. 1995. Who would have thought it? An operation proves to be the most effective therapy for adult-onset diabetes mellitus. *Ann Surg* 222(3):339–350; discussion 350–352.

Porter R. 1997. *The Greatest Benefit to Mankind. A Medical History of Humanity*. New York: W.W. Norton & Company.

Preuss J. 1978. *Biblical and Talmudic Medicine.* Transl. and ed. F. Rosner, MD. New York: Hebrew Publishing Co.

Regan J.P., Inabnet W.B., et al. 2003. Early experience with two-stage laparoscopic Roux-en-Y gastric bypass as an alternative in the super-super obese patient. *Obes Surg* 13(6):861–864.

Ren C.J., Horgan S., et al. 2002. US experience with the LAP-BAND system. *Am J Surg* 184(6B):46S–50S.

Roman S., Napoleon B., et al. 2004. Intragastric balloon for non-morbid obesity: A retrospective evaluation of tolerance and efficacy. *Obes Surg* 14(4):539–544.

Rubenstein, R.B. 2002. Laparoscopic adjustable gastric banding at a U.S. center with up to 3-year follow-up. *Obes Surg* 12(3):380–384.

Ryden A., Sullivan M., et al. 2004. A comparative controlled study of personality in severe obesity: A 2-y follow-up after intervention. *Int J Obes Relat Metab Disord* 28(11):1485–1493.

Salem L., Devlin A., Sullivan S.D., Flum D.R. 2008. Cost-effectiveness analysis of laparoscopic gastric bypass, adjustable gastric banding, and nonoperative weight loss interventions. *Surg Obes Relat Dis* 4(1):26–32.

Salem L., Jensen C.C., Flum D.R. 2005. Are bariatric surgical outcomes worth their cost? A systematic review. *J Am Coll Surg* 200(2):270–278.

Sallet J.A., Marchesini J.B., et al. 2004. Brazilian multicenter study of the intragastric balloon. *Obes Surg* 14(7):991–998.

Sampalis J.S., Liberman M., Auger S., Christou N.V. 2004. The impact of weight reduction surgery on health-care costs in morbidly obese patients. *Obes Surg* 14(7):939–947.

Sapala J.A., Wood M.H., et al. 2003. Fatal pulmonary embolism after bariatric operations for morbid obesity: A 24-year retrospective analysis. *Obes Surg* 13(6):819–825.

Schauer P., Ikramuddin S., et al. 2003. The learning curve for laparoscopic Roux-en-Y gastric bypass in 100 cases. *Surg Endosc* 17(2):212–215.

Schauer P.R., Ikramuddin S., et al. 2000. Outcomes after laparoscopic Roux-en-Y gastric bypass for morbid obesity. *Ann Surg* 232(4):515–529.

Schneider B.E., Sanchez V.M., et al. 2004. How to implant the laparoscopic adjustable gastric band for morbid obesity. *Contemporary Surgery* 60(6):256–264.

Schneider B.E., Villegas L., et al. 2003. Laparoscopic gastric bypass surgery: Outcomes. *J Laparoendosc Adv Surg Tech A* 13(4):247–255.

Schouten R., Rijs C.S., Bouvy N.D., Hameeteman W., Koek G.H., Janssen I.M., Greve J.W. 2009. A multi-center, randomized efficacy study of the EndoBarrier Gastrointestinal Liner for presurgical weight loss prior to bariatric surgery. *Ann Surg*. Oct 24. [Epub ahead of print]

Scopinaro N., Gianetta E., et al. 1996. Biliopancreatic diversion for obesity at eighteen years. *Surgery* 119(3):261–268.

Scott H.W. 1991. A tribute to Edward Eaton Mason. The first Annual Edward E. Mason Founders Lecture. *Obes Surg* 1:13–19.

Shekelle P.G., Morton S.C., et al. 2004. Pharmacological and surgical treatment of obesity. *Evid Rep Technol Assess* (Summ)(103):1–6.

Sherwinter D.A., Ghaznavi A.M., Spinner D., Savel R.H., Macura J.M., Adler H. 2008. Continuous infusion of intraperitoneal bupivacaine after laparoscopic surgery: A randomized controlled trial. *Obes Surg* 18:1581–1586.

Shikora S.A. 2004. Implantable gastric stimulation for the treatment of severe obesity. *Obes Surg* 14(4):545–548.

Sjostrom L. 2004. Surgical treatment of obesity: An overview and results from the SOS Study. *Handbook of Obesity: Clinical Applications*. G.A. Bray and C. Bouchard, eds. New York: Marcel Dekker Inc., pp 359–389.

Sjostrom L., Larsson B., et al. 1992. Swedish obese subjects (SOS). Recruitment for an intervention study and a selected description of the obese state. *Int J Obes Relat Metab Disord* 16(6):465–479.

Sjostrom L., Lindroos A.K., et al. 2004. Lifestyle, diabetes, and cardiovascular risk factors 10 years after bariatric surgery. *N Engl J Med* 351(26):2683–2693.

Sjöström L., Narbro K., Sjöström C.D., Karason K., Larsson B., Wedel H., Lystig T., Sullivan M., Bouchard C., Carlsson B., Bengtsson C., Dahlgren S., Gummesson A., Jacobson P., Karlsson J., Lindroos A.K., Lönroth H., Näslund I., Olbers T., Stenlöf K., Torgerson J., Agren G., Carlsson L.M. 2007. Swedish Obese Subjects Study. *N Engl J Med* 357(8):741–752.

Sjöström C.D., Lissner L., Wedel H., Sjöström L. 1999. Reduction in incidence of diabetes, hypertension and lipid disturbances after intentional weight loss induced by bariatric surgery: The SOS Intervention Study. *Obes Res* 7(5):477–484.

Sjostrom L.H., Jacobson P., Peltonen M., Karason K., Narbro K., Sjostrom C.D., Carlsson L.M. 2009. Bariatric surgery and myocardial infarction: Effect-modification of baseline fasting glucose in the prospective, controlled intervention trial Swedish Obese Subjects. *Obesity Society* (Abs).

Sjostrom L. 2008. Bariatric surgery and reduction in morbidity and mortality: Experiences from the SOS Study. *IJO* 32:S93–S97.

Sjöström L., Gummesson A., Sjöström C.D., Narbro K., Peltonen M., Wedel H., Bengtsson C., Bouchard C., Carlsson B., Dahlgren S., Jacobson P., Karason K., Karlsson J., Larsson B., Lindroos A.K., Lönroth H., Näslund I., Olbers T., Stenlöf K., Torgerson J., Carlsson L.M. 2009. Swedish Obese Subjects Study. Effects of bariatric surgery on cancer incidence in obese patients in Sweden (Swedish Obese Subjects Study): A prospective, controlled intervention trial. *Lancet Oncol* 10(7):653–662.

Sugerman H.J., Sugerman E.L., et al. 2003. Bariatric surgery for severely obese adolescents. *J Gastrointest Surg* 7(1):102–107; discussion 107–108.

Talbot J.H. 1970. *A Biographical History of Medicine. Excerpts and Essays on the Men and Their Work*. New York: Grune & Stratton.

Tarnoff M., Rodriguez L., Escalona A., Ramos A., Neto M., Alamo M., Reyes E., Pimentel F., Ibanez L. 2009. Open label, prospective, randomized controlled trial of an endoscopic duodenal-jejunal bypass sleeve versus low calorie diet for pre-operative weight loss in bariatric surgery. *Surg Endosc* 23(3):650–656.

Thorne A., Lonnqvist F., et al. 2002. A pilot study of long-term effects of a novel obesity treatment: Omentectomy in connection with adjustable gastric banding. *Int J Obes Relat Metab Disord* 26(2):193–199.

Thorwald J. 1956. *The Century of the Surgeon.* New York: Pantheon Books.

Tice J.A., Karliner L., Walsh J., Petersen A.J., Feldman M.D. 2008. Gastric banding or bypass? A systematic review comparing the two most popular bariatric procedures. *Am J Med* 121(10):885–893.

Torgerson J.S., Sjostrom L. 2001. The Swedish Obese Subjects (SOS) study—Rationale and results. *Int J Obes Relat Metab Disord* 25(Suppl 1):S2–S4.

Tritos N.A., Mun E., et al. 2003. Serum ghrelin levels in response to glucose load in obese subjects post-gastric bypass surgery. *Obes Res* 11(8):919–924.

Tsai W.S., Inge T.H., Burd R.S. 2007. Bariatric surgery in adolescents: Recent national trends in use and in-hospital outcome. *Arch Pediatr Adolesc Med* 161(3):217–221.

U.S. Food and Drug Administration. 2001. The lap-band adjustable gastric banding system: Summary of safety and effectiveness data. Retrieved 2 March, 2006, from http://www.fda.gov/cdrh/pdf/p000008.htm.

Uy M.C., Talingdan-Te M.C., Espinosa-Ma W.Z., Daez L.O., Ong J.P. 2008. Ursodeoxycholic acid in the prevention of gallstone formation after bariatric surgery: A meta-analysis. *Obes Surg* 18:1532–1538.

Vetter M.L., Cardillo S., Rickels M.R., Iqbal N. 2009. Narrative review: Effect of bariatric surgery on type 2 diabetes mellitus. *Ann Intern Med* 150(2):94–103.

Westling A., Gustavsson S. 2001. Laparoscopic vs open Roux-en-Y gastric bypass: A prospective, randomized trial. *Obes Surg* 11(3):284–292.

Wittgrove A.C., Clark G.W. 2000. Laparoscopic gastric bypass, Roux-en-Y 500 patients: Technique and results, with 3–60 month follow-up. *Obes Surg* 10(3):233–239.

Zingmond D.S., McGory M.L., et al. 2005. Hospitalization before and after gastric bypass surgery. *JAMA* 294(15):1918–1924.

CHAPTER 9

Postscript

Actuarial Society of America and Association of Life Insurance Directors. *Medico-Actuarial Mortality Investigation.* New York, 1913.

Al Mamun A., Lawlor D.A., Cramb S., O'Callaghean M., Williams G., Najman J. 2007. Do childhood sleeping problems predict obesity in young adulthood? Evidence from a prospective birth cohort study. *Am J Epidemiol* 166:1368–1373.

Angel A., Anderson H., Bouchard C., Lau D., Leiter L., Mendelson R. 1996. *Progress in Obesity Research: 7.* London: John Libbey.

Appel L.J., Moore T.J., et al. 1997. A clinical trial of the effects of dietary patterns on blood pressure. *N Engl J Med* 338:1117–1124.

Atwater W.O., Rosa E.B. 1899. *Description of a New Respiration Calorimeter and Experiments on the Conservation of Energy in the Human Body.* USDA Bull. 63, Washington, D.C.: USDA Office of Experimental Station.

Babinski M.J. 1900. Tumeur du corps pituitaire sans acromégalie et avec de développement des organes génitaux. *Rev Neurol* 8:531–533.

Banting W. 1864. *Letter on Corpulence Addressed to the Public.* London: Harrison, 3rd ed.

Berry E.M., Blondheim S.H., Eliahou E., Shafrir E., eds. 1987. *Recent advances in obesity: V. Proceedings of the 5th International Congress on Obesity.* London: John Libbey.

Bjorntorp P., Cairella M., Howard A.N., eds. 1981. *Recent advances in obesity research: III. Proceedings of the 3rd International Congress on Obesity.* London: John Libbey.

Bouchard C., Bray G.A., Kozak L., Ravussin E., eds. 2009. Twenty most important contributions to obesity in the past 20 years. *Intern J Obes* 32(Suppl 7):S1.

Bray G.A. 1976. *The Obese Patient.* Philadelphia: W.B. Saunders Company.

Bray G.A., ed. 1976. *Obesity in Perspective.* Fogarty International Center Series on Preventive Med. Vol 2, parts 1 and 2. Washington, DC: US Govt Printing Office, DHEW Publication #75–708, Parts 1 and 2.

Bray G.A., York D.A. 1979. Hypothalamic and genetic obesity in experimental animals: An autonomic and endocrine hypothesis. *Physiol Rev* 59(3):719–809.

Bray G.A. 1978. *Recent Advances in Obesity Research: II. Proceedings of the 2nd International Congress on Obesity, 23–26 October 1977, Washington, D.C.* London: Newman Publishing Ltd.

Bray G.A. 1995. Obesity research and medical journalism. *Obes Res* 3:65–71.

Bray G.A, Flatt J.P., Volaufova J., Delany J.P., Champagne C.M. 2008. Corrective responses in human food intake identified from an analysis of 7-d food-intake records. *Am J Clin Nutr* 88(6):1504–1510.

Bray G.A. 2010. Soft drink consumption and obesity: It's all about fructose. *Curr Opin Lipidology* 21:51–57.

Brillat-Savarin J.A. 1994. *The Physiology of Taste or Meditations on Transcendental Gastronomy* (Translated from the French by M.F.K. Fisher; with drawings and color lithographs by Wayne Thiebaud), San Francisco: The Arion Press.

Christakis N.A., Fowler J.H. 2007. The spread of obesity in a large social network over 32 years. *N Engl J Med* 357(4):370–379.

Conrad N.J. 2009. A female figurine from the basal Aurignacian of Hohle Fels Cave in southwestern Germany. *Nature* 459:248–252.

Cushing H. 1912. *The Pituitary Body and its Disorders. Clinical States Produced by Disorders of the Hypophysis Cerebri.* Philadelphia: J.B. Lippincott.

Cushing H. 1932. The basophil adenomas of the pituitary body and their clinical manifestations. Pituitary basophilism. *Bull Johns Hopkins Hospital* L:137–195.

DPP Research Group. 2002. Reduction in the incidence of type 2 diabetes with lifestyle intervention or metformin. *N Engl J Med* 346:393–403.

Farooqi S., O'Rahilly S. 2005. Monogenic obesity in humans. *Annu Rev Med* 56:443–458.

Farooqi I.S., O'Rahilly S. 2007. Genetic factors in human obesity. *Obes Rev* 8(Suppl 1):37–40.

Flier J. Obesity Wars. 2004. Molecular progress confronts an expanding epidemic. *Cell* 116:337–350.

Frohlich A. 1901. Ein fall von tumor der hypophysis cerebri ohne akromegalie. *Wiener Klin Rdsch* 15:883–886.

Guy-Grand B., Ailhaud G. 1999. *Progress in Obesity Research: 8.* London: John Libbey.

Hassall A. 1849. Observations on the development of the fat vesicle. *Lancet* 1:63–64.

Helhmoltz von Helmholtz H. 1847. *Über die Erhaltung der Kraft, eine physikalische Abhandlung: vorgetragen in der Sitzung der physikalischen Gesellschaft zu Berlin am 23sten Juli 1847.* Berlin: G Reimer.

Hirsch J., Van Itallie T.B., eds. 1985. *Recent Advances in Obesity Research: IV. Proceedings of the 4th International Congress on Obesity, 5–8 October, 1983 New York, USA.* London: John Libbey.

Howard A.N., ed. 1975. *Recent Advances in Obesity Research: I. Proceedings of the 1st International Congress on Obesity*, 8–11 October 1974 held at the Royal College of Physicians, London. London: Newman Publishing Ltd.

Hubert H.B., Feinleib M., McNamara P.M., Castelli W.P. 1983. Obesity as an independent risk factor for cardiovascular disease: A 26-year follow-up of participants in the Framingham Heart Study. *Circ* 67:986–977.

King B.M. 2006. The rise, fall, and resurrection of the ventromedial hypothalamus in the regulation of feeding behavior and body weight. *Physiol Behav* 87(2):221–244.

Kissebah A.H., Vydelingum N., Murray R., Evans D.J., Hartz A.J., Kalkhoff R.K., Adams P.W. 1982. Relation of body fat distribution to metabolic complications of obesity. *J Clin Endocrinol Metab* 54(2):254–260.

Kuhn T.D. 1962. *The Structure of Scientific Revolutions.* Chicago: The University of Chicago Press.

Lapidus L., Bengtsson C., Larsson B., Pennert K., Rybo E., Sjöström L. 1984. Distribution of adipose tissue and risk of cardiovascular disease and death: A 12 year follow up of participants in the population study of women in Gothenburg, Sweden. *BMJ (Clin Res Ed)* 289(6454):1257–1261.

Larsson B., Svardsudd K., et al. 1984. Abdominal adipose tissue distribution, obesity and risk of cardiovascular disease and death: 13 year follow up of participants in the study of 792 men born in 1913. *BMJ* 288:1401–1404.

Lavoisier A.L. 1789. *Traité Elémentaire de Chimie, Présenté dans un Ordre Nouveau et d'après les Découvertes Modernes . . . ; avec figures.* Paris: Chez Cuchet.

Leake C.D. 1958. *The Amphetamines: Their Actions and Uses.* Springfield, IL. Charles C. Thomas.

Lichtman S.W., Pisarska K., Berman E.R., Pestone M., Dowling H., Offenbacher E., Weisel H., Heshka S., Matthews D.E., Heymsfield S.B. 1992. Discrepancy between self-reported and actual caloric intake and exercise in obese subjects. *N Engl J Med* 327:1893–1898.

Lifson N., Gordon G.B., Visscher M.B., Nier A.O. 1949. The fate of utilized molecular oxygen and the source of the oxygen of respiratory carbon dioxide studied with the aid of heavy oxygen. *J Biol Chem* 180:803–811.

Mason E.E., Ito C. 1967. Gastric bypass in obesity. *Surg Clin North Am* 47(6):1345–1351.

Medeiros-Neto G., Halpern A., Bouchard C. 2003. *Progress in Obesity Research: 9.* London: John Libbey.

Oomura Y., Tarui S., Inoue S., Shimazu T. 1991. *Progress in Obesity Research 1990.* London: John Libbey.

Pamuk E.R., Williamson D.F., Madans J., Serdula M.K., Kleinman J.C., Byers T. 1992. Weight loss and mortality in a national cohort of adults, 1971–1987. *Am J Epidemiol* 136:686–697.

Pinto S., Roseberry A.G., Liu H., Diano S., Shanabrough M., Cai X., Friedman J.M., Horvath T.L. 2004. Rapid rewiring of arcuate nucleus feeding circuits by leptin. *Science* 304(5667):110–115.

Pollan M. 2008. *New York Times Magazine*, Nov 22.

Prader A., Labhart A., Willi H. 1956. Ein syndrome von adipositas, kleinwuchs, kryptorchismus und oligophrenie nach myotonieartigem zustand im neugeborenenalter. *Schweiz Med Wochenschr* 86:1260–1261.

Quetelet, A. 1835. *Sur l'homme et le developpement de ses facultes, ou essai de physique sociale*. Paris: Bachelier.

Sacks F.M., Bray G.A., Carey V., Smith S.R., Ryan D.H., Anton S., McManus K., Champagne C.M., Bishop L.M., Laranjo N., Leboff M.S., Rood J.C., Levitan L.D., Greenway F.L., Loria C.M., Obarzanek E., Williamson D.A. 2009. Comparison of weight-loss diets with different compositions of fat, carbohydrate and protein. *New Engl J Med* 360:859–873.

Sacks F.M., Svetkey L.P., et al. for the DASH-Sodium Collaborative Research Group. 2001. A clinical feeding trial of the effects on blood pressure of reduced dietary sodium and the DASH dietary pattern (The DASH-Sodium Trial). *N Engl J Med* 344:3–10.

Santorio, Santorio [Sanctorius]. [1624]. *Ars . . . de statica medicina aphorismorum sectionibus septem comprehensa. Accessit Statico Mastrix, sive ejusdem artis demolitio Hippolyti Obicii*. Leipzig: Gregor Ritsch fur Zacharia Schurer und Matthias Gotzen.

Schoeller D.A. 1998. Balancing energy expenditure and body weight. *Am J Clin Nutr* 68(Suppl):956S–961S.

Schwann T.H. 1847. *Microsccopical Researches into the Accordance in the Structure and Growth of Animals and Plants*. Transl. H Smith. London: Sydenham Society.

Sjöström L., Narbro K., Sjöström C.D., Karason K., Larsson B., Wedel H., Lystig T., Sullivan M., Bouchard C., Carlsson B., Bengtsson C., Dahlgren S., Gummesson A., Jacobson P., Karlsson J., Lindroos A.K., Lönroth H., Näslund I., Olbers T., Stenlöf K., Torgerson J., Agren G., Carlsson L.M., Swedish Obese Subjects Study. 2007. Effects of bariatric surgery on mortality in Swedish obese subjects. *N Engl J Med* 357(8):741–752.

Stuart R.B., Davis B. 1972. *Slim Chance in a Fat World: Behavioral Control of Obesity*. Champaign, IL: Research Press Company.

Swinburn B., Sacks G., Ravussin E. 2009. Increased food energy supply is more than sufficient to explain the US epidemic of obesity. *Am J Clin Nutr* 90(6):1453–1456.

Vague J. 1947. La differenciation sexuelle facteur determinant des formes de l'obésité. *Presse Medicale* 55:339–340.

Westerterp K., Speakman J.R. 2008. Physical activity energy expenditure has not declined since the 1980s and matches energy expenditures of wild mammals. *Int J Obes* (London) 32(8):1256–1263.

Zhang Y., Proenca R., et al. 1994. Positional cloning of the mouse obese gene and its human homologue. *Nature* 372:425–432.

Ziman J. 1976. *The Force of Knowledge. The Scientific Dimension of Society*. Cambridge: Cambridge University Press.

Index

C

D

E

F

N

O

P